The Educational Process
in Nursing Staff Development

The Educational Process
in Nursing Staff Development

JoAnn Grif Alspach, R.N., M.S.N., Ed.D., F.A.A.N.

Consultant, Nursing Staff Development and Competency-Based Education
Editor, *Critical Care Nurse*
Annapolis, Maryland

With 38 illustrations

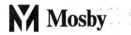 **Mosby**

St. Louis Baltimore Berlin Boston Carlsbad Chicago London Madrid
Naples New York Philadelphia Sydney Tokyo Toronto

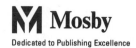

Mosby
Dedicated to Publishing Excellence

Editor: Timothy M. Griswold
Developmental Editor: Jolynn Gower
Project Manager: John Rogers
Senior Production Editor: Helen Hudlin
Designer: Claudia Durrell
Manufacturing Supervisor: John Babrick

Printed in the United States of America
Compositon by University Graphics, Inc.
Printing/binding by Maple Vail Book Manufacturing Group/York

Mosby–Year Book, Inc.
11830 Westline Industrial Drive
St. Louis, Missouri 63146

Library of Congress Cataloging-in-Publication Data

Alspach, JoAnn.
    The educational process in nursing staff development / JoAnn Grif Alspach.
        p.   cm.
    Includes bibliographical references and index.
    ISBN 0-8016-7422-0
    1. Nursing—Study and teaching (Continuing education)   2. Nurses—in-service training.   3. Competency-based education.   I. Title.
    [DNLM: 1. Education, Nursing, Continuing.   2. Nursing—education.
3. Staff Development—methods.   WY 18.5 A462EA 1994]
RT76.A47   1994
610.73'071'5—dc20
DNLM/DLC
for Library of Congress   94-20732
                                                                        CIP

95 96 97 98 99 / 9 8 7 6 5 4 3 2 1

To my mother
Dora Cote Griffin
and
in memory of my father
Joseph Francis Griffin

Preface

The purpose of *The Educational Process in Nursing Staff Development* is to provide nurse educators with a single reference that describes both traditional elements of educational theory and practice together with a competency-based approach for application of that theory and practice to contemporary nursing staff development. My rationale for combining traditional and competency-based approaches to instruction derives from a number of reasons. Some of these reasons account for the book's substantial emphasis on basic principles of education and adult education and others account for its focus on competency-based approaches to nursing staff development.

From 1981 through 1986, I served as chairperson of the American Association of Critical-Care Nurses (AACN) Education Standards Task Force. One of the activities undertaken by this task force was a national survey on critical care nursing education. The findings from that survey* revealed that the individual responsible for nursing staff development was, in the majority (58%) of cases, not an educator but a nurse manager (supervisor, head nurse, or director of nursing) or some other type of practitioner (clinical nurse specialist, staff nurse). Some 40% of these individuals had never taken an academic course in the field of education, 13% had taken only one course, and 22% had received no orientation whatsoever to their position as an educator. One implication drawn from these findings is that a significant number of those who are responsible for

staff development need a foundation in education and adult education to enable them to carry out their responsibilities on the basis of sound educational theory rather than on a trial-and-error basis or the reading of an occasional journal article.

Having consulted in the areas of nursing staff development, hospital-based education, and competency-based education for nearly 15 years, my experience with nurse educators and nurse managers from many clinical specialties, with directors of nursing, and with human resource department personnel also confirmed to me that many individuals who work in these fields would find a comprehensive handbook that combined staff development and competency-based education helpful in their work. In addition, the Joint Commission on Accreditation of Healthcare Organizations' (JCAHO) recent emphasis on the necessity of competency assessment and competency development for all healthcare workers has ignited a need for hospital-based nurse educators to acquire facility in the area of competency-based instruction and evaluation. As a result of these considerations, *The Educational Process in Nursing Staff Development* attempts to provide both a foundation of general educational principles as well as a description of how to apply these principles and those of competency-based education to nursing orientation, in-service, and continuing education programs.

The book is organized into four units. Unit 1 covers the

*Alspach JG, Bell J, Canobbio MM et al, editors: *AACN education standards for critical care nursing,* St Louis, Mo, 1986, CV Mosby.

theoretic, philosophic, and structural basis of nursing staff development. It includes discussions related to the mission, philosophy, goals, educational structure, and organizational structure of a hospital-based nursing education department. Unit 2 includes four chapters that describe the educational process elements common to any nursing staff development program. Each chapter in Unit 2 employs traditional educational theory to cover one phase of the educational process in depth: needs assessment, program planning, program implementation, and program evaluation.

The two chapters in Unit 3 use a competency-based approach to the educational process for each of the distinct components of nursing staff development. Chapter 6 covers the design of competency-based orientation programs and offers special emphasis on preceptorships, the most commonly employed orientation format. Chapter 7 uses principles of competency-based education to describe application of the educational process for in-service and continuing education programs. Unit 4 devotes attention to the management aspects of the nurse educator's role. It covers such areas as quality improvement in nursing staff development, policies and procedures, recordkeeping, budgeting, and program marketing.

The primary audience for this book is nursing staff development educators and managers. Others who will find the book useful include directors of nursing staff development, human resource educators, unit instructors, preceptors, nurse managers, and directors of nursing at small- and medium-sized healthcare facilities. The content is also highly relevant for master's degree programs in nursing that prepare nurse educators, clinical nurse specialists, nurse managers, or other advanced practitioners for their educator role or subrole.

Throughout the book, I have attempted to present material in a clear, direct, and organized manner that will enable readers to readily understand and immediately use the information in their work. Because nursing staff development educators are busy people with a multitude of functions and obligations, I have tried to be both comprehensive and pragmatic in blending theory with reality and in providing sufficient examples so that both aquisition and integration of this material are facilitated.

My thanks to those of you who have enlightened me over the years with your knowledge and experience. I hope you find that *The Educational Process in Nursing Staff Development* assists you in your work.

Grif Alspach

Contents

U N I T   1

Foundations of Nursing Staff Development

C H A P T E R   1   *The Theoretical, Philosophical, and Structural Bases
of Nursing Staff Development,* 2

Theoretical foundation, 2
Philosophical foundation, 2
Structural foundation, 8

U N I T   2

Common Elements in Nursing Staff Development Programs

C H A P T E R   2   *Needs Assessment,* 12

Definition of an educational need, 12
Categories of educational needs, 12
Sources for determining educational needs, 13
Methods for assessing educational needs, 16
Distinguishing between educational and noneducational needs, 19
Setting priorities among educational needs, 19
Validation of educational needs, 20
Tracking educational needs assessments, 22

C H A P T E R   3   *Program Planning,* 23

Specifying instructional outcomes, 23
Curriculum development, 33

CHAPTER 4   *Program Implementation,* 56
                  Guiding principles, 56
                  Teaching methods, 68

CHAPTER 5   *Program Evaluation,* 112
                  Definition of evaluation, 112
                  Functions of evaluation, 112
                  Overview of program evaluation, 113
                  Participants in the evaluation process, 115
                  Timing of evaluations, 116
                  Elements of evaluation, 117
                  Evaluation of learning, 117

UNIT 3
Designing Staff Development Programs: A Competency-Based Approach

CHAPTER 6   *Orientation,* 162
                  Needs assessment, 162
                  Program planning, 177
                  Program implementation, 196
                  Program evaluation, 225

CHAPTER 7   *In-Service Education and Continuing Education,* 237
                  In-service education, 237
                  Continuing education, 249

UNIT 4
Managing Nursing Staff Development Programs

CHAPTER 8   *Managing Selected Staff Development Functions,* 276
                  Monitoring and improving organizational performance, 276
                  Developing policies and procedures, 288
                  Recordkeeping and reports, 290
                  Budgeting, 302
                  Marketing, 320

*The Educational Process
in Nursing Staff Development*

Foundations of Nursing Staff Development

CHAPTER 1

The Theoretical, Philosophical, and Structural Bases of Nursing Staff Development

The continuing professional development of nurses embraces all forms of education they may pursue following their basic nursing education. The scope of professional development in nursing, therefore, embraces academic education, continuing education, and staff development activities. Nursing staff development is distinguished from the other two forms of professional development by its location and focus within the nurse's employment setting. This chapter will address the theoretical, philosophical, and structural framework from which nursing staff development emanates.

THEORETICAL FOUNDATION

The theory base that underlies nursing staff development includes concepts related to nursing and to nursing education. The American Nurses' Association[1] defines nursing as "the diagnosis and treatment of human responses to actual or potential health problems." Benner's[7] widely accepted model of nursing distinguishes five ascending levels of nursing practice, ranging from the novice to the expert nurse. The educational foundation of nursing practice encompasses principles of teaching and learning, principles of adult education, and four interrelated and sequential phases (assessment, planning, implementation, evaluation) of the educational process.

The ultimate goal of both nursing practice and nursing staff development is the provision of quality patient care.

Nursing staff development contributes to quality patient care by ensuring the clinical competency of nursing staff.

Various sets of standards related to nursing practice and nursing staff development afford a mechanism for monitoring the quality and effectiveness of staff development activities. The effectiveness of nursing staff development is determined by evaluating the nurse's knowledge, attitudes, and clinical skills that reflect competent nursing practice and, ultimately, by evaluating the quality of nursing care that the nurse provides to patients. The relationships among these theoretical elements are illustrated in Figure 1.1.

PHILOSOPHICAL FOUNDATION

The philosophical foundation of a nursing staff development program includes its overall purpose and the various sets of beliefs, values, attitudes, assumptions, perceptions, mandates, and goals that influence the structure and process of educational activities. These elements are typically expressed in the mission, philosophy, and goals of the nursing staff development unit. Taken collectively, these statements represent the organizational commitment made to nursing staff development and serve as a means of accountability for the staff development unit. At an operational level, these statements provide the basis for originating, designing, delivering, and evaluating nursing staff development programs.

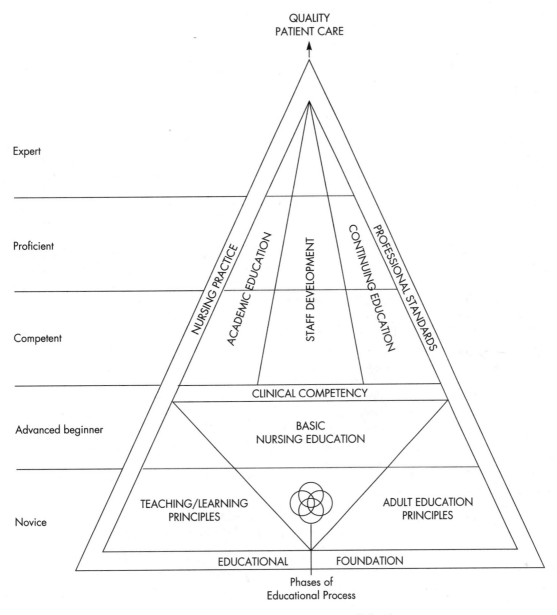

Figure 1.1 Theoretical foundation of nursing staff development.

MISSION

An organization's mission statement defines its *raison d'être* (i.e., its reason or purpose for existence.)[12] Each unit, division, department, or service within that organization shares in the responsibility for achieving this overall mission. Component departments identify how they contribute to attainment of the agency's purpose by means of departmental mission statements. The mission statement of the nursing staff development unit, then, flows from both the agency's mission and the nursing service department's mission. At each organizational level, the mission statement answers the following questions: For what purpose does this organizational unit exist? How does this organizational unit contribute to achieving the overall mission of the agency? For what aspect of the agency's mission is this organizational unit accountable?[11]

A healthcare agency's mission statement typically includes statements related to provision of the highest quality of health care for the community served and provision of quality services by competent professionals who provide state-of-the-art healthcare services. The nursing service department's mission statement then defines how nursing services contribute their part to patient care. If a nursing staff development unit exists within the nursing services department, its mission statement will further delimit how staff development contributes to the provision of nursing services and quality patient care.

Habel[10] states that a mission statement contains four

elements: (1) the purpose of the department/program, (2) the product or service provided, (3) the client(s) served, and (4) the scope of service provided. A nursing staff development unit's mission statement, then, might be written as in Box 1.1. In this mission statement, the purpose is "to promote quality patient care," the product or service provided is "educational programs and services," the clients served are the "nursing staff," and the scope of services provided includes programs and activities related to "acquiring, maintaining, and improving competence in the delivery of patient care services."

If the nursing staff development unit also has responsibilities for areas such as patient/family education and/or mentoring various types of student nurses, mission statements related to each of those areas need to be included.

PHILOSOPHY

A *philosophy* is a statement of the central beliefs and values that direct decisions and activities. A philosophy of nursing staff development is the system of beliefs and values related to nursing and to education that directs the daily operation of nursing staff development programs and the activities of nurse educators. It is important to state these beliefs and values explicitly because they provide the framework within which the nursing staff development unit will operate and educators will carry out their responsibilities. Philosophy statements are important because they represent the system of beliefs that will determine how the nursing staff development unit intends to achieve its mission.

Because nursing staff development is typically located within the nursing services department, its philosophy must be consistent with the beliefs and values of its parent department(s) as well as the agency as a whole. The philosophy of the nursing services department consists of the values and beliefs that underlie nursing practice at that facility. One of these values or beliefs should relate to the nursing department's commitment toward providing opportunities for the professional growth and development of nursing staff.

The philosophy of nursing staff development, therefore, must be consistent with the philosophy of the nursing services department and the philosophy of the healthcare institution. If the staff development unit is organizationally located under a specific nursing division, within a department of nursing education, or in a human resources de-

partment, its philosophy statement needs to be consistent with that organizational unit as well.

What a Philosophy Statement Includes

There is no "correct" form or content for a philosophy statement, but the more clear and inclusive the statement is, the better it will guide the decisions and function of the nursing staff development program. Some institutions have only a few elements in their belief statements; others have a rather extensive listing of beliefs. The length of the philosophy statement is less important than its inclusion of all of the fundamental beliefs that will be used to make decisions regarding the nursing staff development program and its operation.

Presenting the philosophy in an organized fashion will serve to communicate it more clearly to other areas in the nursing department and to other departments and disciplines within the healthcare agency. Some institutions have found it easiest to organize their system of beliefs around some of the major elements involved in nursing staff development: nursing, continuing education, learning, teaching, the educational process, and adult learners. Using these elements as categories, then, the philosophy statement for nursing staff development might include beliefs related to some or all of the areas listed in Box 1.2. Your agency's philosophy statement does not need to include all of these elements, but it should encompass the beliefs that are most important to decision-making for your staff development program.

Who Participates in Developing a Philosophy Statement

Development of a philosophy statement needs to be a joint endeavor for two reasons. First, nursing staff development exists to support nursing practice and patient care. In order to ensure a close and direct linkage between staff development and nursing practice, both nursing staff and nurse managers must be involved with educators in determining the agency's beliefs related to how staff development best contributes to quality patient care. Second, the programs, services, and operation of the nursing staff development unit require the agency's administrative support. If the agency's administrators are actively involved in determining the philosophy statement for nursing staff develop-

---

Box 1.1

SAMPLE MISSION STATEMENT FOR NURSING STAFF DEVELOPMENT

The primary mission of the nursing staff development unit is to promote quality patient care by providing educational programs and services that assist the nursing staff in acquiring, maintaining, and improving competence in the delivery of patient care services.

Box 1.2

ELEMENTS THAT MIGHT BE INCLUDED IN A PHILOSOPHY STATEMENT

BELIEFS ABOUT NURSING

Definition of nursing
Relationship between nursing and quality patient care

BELIEFS ABOUT THE IMPORTANCE OF CONTINUING PROFESSIONAL DEVELOPMENT IN NURSING

Definition and purpose of continuing education in nursing
Definition and purpose of nursing staff development
Relationship among continuing education, staff development, and quality patient care
Relationship between staff development and competence of nursing staff to provide quality patient care
Responsibility of the healthcare agency to provide for staff development and continuing education
Obligation of nursing staff to pursue their own professional development
What staff development is responsible for
Who is responsible for staff development

BELIEFS ABOUT LEARNING

Nature of learning and the learning process
How learning is best facilitated
Importance of the learning environment
How adults learn
Need for lifelong learning
How learning is best evaluated

BELIEFS ABOUT TEACHING

Principles of adult education
Methods and formats that enhance teaching effectiveness
How teaching is best evaluated
Roles and responsibilities of nurse educators
Faculty/instructor qualifications

BELIEFS ABOUT THE EDUCATIONAL PROCESS

How learning needs are best identified
How educational programs are best planned
How educational programs are best delivered
How educational programs are best evaluated
Need for collaboration and cooperation with nursing practice, management, and administration
Need for collaboration and cooperation with other healthcare disciplines
Responsibility of staff development educators to nursing units

BELIEFS ABOUT ADULT LEARNERS

Salient characteristics of adult learners
Learning needs of adults as employees
How adult learners participate in the teaching-learning process
Responsibilities of educators to learners

---

ment, their future support in providing resources for the program is more likely.

Those who should be involved in developing the philosophy statement, therefore, include all members of the staff development unit and as many representatives as possible and appropriate from each of the following groups: staff nurses, clinical nurse specialists, nurse managers, nursing service directors, quality assurance staff, nursing education department, and/or human resource development staff. These groups represent the constituency of the nursing staff development program. Their collective participation in developing the philosophy statement leads to a sense of shared ownership and a greater sense of organizational commitment to actualizing the beliefs and values expressed in the day-to-day operation of the nursing staff development unit.

How a Philosophy Statement Is Developed

The process for drafting, refining, and finalizing the philosophy of nursing staff development can be carried out in a variety of ways but needs to include the following elements:

- Reviewing the agency and parent department philosophy statements
- Drafting a philosophy of nursing staff development:

Determining all relevant categories of beliefs and values to be included
Defining relevant terms
- Soliciting feedback and suggestions from all constituents of the staff development program
- Revising and refining the philosophy statement based on input from constituent groups
- Reaching consensus on the final version of the philosophy statement
- Distributing the philosophy statement to all constituent and relevant organizational groups

In smaller healthcare institutions where there is a single nurse educator, drafting the philosophy statement can best be accomplished by enlisting representatives from other interested groups. If there are numerous educators, they might draft the philosophy statement and then use an advisory committee consisting of representatives from each of the constituent groups to provide feedback on the drafted statement. Distribution of the finished statement will serve as a tangible reminder of the philosophical convictions of the nursing staff development unit.

Uses of a Philosophy Statement

As mentioned earlier, a philosophy statement represents the basis for originating, designing, delivering, and evalu-

---

Box 1.3

USES OF A PHILOSOPHY STATEMENT

- Serves as a source document for guiding development of educational policies, procedures, standards, and position descriptions
- Assists in determining the range of educational services and types of programs provided
- Helps in estimating necessary budget and resources needed for the program
- Establishes priorities and goals for nursing staff development activities
- Aids in allocation of resources to programs
- Clarifies roles and relationships among nurse educators, staff nurses, managers, and administrators
- Clarifies how nursing staff development contributes to quality patient care at that institution
- Assists in developing mechanisms to evaluate all aspects of educational programming

From Austin EK: *Guidelines for the development of continuing education offerings for nurses*, New York, 1981, Appleton-Century-Crofts.

Box 1.4

SAMPLE GOALS FOR NURSING STAFF DEVELOPMENT

- The goal of the nursing **orientation** program is to ensure that all nursing staff acquire the competency necessary to fulfill the responsibilities stated in their respective position descriptions.
- The goal of the nursing **in-service** program is to ensure that all nursing staff maintain and increase competency in their respective position following completion of their orientation and throughout their employment at this facility.
- The goal of the nursing **continuing education** program is to enhance the professional competency and career growth and development of nursing staff beyond the expectations required for fulfillment of their current position description.
- The goal of the **career development** program is to assist nursing staff in identifying their educational needs, planning to meet those needs, implementing their learning plans within or outside the employing agency, and evaluating the outcomes of these experiences.

---

ating the nursing staff development program and affords a frame of reference for nurse educators to carry out their role and responsibilities. A thoughtfully developed philosophy statement affords a practical, working document for making decisions and for clarifying how staff development contributes to quality patient care. Some specific uses for the philosophy statement[6] are enumerated in Box 1.3.

In order for the philosophy statement to maintain its usefulness, it must be reviewed at defined intervals to determine if changes, updating, additions, or deletions are indicated. An annual review by nurse educators and program constituents can ensure that the philosophy statement remains appropriate, timely, and congruent with the organization's needs and related departmental philosophy statements.

GOALS

Goals are statements of broad direction or general intent.[5] The goals of a nursing staff development program are broad statements of what the program is intended to accomplish. These goals are derived from and are consistent with the mission and philosophy statements of the program but are more concrete and specific than either of these. Goals, in turn, serve as a basis for developing more detailed outcomes for each component in the staff development program.

Since the primary mission of nursing staff development is to provide educational programs and services that assist nursing staff to gain, maintain, and improve their competence in patient care, goals related to each of these responsibilities need to be specified. These goals might be stated as in Box 1.4.

PURPOSE   BELIEFS and VALUES   DIRECTION
                                                                      of
                                                               ACCOMPLISHMENTS

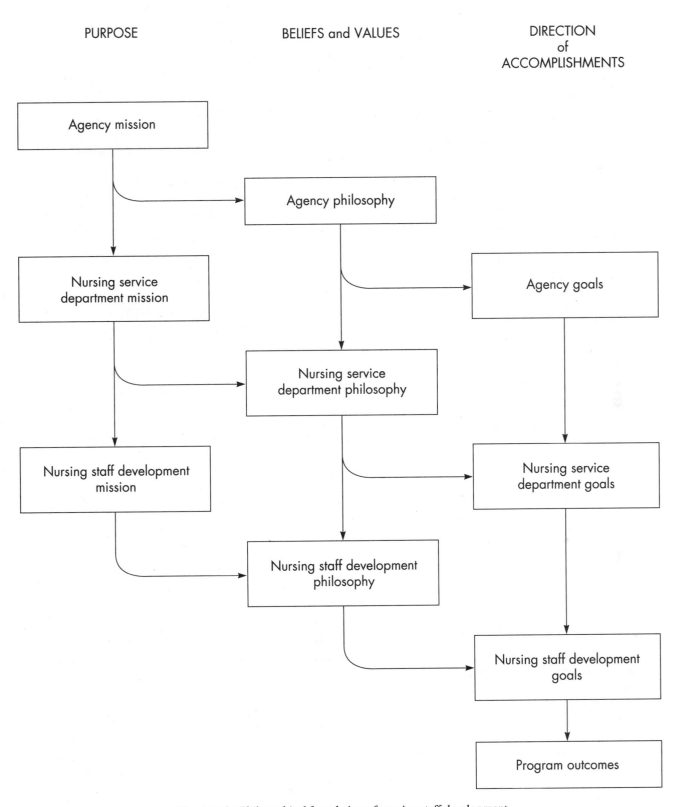

Figure 1.2 Philosophical foundation of nursing staff development.

Other goals could be added to reflect programs for cross training, orientation of float or agency nurses, preceptor training, patient education, community education, and/or precepting nursing students. The agency might also include one or more goals related to specific commitments regarding the effectiveness, efficiency, or accessibility of the nursing staff development program: "The fiscal goal of the nursing staff development program is to maintain the delivery of quality education services at a reduced cost to the facility."

Unlike mission and philosophy statements that tend to endure, the goals of a nursing staff development program are likely to change over time. As needs and priorities evolve within the organization, the staff education program's goals need to reflect these modifications. For this reason, goals need to be systematically reviewed, revised, and updated on a periodic basis to ensure that they are consistent with the organization's needs and goals. Both the ANA *Standards for Nursing Staff Development*[4] and the American Society for Healthcare Education and Training (ASHET) *Standards for Healthcare Education and Training*[5] require that these goals be reviewed and revised at least annually.

The relationships among the various elements in the philosophical foundation of nursing staff development are illustrated in Figure 1.2.

STRUCTURAL FOUNDATION

The structural foundation of nursing staff development includes both an educational and an organizational dimension. The educational structure describes how nursing staff development fits into the overall scheme of professional nursing education. The organizational structure describes how the staff development program is situated within the overall organization of the healthcare facility.

EDUCATIONAL STRUCTURE

The American Nurses' Association[4] distinguishes three components of nursing education: basic, graduate, and continuing education. *Continuing education* is defined as "those learning activities intended to build upon the educational and experiential bases of the professional nurse for the enhancement of practice, education, administration, research, or theory development to the end of improving the health of the public."[2] Continuing education relates to professional growth and development that occurs following completion of entry-level nursing education and is not restricted to any particular setting or provider.

Nursing staff development is defined as "a process consisting of orientation, in-service education, and continuing education for the purpose of promoting the development of personnel within any employment setting, consistent with the goals and responsibilities of the employer."[4] In contrast to continuing education, staff development is specific to the employment setting and to the potential influence that this setting may have on the educational process.[3] The ANA uses the term *provider unit* to describe an individual or department with responsibility for nursing staff development in the employment setting.[4]

In addition to continuing education, nursing staff development includes orientation and in-service education. *Orientation* is defined as "the means by which new staff members are introduced to the philosophy, goals, policies, procedures, role expectations, physical facilities, and special services in a specific work setting."[4] *In-service education* is defined as "activities intended to assist the professional nurse in acquiring, maintaining, and/or increasing competence in fulfilling the assigned responsibilities specific to the expectations of the employer."[4] Both orientation and in-service education are provided in the work setting to assist nursing staff in fulfilling their assigned responsibilities in that agency.

One departure from these ANA definitions used in this book affects the scope of the orientation component of staff development. Although the ANA definition of in-service education includes all aspects of competency development, this book considers the *acquisition* of clinical competency to perform one's assigned responsibilities to be within the scope of the orientation program rather than a part of the in-service program. The rationale for this departure is the fact that most nursing orientation programs are expected to produce staff who are able to perform all major aspects of their job description. Nurse orientees are generally not considered to have completed their orientation to the agency until they have demonstrated this initial level of competency to do their job.

In-service education, then, will be considered primarily as a means for the maintenance and increase of clinical competency related to one's job following completion of the agency's orientation program. There are two dimensions of in-service education. One dimension is concerned with ensuring that new areas of nursing practice added over time to the repertoire of nursing practice (e.g., new policies, procedures, protocols, therapies, equipment, and the like) are acquired by all nursing staff. The other dimension is concerned with ensuring that selected areas of nursing competency are maintained at expected levels of performance over time. These competency areas typically include selected nursing functions of high priority (e.g., cardiopulmonary resuscitation [CPR], infection control measures, or fire safety) or those that involve some concern for patient safety and require advanced training and clinical skills (e.g., defibrillation, endotracheal intubation, and the like). The former group is usually considered "mandatory in-services." The latter are often considered as part of the agency's local certification or credentialing program. In-service education is necessary to ensure that these additional elements of competency are integrated into nursing practice and are maintained over time.

ORGANIZATIONAL STRUCTURE

The responsibility for nursing staff development may be located within any one of three types of organizational structures: centralized, decentralized, or some combination of the two. The most commonly employed organizational structure for the nursing staff development unit is the combined form.[8]

In a *centralized organizational structure,* the responsibility for nursing staff development may exist within a human resources development (HRD) department or within a hospitalwide education department. The educators within these structures are often generalists who report administratively to managers holding either line or staff authority. Human resource development departments usually consist of three major components: job-related staff development, career development of employees, and organizational development.[13] The latter encompasses the facilitation of change and growth within the organization as a whole. If the nursing staff development program is organizationally located within an HRD department, it may represent one small part of a much larger department that is responsible for functions as diverse as staff recruitment, development, and retention; personnel policies; job descriptions and employee benefit plans; career planning; managerial and leadership development; patient and community health education; and community relations. If the staff development program is centrally placed within a hospitalwide education department, the focus will likely concentrate more on education than on personnel issues, but nurses will be only one of many categories of healthcare workers whose learning needs must be accommodated. However, because nurses represent the largest category of healthcare workers, nursing staff development typically draws heavily on such resources allocated within a hospitalwide education department.

Decentralized organizational structures may locate the responsibility for nursing staff development at the level of the nursing department, at some subdivision of that department, or at the unit level. One form of a decentralized structure involves the vestment of responsibility for nursing staff development within a central nursing administration. The individual in charge of nursing staff development might occupy the position of associate director of nursing for education and research, director of nursing staff development, or some other title that reports to the chief executive officer for nursing services. Nurse educators in this type of structure may share or have sole responsibility for various aspects of staff development (e.g., centralized nursing orientation, in-service education, CPR). A second form of a decentralized structure may have some nurse educators assigned to centralized nursing staff development programs while other nurse educators are assigned to various clinical divisions within the nursing services department, such as the maternal/child health division, the critical care division, or the ambulatory care division. The most extreme form of a decentralized structure places all responsibility for nursing staff development on the individual nursing units, where unit-based educators (unit instructors, preceptors) who are specialists in their clinical area are assigned these functions. These unit-based instructors may work as educators full-time or may work as both educators and as staff nurses on their unit. As organizational structures become more decentralized, unit-based learning needs may be met more effectively, but many of the advantages of centralization (such as efficient use of resources, minimal duplication of efforts, provision of clerical support, and opportunities for peer support) are lost in the process.

Combined organizational structures attempt to maximize the advantages and minimize the disadvantages of centralized and decentralized models. Combined structures exist in many forms but typically provide centralized provision of instruction that addresses learning needs common to all or most members of the nursing staff, while affording decentralized provision of programming to address the unique needs of specialty and subspecialty area nursing staff. A combined organizational structure might consist of a core of centralized nurse educators who report to the director of nursing staff development together with a cadre of unit-based nurse educators who report to the nurse manager of their assigned unit. This dual structure allows for greater efficiency in use of educational resources for more generic learning needs without compromising the need to be responsive to the unique needs of individual nursing units. Although the combined model is not without problems,[9] its ability to blend some of the best features of the alternative structures makes it a particularly appealing alternative for many hospitals.

There is no one best way to structure the nursing staff development function within an organization.[5] Each type of structure has its advantages and disadvantages. Although many possible organizational structures and variants of these may be found, the specific structure adopted by the institution is less important than whether the selected model works effectively and efficiently. Clarity in lines of communication, collaboration, authority, and responsibility are more important than the precise positioning of the nursing staff development unit within that facility.

REFERENCES

1. American Nurses' Association (ANA): *Nursing: a social policy statement,* Kansas City, MO, 1980, ANA.
2. American Nurses' Association (ANA): *Standards for continuing education in nursing,* Kansas City, MO, 1984, ANA.
3. American Nurses' Association (ANA): *Standards for nursing continuing education and staff development,* Washington, DC, 1994, ANA.
4. American Nurses' Association (ANA): *Standards for nursing staff development,* Kansas City, MO, 1990, ANA.
5. American Society for Healthcare Education and Training: *Standards for healthcare education and training,* Chicago, 1990, American Hospital Association.

6. Austin EK: *Guidelines for the development of continuing education offerings for nurses,* New York, 1981, Appleton-Century-Crofts.

7. Benner P: *From novice to expert,* Menlo Park, CA, 1984, Addison-Wesley.

8. Blocker VT: Organizational models and staff preparation: a survey of staff development departments, *J Cont Educ Nurs* 23:259, 1992.

9. Cummings C, McCaskey R: A model combining centralized and decentralized staff development, *J Nurs Staff Develop* 8:22, 1992.

10. Habel M: A management blueprint for nursing staff development, *J Nurs Staff Develop* 2:134, 1986.

11. Morton PG: A hospital nursing education manual, *J Nurs Staff Develop* 1:61, 1985.

12. Stein D: Philosophy and mission statement: the framework for hospitalwide education services units. In *Resource manual,* Chicago, 1991, American Hospital Association.

13. Stream T, Chalofsky N: HRD in industry: lessons for health care, *J Healthcare Educ Train* 2(2):13, 1987.

Common Elements in Nursing Staff Development Programs

Hospital-based nursing education programs may be designed for any of the three areas of staff development—orientation, in-service education, or continuing education. Although each of these programs has features that distinguish it from the others, they share certain common features. The chapters in this unit will address a number of common features that characterize nursing staff development programs. Each of the chapters will cover one phase of the educational process for nursing staff development: Chapter 2 discusses needs assessment, Chapter 3 covers program planning, Chapter 4 addresses program implementation, and Chapter 5 reviews program evaluation.

CHAPTER 2

Needs Assessment

DEFINITION OF AN EDUCATIONAL NEED

An educational need may be defined as the difference between what someone presently knows or is able to do and what they need to know or be able to do. It represents an interruption along a continuum between an individual's present level of cognitive, affective, and/or psychomotor performance and the desired or necessary level of performance. Educational needs related to nursing staff development arise from a nurse's assigned role, responsibilities, and/or functions. Moreover, for a need to be a true educational need, it must be one that can be satisfied through some type of instructional experience.

CATEGORIES OF EDUCATIONAL NEEDS

If our working definition of "education" is nursing staff development, then these programs are concerned with one of three categories of educational needs: a need for orientation, a need for in-service education, or a need for continuing education.

NEED FOR ORIENTATION

An educational need for orientation exists for all nursing staff when they enter the institution as new employees. As the ANA definition of orientation[2] reminds us, all new staff members need to be acquainted with the philosophy, goals,

policies, procedures, role expectations, physical facilities, and services of the facility.

If the goal of an orientation program is to ensure that all nursing staff acquire the competency necessary to fulfill their assigned responsibilities, however, it is obvious that many orientees will need more than an introduction to the areas mentioned in order to perform their job effectively. Nurses with many years of experience may require a minimum of additional instruction before they are ready to take a patient assignment. Nurses with years of experience in one clinical specialty may need a moderate amount of instruction to acquire the additional knowledge, attitudes, and skills necessary to working in a different clinical specialty area. New graduates who have no professional nursing experience will demand a maximum of instructional support before they will be able to function safely, effectively, and independently in the clinical area.

Although the need for orientation is universal, the depth and scope of instructional support that individual orientees require before they are able to perform competently is highly individualized and variable. This variability exists even among nurses with comparable amounts and types of nursing experience: some will adapt and become functional quite readily, others will need more instruction and time to integrate as staff, and a few may never be fully successful in changing poor work habits and clinical skills brought from their previous employment. Every orientee needs to be evaluated and supported on an individual basis.

NEED FOR IN-SERVICE EDUCATION

As with the need for orientation, a need for in-service education arises from the job requirements of a particular work setting. As discussed in Chapter 1, in-service needs arise as requirements for competency in a particular role and setting change over time. In-service education is primarily concerned with either the addition of new areas of competency (new or revised policies, procedures, protocols, drugs, therapies, technologies, treatments, and the like) or the validation that one's performance in a particular competency area (CPR, defibrillation) has been maintained. In contrast to the need for orientation that arises at a nurse's entry into employment or on entry into a new position, the need for in-service education arises following orientation and occurs throughout the nurse's employment at that agency. Whereas orientation is directed at ensuring that nurses have acquired basic competency to do their assigned job, in-service education is directed at ensuring that competency remains current and complete for assigned responsibilities.

NEED FOR CONTINUING EDUCATION

Continuing education may be broadly construed as any planned learning experience that is provided following basic nursing education. Within the context of staff development, however, the need for continuing education arises from a nurse's interest in professional or career development in areas that extend beyond the specific requirements of the currently assigned position. For example, staff nurses in a coronary care unit might wish to become certified in advanced cardiac life support (ACLS) or might want to begin development of the management skills necessary to be a head nurse. Because their current positions as staff nurses do not require these areas of capability, these learning interests represent a need for continuing education.

In summary, then, the need for orientation and for in-service education reflects the educational needs related to a nurse's assigned job description. The need for continuing education reflects learning interests that exist beyond the scope of a nurse's current job description.

SOURCES FOR DETERMINING EDUCATIONAL NEEDS

Once educators can recognize and categorize educational needs, they will have a clearer understanding of the kind of information that needs to be acquired during the assessment phase of the educational process. The next step in the assessment process is determining the information sources for identifying nurses' educational needs.

In general, educators will want to use as many sources of input as time and resources allow. The major reason for securing information from multiple sources is to obtain an adequate amount of information for decision-making and

to obtain input from a diversity of perspectives that may view educational needs quite differently. The various sources of information can be divided into primary, secondary, and combined sources.

PRIMARY SOURCES

Primary sources of information related to the educational needs of nursing staff include the agency's written documents, such as the position description for nurses, standards of patient care, standards of nursing practice, other written protocols, and the nursing staff itself, preceptors, and nurse managers. These sources are designated as primary because they afford the most direct, valid, and reliable information that can be used for planning instruction of nursing staff.

Position Descriptions

The single most important document for determining educational needs related to nursing orientation and in-service education is the written job/position description. Every position within the nursing service (staff nurse, head nurse, clinical specialist, etc.) should have its own position description that details the roles, responsibilities, and expectations of anyone who is hired for that position. The position description represents the basis for employment and should make explicit what the agency expects in the area of performance for all employees who are hired for that position.

Some healthcare institutions have a single job description for each position within the nursing service department. Others may have extensive, detailed, clinical ladders that define progressive expectations at successively higher levels within the same position (e.g., Staff Nurse I for new graduates, Staff Nurse II for nurses with 1 year of clinical experience, etc.).

Position descriptions are not always written in a form that facilitates their usefulness in educational needs assessment. Some of these documents are written in vague, nonspecific language that is too generalized to be helpful in suggesting instructional needs. Others may not reflect current roles, responsibilities, or functions of nursing staff on one or more nursing units. Despite these possible limitations, position descriptions represent the customary "starting point" for determining the educational needs of all nursing staff.

Standards

Standards are statements of quality related to some aspect(s) of performance. *Standards of patient care* reflect patient outcomes that nurses attempt to provide, whereas *standards of nursing practice* (such as those promulgated by the American Nurses' Association or numerous specialty nursing organizations) reflect the interventions that nurses carry out to assist patients in achieving those expected outcomes.[13] Accreditation standards such as those of the Joint Commission on Accreditation of Healthcare Organizations (JCAHO)[12] reflect structures, processes, or outcomes that are considered necessary attributes of quality patient care. These are relevant documents for determining educational needs because hospital, nursing department, and nursing unit standards represent the quality of performance expected of nursing staff. To a great extent, a nurse's position description describes what the nurse is expected to do in the job, and various sets of standards represent how those responsibilities are to be fulfilled.

Protocols

Some institutions have established written protocols, unit routines, or other guidelines that indicate how certain nursing responsibilities are to be performed. Although they may not be referred to as a "standard," these established ways of doing things function very similarly to standards and have a comparable degree of usefulness for determining nurses' educational needs.

Nursing Staff

The most relevant and direct source of information regarding nurses' educational needs is the nursing staff itself. As adult learners, the nursing staff can be expected to actively participate in identifying its own learning needs relative to unit assignments. The validity and reliability of those appraisals, however, may be influenced to some extent by the individual nurse's knowledge and experience in nursing. Educators should not assume that all nursing staff are equally proficient at identifying educational needs.

Experienced nurses are more likely to be adept at identifying the precise nature of their educational needs. A thorough foundation in the core knowledge, attitudes, and skills of the clinical practice area affords seasoned practitioners with a sound basis for distinguishing what they know from what they do not. Recent graduates and other beginning practitioners, on the other hand, may be less able to specify the true nature and scope of their educational needs. Indeed, a concern that often exists regarding the orientation of new graduates is that they may fail to recognize when they should seek information and resources to make sound clinical decisions. If inexperienced nurses claim that "I don't know enough yet to know what I *don't know*," then they are not likely to provide valid and complete assessments of their own educational needs.

Even experienced nurses may need some help in identifying their learning needs. For nursing staff with limited or no experience, it may be more helpful to seek information regarding their needs from others who have observed their clinical performance—for example, from their preceptors and/or nurse managers.

Preceptors

In hospitals that use a preceptorship for their orientation program, each preceptor represents a prime source of information regarding the educational needs of the orientee. The preceptor's close rapport with the orientee and firsthand appraisal of the orientee's knowledge, attitudes, and clinical skills afford a direct avenue for identifying that orientee's need for instruction. In addition, highly experienced preceptors are also in a position to compare and contrast the individual orientee's needs with the educational needs of other orientees they have worked with over the years. Their insights and appraisals are often invaluable in appraising the educational needs of nursing staff on their unit.

Nurse Managers

Head nurses have access to many forms of information related to the educational needs of their staff. The head nurse's formal and informal monitoring of nursing practice and patient care on the unit elicits a wide array of both objective and subjective indicators of where instructional support has been, is, and will be needed. Their interactions with all members of the nursing staff give them a broad overview of educational needs on their unit. Their communication with preceptors and orientees affords insight into the need for orientation of their staff. Their awareness of future intended changes on the unit enables them to project in-service educational needs. Finally their acquaintance with the interests and career plans of the staff provides information related to needs for continuing education. Many healthcare agencies require all nursing staff to complete self-assessments annually in conjunction with their performance evaluation. These self-appraisals usually include identification of their educational needs and goals for the year. Head nurses can forward this information to the staff development educator so that staff may be notified of future offerings related to their areas of need. The nurse manager's perspective is, then, both unique and encompassing. In addition, the head nurse's managerial vantage point often reveals insights and appraisals of educational needs that are strikingly dissimilar to those offered by staff nurses, educators, and others.[9,16]

At many smaller healthcare agencies, there may be no individual designated as a staff development educator. Instead, all staff development functions may be performed by the head nurse/nurse manager of each unit.[4] At these institutions, the head nurse's appraisal regarding the educational needs of unit staff is of paramount importance.

SECONDARY SOURCES

Secondary sources of information regarding the educational needs of nursing staff include other professional groups on the healthcare team, related professional literature, and local schools of nursing. These sources are designated as secondary because the information they provide tends to be more indirect and at times less immediately applicable than the information provided by the primary sources.

Other Professional Groups on the Healthcare Team

A recent survey on critical care orientation programs[1] indicated that a number of other professional groups commonly participate in educational programs for nursing staff. These collaborative groups include dietitians, clinical pharmacologists, social workers, respiratory and physical therapists, and physicians. Although it is not appropriate for these individuals to assess educational needs related to nursing practice per se, they may be able to offer insights and suggestions on facets of patient care that overlap with their own professional responsibilities. Because these professionals work collaboratively with the nursing staff, their perspectives on patient care deserve serious consideration. Involving relevant professional groups fosters open communication and a more collaborative approach to patient care.

Related Professional Literature

Many specialty nursing organizations such as the American Association of Critical-Care Nurses, the Emergency Nurses Association, the Association of Women's Health, Obstetric, and Neonatal Nurses, and the American Association of Neurological and Neurosurgical Nurses publish core curriculum texts that offer the knowledge base for nursing practice in their respective clinical area. Depending on the type of clinical units the educator is responsible for, one or more of these core curriculum references may be useful for determining educational needs of nursing staff who work in that area.

In addition to these core textbooks, a multitude of other book references on nursing practice provide a wealth of information on the educational needs of nurses. Professional nursing journals publish an ongoing source of information related to trends in nursing practice and education. These and other references and periodicals offer a fund of information to the staff development educator regarding the present and future educational needs of practicing nurses.

The professional literature derived from healthcare fields other than nursing (e.g., books and periodicals from medical, biomedical, pharmacological, and basic scientific research) may all be useful as references for identifying nurses' current and future needs for education. As discoveries and developments arise in the sciences that underlie and affect nursing practice, learning needs emerge from the necessity to keep abreast with new information.

Local Schools of Nursing

The type and quality of basic nursing education programs in a geographic area may suggest educational needs likely to exist in the graduates of these programs. Because the scope, depth, curriculum components, and expectations of students may vary somewhat from one academic institution to another, nurses recently graduated from these institutions can be expected to vary in their clinical competency as they leave school and enter employment. As the healthcare agency gains experience with integrating graduates from each of these programs into their staff, educators will become increasingly able to project the educational needs and amount of instructional support that graduates from each program will require. Faculty from these schools of nursing may also be able to share their knowledge of a particular graduate's strengths and weaknesses and the types of learning experiences their graduates usually need for successful employment. Ongoing two-way communication between the healthcare facility and nearby schools of nursing can not only enhance cooperation and collaboration but improve the employability of new graduates who enter the workplace. Cooperative relationships may be fostered by a number of mechanisms, including joint appointments, guest lectures, and use of the healthcare facility as a clinical site for students.

COMBINED SOURCES

Rather than consulting with each of these separate sources every time an educational program is being considered, some healthcare institutions have found it more realistic and efficient to use an advisory committee for nursing staff development. A well-constituted advisory committee, with representatives from all relevant sources of information, can then serve as the primary vehicle for assisting the educator in determining the educational needs of nursing staff.

The purpose of the advisory committee may be limited to identifying nurses' educational needs but may also encompass conceptualizing, promoting, planning, providing, and evaluating these programs. The range of functions that this committee may assume includes the following:

- Identifying and verifying educational needs and ideas for programs
- Determining long-range goals for staff development
- Defining program outcomes and formats
- Specifying program content
- Securing faculty and material resources
- Resolving problems that arise in conjunction with programs
- Communicating with all relevant professional groups
- Supporting and publicizing programs within and outside the hospital
- Evaluating educational programs

- Promoting a shared responsibility and commitment to nursing staff development

Advisory committee meetings provide an opportunity for discussion that can assist in reaching a consensus on the educational needs of nurses. The greater the variety and scope of perspectives, the more potential this group has for providing meaningful assistance to the educator. Committee members should be able to represent their constituents responsibly and express clearly the viewpoints of their respective groups.

Although such a committee may be instrumental in offering perceptions and recommendations related to educational needs, the advisory committee should neither usurp the nurse educator's perogative nor be used by the educator to abdicate responsibility. The educator should retain responsibility and accountability for the outcomes and actions that follow from the committee's deliberations.

METHODS FOR ASSESSING EDUCATIONAL NEEDS

In addition to consulting multiple sources to assess educational needs, the educator should employ several methods to appraise those needs.[3] The rationale for using multiple sources is the fact that no one method is likely to reveal all of the important needs in a given area.

In a classic paper, Bell[6] described the variety of methods available to the staff development educator for determining the educational needs of nursing staff. Each method has its advantages and disadvantages for gathering information. The methods employed may be direct or indirect in their approach.

DIRECT METHODS

Direct methods provide information by means of a straightforward solicitation of educational needs. Examples of direct techniques include interviews, focus groups, and written questionnaires.

Interviews

Interviewing nursing staff to elicit their perceived educational needs is a necessary part of the adult education process. As mentioned earlier, however, this self-appraisal may be more accurate for the experienced nurse than for a nurse new to a particular clinical field or a new graduate. Personal interviews with an experienced nurse can provide a detailed enumeration of specific, concrete educational needs as that nurse perceives them. These "felt needs" are important to determine because they often provide the basis of that nurse's motivation for participating in a staff development program. The educator needs to keep in mind, however, that to be relevant as an educational need, the perceived needs must coincide with the agency's job expectations for that nurse.

Experienced nurses who are new to a particular clinical area (e.g., those with medical-surgical nursing experience who wish to transfer to a critical care unit) and recently graduated nurses may require various amounts of assistance to identify their specific educational needs. Structuring the interview by citing some specific questions related to orientation, in-service, and continuing education areas may be helpful for this process.

Interviews with staff need not be formally scheduled. In fact, interviews may be as effective when they occur spontaneously during lunch, breaks, or during or after work. If informal gatherings do not afford adequate information, scheduling the interview at a mutually convenient time may be a reasonable alternative.

The educator's personal contact with the nursing staff offers an opportunity to clarify and verify the nature, scope, depth, and priority of the individual nurse's perceived need for instruction and the perceived level of competency in relation to those needs. Interviews also afford an opportunity for the educator to establish rapport with staff[3] and to communicate interest, accessibility, and willingness to assist in meeting that nurse's needs.

Focus Groups

In addition to gathering information on each nurse's individual educational needs, focus groups can be used to solicit information related to common or recurring educational needs that exist among nursing staff as a whole or among nurses who work in the same specialty area. The focus group need not include every member of the nursing staff but should represent all units, all shifts, and as many formal and informal subgroups within the staff as possible (e.g., staff with many, moderate, and few years of clinical experience; preceptors and nonpreceptors; long-time and new employees; satisfied and dissatisfied staff; leaders and followers; younger and older staff). For focus group meetings to be successful, the educator needs to prepare an introduction to the meeting, plan an agenda of questions to be considered and/or issues to be resolved, and manage a group discussion toward consensus.

Written Questionnaires

Written questionnaires or surveys represent another commonly employed method for eliciting educational needs. One advantage to this method of needs assessment is that it provides a written record of responses to predetermined inquiries that can be readily tabulated for interpretation. A second advantage of the method is that, like the structured interview, the focus of the responses can be made highly specific for answering certain questions regarding learning needs.

The questionnaire or survey format also has some inherent disadvantages.[16] Constructing a valid survey document that asks all of the "right questions" in a clear and unambiguous manner takes time to do well.[6] Constructing a questionnaire that elicits true educational needs rather than mere learning interests takes practice. Constructing a questionnaire that is neither too long nor too short can be challenging. A lengthy and/or confusing survey form will very likely be left incomplete or ignored by busy staff and can be agonizing and time-consuming to tabulate by hand. A cursory survey may be completed but will not provide answers to all of the necessary questions. Motivating staff to complete and return these devices in a timely manner can be a daunting task at times. If fewer than half of the staff of a given unit return the survey, the information obtained will not be truly representative of the staff on that unit.

Questionnaires and surveys can be prepared in a number of different formats.[3,6] These formats include open-ended questions, direct questions, projective questions, and checklists.

Open-Ended Questions

Open-ended questions are most useful for nurses who are experienced, highly motivated to learn, well attuned to their own educational needs, and articulate in expressing their needs clearly and fully. For these nurses, an open-ended question such as "To provide better care for patients in acute respiratory failure, I need to learn more about ..." may be all that is necessary for enumerating their specific needs.

Open-ended (nondirective) questions require minimal preparation time for the educator. The effectiveness of this format, however, is highly dependent on the nurse's willingness to invest the time and energy necessary to provide thoughtful, relevant, and accurate information. Busy and tired staff may not be interested in making this investment.[14] In addition, the data provided may be difficult to tabulate, collate, and analyze. If the questions are too broadly stated, they may not elicit the specific responses desired. To avert these problems and to provide a means for gathering information from the less than highly introspective nurse, more structured formats may be preferable.

Direct Questions

Directly questioning nursing staff about their educational needs may be more efficient than using open-ended questions when one is attempting to elicit information about specific aspects of nursing practice. For example, a question such as "Do you need to learn more about titrating vasoactive drugs?" is more direct than "Areas of coronary care nursing I need to learn more about are. . . ."

One disadvantage of direct questioning is that it assumes the educator has a thorough knowledge of the range of potential areas of educational needs. If all of the possible

areas of educational need are not included in the questionnaire, the information obtained may be incomplete. A second possible disadvantage is that this type of survey can generate a large volume of data that is difficult and unwieldy to tabulate manually. If computer tabulation is not available, the educator may use a more restricted or abridged form for surveying purposes and survey more frequently during the year. The obvious advantage of this format is that it can produce straight yes/no answers to any question posed.

Projective Questions

Projective questions or statements require respondents to imagine themselves in certain situations and then relate their reaction. These responses can uncover educational needs specific to the given context. For example, the educator might ask for responses to the following:

- "When I am assigned to a patient with head trauma, the aspect of nursing care I feel least secure in is _____."
- "In attempting to support the family of a patient who is dying, my biggest problem is usually _____."
- "In assessing a patient with a pacemaker, I often have questions about _____."

Especially for nurses who need some assistance in specifying their educational needs, providing a clinical context for reflection may be very helpful in focusing their responses. New graduates and nurses unfamiliar with a new clinical specialty are not likely to be aided by projective questions until they have had sufficient exposure to these practice areas.

Checklists

Rather than directly questioning staff on the full spectrum of educational needs they might have, educators could construct a simple checklist that contains the listing of potential learning needs and asks staff to indicate their need to learn about that topic. Designing such a list is a relatively simple and straightforward process and completing it is fast and easy for staff. The checklist can be limited to a particular area of inquiry or can attempt to cover an entire range of potential educational needs. Other advantages of the checklist are that it does not demand the educator's time to complete, its data can be readily tabulated, and it permits a written record of responses. Its disadvantages are its impersonal nature, the potential that staff will not be willing to invest the time to complete it, the large volume of data produced, the possible omission of important topic areas, and wording of items such that responses are too general for definitive program planning.

A *reiterated checklist* can overcome some of the potential limitations of the standard checklist. After a standard checklist is used, a follow-up reiterated checklist is constructed to verify the results and more narrowly define the responses. Based on the initial checklist responses, the reiterated checklist may ask nursing staff to rank the importance of the needs that were mentioned most often, to further specify aspects of the topic areas that warrant instruction, to establish a personal priority among the identified needs, or to offer additional description of those needs.[7]

INDIRECT METHODS

Direct methods of needs assessment assume that nursing staff can, to some degree, recognize and articulate their educational needs. Educational needs are not always so visible to learners and, as mentioned earlier, not all nursing staff may be ready or able to accurately appraise their own needs. Under these circumstances, gathering information from less subjective and more indirect sources can be helpful.

Indirect methods of needs assessment use analyses of the work situation and various hospital records to yield information related to nurses' educational needs. Examples of indirect techniques include observation, listening, and review of hospital documents.

Observation

Observation of staff performance on-the-job or in a simulated clinical setting can provide meaningful and specific information regarding the nature and quality of clinical performance. Observation is very helpful in appraising psychomotor and affective components of performance and may be most useful when used in conjunction with other assessment methods to confirm or disconfirm those findings. At times, nurses may not be aware of areas where refinement or correction are necessary, but their clinical performance may suggest areas needing improvement.

To be valid, observations of staff performance need to be guided by objective, measurable, and behavioral indices of "satisfactory performance." These behavioral criteria then serve as the standards against which clinical performance is compared to determine if it meets the agency's expectations. If these performance criteria are clear, unambiguous, and inclusive of all essential aspects of performance in a given area, they will provide an immensely valuable tool to identify clinical practice deficits or deviations that may be amenable to improvement by instruction.

The observer may be the staff development educator, a preceptor, head nurse, or any member of the staff who has been trained to use the observation guide and is knowledgeable regarding the performance standards. Observation may be random or systematic. Planned observations may be incorporated as part of the orientation program, and spontaneous observations may be used as part of a quality assurance monitoring program. By systematically comparing observed performance with the standards established for performance in that area, many educational needs can be detected that might otherwise go unnoticed.

Listening

Purposeful listening during change-of-shift reports, nursing rounds, patient care conferences, or staff meetings can be a fruitful mechanism for uncovering educational needs that may be imbedded in these processes. For example, nursing rounds may reveal that a diabetic patient admitted for acute ketoacidosis is developing gangrene in the right foot. If none of the nursing staff on the evening shift has had experience providing nursing care for a patient with gangrene, some instruction in this aspect of care is warranted. Serendipitous needs such as this will only be met if someone is listening for them.[5] Thinking through situations, problems, implications, and daily occurrences for their educational ramifications requires a sensitivity to subtleties and a genuine interest in meeting educational needs. Purposeful listening also affords an opportunity to provide relevant and timely instruction when it is most needed and to identify patient case studies that can be used for teaching skills in critical thinking.

Review of Hospital Documents

Reviewing hospital documents and forms represents another method for collecting data on nurses' educational needs. Periodic appraisal of documentation forms (flowsheets, plans of patient care, and nursing notes; accreditation reports; minutes of staff meetings and summaries of performance evaluations; audit reports from quality monitoring mechanisms; and incident reports) can illuminate areas of educational need among staff. Reviews need not be formal and time-consuming, but they should be periodic, unannounced, and thorough enough to determine if educational implications exist. They can also provide a means to give praise and positive feedback to staff for exemplary performance in the areas reviewed.

Numerous other needs assessment methods are available for the educator to consider. These include pretests, the Delphi method,[8] the critical incident technique, matrix assessment, pyramid assessment, nominal group technique,[10,11] brainstorming, job analysis, and performance inventories.

The outcomes of an educational needs assessment may not always afford clear directions for planning staff development programs. Rather, the educator must analyze the information to determine the extent to which the results indicate true educational needs as opposed to other types of needs or problems, must establish priorities among the educational needs, and must verify that the needs were communicated effectively and accurately.

DISTINGUISHING BETWEEN EDUCATIONAL AND NONEDUCATIONAL NEEDS

As the educator gathers information related to the learning needs of nursing staff, it may become obvious that not all of the identified needs are truly "educational" needs. Remember that for a need to be an *educational* need, it must be one that can be met through some form of instruction. Many staff performance problems are not attributable to educational needs and, therefore, do not warrant educational remedies.

For example, the director of nursing may send you a memorandum indicating that the coronary care unit nursing staff need an educational program on cardiac drugs. The basis for this memorandum was the occurrence of two medication errors by nurses on that unit within a 4-week period. If you fail to investigate further, you might not find out that the first incident involved an exhausted but competent staff nurse who was working a double shift necessitated by short staffing. In the midst of completing her second shift, one of her patients experienced a lethal ventricular dysrhythmia and lost consciousness. The nurse reflexly administered lidocaine to the patient rather than the procainamide that had been ordered. Without investigating this, you would also not know that the second incident involved a new graduate who administered dopamine instead of dobutamine because she thought that they were the generic and trade names for the same medication and did not know their comparative similarities and differences.

Assuming that both incidents can be remedied through instruction is obviously erroneous. The first incident may have been attributable to any number of reasons: not taking the time to check the physician's order, confusion and anxiety over the patient's sudden deterioration, inadequate staffing to allow for a rest break to sharpen the clarity of her judgment, a lack of clear thinking from not having eaten lunch or dinner that day, or simple exhaustion. Whatever the precipitating cause, it was functional rather than educational in origin. The second nurse's error, by contrast, was directly attributable to her lack of knowledge regarding the differences between two drugs. Her error represents a true educational need.

Staff development educators need to make a clear distinction between needs that arise from a lack of knowledge, attitudes, and/or skills and those that arise because of attendant or associated problems in the execution of a known task or function. These potential causes of performance problems include inadequate supplies, malfunctioning equipment, insufficient staffing, inadequate administrative and/or peer support systems, lack of guidelines for performance, ambiguous or unrealistic expectations, and administrative or operational obstacles to performance.[15] Educational bandaids will not heal performance problems that are noneducational in origin. Before an educator takes action on a perceived need, the educator needs first to verify that the need represents a true educational need.

A second necessary distinction is to differentiate among educational interests or desires, perceived educational needs, and true educational needs. *Educational interests* reflect a learner's desires or preferences for learning. These interests may influence a nurse's motivation to pursue learning but do not necessarily coincide with the hospital's interests or that nurse's assigned job. *Perceived educational needs* (or "felt needs") represent a learner's perceptions or insights regarding their need for instruction in some area. As with educational interests, felt needs may or may not represent true educational needs. Educators must remember that felt needs only include educational gaps of which the learner is aware. In these days of limited budgets and downsizing of staff development departments, it is increasingly imperative that educators devote their limited resources to meeting true educational needs. Before any felt needs are designated as educational needs, they must pass the litmus test of a direct relationship to the agency's expectations of that nurse's performance on the job.

SETTING PRIORITIES AMONG EDUCATIONAL NEEDS

Ordering educational needs according to their relative importance is a pivotal step in the educational process. The rationale for setting priorities among educational needs is based on three interrelated factors:

- *Not all educational needs are of equivalent importance.* Some directly affect the quality of patient care that nurses deliver and others do so to a much lesser extent.
- *Educational needs are more or less infinite.* They exist along a continuum of importance that can vary among learners and change over time.
- *The resources available to meet educational needs are more or less finite.* The time, money, personnel, equipment, facilities, and other requirements available to the educator rarely approximate the full extent of the need for such resources.

Because of these realities, the staff development educator must be able set priorities that are appropriate to the situation, realistic in relation to the demands of nursing practice and patient care, and feasible in regard to the resources they require. To accomplish this, educators must be able to balance the priority educational needs, time, and resources with the needs of the staff, the unit, and the institution.

To appreciate this notion more fully, consider the following list of educational needs:

- An orientee needs to learn how to assist with transferring a neonate to the operating room 1 hour from now.
- A recently hired staff nurse is not performing CPR correctly on a patient.
- A critical care orientee needs supervised practice in obtaining and documenting hemodynamic parameters.
- Nursing staff have requested that a program on ethics be planned for next year's celebration of Nurses' Week.
- An orientee needs guidance in how to admit patients to her unit.
- A new preceptor would like some assistance in how to teach clinical skills more effectively.
- An emergency department nurse is not following universal precautions or hospital policies regarding the use of gloves, protective shields, and handling of potentially contaminated materials.

After reviewing this list, you can see how some educational needs take priority over others. Some needs (incorrect performance of CPR, not using universal precautions) demand the educator's full and immediate attention and intervention. Some needs (admitting patients) are important because they represent an essential element of nursing practice on a particular unit. Some (obtaining and documenting hemodynamic parameters) are important because they represent an aspect of nursing practice that is performed often on that unit. Others (learning how to assist with patient transfers to the OR) are important because they have a time frame that is definite or very pressing.

To summarize, then, at least four factors influence the priority of an educational need. These can be characterized as the "four F-filters of educational priority":

FATAL   This educational need represents a potentially life-threatening priority because failure to meet the need could result in serious harm or death to a patient or staff member.

FUNDAMENTAL   This educational need represents a fundamental or essential aspect of nursing practice on a particular nursing unit.

FREQUENT   This educational need represents an aspect of nursing practice that is performed numerous times and for virtually all patients on that unit.

FIXED   This educational need is important because it must be met within a very specific time frame.

Staff development educators can use these four filters to screen educational needs and determine their relative priority as well as to allocate resources accordingly.

VALIDATION OF EDUCATIONAL NEEDS

When multiple sources and numerous methods are employed during the needs assessment process, it is almost inevitable that some breakdown will occur in sending, receiving, or interpreting communication of those needs. In order to avoid miscommunication, misunderstanding, and misinterpretation, educators need to validate the compiled list of educational needs with those who originally identified those needs.[3] Without this validation check, educa-

---

Box 2.1

JCAHO Standard SE 2.1

SE 2.1 The needs identified for training and education are based on, as appropriate:

SE 2.1.1   The patient population served and type and nature of care provided by the hospital and the department/service

SE 2.1.2   Individual staff member needs

SE 2.1.3   Information from quality assessment and improvement activities

SE 2.1.4   Needs generated by advances made in healthcare management and healthcare science and technology

SE 2.1.5   Findings from department/service performance appraisals of individuals

SE 2.1.6   Findings from review activities by peers, if appropriate

SE 2.1.7   Findings from the organization's plant, technology, and safety management programs

SE 2.1.8   Findings from infection control activities

From Joint Commission on Accreditation of Healthcare Organizations: *Accreditation manual for hospitals*, Oakbrook Terrace, IL, 1994, JCAHO.

Identification of staff educational needs

Name:* _____   Date: _____

Position: _____

Unit/Department: _____   Telephone: _____

* Please indicate if you are representing a group:

☐ Task Force: _____   ☐ Committee: _____

☐ Council: _____   ☐ Some other group (name): _____

Description of the educational need(s):

_____

_____

_____

Category of staff this need pertains to (check all that apply):

☐ RN   ☐ Nurse managers   ☐ Other professional staff: _____

☐ LPN   ☐ Clinical specialists   ☐ Other ancillary staff: _____

☐ Unlicensed nursing staff   ☐ Other nursing staff: _____

Category of educational need:

☐ Orientation   ☐ In-service education   ☐ Continuing education

---

Source of educational need (Indicate how this need was identified. Check all that apply.)

(01) ☐ Needs of patient population served (the types and nature of care required)

(02) ☐ Needs of an individual staff member

(03) ☐ Information from QA/QI activities

(04) ☐ Advances in healthcare management, science, or technology

(05) ☐ Department/service performance appraisals of staff

(06) ☐ Findings from peer review activities

(07) ☐ Findings from plant, technology, or safety management programs

(08) ☐ Findings from infection control activities

(09) ☐ Other source(s): _____

Action(s) taken   (Staff development unit completes):

Disposition: ☐ Investigate   ☐ Cease action (not a need/   ☐ Add to an   ☐ Develop new program
                    further   not true educational need)   existing program

Date: _____   _____   _____   _____

Figure 2.1 Identification of staff educational needs.

tional planning may be off target, unnecessary, or based on erroneous assumptions. Before educators invest time and energy toward meeting educational needs, they should first verify that what they believe to be the need is the same as what the individual who identified the need perceived it to be.

TRACKING EDUCATIONAL NEEDS ASSESSMENTS

In order to comply with current JCAHO accreditation standards related to orientation, training, and education of staff,[12] healthcare institutions must provide evidence that staff education and training needs are based on information derived from one or more of the sources specified in standard SE 2.1 (Box 2.1). Although educational needs may originate from sources other than the eight identified in SE 2.1, the Joint Commission surveyors will be looking for documentation related specifically to those sources.

One fairly simple way to capture and track this data is to include these eight source categories in the forms used for soliciting and reporting educational need assessments. A form that could be used for this purpose is illustrated in Figure 2.1.

When staff educational needs are communicated to the nursing staff development unit, the data necessary for compliance with standard SE 2.1 would then be readily available for tracking and tabulation either manually or by a computerized recordkeeping system (discussed in Chapter 8). The latter could be accomplished by simply adding a field to designate the needs assessment source and then coding each of the eight JCAHO-monitored sources so that these can be distinguished in printed reports related to assessment data. As educational programs are generated, this source field and code would then automatically be included as part of the course information, just as areas such as the course title, dates, content, and faculty are already included. Tracking the source of educational needs assessments would not only serve to facilitate compliance with JCAHO standards but would also aid in compilation and management of the assessment data to drive program planning efforts in the appropriate direction.

This chapter has focused on the process of educational needs assessment. For any type of staff development pro-

gram, the educator must be able to identify sources of information related to educational needs; select methods to elicit those educational needs; distinguish between educational and noneducational needs; categorize educational needs according to their staff development component (i.e., as a need for orientation, in-service education, or continuing education); set priorities among educational needs, and validate perceptions of expressed needs. A thorough and organized needs assessment sets the foundation for the planning stage of the educational process, the subject of the next chapter.

REFERENCES

1. Alspach JG: Critical care orientation programs: reader survey report, *Crit Care Nurse* 10(5):22, 1990.
2. American Nurses' Association (ANA): *Standards for nursing staff development,* Kansas City, MO, 1990, ANA.
3. American Society for Training and Development: Be a better needs analyst, *Info-line* 502(2), 1985.
4. A national survey of critical care nursing education: final report. In Alspach JG, Bell J, Canobbio MM et al, editors: *Education standards for critical care nursing,* St Louis, 1986, Mosby.
5. Ballard AL: Learning needs assessment, part 1, *J Nurs Staff Develop* 5:91, 1989.
6. Bell DF: Assessing educational needs: advantages and disadvantages of eighteen techniques, *Nurs Educ* 3(5):15, 1978.
7. Bell EA: Needs assessment in continuing education: designing a system that works, *J Cont Educ Nurs* 17:112, 1986.
8. Chaney HS: Needs assessment: a Delphi approach, *J Nurs Staff Develop* 3:48, 1987.
9. Chatham MA: Discrepancies in learning needs assessments: whose needs are being assessed? *J Cont Educ Nurs* 10(5):18, 1979.
10. Farley JK, Fay P: A system for assessing the learning needs of registered nurses, *J Cont Educ Nurs* 19:13, 1988.
11. Harrison EL, Pietri PH, Moore CC: How to use nominal group technique to assess training needs, *Training/HRD* 20(3):30, 1983.
12. Joint Commission on Accreditation of Healthcare Organizations: *Accreditation manual for hospitals,* Oakbrook Terrace, IL, 1994, JCAHO.
13. Joint Commission on Accreditation of Healthcare Organizations: *An introduction to Joint Commission Nursing Care Standards,* Oakbrook Terrace, IL, 1991, JCAHO.
14. Schwab CZ: Assessing learning needs of the experienced critical care nurse, *J Nurs Staff Develop* 4:133, 1988.
15. Sovie MD: Investigate before you educate, *Nurs Educ* 6(2):17, 1981.
16. Sullivan P, Saver C, Moyer D et al: Needs assessment: process and application, *J Nurs Staff Develop* 7:31, 1991.

CHAPTER 3

Program Planning

The needs assessment process provides the educator with an enumeration of educational needs that have been:

- Solicited from all of the major participants in the education of nursing staff
- Scrutinized to ensure that they are truly educational in nature
- Categorized as a need related to orientation, in-service, or continuing education
- Prioritized in relation to their relative importance, potential consequences, and immediacy
- Validated by those who identified them

Once consensus on these educational needs has been reached within the institution, the educator is ready to begin the planning phase of the educational process.

The major elements in planning staff development programs include the specification of instructional outcomes and development of the curriculum.

SPECIFYING INSTRUCTIONAL OUTCOMES

As discussed in Chapter 1, the philosophy, mission, and goal statements related to nursing staff development are used as the basis for determining all aspects of instructional planning. The mission statement for the nursing staff development unit describes its purpose, product, clients, and scope of services. The goals are then specified for each element in the scope of services. For example, if the scope of services is limited to the three traditional components of staff development, there will be three program goals described: one goal for the nursing orientation program, one for the in-service program, and one for the continuing education program. It is from these broad goals (i.e., descriptions of what each program as a whole is intended to accomplish) that the instructional outcomes for nursing staff development are derived.

LEVELS OF INSTRUCTIONAL OUTCOMES

The instructional outcomes* for nursing staff development are typically defined at two distinct levels, a general level and a specific level. The *general instructional outcome* for each program goal is defined as a *program objective*. Program objectives reflect the terminal objective of an instructional program—i.e., what general behavior the learner should be able to demonstrate at the end of the program.

The *specific* instructional outcomes for each program are defined as *instructional objectives*. Instructional objectives reflect the specific cognitive, affective, and psychomotor behaviors that are encompassed by the program objective. Figure 3.1 illustrates the relationship among program goals, program objectives, and instructional objectives for a nursing staff development unit where the scope of services includes only the three custom-

---

*This chapter uses the traditional approach to instructional planning and specification of outcomes. An alternative (competency-based) approach will be used in Unit III to describe outcomes for an orientation program.

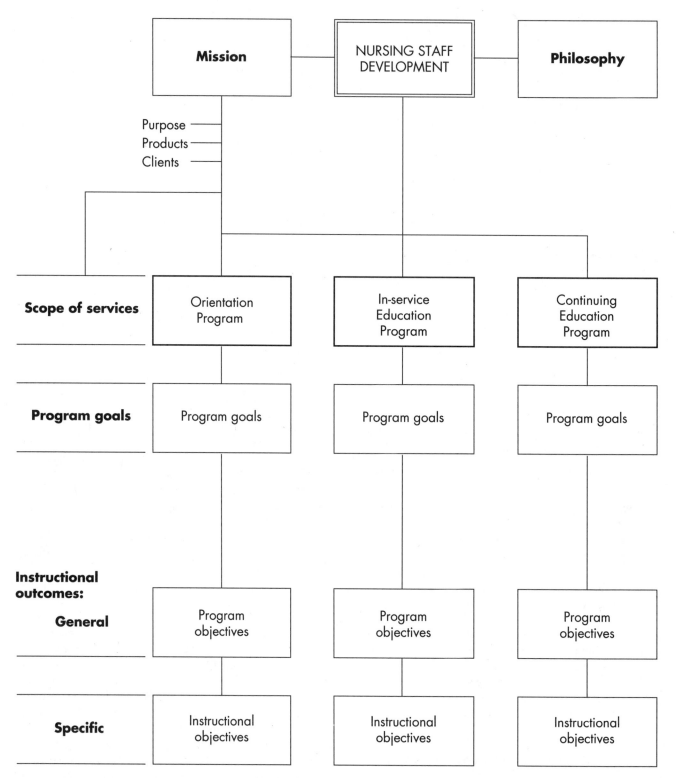

Figure 3.1 Relationship among program goals, program objectives, and instructional objectives for a customary scope of staff development services.

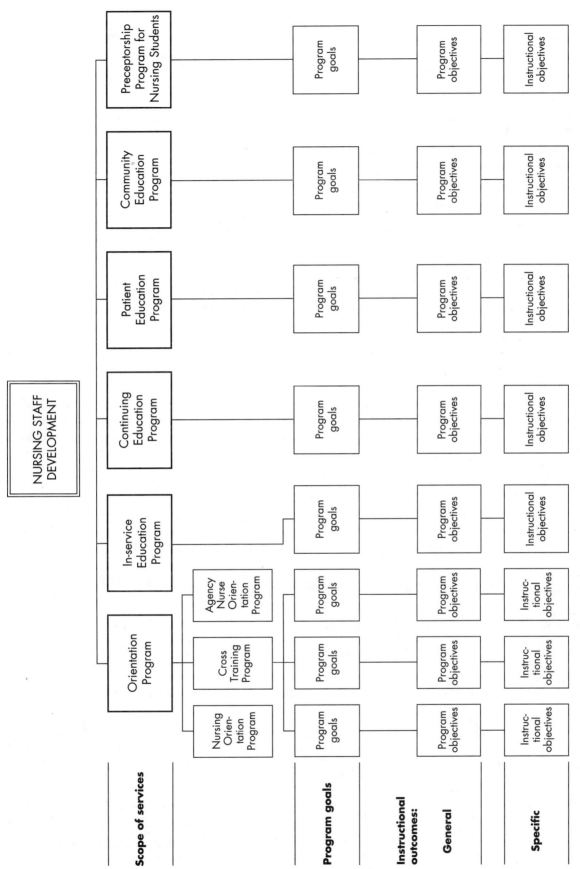

Figure 3.2 Relationship among program goals, program objectives, and instructional objectives for an expanded scope of staff development services.

ary components of staff development: orientation, in-service education, and continuing education.

As mentioned in Chapter 1, the scope of services offered by the staff development unit may include programs beyond traditional employee staff development. These additional programs might include cross training and agency nurse orientation, patient education, or a preceptorship for nursing students. When this expanded scope of services exists, program goals, program objectives, and instructional objectives need to be developed for each program offered (Figure 3.2).

FORMULATING INSTRUCTIONAL OUTCOMES

Developing program and instructional objectives can be a reasonably straightforward process if the educator keeps a few things in mind: the definition of learning, the kinds of learning behaviors, and the purpose of program and instructional objectives.

Learning is defined as a change in behavior. Learners may evidence a change in what they know (their cognitive behavior), in a skill they are able to perform (their psychomotor behavior), or in attitudes (their affective behavior). In order to detect changes in any of these three domains, the behavior must be overt or observable and measurable.

If the purpose of program objectives is to describe in general terms what behavior a learner should be able to demonstrate at the end of an educational program, they need to be written at a fairly broad level that encompasses what the program in its entirety is intended to accomplish. If the purpose of instructional objectives is to describe the cognitive, affective, and/or psychomotor behaviors that are encompassed by the program objective, they need to be written at a more detailed level that distinguishes these cognitive, affective, and psychomotor components.

Writing Program Objectives

Program objectives are, to a great extent, derived directly from program goals. To illustrate this direct relationship, Table 3.1 borrows the program goals used in Chapter 1 for the three components of staff development and suggests one way to write the program objective for each of these goals.

As Table 3.1 demonstrates, each program objective is a translation of a program goal into a broadly stated instructional outcome for that program. Nursing staff development units that offer a more expanded scope of services (see Figure 3.2), need to supply objectives for each program offered.

Writing Instructional Objectives

Once the goal and terminal objective for a program have been determined, the educator's next challenge is to prepare a set of instructional objectives for that program. As mentioned earlier, instructional objectives reflect the cognitive, affective, and psychomotor behaviors that are embodied by the program objective.

Definition of an Instructional Objective

An *instructional objective* is a statement that describes what a learner will be able to do as a result of an educational experience.[2] Mager[43] defines an instructional objective as a description of a performance that the educator wants learners to be able to exhibit as a result of instruction.

The major difference between a program objective and the set of instructional objectives for the program is a matter of specificity. Program objectives are, by definition, broad descriptions of what the whole program is directed toward. Instructional objectives, by contrast, are highly

TABLE 3.1 • SAMPLE PROGRAM OBJECTIVES FOR THE THREE COMPONENTS OF STAFF DEVELOPMENT		
Staff Development Program	**Program Goal**	**Program Objective**
Orientation	The goal of the nursing orientation program is to ensure that all nursing staff acquire the competency necessary to fulfill the responsibilities stated in their respective position descriptions.	By completion of the orientation program, the nurse will be able to fulfill all of the responsibilities described in the Staff Nurse I position description.
In-service education	The goal of the nursing in-service program is to ensure that all nursing staff maintain and increase competency in their respective position following completion of their orientation and throughout their employment at this facility.	By the end of each calendar year, all nursing staff will have met the performance expectations for all scheduled in-service offerings and credentialing programs designated for their assigned unit.
Continuing education	The goal of the nursing continuing education program is to enhance the professional competency and career growth and development of nursing staff beyond the expectations required for fulfillment of their current position description.	By the yearly anniversary of their entry into employment, all nursing staff will fulfill their annual personal objectives related to professional and career growth and development.

specific; they detail the cognitive, affective, and psychomotor behavioral "parts" that the learner should be able to demonstrate to attain the "whole" represented by the program objective.

Purpose of Instructional Objectives

Instructional objectives represent a focal point in all educational programs because they afford direction to the educator, to the learner, and to the program as an entity. In this regard, instructional objectives have at least three purposes:

- They indicate to the educator what needs to be taught. Instructional objectives provide the educator with a means for determining the content and learning experiences that instruction should provide.
- They indicate to the learner what needs to be learned, i.e., the expectations for learning. Instructional objectives provide the learner with a means for determining what needs to be accomplished during the program.
- They provide guidance for all remaining aspects involved with planning, implementing, and evaluating the instructional program.[2,43]

Components of Instructional Objectives

If instructional objectives are to be maximally effective in guiding both learners and educators through an educational program, they need to describe four components:

- A *performance* that indicates what the learner is *doing* when demonstrating achievement of that objective
- A *content area* that specifies what subject matter the performance is *directed at*

- The *criterion* by which the qualitative or quantitative *level of acceptable performance* is identified
- Any necessary *conditions* or *circumstances* under which the performance must be demonstrated[43]

PERFORMANCE The performance contained in the instructional objective should be observable, measurable, and stated in terms of the learner.[52] If the learner is to offer behavioral evidence of the ability to meet an objective and if the educator needs to see this behavioral evidence, then the performance included in the objective must be observable and measurable. Thus behaviors such as "understands," "knows," or "appreciates" are not useful in instructional objectives because the educator cannot observe these behaviors. In stating instructional objectives, therefore, the educator needs to remember that learning cannot be directly observed but must be inferred from overt behavioral evidence. In order to measure that behavior, the educator must be able to see some visible evidence of it in a learner's actions.[7] In selecting behaviors to use in instructional objectives, then, educators need to avoid using behaviors such as those in Box 3.1, which cannot be directly observed. For example, an objective that said "Understands 12-lead ECGs" or "Knows how to interpret a 12-lead ECG" is virtually impossible to evaluate because the educator cannot see someone "understanding" or "knowing." Wording of the objective such as "Identifies a 12-lead ECG that contains evidence of an acute MI" provides much clearer behavioral evidence because it explicitly specifies an observable behavior.

The performance in an instructional objective should always be stated in terms of what the *learner* is doing. Thus an objective such as "Provides opportunities for practicing problem-solving skills" would not be appropriate as an instructional objective because it describes what the educator

---

Box 3.1

**BEHAVIORS THAT SHOULD BE *AVOIDED* FOR INSTRUCTIONAL OBJECTIVES
(ARE NEITHER OBSERVABLE NOR MEASURABLE)**

appreciate
be acquainted with
be aware of
be familiar with
believe
comprehend
know
learn
perceive
realize
remember
think
understand

From Ballard, AL: Writing behavioral objectives, *J Nurs Staff Develop* 6:40, 1990, and Dyche J: *Educational program development for employees in healthcare agencies*, Calabasas, CA, 1982, Tri-Oak Education.

will be doing during the course rather than what the learner is expected to do.

Insofar as possible, the behaviors selected for the performance should relate closely to the performance that will actually be required on the job. Thus a performance such as "Recognizes abnormal breath sounds" would be a more clinically relevant performance than one such as "Describes the characteristics of adventitious breath sounds." The former is an important element of nursing practice, but the latter only represents information without any clinical context.

Performance Domains   Instructional objectives can be grouped into three broad categories or *domains* of behavior: cognitive, affective, or psychomotor. Behaviors in the **cognitive** domain refer to intellectual processes such as comprehending, understanding, explaining, or defining. The cognitive domain includes all objectives related to the acquisition, processing, and application of knowledge.

Behaviors in the **affective** domain relate to feelings, emotions, attitudes, or values. Affective behaviors include conduct such as accepting, respecting, cooperating, and defending beliefs and values.

Behaviors in the **psychomotor** domain refer to manual skills and the performance of tasks or procedures. Psychomotor skills include behaviors such as assembling, auscultating, injecting, calibrating, or demonstrating. Psychomotor behaviors involve the use of knowledge in performance of motor skills.

Performance Levels   In addition to categorizing instructional objectives according to the domain of learning they refer to, instructional objectives can be written at various levels of performance complexity. A number of authors have devised ways to systematically order behaviors within each of the domains of behavior. These classification systems, called *taxonomies,* enumerate successive levels of performance within each domain that range from simple to complex. In each taxonomy, higher levels of performance subsume mastery of the levels below them.

The classic taxonomy of cognitive behaviors was devised by Bloom[12] and includes six levels of performance ranging from knowledge to evaluation. A description of these levels with examples of instructional objectives for each level are provided in Table 3.2. Some of the performance verbs that might be used for each of these levels are provided in Figure 3.3.

A classic taxonomy for the affective domain was designed by Krathwohl, Bloom, and Masia[40] and includes five levels of performance. A description of these levels with examples of instructional objectives at each level is provided in Table 3.3.

Unlike the taxonomies for the cognitive and affective domains, which have enjoyed virtually universal acceptance for many years, the various taxonomies proposed for the

TABLE 3.2 • EXAMPLE OF INSTRUCTIONAL OBJECTIVES FOR EACH COGNITIVE LEVEL		
Cognitive Level	**Description**	**Sample Instructional Objective**
1.0 Knowledge	The lowest and least complex level of cognitive behavior. Includes performances involving remembering by either recall or recognition, memory, and relationships.	The nurse will be able to define the term *cyanosis.*
2.0 Comprehension	The lowest level of understanding. Includes performances involving paraphrasing or interpreting something via translation, interpretation, or extrapolation.	The nurse will be able to describe what cyanosis means in his/her own words.
3.0 Application	The use of information in practical ways. Includes performances involving the use of theories, concepts, or ideas.	The nurse will be able to interpret the clinical significance of cyanosis.
4.0 Analysis	The breaking down of information into its constituent parts and detection of relationships among the component parts. Includes performances involving distinguishing, comparing, and differentiating.	Given two sets of patient laboratory data, the nurse will be able to distinguish whether either patient would be expected to manifest cyanosis.
5.0 Synthesis	The reorganizing of information from a variety of sources into a meaningful whole. Includes performances involving arranging, creating, constructing, and proposing.	Given two case studies of patients with varying degrees and severity of cyanosis, the nurse will be able to devise a plan of nursing care specific for each patient.
6.0 Evaluation	The highest and most complex cognitive level. Represents value judgments and includes performances involving appraisal or critique of ideas, processes, or products.	Given an actual patient case, the nurse will validate the effectiveness of nursing care for a patient with cyanosis.

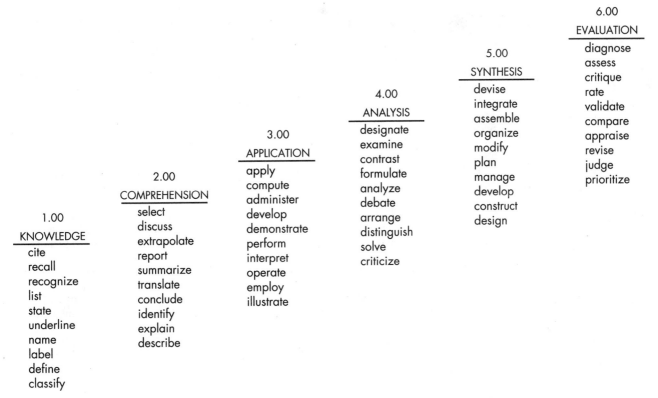

Figure 3.3 Performance verbs for various levels in the taxonomy for the cognitive domain.

psychomotor domain have considerably less widespread acceptance. Dyche[29] refers to a three-level taxonomy of psychomotor behaviors that ranges as follows:

1.0 IMITATING	Performing a procedure as demonstrated
2.0 PRACTICING	Repeated, habitual, trial-and-error movements in performance of a task or procedure
3.0 ADAPTING	Ability to adjust or modify a procedure as required by a situation

Boyle[14] refers to another psychomotor taxonomy proposed by House[37] that includes five levels of performance:

1.0 PERCEPTION	Learner gains awareness of an activity via the senses
2.0 SET	Learner acquires a mental, physical, or emotional readiness for learning
3.0 GUIDED RESPONSE	Trial-and-error performances
4.0 MECHANISM	Habitual performance
5.0 COMPLEX OVERT RESPONSE	Performance without hesitation

Cranton[24] attributes a similar but more complex taxonomy for psychomotor behaviors to Simpson,[55] whose system comprises the seven levels indicated in Table 3.4. Other psychomotor taxonomies have been proposed by Dave,[25] Harrow,[34] and Kibler, Barker, and Mires.[39]

The various domains and levels of performance are useful to the educator in planning for instruction that will best achieve the learning outcomes necessary for nursing practice. Often, instructional outcomes tend to be confined to only the cognitive and psychomotor domains and tend to be written at only the lower levels of performance within those domains. Our clinical expectations of staff, by contrast, tend to be found among the higher levels of performance in all three domains.

One way to use the performance domains and taxonomy levels, then, is to select from among the domains and levels the most appropriate category and level of performance. A second way is to select the performance domain and level that corresponds best to the performance domain and level that the nurse's job will require. A third way is to use the performance levels to structure sequential offerings on the same topic area.[6] For example, the educator might use the lower-to-middle range of performance levels in each domain for the orientation program and use higher levels for in-service and continuing education offerings. The educator's task is to scan all three domains and all levels of performance within each domain to determine the performance level that best approximates the behavior that clinical practice will require of the nurse.

TABLE 3.3 • EXAMPLE OF INSTRUCTIONAL OBJECTIVES FOR EACH AFFECTIVE LEVEL		
Affective Level	**Description**	**Sample Instructional Objective**
1.0 Receiving/attending	The lowest level of affective behavior. Includes performances involving sensitivity and/or awareness of situations or conditions.	The nurse will identify a clinical situation that may represent a crisis to the patient or family.
2.0 Responding	The active reaction to a situation. Includes performance involving responses such as compliance, inquiry, or adaptation that indicate active involvement with the situation.	The nurse includes potential crisis situations for the patient or family in the plan of nursing care.
3.0 Valuing	Refers to behaviors that reflect a value or belief. Includes performances involving supporting, rejecting, defending, and accepting a value or belief.	The nurse initiates the crisis intervention process with patients or family whenever this is indicated
4.0 Organizing	The incorporation of an integrated and systematic belief or value into a situation or experience. Includes performances involving making commitments or operationalizing values into a coherent system.	After reading three different approaches to crisis intervention, the nurse will identify which approach or combination of approaches best suits the patient's/family's need.
5.0 Characterizing	The full internalization of a belief or value. Includes performances involving behaving in a manner consistent with beliefs and values.	The nurse demonstrates the ability to recognize and manage patient/family crises that occur commonly in the assigned unit.

TABLE 3.4 • SIMPSON'S TAXONOMY FOR THE PSYCHOMOTOR DOMAIN		
Psychomotor Level	**Description**	**Sample Instructional Objective**
1.0 Perception	The basis for all psychomotor learning; learner needs perceptual skills to master more complex psychomotor skills; gains awareness of objects through the senses.	The nurse will be able to distinguish among the various components of a chest tube drainage system.
2.0 Set	Readiness for action; includes mental set (knowing the steps in performance), physical set (body positioned correctly to perform), and emotional set (willingness or desire to perform).	The nurse will verbally relate the steps included in setting up a chest tube drainage system.
3.0 Guided response	Replication of the components of a complex task; performance is guided by imitation and feedback from an observer.	The nurse will return demonstrate how to set up a sterile thoracotomy tray for chest tube insertion.
4.0 Mechanism	Performance becomes proficient, habitual, and independent.	The nurse will demonstrate how to set up a waterseal chest drainage system according to unit procedure and without preceptor assistance.
5.0 Complex overt response	Ability to perform more complex patterns or sequences of behavior automatically.	The nurse will demonstrate how to manage a patient with a chest tube drainage system, including initiation, maintenance, and discontinuation of the system.
6.0 Adaptation	Ability to modify motor activities to meet unanticipated demands of the situation.	The nurse will demonstrate how to manage occlusion of a chest tube.
7.0 Origination	Ability to devise new motor activities based on previously developed skills.	The nurse will modify management of the chest tube drainage system for a patient who needs to ambulate with a chest tube in place.

From Simpson EJ: *The classification of educational objectives: psychomotor domain,* Chicago, 1966, University of Illinois (research project N. OE 5).

CONTENT AREA The content area of an instructional objective identifies what topic the performance is directed at. For example, the performance of "recognizes" might be directed at a variety of topic areas: recognizes lethal dysrhythmias, recognizes acute airway obstruction in a neonate, recognizes a malfunctioning IV infusion device, recognizes a need for emotional support, and the like. Each instructional objective should have a clearly defined content area that both the learner and educator can readily identify.

CRITERION A criterion is the standard against which performance is compared to determine if that performance is "acceptable." Including a criterion in the instructional objective provides both the learner and educator with a basis for determining whether the learner's demonstrated performance matches the desired performance. The criterion specifies *how* the performance must occur just as the content area specifies *what* the performance is directed at. The criterion in an instructional objective may relate to the time in which a performance must occur, the accuracy of that performance, or the quality of the performance.[7,43]

Although we are usually less concerned with how quickly or slowly a performance occurs than with the quality of that performance, there are situations in which the **time** frame of the performance is important. In some instances (e.g., establishing an open airway or beginning cardiac compressions) the desired performance must occur within certain minimum times. In other instances (e.g., placing an arterial blood gas specimen on ice, applying endotracheal suction), the desired performance should not exceed certain maximum times. Whenever time frames are crucial to the desired behavior, these should be stated explicitly and clearly in the instructional objective. For example, the objective might read as follows: "The nurse will perform endotracheal suctioning with the suction applied for *no more than 15 seconds.*"

Accuracy is a more commonly employed criterion of performance. The accuracy of a performance relates to the expected degree of correctness (or conversely, to its freedom from errors or mistakes). For example, it might be important to delineate how precise the calculations of intravenous infusion rates must be to be considered acceptable, to establish how precise a manometer central venous pressure reading must be, or to require that staff correctly identify no less than 18 of 20 cardiac dysrhythmias. All of these examples establish a criterion that controls for the acceptable accuracy limits of the performance.

A third possible criterion of performance is the **quality** of that performance. Quality refers to the nature or characteristics of performance, its distinctive attributes. For example, an instructional objective might require that the nurse be able to demonstrate how to assess a patient *systematically,* how to plan nursing interventions *based on a priority of patient care needs,* or how to provide care for patients receiving total parenteral nutrition *according to the unit's nursing procedure.*

Each of these possible criteria of performance—time, accuracy, and quality—are included in the instructional objectives to clarify the standard required for the performance to be considered acceptable. The criterion is included to assist learners in attaining the instructional outcomes and to assist educators in evaluating learner performance.

CONDITION(S) Conditions of performance refer to any special circumstances in which the performance must be demonstrated for it to be considered satisfactory or acceptable.[7] Two questions can be posed to determine if conditions are important to the desired performance:

- What will the learner be allowed to use during the performance?
- What will the learner be denied use of during the performance?[43]

The first question may generate a list of "givens" that are relevant to performance. Some examples of these "givens" include:

- *Given ten sample sets of laboratory findings,* the nurse will interpret all findings correctly.
- *Given five written case studies of obstetric patients,* the orientee will identify the top three priority nursing diagnoses for each case.

The second question could generate a list of "withouts" that are often imposed as restrictions on performance. Some examples of these "withouts" include:

- The nurse will be able to determine the correct infusion rate for three sets of sample vasopressor medications *without the aid of a calculator.*
- The nurse will complete a neurological assessment of a trauma patient *without preceptor assistance.*

Examples of Instructional Objectives

Table 3.5 provides some examples of how instructional objectives are written to incorporate the four components described previously. Box 3.2 provides an example of a set of instructional objectives developed for an in-service program on "Nursing Care of the Patient With Acute Thoracic Trauma." It shows the relationship between the broad program objective and the set of instructional objectives that define the specific cognitive, affective, and psychomotor behaviors that learners need to demonstrate to successfully complete the in-service program.

As with other aspects of program planning, program and instructional objectives are not static and fixed but need reappraisal and modification over time to remain relevant, timely, and effective. Because of their centrality to the educational process, the instructional outcomes prepared for a particular educational program should also be scrutinized each time they are used to determine if they are

TABLE 3.5 • EXAMPLES OF INSTRUCTIONAL OBJECTIVES

Performance	Content Area	Condition(s)	Criterion
Develops	nursing diagnoses	without preceptor assistance	according to unit standards of nursing practice
Suctions	a patient's endotracheal tube and nasopharynx	without breaking aseptic technique	according to nursing department procedure
Completes	assessment documentation of a postanesthesia recovery (PAR) patient	within 10 minutes of the patient's arrival in the PAR unit	that includes all areas on the PAR assessment flow sheet
Provides	informational support to the family of an emergency department (ED) patient	that supplements the physician's communications	while following ED crisis intervention guidelines
Demonstrates	how to troubleshoot IV infusion device alarms	given three simulated alarm situations	according to the skills checklist criteria

---

Box 3.2

SAMPLE SET OF PROGRAM AND INSTRUCTIONAL OBJECTIVES

In-Service Program: "Nursing Care of the Patient With Acute Thoracic Trauma"
Program Objective: By the end of this in-service offering, the nurse will be able to describe how to provide nursing care to a patient with acute thoracic trauma.
Instructional Objectives: The nurse will be able to:
- Distinguish between the two major categories of chest trauma as described on page 1 of the handout.
- Describe the pathophysiology associated with pneumomediastinum; closed, open, and tension pneumothorax; hemothorax; pulmonary contusion; and myocardial contusion as presented in the lecture.
- Compare the clinical features of tension pneumothorax with the features of flail chest as reviewed in the discussion.
- Explain the purpose of the "plunger test" for tension pneumothorax as illustrated in the readings.
- Identify the clinical parameters found in esophageal laceration as described in the lecture.
- Compare and contrast the clinical problems associated with open, closed, and tension pneumothorax; hemothorax; flail chest; and esophageal laceration as distinguished in the slide presentation.
- Demonstrate how to set up a waterseal drainage system with suction according to nursing department procedure and without preceptor prompting.
- Demonstrate how to assist with chest tube insertion and removal in a simulated laboratory setting according to hospital procedure.
- Specify the nursing diagnoses most often associated with acute thoracic trauma, based on the unit's standard nursing care plans.
- Identify the priorities of nursing care for patients with acute thoracic trauma, based on three written case studies and according to the criteria identified on the handouts.

---

meaningful to learners and fulfilled by the educator. Alexander[4] suggests one simple and straightforward way to accomplish this.

USES OF INSTRUCTIONAL OUTCOMES

In addition to their utility in establishing the intended outcomes of instruction, program and instructional objectives are useful for the following activities:

- Defining the content (subject matter) necessary for instruction
- Selecting the most appropriate teaching methods (learning experiences must provide opportunities for performing the same behavior as that which is stated in the instructional objective; this may require practice with behaviors on lower levels of more than one domain initially with gradual progression up the taxonomic hierarchy to the final domain)

- Guiding decisions related to the human and material resources required for instruction (e.g., selection of faculty, media, audiovisuals; writing case studies and worksheets)
- Establishing guidelines for developing an evaluation plan for the program (types of evaluation instruments, items appearing in each instrument)

In short, development of program and instructional objectives sets the stage for all subsequent steps in the educational process: continuation of program planning, implementation, and evaluation. The next section will address the second aspect of program planning—using the instructional outcomes to develop a curriculum.

CURRICULUM DEVELOPMENT

A *curriculum* consists of a systematic plan of learning experiences that will facilitate learners' attainment of established instructional outcomes. *Curriculum development* is the process of determining and arranging the various components of the curriculum so that they facilitate learning. A curriculum includes all aspects of the instructional plan: selection of content or subject matter, planning the order and timing of instruction, selecting instructional media, designating and managing faculty, and preparing instructional schedules.

SELECTION OF INSTRUCTIONAL CONTENT

The subject matter or content for an educational program is determined by the content area(s) contained in the instructional objectives for the program together with any prerequisite knowledge, attitudes, or skills that learners do not currently possess. For example, in an introductory course on interpreting cardiac dysrhythmias, one objective might be: "Recognizes lethal cardiac dysrhythmias." The primary content area for this objective would be "lethal cardiac dysrhythmias."

Before learners could recognize what a *lethal* dysrhythmia is, however, they would first need to know the fundamentals of electrocardiography, some basic information related to cardiac monitoring and lead systems, basic electrophysiology of the cardiac cycle, the ECG attributes of normal sinus rhythm, a systematic approach for dysrhythmia interpretation, parameters that make a dysrhythmia "lethal," and the like. If pretesting or completion of a previous course had not verified that learners already knew these prerequisite areas, then the content selection process would need to include them.

This point reinforces the notion that educators must know learners' current capabilities before they can plan instruction. If educators assume that the audience already knows the prerequisites, they may fail to include content that is necessary for meeting the instructional objective. As

a result, the audience may find learning the material very difficult because they are missing knowledge and skills from lower levels of each domain that are necessary for understanding higher levels. If educators mistakenly assume that the audience does not know the prerequisites, they may waste their time and the learners' time by including content that was not necessary. Ideally, the educator uses pretests, the results of a previous course, or their personal knowledge of the learners to verify what capabilities learners already possess related to each objective. Without some basis for judging these capabilities, the educator is vulnerable to misjudging the amount and nature of content necessary for a program.

ORGANIZING AND SEQUENCING THE CURRICULUM

Regardless of the time available for instruction, the educator cannot teach and learners cannot learn everything all at the same time. Some things have to be learned first, some later, and some at the end. Part of the educator's responsibility is to decide the order of learning experiences. This process of chronological organization of the curriculum is called *sequencing*.

The order in which material is presented and learned can greatly affect a learner's ability to understand, integrate, retain, and transfer learning. At one time or another, each of us has wrestled with a concept we found difficult to comprehend. Much later, after discovering the missing links in our understanding, we were finally able to understand the concept. In general, the educator should cover prerequisite knowledge, attitudes, and skills first and then cover content related to higher performance levels (such as application, analysis, synthesis, and evaluation).

When sequencing is well planned for a group of learners, facts, concepts, and principles are gradually introduced and interrelated. This creates a comfortable, meaningful, and progressive flow of learning that affords continuity and integration over time.

The effect of appropriate sequencing for a 60-minute class is no less significant than it is for a 6-month curriculum. Learning from a speaker who is totally disorganized can be virtually impossible, whereas even very complex material can be readily learned if it is presented in a logical, orderly fashion that reflects sound and thoughtful sequencing of the curriculum.

As you attempt to decide on the best order for presenting material, try to remember the following:

- The optimal sequence pattern is the one that most enhances learning. No one "right" sequence exists for any curriculum.
- As the composition and the characteristics of the learner group vary, the composition and the order of the sequence are also likely to change. A sequence for planning learning experiences must reflect the learner's background, prior education, and experience,

knowledge, and abilities. The same sequence may not be appropriate for all groups of learners.

- The ultimate purpose of sequencing is in its cumulative effect, that is, attaining smaller elements of learning at the appropriate times and in the appropriate order so that a meaningful whole is gradually formed that is reflected by learners' attainment of the instructional and program objectives.
- The ability to sequence learning requires that the educator be familiar with both the material to be learned and the characteristics of the intended learners. Unless educators understand the subject matter and know what learners already know and what they yet need to know, the sequence of instruction may both begin and end in inappropriate content locations.
- Experience and experimentation with various sequencing patterns provide a wealth of valuable insights into what is best for each particular group of learners.

Armed with a knowledge of the material, the instructional objectives for the program, and an understanding of the characteristics of a particular group of learners, the educator has the raw materials for deciding how to put the components of the curriculum into the most beneficial sequence.

A wide variety of approaches is available for planning a curriculum sequence. Some approaches are rather complex and time consuming.[24] Some alternative approaches for sequencing the curriculum include arranging learning on the basis of one or more of the principles listed in Box 3.3.

Although the overall sequence typically incorporates only one or two major approaches, sequencing is usually determined by using a combination of these approaches. Even the approach of presenting the content in "the way it has always been presented" is valid if this is truly the way that most facilitates learning.

Nursing has often followed a medical model when presenting material related to patient care: definition of the disease or disorder, pathogenesis and pathophysiology, signs and symptoms, medical treatment, and nursing care. Rather than rigidly adhering to this sequence pattern, the educator can attempt to modify, adapt, or create his/her own approach for presenting the material. Experimentation and learner feedback will help determine the best approach. Educators will know that the sequencing is effective when the audience reports that learning complex material was relatively painless and that they can readily apply what they have learned in their daily practice.

ALLOTTING INSTRUCTIONAL TIME

Once content areas have been arranged in a meaningful sequence, the educator must distribute various amounts of time to specific content components. Because the time available for instruction is usually limited, care must be taken in deciding how much time will be devoted to each content element within the total program.

Just as no magical formula exists for sequencing, no foolproof approach exists to allotting instructional time. One guideline to keep in mind is that time is a valuable resource available in a limited supply; it is a resource that the educator will want to use in the most effective and efficient way possible.

One way to approach allotting instructional time is by first considering the total amount of time available for instruction as 100% and then allocating decremental percentages of time to each objective, based on its priority, complexity, and prerequisite subject matter. In general, the percentages of time given to each objective should reflect its relative priority, complexity, and prerequisites. Objectives that are of higher priority, that are more complex, and that have greater amounts of prerequisite content should be given more instructional time.

Box 3.3

PRINCIPLES FOR SEQUENCING INSTRUCTION

- General to specific
- Known to unknown
- Concrete to abstract
- Simple to complex
- Facts to principles
- Principles to applications
- Most to least important
- Most to least interesting
- Part to whole (or whole to part)
- Chronological order
- The inherent or natural logic of the subject matter
- The established order of steps in a procedure
- The customary or traditional way of teaching the content

Box 3.4

FACTORS THAT MAY INFLUENCE HOW ALLOTMENTS OF INSTRUCTIONAL TIME ARE APPORTIONED

- Total time available for instruction
- Total number of objectives
- Priority of importance assigned to each objective
- Nature and complexity of objectives
- Learners' present knowledge, skills, attitudes, and experience related to the objectives
- Nature and complexity of the subject matter
- Types of teaching methods to be used
- Availability of resources (facilities, personnel, etc.)
- Instructor's experience in teaching the subject matter

A number of factors may influence how allotments of instructional time are apportioned. Some of these factors are included in Box 3.4.

In attempting to allot instructional hours, remember that the educator's purpose is to distribute the time available in a manner most efficient for assisting learners to attain the instructional outcomes. Because the instructional process is largely a human social interaction, it is not readily amenable to rigid scheduling. Educators need to be sure to build some flexibility into the instructional time so that questions, reviews, clarifications, practice, and the stress and fatigue level of learners can all be accommodated.

SELECTING INSTRUCTIONAL MEDIA
Rationale for Using Instructional Media

Instructional media such as slides, films, and videotapes serve a number of useful purposes in the teaching-learning process. Audiovisual media are generally thought to enhance the effectiveness and retention of learning by their recruitment of alternative and multiple sensory avenues through which to provide instruction. If it is true that we retain

10% of what we read
20% of what we hear
30% of what we see
50% of what we both see and hear
80% of what we say, and
90% of what we say as we perform something

then it should be apparent that using only a single sensory medium (e.g., only hearing a lecture or only reading an article) may not be the most effective way to learn.

Individuals differ with respect to the sensory learning mode(s) they prefer for learning. Some prefer to learn by hearing, others by seeing, and others by touching or manipulating objects. Some prefer to use combinations of one or more of these sensory avenues. Instructional media, then, can also be useful for accommodating these individual differences among learners.

Media are generally used to complement or supplement other teaching activities. They can be used to stimulate and control learner attention; to introduce creativity, variety, and flexibility in approaches to learning; to provide cues or stimuli for learning; to stimulate recall of previous learning; to allow for repetition, expansion, reinforcement, and new applications of learned material; and to evaluate the extent of learning.

From a practical viewpoint, instructional media allow for greater flexibility and adaptability to time constraints placed on both learners and instructors in hospital-based settings. They offer a pragmatic approach for providing a means of self-instruction for nurses on all shifts. Media can accommodate the limited amount of time that nurses can be away from the patient's bedside or can more effectively and efficiently use those rare quiet periods when patient care demands are temporarily diminished.

Media offer the flexibility of making instruction available at any hour it is needed or desired. Many forms of media can be readily transported to any desired location in the workplace or at home where they can be used at the learner's own pace during one or several sessions.

From the instructor's vantage point, media may afford additional time for expanding on the material covered in the program or for working individually with learners who are experiencing learning problems. Use of media can reduce repetition of frequently needed instruction and extend the capabilities of a single instructor for reaching a larger audience. When staff nurses with widely varying capabilities and backgrounds join the staff, the instructor responsible for in-service education can use a multimedia program to provide a "core course" of essentials rather than repeating the same information each month or every few months as new staff nurses enter the unit. In this manner, all new nursing staff can be prepared at a comparable level of performance. This also affords the instructor more time to reinforce the material, follow through with its transfer and application in the clinical setting, and validate that the essentials have indeed been learned.

Developing vs. Purchasing Instructional Media

Until rather recently, hospital-based staff development programs were nearly universally developed "in-house" by a group of educators. After many hours of planning, designing, script-writing, pilot-testing, evaluation, and refinement, a single program was finally developed. The format was generally limited by the educators' collective knowledge, experience, and resources and often resulted in a written module or an audio tape. Some of the instructional aids were effective, engaging, and efficient, and others—many others—were not.

Over the past two decades, the budgetary and staff resources available to educators have dwindled, while the time frames required for programs have often become more pressing. During this period, however, hundreds of commercially produced instructional aids have become available to healthcare educators. These off-the-shelf programs can offer educators and learners many conveniences and advantages as well as a multitude of audiovisual formats. Although commercial media may ameliorate many of the educator's needs in some areas of instruction, they are

no panacea. Educators are still faced with the dilemma of whether to develop their own instructional media or to purchase off-the-shelf products.[47,49]

The decision to internally develop instructional media or to purchase external products depends on a number of factors. Some of these factors favor internal development and others support purchasing programs. Table 3.6 compares these two sets of factors to aid educators in their decision.

Criteria for Evaluating and Selecting Instructional Media

If the hospital decides to develop instructional media internally, the resulting programs will need to be critiqued both during and after their design. If the hospital determines that it will purchase instructional media, a comparable set of considerations must be employed to examine, compare, and select among the multitude of programs available.[47] Figure 3.4 provides a checklist for the educator to compare, select, or evaluate instructional media.

Guidelines for Using Instructional Media

Because instructional media may be inappropriately used, overused, or underused, their proper employment warrants some mention. The following guidelines are presented to ensure optimal use of instructional resources.

TABLE 3.6 • FACTORS INFLUENCING DECISION TO DEVELOP VS. PURCHASE INSTRUCTIONAL MEDIA		
Factor	**Favors Developing Your Own Media**	**Favors Purchasing Media**
Content and objectives	Content and objectives are unique to the hospital and are not available in commercial programs	Content and objectives of commerical products are compatible with needs and cover all essentials
Need for updating/revising content and/or objectives	Content and/or objectives will need to be updated and revised frequently	Content and/or objectives are not subject to frequent updating or revision
Percentage of program needing modification	Over 25% of program would need to be modified to meet needs	Less than 25% of program would need to be modified to meet needs
Available audiovisual support	Agency has an adequate supply of skilled media experts to design, edit, and produce program(s)	Agency has limited or no media developers available and educator lacks skills to design program(s)
Technical quality of commercial program	Is less than or not better than what could be produced internally	Is much better than what the agency could produce internally
Budget	Funds not available to purchase programs or to pay media consultants	Funds available to purchase programs
Number of users	Relatively few learners will use the program; high cost per user	Substantial number of learners will use the program; low cost per user
Administrative support	Administration more likely to support internal development; views program development as an educator function	Administration will support the most cost-effective means of providing the program
Time before need for program	Extended period of time is available before program must be provided	Limited time is available before program must be provided

From Parry S: Make or buy? *Training* 28(10):14, 1991, and Reilly DE: *Behavioral objectives in nursing: evaluation of learner attainment,* New York, 1980, Appleton-Century-Crofts.

FEATURE	YES	PARTIALLY	NO	NOT APPLICABLE
INSTRUCTIONAL OBJECTIVES				
Provided	☐	☐	☐	☐
Stated in behavioral terms	☐	☐	☐	☐
Match/are compatible with hospital's objectives	☐	☐	☐	☐
CONTENT				
Is accurate	☐	☐	☐	☐
Is up to date	☐	☐	☐	☐
Relates to objectives	☐	☐	☐	☐
Is clinically relevant	☐	☐	☐	☐
Is free of bias	☐	☐	☐	☐
Is validated	☐	☐	☐	☐
Has appropriate scope	☐	☐	☐	☐
Has sufficient depth	☐	☐	☐	☐
PRESENTATION				
Is clear	☐	☐	☐	☐
Is well organized	☐	☐	☐	☐
Is easily understood	☐	☐	☐	☐
Can be individualized	☐	☐	☐	☐
Includes feedback to learner	☐	☐	☐	☐
Provides practice for learner	☐	☐	☐	☐
Provides evaluation of learning	☐	☐	☐	☐
Covers all objectives	☐	☐	☐	☐
AUDIENCE				
Is appropriate for large groups	☐	☐	☐	☐
Is appropriate for small groups	☐	☐	☐	☐
Is appropriate for individualized use	☐	☐	☐	☐
Level of instruction is appropriate for intended audience	☐	☐	☐	☐
Program uses adult education principles	☐	☐	☐	☐

Figure 3.4 Checklist of criteria for evaluating instructional media. *Continued*

FEATURE	YES	PARTIALLY	NO	NOT APPLICABLE
TECHNICAL QUALITY				
Uses good quality text	☐	☐	☐	☐
Illustrations are clear, accurate, and enhance learning	☐	☐	☐	☐
Uses high quality soundtrack	☐	☐	☐	☐
Uses color effectively	☐	☐	☐	☐
EASE OF USE				
Directions are provided and are easy to follow	☐	☐	☐	☐
Material or equipment is easy for learners to use	☐	☐	☐	☐
Material or equipment is easy for instructors to use	☐	☐	☐	☐
Program is easy for learners to use	☐	☐	☐	☐
Program is easy for instructors to use	☐	☐	☐	☐
Components are packaged for easy use and storage	☐	☐	☐	☐
TIME				
Program can be completed within a reasonable time	☐	☐	☐	☐
Program can be completed at the learner's pace	☐	☐	☐	☐
Program saves instructor's time	☐	☐	☐	☐
COST				
Initial purchase price is within budget	☐	☐	☐	☐
Cost of continued use is reasonable	☐	☐	☐	☐

Figure 3.4, cont'd.   Checklist of criteria for evaluating instructional media.

- Be certain that the media selected are consistent with the instructional outcomes established for the educational program. The program's instructional outcomes should not be revised to match the media's objectives; rather, the media's objectives must coincide with the intended outcomes of the program.
- Ensure that the level, depth, and scope of instruction provided in the media are compatible with the background, knowledge, and skills of the intended audience.
- If necessary, demonstrate to learners how to operate and troubleshoot the audiovisual equipment.
- Prepare the audience or users for the presentation by identifying the purpose, content outline, significance, and objectives of the program before showing it. For self-instructional media, this information may be provided in a written form that is distributed or otherwise made available to learners.
- Anticipate the need for clarification, application, supplementation, or correction before the presentation. Provide these as necessary during and following the audiovisual presentation.
- Make every effort to relate concepts and facts from the media's theoretical or hypothetical considerations to their application on the clinical unit or to a situation with which the audience is familiar.
- Give learners responsibility for actively participating in the learning experience by noting points for them to watch or listen for, noting the purpose of their using the program, and noting the accuracy or consistency of the presentation with their own clinical experience.
- Review and summarize major points made in the presentation and validate the learner's understanding of the material from the program.
- Provide a period following the presentation for audi-

ence and instructor to critique the media—its content, format, pace, accuracy, and technical quality.

This section has reviewed the potential value of using instructional media, outlined criteria for evaluating and selecting media, and listed some guidelines for use of instructional aids. The following section summarizes the characteristics of various categories of media that are currently available.

Characteristics of Instructional Media

This section provides an overview of some of the most commonly used instructional media. For each type of instructional aid, its usefulness, limitations, and cost considerations will be presented.

Audio Tapes

USEFULNESS

- An alternative to printed media that is readily available and highly mobile.
- Tapes can be advanced, replayed, or stopped at any point. Can be readily coordinated with other media such as slides.
- Hardware is easy to operate and familiar to learners.
- Can present brief vignettes for analysis and for learning communication skills.
- Can be used to preserve experts' presentations from local or national meetings.
- Can be used to share verbatim programs with staff who were not able to attend outside educational programs.
- Useful for individual or group study.
- Capable of providing instruction in the cognitive and affective domains of learning.
- Can be reused indefinitely. Provides consistent content to learners.
- Even novice instructors can learn to record and edit with relative ease to tailor instruction.

LIMITATIONS

- Can be boring if lengthy, if using only a single speaker, or if delivery is monotone.
- Lack of a visual focus during the program can result in audience losing attention and having diminished retention of learning.
- May be frustrating or confusing if visuals are not available for illustration, reinforcement, and clarification of content discussed.
- May be confining if acoustics or amplification distorts or diminishes quality of sound.
- Inappropriate and generally ineffective for teaching psychomotor skills.
- Quality of locally produced tapes may vary widely.

- Some sounds (such as heart sounds, breath sounds) can be distorted in the recording process, resulting in a product that does not sound true or lifelike.
- Tapes recorded at professional meetings may contain extraneous and distracting sounds; may be missing slides or handout supplements; questions from audience may not be audible.

COST CONSIDERATIONS

- Depends on producer (local hospital, professional audio tape service at meetings, professional media company), length of tape, whether other instructional materials (such as study guide or instructor's guide) are provided with tape, and whether sold as single copy or as part of a set.
- Cost of a single blank audio tape is nominal—less than one dollar; better quality tapes cost $2 to $4 each.
- Cost of a single tape for a 30- to 45-minute prerecorded program may range from $20 to $90.
- Hardware cost for cassette player/recorder varies by model, manufacturer, and features. Cost ranges from $50 to $150.

Chalkboard

USEFULNESS

- A familiar medium to learners and instructors.
- Readily available and easy to use.
- Infinitely reusable.
- Colored chalk can enhance visual effects.
- Instruction can modify written information while teaching to tailor for immediate needs.

LIMITATIONS

- Space for writing can be inadequate at times and require frequent erasures to complete presentation.
- Is a static display; unable to illustrate motion.
- Chalk dust may be bothersome to persons with allergies.
- Visibility may be diminished by sunlight shining on board, by learner's location in room, or by instructor using very hard chalk or some colors of chalk.
- Instructor must turn away from learners to use.
- Time is lost while instructor is writing on board.
- Difficult to teach while simultaneously writing or erasing.
- Instructor's handwriting may be illegible.
- Instructor's artistic and graphic abilities may be poor.
- Learners tend to focus on copying notes from board rather than on listening to presentation.

COST CONSIDERATIONS

- Varies with size, quality, and characteristics of the board. Special board features such as color or texture will increase cost.
- Cost of freestanding chalkboard with dual writing sur-

face is approximately $125 to $135, depending on size. Large, wall-mounted boards are considerably more expensive.

Markerboard

USEFULNESS

- Similar in general features to chalkboard, except that surface is white Melamine® or porcelain.
- Bright, vivid, and erasable marker colors are more eye-catching and visible than powdered chalk.
- Liquid marker pens are erasable, dust free, and wash off.
- Nonglare surfaces enhance visibility even in sunlit rooms.
- Nonreflecting matte finishes enable using board as a projection screen.
- Can be mounted on a wall or in a movable frame; framed boards may be double surfaced with magnetic surface feature.
- Available in a wide variety of sizes.

LIMITATIONS

- Board surface requires more care in cleaning and maintenance than chalkboard.
- Space for writing can be inadequate at times and require frequent erasures to complete presentation.
- Is a static display; unable to illustrate motion.
- Instructor must turn away from learners to use.
- Time is lost while instructor is writing on board.
- Difficult to teach while writing or erasing.
- Instructor's handwriting may be illegible.
- Instructor's artistic and graphic abilities may be poor.
- Learners tend to focus on copying notes from board rather than on listening to presentation.

COST CONSIDERATIONS

- Boards and writing media are more expensive than with chalkboard system.
- Cost of board varies with size and ranges from $50 to $250.
- Set of four marking pens costs approximately $5.

Flip Charts (Pads of Paper Secured to an Easel)[13,19,30]

USEFULNESS

- Are portable and reusable.
- Instructor can tailor to immediate needs and use more than one simultaneously.
- Simple to use and have none of the potential problems associated with media that require electrical hardware.
- Can prepare ahead to structure presentation or use as session progresses.

- Can remove and tape important pages for later reference or to view results of group work.
- If notes on charts are used frequently, can have a graphic artist prepare professionally done series for subsequent use.
- Available with plain or grid paper (nonerasable) easel pad or with reusable and washable sheets; some varieties have static cling feature that allows pages to be temporarily mounted to cement, glass, or wood surfaces.
- Grid paper is useful for spacing characters and lines evenly.

LIMITATIONS

- Shares marker board limitations.
- Paper variety is not reusable, and ink may bleed through to sheets below.
- Easel stand may be unstable and cumbersome to transport.
- Visibility (especially toward the lower half of pages) may be limited when used with larger audiences.
- Instructor may flip pages too quickly, leaving insufficient time for reading, retention, and note taking.

COST CONSIDERATIONS

- Cost of easel varies with material (aluminum, wood, steel) and size. Cost ranges from $30 to $60.
- Cost of 50-page paper easel pads is approximately $10 per pad. Reusable varieties may cost two to three times that amount.

Posters*

USEFULNESS

- Portable; their location can be changed and they can be mounted on many different surfaces.
- Reusable; may be useful for roving in-services.
- Relatively inexpensive to produce and purchase.
- Can attract attention and convey messages efficiently.
- Used to inform, instruct, inspire, or incite.
- May be used to teach or review policies and procedures; to practice selected clinical skills; to stimulate thinking about values and beliefs; or to share new ideas or research findings in a concise format.
- Provide a constant and repeated message simply and efficiently.
- Can be used for self-instruction or with supplementation by the author.

LIMITATIONS

- Design, content, or layout may not be attractive to potential viewers.
- May be placed in an unobtrusive location where they will not be noticed.
- May not be sufficiently self-explanatory; when author

*See references 15, 17, 19, 21, 27, 53.

is not nearby to offer explanations and answer questions, their instructional value may be diminished.
- May be difficult to store if large.

COST CONSIDERATIONS
- Colored poster board sheets cost approximately $20 for a package of 25 sheets.
- Sheets of lighter weight cost less than heavier, stiff boards.
- May be able to secure professionally prepared posters without cost from professional societies such as the American Heart Association or American Lung Association.

Overhead Transparencies*

USEFULNESS
- More dynamic and versatile than slides because they can be altered during the presentation.
- Are easy and inexpensive for novices to produce. Production involves either photocopying images onto acetate transparency sheets or adding lettering and/or images directly onto sheets.
- May be prepared ahead of time or as presentation progresses.
- May use with individual acetate sheets or a roll of acetate film that can be advanced as needed. Both types are relatively easy to use.
- Ink from water-soluble marking pens can be washed off for reuse; permanent ink can be used for repeat presentations.
- More readily visible to larger group than chalkboard or models.
- Add intensity, color, clarity, emphasis, and additional information to presentations.
- Can focus learners' attention on desired amount of information by using covers or overlays with progressive disclosure of transparency content.
- Versatile means of production via colored marking pens, computer-generated transparencies, wax pencils, or photocopies.
- Can be produced in variety of colors or color combinations by using color transparency film, color film overlays, and/or color tapes and markers.
- Instructor able to maintain face-to-face contact with learners even while writing.
- Can reuse materials multiple times.
- Can use with normal room lighting that enables audience to take notes and ask questions more readily.
- Hardware is easy to operate.
- Projectors come in three varieties: classroom, portable, and low-profile ("sit-down"). Low-profile model enables instructor to sit during presentation, allowing for a more informal and interactive relationship with audience. Liquid crystal display (LCD) panels can be used to project images onto a screen from the overhead projector's stage (glass plate).
- Can purchase professionally prepared commercial transparencies.

LIMITATIONS
- Requires an instructor's presence.
- Process of changing transparency sheets may be time-consuming and distracting to audience if white light flashes of blank screen are not avoided.
- Instructor may have illegible handwriting and/or be a poor illustrator. Typed lettering and most journal article printing will not be legible to audience.
- Hand lettering is often of poor quality for projection.
- Continuous pages of typed copy are boring and difficult to read.
- Instructor may distract learners' attention by showing transparencies too soon or by leaving them on too long after topic of discussion has changed.
- Some instructors fail to adequately focus images, keep image within boundaries of screen, or angle the lamp to avoid keystone-shaped projections.
- Acetate transparency film requires some care in handling and avoidance of high heat and humidity. Transparency mounts (press board, plastic, paper) can simplify handling and storage.
- Visibility is usually very poor with large groups.

COST CONSIDERATIONS
- Price of overhead projectors varies with manufacturer, model, and features. Cost ranges from $200 to $300, with portable projectors ranging from $500 to $700. Average price is $550.[32] Computer projection systems are considerably higher, ranging from $1200 to $5000 or more.
- Marking pens are inexpensive: $10 for a package of twelve pens. Colored transparency adhesive film is about $6 per sheet.
- Cost of overhead transparency film varies by type of printer/photocopier used. Clear film for plain paper copiers ranges from $30 to $40 for 100 sheets. Clear film for laser copiers is more expensive, about $25 for 50 sheets. Tinted film for both costs a few dollars more.

Print Media (Books, Journals, Handouts, Reprints)

USEFULNESS
- Most familiar medium of learning.
- Easy to obtain; readily available in virtually all topic areas.
- Easy to duplicate or obtain from publisher.
- Learners may refer to as often as necessary for reinforcement and clarification.

*See references 16, 18, 20, 21, 28, 36, 44.

LIMITATIONS

- Information may be outdated or incomplete.
- Usefulness may be limited by learners' reading ability, comprehension, reading speed, and retention of information over time.
- May afford too much or too little information on a given topic.
- Usually require supplementation by instructor but offer large potential for self-instruction on a topic.

COST CONSIDERATIONS

- Cost of photocopied and reprinted materials is nominal.
- Journal subscriptions and books are more expensive, but costs can be spread over many users.

Slides (2″ x 2″, 35 mm)[22,31,44,59]

USEFULNESS

- Versatile and flexible medium; can arrange in any sequence; can alter sequence readily; can combine locally made and commercially made slides; can pace use to any desired rate.
- Attractive and eye-catching multicolor slides can include text, graphics, and visual effects that focus learners' attention.
- Can use text and graphics alone or in various combinations.
- Are easy to store and maintain; projectors are portable and easy to use.
- Can be used and synchronized in conjunction with other media such as audio tapes.
- Can be used with audiences of any size.
- Can be produced by novice photographers or professional slide production services; computer-generated slides can be readily produced and tailored to individual needs.
- Related sets can be updated readily by changing, adding, deleting, or reorganizing slides.
- Slide-tape systems combine the usefulness of slides and audio tape. Systems can be set to operate automatically and repeat programs for as long as desired. Afford multisensory learning avenue that is useful for self-paced instruction at any time and location.

LIMITATIONS

- If a viewing system is not available, instructor may expend substantial time in arranging and sequencing a set of slides from multiple programs.
- Instructor may insert slides incorrectly into slide tray, resulting in annoyances to learners such as inverted or reversed slides or having slides out of correct order.
- Design flaws (too much information, poor color contrasts, complicated graphs, small typeface, all-text slides, and the like) make slides difficult to read.
- Slides that lack titles tend to initially confuse audience.

- Strong visual focus may distract learners from listening to presentation.
- Slides may not project well if room has too much sunlight or if room lighting is not adequately dimmed.
- Projector malfunctions, burned out lamps, jammed slides, or a remote control that is not working can delay presentations and annoy audience.
- Darkened room interferes with note taking and asking questions; diminishes learners' attention.
- Slides can be damaged by misuse, exposure to heat, bending, or humidity.

COST CONSIDERATIONS

- Cost of locally produced slides is nominal (less than $.50 per slide). Black and white slides are less costly than color.
- Cost of professionally prepared slides varies with manufacturer, number of slides in set, and whether accompanying materials (such as workbooks, instructor's guide, storage case) are included.
- Custom-made computer-generated slides prepared by hospital's media department can be secured for nominal cost ($1 to $3 or less per slide).
- Custom-made computer-generated slides prepared by outside vendors can be expensive (about $25 to $50 per slide), depending on content and graphics desired and whether slide copy is provided via modem by client ($6 to $10 per slide).
- Cost of slide projectors varies with model and features desired. Standard projectors range from $250 to $450, with lenses sold separately at $75 for a standard lens and $150 to $200 for a zoom lens.
- Slide-tape systems retail for approximately $1000.
- Slide trays are fairly nominal in price, ranging from $7 to $10 each.
- Screens for projection vary in cost, depending on size, whether wall mounted or freestanding, composition of screen material, and screen features. Cost of tripod portable screens ranges from $100 to $150 for a small screen to $185 to $375 for larger models. Wall-mounted electrical screens are considerably more expensive.

Models (Simulated Objects)

USEFULNESS

- Provide three-dimensional replica of reality for learners to manipulate objects and observe how they interrelate functionally.
- Afford hands-on simulated practice in learning procedures and skills.
- May be scaled to real size for illustration, be larger than reality for clarification, or be smaller for experiencing an entire object and its related parts.
- Most are portable, easy to maintain, and infinitely reusable.

LIMITATIONS

- Generally unsuitable for use with large group when model is small; to use with large group, need to repeat explanations with each segment of group.
- Appearance of object may be lifelike, but features such as texture and elasticity may be lacking.
- Some include numerous small components that can be lost or broken; others are fragile and require great care to use.
- May be large and bulky to manipulate, transport, and store.
- Some (e.g., mannequins) require special cleaning, maintenance, and storage procedures or have parts that require replacement at given intervals.

COST CONSIDERATIONS

- Varies markedly with the specific model.

Films (3/4″ U-matic or 1/2″ VHS Videocassettes)

USEFULNESS

- Can be used to teach instructional objectives in all three domains of learning.
- Particularly useful for teaching psychomotor and affective areas, where other media have much more limited applicability.
- Can be used to make the abstract concrete, to animate and focus attention on desired images and aspects.
- Best used for small groups or one-on-one, when learners can control the progress of the film.
- Action can be slowed, stopped, or repeated to demonstrate and reinforce sequence of motions or behaviors to be learned.
- Simultaneous use of color, movement, and sound commands learners' attention and stimulates interest.
- Versatile for all phases of the educational process: for stimulating initial discussions, teaching principles and their application, reinforcement of learning, supplementation of instruction, and evaluation of learning.
- Provide consistency and control over instructional content.
- Hardware can also be used for patient and family education.
- Can be made locally to meet institutional needs or can be purchased as prerecorded videos from outside vendors.
- A wide diversity of topics is readily available from nonprofit healthcare agencies and associations as well as from proprietary vendors.
- Videocassettes are self-contained and easy to use, organize, and store.
- Ease of use for learners facilitates self-instruction.
- Can rent rather than purchase programs if desired use is limited.

LIMITATIONS

- Portions of prerecorded films may become obsolete, reducing their overall value and requiring disclaimers and clarifications by instructor.
- Commercially prepared films cannot be edited or updated.
- Can rarely be used as a stand-alone instructional tool; usually needs viewer's guide or other printed materials to supplement.
- Damage or breakage to the cassette precludes use of any portion of the product.
- Local production requires substantial planning time, skilled personnel, appropriate facilities, and relatively expensive equipment; resources for local production of films may be lacking at smaller healthcare agencies.
- Flaws in design, enactment, or production may detract from the quality of the program.
- Selecting a commercial video producer requires considerable preplanning.[38]
- Audience attention may wane with long videos. After 10 to 15 minutes, a substantial proportion of the audience may lose interest in the film unless it continues to captivate their full attention.[48]

COST CONSIDERATIONS

- Rental and purchase are relatively expensive compared to other media.
- One- to three-day rentals are priced from $60 to $140 for a 22- to 30-minute videocassette, with higher fees for newer releases.
- Purchase prices for 30-minute cassettes range from $275 to $600, depending on the vendor and whether the film is an old or new release. Some multiple-order discounts are available.
- Videocassette recorders/players (VCRs) for industrial use range in price from $400 for basic models to $8000 for top-quality machines. The average price is $1000.[32]
- Quality video cameras cost approximately $3000 for monochrome and $5000 for color.

Television (Video Teleconferencing via Closed-Circuit Television, Cable Network, or Satellite)[11,17,42,46,54,56,61]

USEFULNESS

- Extremely versatile and sophisticated medium for providing all components of staff development, for teaching in all three domains of learning, and for reaching audiences of any size in multiple locations.
- Conferences are conducted in a studio setting having broadcast capabilities and are transmitted to reception sites ("downlinks") locally, regionally, or nationally. Viewers at reception sites can participate in conference by means of talk-back systems that permit conversations with presenters in the broadcast studio.

- Provides an effective and efficient way to deliver and disseminate important and timely information quickly and consistently to large and dispersed audiences.
- Staff can view live programs when they are offered or view taped copies at their convenience 24 hours of the day at work or at home. Accommodates flexible work schedules and variations in workload during shift. Learners able to pace and control their own learning.
- Use of programs can enable staff to secure continuing education and staff development, obtain continuing education units (CEUs) without the time losses or costs (e.g., airfare, lodging, meals, ground transportation) associated with travel to distant meetings.
- Programs can be produced locally, rented, subscribed to on an ongoing basis, or purchased.
- Equipment (tape players, VCRs) is familiar to users and relatively easy to use. Tapes may be played at work or home.
- Increases access to national experts on a topic. Can be used to preserve and disseminate information from experts on a topic to many who would not otherwise have had access to the expert or the program.
- Programs may be broadcast live or taped for rebroadcast at viewers' convenience. Tapes can be centrally located in a learning library or placed on mobile carts for use on clinical units, in learning laboratories, skills laboratories, or classrooms.
- Interactive teleconferencing in conjunction with live broadcasts enables learners to actively participate in discussions and ask questions.
- Local educational facilitators can enhance program effectiveness at downlink sites by introducing programs; managing questions, discussions, and interactions; coordinating on-site segments; and summarizing and evaluating the event. This local educational "wraparound" can make the program more relevant and meaningful for learners.[5]
- Reduces the time and expenses associated with staff traveling to distant sites for continuing education.
- Programs can be integrated with formal or self-directed learning formats in any area of staff development.
- Closed-circuit television (CCTV) networks are dedicated systems accessible to any component part of the network circuit. Hospitals may have their own cable network or be part of a local or regional network that includes multiple healthcare facilities. A central computer can then control and distribute programs to desired points within the network for viewing at specific times or when desired 24 hours a day, making programs available to all staff on all units and all shifts. CCTV programs can be broadcast for simultaneous viewing by a group of any size or can be viewed by one individual at his/her convenience. Resources and faculty may be shared by users. Sophisticated systems can also monitor use and survey various groups of users.
- Cable access networks may interconnect multiple facilities and private residences within one or more communities to provide a wider viewing area than CCTV typically affords. Nurses within those communities can avail themselves of programs at work or at home; many receiving sites will likely already have connections to the cable system. Larger viewing audiences may be reached by purchasing air time through the Public Broadcast System (PBS).
- Satellite teleconferences involve the transmission of broadcast signals to a telecommunications satellite orbiting the earth. Signals are then beamed from the satellite to television sets located in the downlink sites. One-way video transmissions and two-way audio transmissions afford interactive programming.[11] Satellite network conferences have the potential to reach thousands of viewers at numerous locations throughout the country simultaneously.

LIMITATIONS

- Is a significantly more complex medium for instruction.
- Equipment necessary for production and viewing is elaborate and expensive.
- The number of programs available in specific areas of need may be limited; available programs may not be tailored to meet institution's needs.
- Production of local programs may not be feasible for small facilities because such production requires special facility and equipment as well as technical and media experts.
- Faculty may lack experience in working in this medium. Educators need to adapt teaching plans specifically for video presentation, prepare and distribute teaching materials well in advance of conference, coordinate plans at each downlink site, and gain facility in working with scripts and camera system. Additional time must be allotted for planning course offerings, identifying target markets, developing a budget, designating a conference coordinator, designing the logistics for each reception site, selecting and preparing faculty, registering of learners, and evaluating the conference program.[11]
- The time staff has available for viewing programs may be limited, making short (15- to 20-minute) programs desirable. Multiple, brief tapes may be necessary rather than a single long tape.
- Individual use of programs can be perceived as impersonal and devoid of faculty-learner interaction.
- CCTV: Unless cable and hardware for the system are already in place, the purchase and installation costs are considerable. Service calls for repair of system malfunctions can be expensive and may require shutting the system down.
- Live programs must start and stop on schedule and have limited flexibility for learners who cannot slow, stop, or take a break from program. Interactions with

presenters are not purely natural; time lags from transmission delays leave long, unnatural pauses in communication.

- Not all experts present well in this medium. Presenters may have limited experience in teleconferencing technique or may not be skilled at reading from a teleprompter while looking into a camera. Speakers' movements are restricted so they can stay within the camera's view; this may reduce their spontaneity. Presenters cannot see or interact with audience as in a classroom setting.

COST CONSIDERATIONS

- Costs per institution and per viewer need to be considered in calculating true cost.
- CCTV: Relative costs can be reduced if system can also provide programming to other professional and allied health practitioners at the facility as well as provide patient/family education programs. Other facilities in the area may be willing to share the costs of producing or purchasing tapes.
- Cable access networks: Viewing time is more costly than CCTV since air time must be purchased from outside source.
- Fees for satellite networks vary with the network subscribed to and the range of services desired. Costs are often based on the number of occupied beds per day or the number of staff in particular fields such as nursing.
- Construction of videoconferencing rooms is expensive, depending on the equipment capabilities, audience size and features desired ($100,000 to nearly $1,000,000).
- Cost of video cameras varies widely, depending on manufacturer, model, and features.
- Televisions and television/VCR unit prices vary with manufacturer, model, screen size, and features ($800 to $1300). Videodisc players range from $600 for basic models to more than $8000 for top-quality models.
- Blank color videocassette prices vary with manufacturer, quality, tape length, and range from $5 to $10 each, with volume discounts usually available.
- Cost of professionally produced, prerecorded programs varies widely with vendor, length of program, and inclusion of other instructional materials or options such as CEUs.

Computer (Computer-Assisted Instruction, Interactive Videodisc, and Laser Disc)

USEFULNESS[9,33,51,57,60]

- Computer-assisted instruction (CAI) can provide consistent, high-quality instruction that is multisensory (color, graphics, animation, video, audio, and text), interactive, learner driven, individualized, and well retained over time.

- CAI can provide a variety of instructional forms[23,51]: drill and practice that supplement the customary teaching process, tutorials that provide for basic understanding and application of concepts, problem-solving sessions that require judgment and critical thinking, and simulations of clinical practice that portray real-life situations requiring management.
- CAI can be used for initial or remedial instruction, self-assessment, or evaluation of learning. It is particularly amenable to providing experiential and real-life learning related to affective and psychomotor domains and simulation of situations, such as malfunctioning equipment or development of clinical complications, that other formats cannot readily provide.[23,51]
- For learners, CAI is self-paced, self-sequenced, compelling, private, nonpunitive, and convenient in time and location to work or home schedules.
- CAI is consistent with the principles of adult education because learners are active and interactive participants in learning who can control the pace and sequence of learning as their needs dictate.
- For instructors, CAI supplements time for teaching, provides remedial instruction tailored to learner needs, allows learners to make mistakes with no harmful consequences to patients, reinforces or supplements content provided in other settings, and provides for validation and evaluation of learner performance in a reliable and objective manner.
- CAI can enhance instructional efficiency by avoiding unnecessary instruction for both learners and instructors (learners can pretest out of program segments); by individualizing instruction to learner's needs; by removing dependency on instructors; by saving instructors time in developing teaching plans and in repetitive teaching; by enabling learners to progress through programs as rapidly as they can; by providing instruction on all work shifts; by using slower periods during shift (vs. overtime) for continuing education; and by bringing instruction to wherever learners are when they are ready to learn.
- For instructional management, CAI affords record keeping on staff development participation for later summary and tabulation as required by agency and accrediting organizations. Computerized records also provide a means for dynamic record keeping related to budgets and quality assurance.
- Computer-assisted interactive videodisc (IVD) programs are menu-driven, easy-to-use, learner-paced and learner-sequenced means of instruction that provide immediate feedback to learners on their performance.[35] Learners are often familiar with videodisc technology from their home VCRs. Input devices are easy to use and come in a variety of forms: computer keyboard, key pad, light pen, or touch screen. Videodisc media can improve learner achievement and retention and save instructional time in comparison with more traditional teaching methods.[41,46] The discs

are virtually indestructible, easy to store, not subject to damage by electrical interference nor are they vulnerable to the temperature and humidity problems associated with tape media.

- IVD can simulate hands-on experience with concepts, skills, equipment, or clinical situations. Unlike video tapes that are passively viewed and listened to, interactive videodisc programs actively involve learners in learning. IVD can simulate psychomotor and affective skills equally well or better than many other teaching methods.[50] Clinical skills such as decision making, patient assessment, and priority setting can be taught effectively.[45]

LIMITATIONS [8-10,23,33,51,60]

- Hardware and software are not universally standardized. Programs that run on one type of system may not be usable on another.
- Hardware and software (both initial and ongoing) costs are generally more expensive than for many other media.
- Requires one keyboard and monitor per learner. Stand-alone computers can serve only one learner at a time.
- Software selection requires a thorough and systematic evaluation.[10] Some software for nursing is of poor quality.[33]
- CAI is an impersonal and mechanistic medium of instruction for both learners and educators. Learners may miss interactions with peers and the instructor.[26,51]
- Computers may create an unrealistic environment where there is a solution to every problem. Reality may be considerably less clear in its solutions.
- Both instructors and learners may resist use of computers because this medium may not be consistent with their philosophy and preferences for teaching and learning. Educators may lack facility in using computers and/or expertise in developing programs.
- Few commercial programs are available on advanced specialty nursing area topics.[9]

COST CONSIDERATIONS

- The cost of developing an interactive videodisc program, while decreasing, is still expensive (estimated to be between $100,000 and $200,000[42] or $20,000 to $65,000 per module.[62] One hour of CAI may require 50 to 700 hours to create.[10]
- Local production of interactive CAI is usually feasible and cost effective only if there will be many users, if users are geographically dispersed, if content experts are not available, if the content is intrinsically visual in nature, if live demonstration is inappropriate, if users vary in experience or skill, or if the program can

be used repeatedly and its content will remain relatively stable over time.[50]

- Costs per learner must be viewed in relation to costs saved by lowering travel costs and time away from work, and cost of instructors' salaries.
- Commercially available CAI programs can be rented, contracted through a vendor, or purchased.

Securing Instructional Media

Instructional media are available from a wide array of sources. Some of these sources will provide media free of charge and others will lend it free or at a nominal charge. Some sources will allow preview or rental of programs for varying periods of time; others will contract provision of specific forms of media, and still others will offer purchase of media.

The various sources of instructional media can be grouped into the following nine categories:

- Federal government agencies
- Educational institutions
- Publishing companies
- Pharmaceutical companies
- Healthcare equipment vendors
- Healthcare institutions
- General healthcare associations and organizations
- Professional nursing associations
- Proprietary media vendors

The National Audiovisual Center serves as a central distribution source for more than 600 audiovisual programs produced by the federal government. Their collection of audiovisuals is divided among some 28 subject areas and over 100 subsections, including the topics of health, medicine, safety, and surgery. Under the topic of health are found 48 media related to nursing and patient care and programs related to drug and alcohol abuse, geriatrics, nutrition, and public health. Media formats include 16-mm films, ¾" and VHS videocassettes, filmstrips, slide sets, and multimedia kits.* The cost of programs is very reasonable.

A secondary source of information on audiovisuals through the federal government can be tapped through the National Library of Medicine's AVLINE (audiovisuals online) database, which has catalogued audiovisuals in the health sciences since 1975. Any facility with access to MEDLINE should be able to tap into the AVLINE database as well. In this database can be found listings of media (by subject and author), reference citation information, and brief descriptions of the program. Although media cannot be ordered through AVLINE, the database provides information on the procurement sources for all catalogued audiovisuals in the healthcare field.

Media may also be obtainable through shared consortia library arrangements with local educational institutions.

---

*Orders can be placed by telephone (800-638-1300) or by mail (National Audiovisual Center, 8700 Edgeworth Drive, Capital Heights, MD 20743-3701).

Area community colleges, colleges, and universities, including local schools of nursing, may be willing and able to lend programs for use at a healthcare agency. These schools may allow access to their library, learning center, or audiovisual department media hardware and program holdings.

Numerous healthcare publishing companies offer audiovisual media in addition to books and periodicals. Slides, films, audio tapes, filmstrips, a multitude of print media, and videocassette programs are readily available. Computer-assisted learning programs are obtainable on an ever-increasing number of clinical topic areas. Some instructional packages include multiple media, such as printed materials, lecture notes, handouts, transparencies, slides, and computer-managed evaluation of learning, available in a single set.[3] Catalogs of these materials may be secured from the publisher.

Pharmaceutical companies continue to be major sources for high-quality audiovisuals related to the drugs that they market. A number of pharmaceutical houses will supplement their customer in-service education programs with printed materials, slide sets, videocassettes, or computer-assisted instruction on their drugs. Many of these are available by simply requesting them through the drug company representatives who work in your region. Healthcare equipment vendors are equally helpful in providing this type of material related to their products. A majority of these media are available at no cost or for a nominal charge.

Neighboring healthcare institutions in a geographic region may be willing to pool their collective instructional resources by cooperatively renting or purchasing programs for use by multiple hospitals and healthcare agencies. Savings can be realized by sharing costs, planning cooperative use schedules, and avoiding duplication of purchased programs. Some healthcare agencies may share the costs of producing a needed program or pay nominal fees to borrow a program developed at another institution.

Numerous general healthcare associations and organizations such as the American Hospital Association, the American Heart Association, the American Lung Association, the American Cancer Society, and innumerable other civic and social agencies have produced media related to their area of interest. Many of these programs are made available for use free by healthcare professionals and the public on a loan basis or at a very reasonable cost.

Virtually all professional nursing associations provide one or more forms of media for their members. Smaller associations may provide only printed media, whereas larger associations offer an array of print, audiovisual, and CAI programs. Some of these products are available directly from the association and others must be secured from the publisher or producer. These instructional resources are often available to members at a discount. In addition, the National League for Nursing offers an annual directory of educational software related to nursing.

An increasing number of proprietary media vendors have emerged over the past decade. These companies develop and produce instructional media or distribute it through institutions that pay a fee to enter their media system or network. Professional nursing conferences are a good place to meet with representatives of these companies who often exhibit there to reach their program audiences. Even the best instructional media, however, cannot replace the skilled instructor. The following section considers this irreplaceable instructional resource.

MANAGING PROGRAM FACULTY
Securing Program Faculty

Budget cuts, corporate mergers, and the downsizing or elimination of hospital staff development departments have left fewer prospective staff to assist in providing instruction for nurses. At some healthcare institutions, one or two educators are responsible for numerous nursing units or an entire service or division. At other agencies, all of the responsibilities formerly borne by a nurse educator are now vested among the multitude of duties of the nurse manager or nursing coordinator. Since it is not feasible that one or two individuals can possibly provide all of the instruction necessary for large numbers of nursing staff, other nursing staff are often recruited to assist in providing this instruction. In addition, the multidisciplinary nature of nursing practice suggests that other professional groups besides nurses should participate in educational programs for nursing staff.

Which staff might be recruited to serve as program faculty? In general, suitable candidates will demonstrate two common traits: (1) thorough knowledge and experience in their clinical area and (2) an ability and willingness to help others learn. Possible instructor candidates from within the nursing service include clinical nurse specialists, nurse managers, experienced staff nurses, quality assurance coordinators, and nurses who work in special departments such as the electrophysiology laboratory, the emergency department, infection control, or parenteral support team. Outside the nursing service, instructors from the following professional groups are often recruited: pharmacologists, dietitians, social workers, respiratory and physical therapists, and physicians.[1]

Some teacher characteristics are thought to facilitate the learning process. The traits listed in Box 3.5 can be considered in determining whether a particular individual might be a good instructor for adult learners. Other instructor characteristics are believed to inhibit the learning process. Individuals who exhibit the traits found in Box 3.6 should likely be dropped from consideration as prospective faculty if these characteristics do not seem amenable to improvement.

Many nursing staff development programs require classroom, laboratory, and clinical instructors. Although many faculty will be equally adept in all three instructional settings, this is not always the case. Some faculty may be very effective in the classroom or skills laboratory but not in the clinical setting. Others may be very relaxed in their clinical

---

Box 3.5

TEACHER CHARACTERISTICS THAT FACILITATE THE LEARNING PROCESS

- Enthusiasm for the subject matter
- Enthusiasm for teaching
- Clarity, audibility, and organization in expression
- Interest, concern, and respect for learners, their views and experiences
- Fairness and impartiality toward learners
- Flexibility and openness to others' opinions and ideas
- Sense of humor, friendliness, and permissiveness toward others
- Ability to admit mistakes
- Generous use of positive reinforcement
- Understanding and ability to adapt knowledge and expertise to audience needs
- Facility in applying principles and theory to practice realities
- Adeptness at problem solving and decision making
- Ability to facilitate learner participation in learning
- Ability to provide instruction consistent with instructional outcomes
- Innovation and creativity in teaching methods

Box 3.6

TEACHER CHARACTERISTICS THAT INHIBIT THE LEARNING PROCESS

- Intolerance for the views of others
- Disinterest in learners
- Disinterest in teaching
- Disorganized, boring, or too rapid in providing instruction
- Tendency to discount or patronize learners
- Tendency to read lecture notes or procedures to learners
- Inability to respond effectively to questions
- Tendency toward rigidity and defensiveness in instruction
- Marked insecurity or anxiety with the educator role
- Feedback on performance tends to be ambiguous or negative
- Domineering and controlling in relationships with learners

---

unit but be extremely self-conscious and disorganized in a classroom situation. The educator needs to know prospective instructors as individuals and determine their preferences and abilities for each instructional setting.*

Developing Program Faculty

The educator's responsibility for faculty does not stop at designating and scheduling instructors for topics. Because many nurses may serve as instructors who have little or no preparation in the fields of education or adult education, the educator has an obligation to assist would-be faculty in developing their teaching skills. Two other benefits of helping nursing staff learn the fundamentals of instruction are: (1) such help will afford a larger cadre of more highly skilled faculty and (2) a better-prepared faculty will ultimately improve learners' abilities to attain the instructional outcomes for the program. A capable and confident faculty can help to ensure a more effective, efficient, and satisfying learning experience for both learners and instructors.

Weaknesses in instructor performance generally emanate from shortcomings either in preparing for or in providing instruction. Once a teaching deficiency is defined and related to one of these two areas, the approaches necessary to resolve the inadequacy become more clearly apparent. Box 3.7 lists areas in which beginning instructors commonly need improvement. These areas can serve as the basis for developing instructors for your programs. Some suggested approaches for assisting instructors in each area are discussed in the following sections.

Areas Related to Preparation for Instruction

PLANNING RELEVANT LEARNING EXPERIENCES   Review the instructional outcomes to be addressed. Work with the instructor on suggesting a range of possible learning activities

---

*Chapter 6 will describe how to secure and prepare preceptors.

Box 3.7

AREAS COMMONLY NEEDING IMPROVEMENT IN NEOPHYTE INSTRUCTORS

AREAS RELATED TO PREPARATION FOR INSTRUCTION
- Planning relevant learning experiences
- Thorough and current knowledge of the subject matter
- Appropriate level of instruction
- Organization of the presentation
- Clarity in presentation
- Consistency between learning experiences and instructional outcomes
- Total time and pacing of instructional segments
- Distinguishing major points of emphasis

AREAS RELATED TO PROVISION OF INSTRUCTION
- Establishment of rapport with learners
- Quality of performance as role model
- Ability to respond to questions
- Technical qualities of presentation
- Demonstrations of how to apply theory and principles to clinical practice
- Involvement of learners in learning experiences
- Creation of a comfortable (psychological, physical) learning environment
- Nature and quality of feedback provided to learners

(such as background readings, written case studies, skills practice, simulations, role playing, etc.) that could lead to attainment of those objectives. Help the instructor identify actual unit and patient situations as examples that learners can relate to for illustrating points of emphasis and application. Ask questions that the audience may pose to give the instructor practice in showing how the material being covered relates directly to clinical practice. Remind the instructor that adult learners are pragmatic and problem oriented; help the instructor anticipate clinical problems the audience may identify and some ways to offer solutions to these.

THOROUGH AND CURRENT KNOWLEDGE OF THE SUBJECT MAT-TER Depending on the time and resources available to the educator, assistance can vary from directing the instructor to avenues for securing recent literature to actually providing this material. Instructors may be better served by learning how to obtain this information on their own so that they are able to do this independently in the future. Thus the educator could teach instructors how to access the National Library of Medicine's MEDLINE literature search services or teach them how to use the Grateful Med software to access the MEDLINE database themselves. Other alternatives are to provide the instructor with either a bibliography of recent journal articles or actual copies of the most current literature available in the assigned topic area. Regardless of the degree of support given to the instructor in obtaining recent literature, the educator can then work with the instructor to summarize major developments in the topic

area and identify the relevance and implications for nursing.

APPROPRIATE LEVEL OF INSTRUCTION If the instructor is a nurse, provide the instructor with descriptions of what learners have already mastered in knowledge and skills related to the topic. Share copies of the assigned readings with the audience and summarize audience characteristics, such as age range, amount and types of clinical experience, instructional outcomes already attained, strengths and weaknesses, and the like. Distinguish what learners already know about that topic and what, if anything, they will later learn about that topic. If the instructor is not a nurse, familiarize the individual with relevant nursing issues (e.g., nursing diagnoses, the nursing process, standards of nursing care) so that nursing's frame of reference is understood and the subject matter can be approached in relation to its implications for nursing practice. Review the depth and scope of what the instructor plans to provide to verify that it coincides with an appropriate instructional level for the intended audience.

ORGANIZATION OF THE PRESENTATION Ask the instructor to prepare a detailed content outline for the presentation. Review the outline with the instructor in relation to the appropriateness of its organizing theme, smoothness of instructional flow, and transitions between subtopics. Verify that the instructor understands how concepts relate to one another in some logical fashion. If the instructor needs additional practice, review fundamental organizing themes (such as those mentioned for sequencing a curriculum) and provide practice selecting appropriate organizational systems for a variety of topic areas.

CLARITY IN PRESENTATION   Verify that the instructor is familiar with relevant attributes of the audience in relation to the topic: learners' knowledge, skills, clinical experiences, and the like. Verify that the instructor thoroughly understands the topic area, its concepts and complexities. Clear up any misconceptions or misunderstandings that may be evident. Have the instructor describe how he/she will explain and link various points into a logical whole for the presentation. Provide guidance in identifying concrete illustrations and applications of abstract ideas that the audience will find meaningful. Play the role of a learner by asking the type of questions the audience will likely pose and by anticipating concepts that nurses typically have some difficulty understanding. Have the instructor demonstrate how he/she would respond to each. Assist the instructor in identifying alternative ways to explain and portray concepts. Help the instructor locate audiovisual support for elucidating, simplifying, and/or amplifying points.

CONSISTENCY BETWEEN LEARNING EXPERIENCES AND INSTRUCTIONAL OUTCOMES   Review the desired relationship between instructional outcomes and learner evaluations. Verify that the instructor is aware of the specific instructional objectives or performance criteria that relate to the topic area. If evaluation tools are already developed for that area, show these to the instructor so that there is awareness of how learners will be evaluated in that topic area. If evaluation items are not yet developed, work with the instructor to design these as direct reflections of the content and behaviors contained in the instructional objectives or performance criteria.

TOTAL TIME AND PACING OF INSTRUCTIONAL SEGMENTS   Be sure that the instructor understands the starting and stopping times planned for his/her teaching segment. Ask the instructor to indicate how he/she plans to allot instructional time for each element in the content outline. Review the soundness and feasibility of that time distribution plan. If necessary, remind the instructor of the two major determinants of how instructional time is apportioned (importance of content and complexity of content) and suggest alternative ways to allot time. Attend session(s) taught by the instructor. If the plans for time allotment were satisfactory but are now exceeded, review factors (such as straying from the topic, using too many examples, or allowing a few learners to monopolize discussions) that may have caused this problem. Suggest ways to manage problems that tended to interfere with completing the instruction on time. Suggest that instructor mark notes to signal the time needed to complete each of the subtopics. If possible, have room clock face instructors so that they may pace themselves unobtrusively. Remind instructors that if they plan to use audiovisuals, they will need to preview the program and its time requirements and have all equipment ready beforehand.

DISTINGUISHING MAJOR POINTS OF EMPHASIS   Suggest that the instructor peruse entire content outline and then summarize the five most important points of the learning experience. Review the relationship between major points of emphasis and instructional outcomes for the presentation. Some instructors may find it helpful to highlight these points in their notes to be certain they are emphasized and to include them in audiovisuals or handouts for learners.

Areas Related to Provision of Instruction

ESTABLISHMENT OF RAPPORT WITH LEARNERS   Explore how instructor views his/her relationship with learners. Determine if this relationship tends toward being pedagogical (viewing the teacher as supreme, the source of all knowledge) or andragogical (viewing the teacher more as a peer, a facilitator of learning). If the instructor's approach seems to be pedagogical, review or role play the adult learner's responses to this type of relationship. Assist the instructor in understanding that adult learners need to be respected as persons with valuable life and professional experiences. Help instructor gain insight into any tendencies toward being dogmatic in instructional settings.

QUALITY OF PERFORMANCE AS ROLE MODEL   Distinguish between instructor's weaknesses in knowing how to perform and faulty demonstration of clinical practice caused by some other factor(s). Review procedure performance elements and differentiate between important and trivial performance details. Verify that instructor recognizes critical procedural elements that need emphasis with learners. Provide practice in role performance through informal sessions in learning laboratory or by videotaping the performance and then reviewing strengths and weaknesses.

ABILITY TO RESPOND TO QUESTIONS   Remind instructor that fear of learners asking them questions is usually unwarranted. Even the most experienced and expert instructors will occasionally encounter questions that they cannot answer. When this situation occurs, it is best just to say that they do not know the answer or that they will find the answer and get back to the requester. Most novice instructors are pleasantly surprised to find that they can provide answers to a vast majority of questions raised if they can remain poised, listen fully to the question, repeat or paraphrase the question, ask for clarifications as necessary, and give themselves a few moments to reflect and formulate a response. Most importantly, before continuing with the learning experience, instructors need to verify that the learner's question has been adequately addressed. Remind instructors that most inappropriate responses to questions occur because the question was not clearly or correctly understood, because they did not listen fully to the question, or because they did not think longer before responding. All of these abilities are refined with experience. If time permits, role play as a student asking questions so that the instructor gets practice in formulating suitable responses.

Technical Qualities of Presentation Assist instructors in gaining insight into how their vocal qualities and visibility affect communication with learners. Offer suggestions on how better to project voice, vary modulation, improve enunciation, and enhance visibility for the audience. Use role-playing simulations or videotaping of teaching sessions to identify mannerisms (e.g., nervously pacing back and forth while presenting) or habits (repeating certain words such as "you know" or "like" or turning away from the audience while speaking) that might detract from the presentation. Help instructors identify these areas and concentrate on minimizing them.

Demonstrations of How to Apply Theory and Principles to Clinical Practice Emphasize the necessity for relating abstract concepts and basic scientific principles to bedside patient care. Review principles of adult education related to meaningfulness and immediacy of application to the work setting. Provide practice for instructor in describing how concepts and principles related to the presentation could be correlated with nursing practice. Verify that instructor understands all relevant theoretical and scientific precepts that underlie nursing care in the topic area.

Involvement of Learners in Learning Experiences Review the principles of adult education that relate to the types of learning experiences that adults prefer. Explain how experiential learning differs from passive, rote memorization of facts. Explore the notion of preferred learning styles* with the instructor and the implications of this notion in planning instruction for adult learners. Provide instructors with an enumeration of possible teaching methods and work with them in designating which methods actively involve learners in the learning experience and which do not. Ask instructors to consider their tentative teaching plans and to propose alternative teaching methods that might involve learners more actively in these experiences. The educator might also provide some readings on adult education methodologies and creative teaching techniques to stimulate thinking.

Creation of a Comfortable (Psychological, Physical) Learning Environment Distinguish between the psychological and physical aspects of the learning climate. Have instructors reflect on elements that influenced their own psychological comfort in a learning situation. Have them

*Discussed in Chapter 4.

also identify elements that induced stress, anxiety, and/or withdrawal during learning sessions. Once these contrasting factors are enumerated, explore how the instructor might facilitate a comfortable psychological environment for learners and minimize psychological detractors. Remind instructors that their own behavior can be defensive, dogmatic, and intimidating toward learners.

In relation to the physical climate for learning, review relevant aspects of the learning environment for adult learners, including factors such as lighting, seating arrangements, room temperature, distractions and noise, visibility of instructional materials, and acoustics. Remind instructor that creature comforts are a necessity for adults, as are access to telephones, restrooms, and nourishment. Review how the all-important physical needs will be attended to before, during, and after the presentation.

Nature and Quality of Feedback Provided to Learners Inquire about the instructor's past experiences as a learner, highlighting situations in which the individual received both positive and negative feedback on performance. Ask the instructor to identify which approaches best served to improve performance while simultaneously leaving ego and self-concept intact. Help instructors distinguish among the various effects of positive, constructive, and negative feedback on performance and self-concept. Use written material, prerecorded videotape, or role-playing simulations to illustrate the effects of different types of feedback on learner performance. Assist the instructor in differentiating how timing, tone, and specificity of the feedback can influence learner performance.

Supporting Program Faculty

In order for program instructors to function effectively in their role, the educator must be prepared to support faculty before, during, and following their teaching assignments. Some ways in which the educator can lend support for faculty are described in the following sections.

Before the Presentation

Before each faculty member's presentation, the educator needs to provide the instructor with certain information related to the teaching assignment. Faculty will be better able to fulfill expectations if they are provided beforehand with the information listed in Box 3.8.

Although some of these items may only need to be mentioned verbally, it is usually a better idea to provide faculty with a written letter or form that contains and confirms this information. Busy professionals have many responsibilities that compete for their time and attention. Putting these areas in writing can help to ensure that the right instructor appears at the right time and location to provide instruction on the topic area(s) desired. Figure 3.5 illustrates an example of a faculty confirmation form. If the educator has many faculty members to coordinate, it may also be helpful to ask faculty to acknowledge their receipt of and concurrence with these arrangements. A means for accomplishing this is illustrated in the lower panel of Figure 3.5, where a faculty RSVP form is provided for return to the educator. As you can see, this RSVP form also affords the instructor with a means for making the audiovisual needs known to the educator so that this equipment can be provided on site.

During the Presentation

The educator has a responsibility to the learners not only to schedule instructors but also to monitor the effectiveness and quality of instruction they provide. The educator also has a responsibility to attend presentations of novice instructors in order to offer any support or assistance they may need and be present to hear faculty who have not been heard before to verify the instruction provided. If the presentation seems to be getting off on a tangent, is progressing too rapidly or too slowly, or is not focusing on the intended outcomes, the educator may be able to subtly reconstruct, reorganize, or refocus the discussion, fill in information gaps, or offer clarification. Whenever possible, this should be done as unobtrusively as possible so that no embarrassment or undermining of the instructor's confidence occurs. Even when using instructors with well-established teaching reputations or those whom the educator has observed many times before, intermittent monitoring is a good way to ensure that the quality of these educational sessions is being maintained.

Following the Presentation

Following the faculty member's presentation, the educator provides feedback to the instructor regarding their contribution to the program. Educators can accomplish this by sharing learners' evaluations of the instructor's performance, by sharing their own impressions of the presentation, and by offering an analysis of the instructor's strengths and weaknesses. Instructors need to be aware of their strengths so that these areas can be reinforced for continued use. They need to be aware of their weaknesses in order to obtain support to improve those areas. Few instructors are so expert that they cannot improve in at least some aspects of their teaching role.

Virtually all faculty will want to know these evaluation results. Neophyte instructors may initially fear them until their skills and self-confidence have developed. Even seasoned instructors will appreciate the input and suggestions of others regarding their performance but will tend to be less intimidated by the evaluation process itself. When sharing feedback on performance, the educator should be mindful that all individuals are sensitive to critiques of their performance. Everyone likes to hear complimentary reviews and no one really wants to hear highly critical reviews, as necessary as some of these may be. The educator's sensitivity to the instructor receiving negative feedback is vitally important to how that type of input is perceived and responded to. A supportive educator can cushion the impact of critical feedback and use it to lay the groundwork for improving the instructor's skills. The performance areas used in the discussion on developing faculty can be helpful in making these refinements. It may also be useful to mention that even very experienced and effective instructors will at times receive negative feedback from learners and that no instructor pleases all learners all of the time.

PREPARING INSTRUCTIONAL SCHEDULES

The final phase in curriculum design is the practical outcome of all the preceding phases. A class schedule reflects the instructional plan of learning activities aimed at meeting the program and the instructional objectives estab-

---

Box 3.8

INFORMATION PROVIDED TO FACULTY BEFORE THEIR PRESENTATION

- The topic and major subtopics to cover
- The specific instructional outcomes for the session
- The time, date, and location for the presentation
- The composition, number, and general characteristics of the audience that will be addressed
- Topics related to the assigned area that have already been covered and any that will be covered after the presentation by other instructors
- References or bibliography provided to learners for the topic to be presented
- Any instructional media available for the topic area
- Instructions on how to secure audiovisual or logistical support for the presentation
- Any handouts that can be made available for the presentation
- A general description of how learners will be evaluated on the subject matter of the session

FACULTY CONFIRMATION FORM

Dear _____:

This is to confirm your agreement to serve as faculty for our _____ program according to the following arrangements:

Date: _____   Time: _____ am/pm
Topic: _____   Location: _____
The audience for your presentation will be _____.

Attached please find the following materials related to your session:

1. an outline of the major content areas we would like you to cover

2. a list of the instructional outcomes for your session

3. copies of the handouts, reading assignments, and evaluation items, and

4. a list of audiovisual and CAI programs available for your topic.

Prior to your presentation, the participants will already have received instruction on _____
_____. Related areas that will be covered in *future sessions*
include: _____.

If you will need any audiovisual equipment or programs for your presentation, please indicate these below when you RSVP this confirmation. Thank you for your contribution to this program. If you have any questions regarding your presentation, please call Nursing Staff Development at extension 5305.

FACULTY RSVP FORM

This is to confirm my agreement to serve as faculty for the _____ program scheduled for

[time]___ am/pm on ___[day]___ , ___[date]___ . I will be presenting on the topic of _____.

I will need the following audiovisual program(s) for my presentation:_____

I will need the following audiovisual equipment for my presentation (check all that apply):

_____	35 mm slide projector	_____	overhead projector	_____	marker board
_____	videocassette player	_____	audiocassette player	_____	podium
_____	videodisc player	_____	chalkboard	_____	lavaliere microphone
_____	videotape player	_____	electric pointer	_____	podium microphone

Figure 3.5 Faculty confirmation and RSVP forms.

lished for the educational program. It delineates the timely and orderly sequence of planned instructional activities.

In formal academic settings, the class schedule is incorporated into a course or program syllabus that includes a course description; an outline of course content; specific dates, times, and locations of all learning experiences; and, possibly, an enumeration of due dates for assignments, evaluation dates, and required readings. The educator may adopt this syllabus approach for extensive educational programs that span weeks and/or months. But even when the program only requires a few hours of instruction, both the instructors and participants will find it helpful if they are mutually informed about how the teaching-learning process will proceed.

NAME OF PROGRAM

Class Schedule

Day	Date	Time	Location	Topic	Instructor	Teaching Method	Assigned Readings

Figure 3.6 Sample class schedule format.

Participants will find the class schedule useful in organizing their preparation and work time, in seeing when certain learning outcomes will likely be achieved, and when assignments and evaluations will occur. Instructors responsible for providing these learning experiences will find the schedule useful in understanding how their session fits into the overall program and in making arrangements for any logistical support they may need.

The amount of information that needs to appear on a class schedule should be dictated by what is necessary and most helpful for both instructors and learners. Overly detailed schedules may be more confusing than helpful, whereas those with insufficient detail will not afford much direction.

It is often helpful to first devise a rough draft of the schedule. Before the draft can be transformed into a final draft for distribution, it needs to meet the following criteria:

VALIDITY The learning experiences planned directly reflect the instructional outcomes for the program

CLARITY Anyone reading the schedule can easily understand it

CONTINUITY The flow and sequence of learning activities, assignments, and evaluations are appropriate

FEASIBILITY Time allotments and logistical arrangements are realistic and appropriate for the subject matter to be covered and for the outcomes to be attained

CONFIRMATION All faculty participation details have been verified; media, facilities, and support have all been arranged and scheduled in advance

UTILITY Both faculty and learners find that the schedule serves as a useful map of planned learning activities

VARIETY Planned learning experiences and teaching methods vary to promote interest, attention, retention, and transfer of learning to practice; a variety of learning experiences are incorporated that involve learners as active participants in instruction

Figure 3.6 illustrates one way to format the information for a class schedule.

Curriculum design is not a mystical process. If anything, it is a rather pragmatic and methodical art that blends and matches desired instruction with the resources available for providing it. When designed well, a curriculum is successful in bringing to fruition the planned learning activities necessary for participants to attain the program's instructional outcomes. Curriculum design, in short, makes instruction operable. Actualizing the curriculum plans is the subject of the next chapter.

REFERENCES

1. Alspach JG: Critical care orientation programs: reader survey report, *Crit Care Nurse* 10(5):22, 1990.
2. Alspach JG: *From staff nurse to preceptor: a preceptor training program,* Aliso Viejo, CA, 1988, American Association of Critical-Care Nurses.
3. Alspach JG, editor: *Instructor's resource manual for the AACN core curriculum for critical care nursing,* Philadelphia, 1992, WB Saunders.
4. Alexander MA: Evaluating the behavioral objectives, *J Cont Educ Nurs* 16:63, 1985.
5. American Society for Healthcare Education and Training: The role of video teleconferencing in education, *Healthcare Educa Dateline,* Winter:10, 1991.
6. Austin EK: *Guidelines for the development of continuing education offerings for nurses,* New York, 1981, Appleton-Century-Crofts.
7. Ballard AL: Writing behavioral objectives, *J Nurs Staff Develop* 6:40, 1990.
8. Billings DM: Advantages and disadvantages of computer-assisted instruction, *Dimen Crit Care Nurs* 5:356, 1986.
9. Billings DM: Integrating computer-assisted instruction into your educational programs, *Trendlines* 3(2):6, 1992.
10. Billings DM: Selecting CAI software, *Dimen Crit Care Nurs* 7:118, 1988.
11. Billings D, Frazier H, Lausch J et al: Videoteleconferencing: solving mobility and recruitment problems, *Nurs Educ* 14(2):12, 1989.
12. Bloom BS, editor: *Taxonomy of educational objectives: handbook I—cognitive domain,* New York, 1956, Longman.
13. Bloomwell AE: 47 Tips for flip-chart users, *Training* 20(6):35, 1983.
14. Boyle PG: *Planning better programs,* New York, 1981, McGraw-Hill.
15. Carlson DS: Self-produced programs as an alternative to purchasing audio-visual materials, *J Cont Educ Nurs* 19:76, 1988.
16. Chermak D: Overheads that blow the roof off, *Training-Presentation Technologies,* Suppl 27(9):22, 1990.
17. Clark CE: Telecourses for nursing staff development, *J Nurs Staff Develop* 5:107, 1989.

18. Clark CE: Transparencies: let them work for you, *Nurs Educ* 13(2): 21, 1988.
19. Cooper SS: Methods of teaching revisited—visual materials, *J Cont Educ Nurs* 21:148, 1990.
20. Cooper SS: One more time: the overhead projector, *J Cont Educ Nurs* 21:141, 1990.
21. Cooper SS: Teaching tips, *J Cont Educ Nurs* 17:66, 1986.
22. Cooper SS: Teaching with slides, *J Cont Educ Nurs* 18:68, 1987.
23. Cordell BJ, Greaf WD: Computer-assisted instruction: is it right for you? *J Cont Educ Health Prof* 8:97, 1988.
24. Cranton P: *Planning instruction for adult learners,* Toronto, 1989, Wall & Thompson.
25. Dave RH: Psychomotor levels. In Armstrong RJ, editor: *Developing and writing behavioral objectives,* Tucson, AZ, 1970, Educational Innovators Press.
26. Day R, Payne L: Computer-managed instruction: an alternative teaching strategy, *J Nurs Educ* 26(1):30, 1987.
27. Duchin S, Sherwood G: Posters as an educational strategy, *J Cont Educ Nurs* 21:205, 1990.
28. Duncan J: How to use transparencies: a refresher course, *Training* 22(7):27, 1985.
29. Dyche J: *Educational program development for employees in healthcare agencies,* Calabasas, CA, 1982, Tri-Oak Education.
30. Facilitator GJ: Dead men don't use flip charts, *Training* 21(2):35, 1984.
31. Farace J: 10 Steps to better slide shows, *Training* 21(7):52, 1984.
32. Filipczak B: Make room for training, *Training* 28(10):76, 1991.
33. Greipp ME: A plan for implementing computer-assisted instruction, *Nurs Educ* 13(2):17, 1988.
34. Harrow AJ: *A taxonomy of the psychomotor domain: a guide for developing behavioral objectives,* New York, 1972, Longman.
35. Hekelman FP, Phillips JA, Bierer LA: An interactive videodisk training program in basic cardiac life support: implications for staff development, *J Cont Educ Nurs* 21:245, 1990.
36. Hofland SL: Transparency design for effective oral presentations, *J Cont Educ Nurs* 18:83, 1987.
37. House G: *The psychomotor domain,* Washington, DC, 1972, National Special Media Institute.
38. Ingrisano JR: A guide to cost-effective video, *Training* 22(8):41, 1985.
39. Kibler RJ, Barker LL, Miles DT: *Behavioral objectives and instruction,* Boston, 1970, Allyn.
40. Krathwohl DR, Bloom BS, Masia BB, editors: *Taxonomy of educational objectives: handbook II—affective domain,* New York, 1964, Longman.
41. Land L, Leedom CL, Persaud D et al: Computer-assisted interactive video instruction in nursing (CAIVIN), *J Nurs Staff Develop* 5:273, 1989.
42. Lewis BJ, Levinson L: Hi-tech education: teleconferencing in a hospital setting, *J Healthcare Educ Train* 4(3):28, 1990.
43. Mager RF: *Preparing instructional objectives,* ed 2, Belmont, CA, 1984, Pitman Learning.
44. Meilach D: Visually speaking, *Presentation Products* 7(6):A, 1993.
45. Mirr MP, Sparks RK, Golembiewski IW: Using interactive video to supplement student experience in critical care nursing, *Focus Crit Care* 13(4):28, 1986.
46. Nierenberg J: New technology for educating nurses, *J Cont Educ Nurs* 18:17, 1987.
47. Oermann MH: Analyzing and selecting audiovisual materials, *Nurs Educ* 9(4):24, 1984.
48. O'Grady T, Matthews M: Video through the eyes of the trainee, *Training* 24(7):57, 1987.
49. Parry S: Make or buy? *Training* 28(10):14, 1991.
50. Pribble R: Enter the videodisc, *Training* 22(3):91, 1985.
51. Quinn CA: Computer-assisted instruction: is it really your best choice? *Nurse Educ* 11(6):34, 1986.
52. Reilly DE: *Behavioral objectives in nursing: evaluation of learner attainment,* New York, 1980, Appleton-Century-Crofts.
53. Rosier PK, Wall B, Discoe A: Posters: valuable educational tool, *J Cont Educ Nurs* 20:238, 1989.
54. Sheridan D: Off the road again training through teleconferencing, *Training* 29(2):63, 1992.
55. Simpson EJ: *The classification of educational objectives: psychomotor domain,* Chicago, 1966, University of Illinois (research project No. OE 5).
56. Tribulski JA, Frank C: Closed circuit TV: an alternate teaching strategy, *J Nurs Staff Develop* 3:110, 1987.
57. Umlauf MG: How to provide around-the-clock CPR certification without losing any sleep, *J Cont Educ Nurs* 21:248, 1990.
58. Van Ort S: Evaluating audiovisual and computer programs for classroom use, *Nurs Educ* 14(1):16, 1989.
59. Young S: Cost-effective slide production for the small education department, *J Cont Educ Nurs* 21:93, 1990.
60. Zemke R: Evaluating computer-assisted instruction: the good, the bad and the why, *Training* 21(5):22, 1984.
61. Zemke R: The rediscovery of video teleconferencing, *Training* 23(9): 28, 1986.
62. Zemke R: Shell scores with interactive video, *Training* 28(9):33, 1991.

CHAPTER 4

Program Implementation

The implementation phase of the educational process puts the curriculum plan into action. Implementation of a curriculum consists of providing learning experiences that will enable learners to meet the instructional outcomes established for that program. The heart of the implementation phase, then, involves the interaction of teachers and learners in the instructional process.

In order to provide effective instruction, the educator needs to consider the interacting elements of the instructional process. These interacting elements consist of the following:

- The teaching-learning process: how teachers and learners interact
- The adult education process: how the teaching-learning process is influenced when the learners are adults
- How adults process information
- How different learners prefer to learn
- How different teachers prefer to teach

The first section of this chapter will use these interacting elements to provide some guiding principles for understanding the fundamental precepts that underlie the instructional process. The latter section will then describe a variety of teaching methods available to the educator for implementation of staff development programs.

GUIDING PRINCIPLES

PRINCIPLES OF TEACHING AND LEARNING

The teacher's primary mission is to facilitate learning. In the teaching-learning process, teaching is only a means to learning, not an end in itself. Whatever teaching activities the educator undertakes, they are only effective and successful to the extent that they contribute to learning.

Certain principles constitute the mainstay of the teaching-learning process. The following section discusses some of these principles and describes their implications for the teaching-learning process.[18,32,49,113]

Learning Is a Self-Activity of the Learner

Even the best teaching does not ensure that learning will occur. The learner's willingness to attend, listen, reflect, recall, associate, visualize, memorize, reason, judge, and assimilate what is to be learned will determine the amount and extent of learning. Unless the learner is willing and able to engage in these activities, learning will not occur. The learner who invests energy in learning is likely to learn more, to learn faster, and to better retain what has been learned.

In order to learn, the learner must actively participate

in the teaching-learning process. The educator's responsibility includes eliciting and incorporating learners' participation in assessing their own learning needs, in determining the instructional objectives, in partaking in the scheduled learning activities, and in evaluating their success in attaining the instructional outcomes of the program. The teacher needs to ensure that learners are provided with these opportunities to contribute to each phase of the educational process if potentially passive learners are going to be transformed into active agents in this process.

Learning Is Intentional

Learning does not typically occur by accident, but, rather, through a concerted, focused, and purposeful effort by the learner. The extent of learning is determined by learners' perceptions of their own learning needs. Learning is, therefore, a goal-directed activity of learners, aimed at meeting their own perceived needs.

Learning is most effective when it is directed toward goals the learners can personally identify with; that is, toward goals they perceive as meaningful and worthwhile. Unless learners know what the goals of instruction are and agree those goals are worthwhile for them personally, they will likely expend little energy toward meeting them. The goals for learning may originate with learners or be adopted by them, but at some point learners must "buy in" to those goals before they will become active and willing participants in the learning process. Unless learners already want to learn or unless teachers can catalyze this desire, learners will not learn.

In order to heighten learners' resolve toward learning, educators need to consider the learners' goals in relation to the program objectives and determine the degree of concordance between them. It may be helpful to indicate to learners how their personal goals for learning can be attained in the program. Educators can enhance a learner's convictions by indicating the value of the material to the learners' present or future clinical assignments. Explaining the overall purpose of the program, its instructional outcomes, and what learners can expect to be able to do by the end of the program assists in clarifying goals so that learners can more clearly visualize what they are striving for and why it is important.

The teacher's responsibility is to promote learners' intentions by making instructional activities meaningful, by supplementing or assisting learners to acquire the knowledge, skills, or attitudes needed, and by providing the resources and support necessary for learners to achieve their personal goals during the program.

Unless learners purposefully intend to learn, no amount of coercion will produce the desired result. Requiring learners to attend "mandatory classes" may alienate their interest and significantly diminish the likelihood that they will learn.

Learning Is an Active and Interactive Process

If learning requires active participation and a desire to learn, then the degree to which learners participate in learning experiences will largely determine what and how much they learn. Learning is dynamic; it does not take place without the learner becoming actively engaged in the process. Dewey's[32] maxim that "we learn by doing" underscores the importance of actively involving the learner in instructional activities.

Learning experiences such as simulation exercises, role playing, and return demonstration of clinical skills afford a substantial amount of interaction in instructional activities and increase the probability that learning will occur. Learning experiences that are primarily passive, such as listening to an audio tape, usually minimize the extent of learner interaction in the learning experience. The more that learners can be involved in learning, the more they are likely to acquire, retain, and transfer what they have learned.

Rather than merely discussing how to admit a patient, how to perform an arterial puncture, how to support a grieving family, or how to operate new equipment, educators need to provide opportunities to experience, practice, and refine these abilities.

Learning Is a Unitary Process

The learner responds to the teaching-learning process and to the learning situation as a whole. The composite of features that distinguish one individual from another—those physiological, psychological, emotional, intellectual, hereditary, maturational, and experiential aspects of the learner—function simultaneously in influencing the learner's interaction with and response to the learning experience.

Learning has its physical basis in the functioning of physical structures, including the sensory apparatus and the intellect. The entirety of the learning situation itself also operates during the learning experience: the psychological climate and physical comfort of the learning environment, the subject matter being addressed, and the instructor's influence. All of these factors influence the teaching-learning process and affect the outcomes of learning. Because learning occurs in relation to the collective and cumulative effect of these many disparate features, the outcomes of the teaching-learning process are characterized as a functional unity.

Insofar as possible, individual differences among learners should be taken into account in planning learning experiences. Educators may respond to these differences by varying the focus of teaching on the differing perspectives and interests of learners, adjusting the level of instruction for different audiences, relating content to areas of applicability or the experiences of various learners, or by modifying the pace of instruction to better meet learners' needs.

Learners' weaknesses or physical limitations may be accommodated by offering multiple options for learning similar information. Providing comparable material in different media formats can provide learners with choices for determining how they wish to learn. Shy learners or those who find public speaking unnerving will not likely favor group discussions or presenting case studies at a patient care conference as beneficial learning experiences. Older learners with diminished sight or hearing will not likely find large group lectures with overhead transparencies helpful. Learners who are in the midst of personal crises or serious financial or health problems at home may find themselves easily distracted by those problems when passive learning experiences are used. Learners who have difficulty conceptualizing ideas and applications of principles will not likely gain much from instruction unless it provides them with very concrete examples and some hands-on practice.

The learning environment created by the teacher can have a profound effect on learning. A comfortable, informal, relaxed, and non-judgmental atmosphere facilitates learning and creates a climate conducive to the learner's active participation. If learners are preoccupied with how cold the room is, if they sense a personal gulf between themselves and the instructor, if they are anxious about whether a surprise quiz will be unleashed upon them, or if they fear the instructor's critical remarks about their performance, they won't gain much from an instructional activity. Because learners respond as a whole to learning situations, all of the factors that comprise that whole must be taken into account when instruction is planned and provided.

Learning Is Influenced by the Motivation of the Learner

Learning is more easily acquired and retained when learners have a strong desire to learn; when they genuinely want to learn, they will put forth the effort required. Learners' degree of commitment to participate in the learning process will largely depend on their level of learning aspiration. In its most basic terms, the motivation for learning is generated by the incompleteness learners acknowledge in attaining their learning needs or goals. Once learners have attained their personal goals for learning, their need for learning is satisfied and continued motivation wanes unless additional needs for learning are perceived.

When a person truly wants to learn something, negative extrinsic motivators, such as criticism, threats, or denial of merit increases, or positive external motivators, such as salary incentives or awards, are unnecessary. In this situation, intrinsic motivators such as feelings of adequacy, competence, prestige, and self-satisfaction are more than adequate to ensure that the learner will attend and successfully complete educational programs. Only in the least desirable situation, that is, when learning is necessary but not personally desired by the learner, do external forms of motivation become operative.

In the ideal situation, the educator can simply devote attention to facilitating learning among learners who are already highly motivated to learn. In reality, however, aspirations toward learning may wax and wane. Even if learners are highly motivated for attaining the terminal program outcomes, they may not be equally motivated to work through all of the prerequisite stages that culminate at that end.

To enhance a sustained motivation to learn, the educator can attempt to stimulate the learner's attention, activate intrigue, and provide intermittent incentives for learning by emphasizing the relevance and applicability of the material and the importance and value of the learning outcomes. Interest in learning can be rekindled by pointing out specific and realistic clinical applications and demonstrations of the usefulness of the material and by offering examples with which learners are familiar.

Insofar as possible, educators should always attempt to generate intrinsic motivation in the learner. Negative extrinsic motivators should only be employed when all other alternatives have been exhausted.

Learners' experience of success in learning is one of the single most important motivating forces for learning. Especially for individuals who have perceived or experienced a history of failure and duress in past learning situations, developing intrinsic motivation for learning can be a particular challenge. If educators can demonstrate that learning is not only possible but brings with it success and self-satisfaction, they will encounter fewer problems with motivating learners. If and when negative motivators become necessary, the educator needs to use them judiciously, hesitantly, and sparsely for they rarely create lasting positive results.

Learning Is Influenced by the Readiness of the Learner

Learning readiness denotes a complex state of physical, psychological, and intellectual preparedness for acquiring some specific knowledge, skills, or attitudinal change. Readiness requires the aggregate presence of physical and emotional maturity, mastery of prerequisite learning, and, most important of all, a perception that the material to be learned is somehow necessary, important, desirable, or otherwise worthwhile. The learner who demonstrates readiness is, in short, primed for learning; learning is now both timely and meaningful.

A learner's readiness for learning can be determined in a number of ways. Individuals who voluntarily participate in educational offerings and others who notify educators of topics they would like to learn about exhibit their readiness for learning overtly. New staff nurses who want to learn all that is necessary to function competently or experienced staff who would like to expand their roles are both indicating readiness for certain types of learning. Others may communicate their readiness for learning more covertly by inquiring about how to solve a patient care problem or by relating some error or omission in their patient care.

The most direct way to elicit readiness is by asking prospective learners what they would like to learn more about. Nurses who are introspective, reflective, and experienced often possess much insight into what they would like to or need to learn about. As mentioned in Chapter 2, however, a nurse's perceived learning needs ("felt needs") are not always a reliable measure of their true educational needs.

Educators need to be mindful that readiness is an attribute of the learner not the instructor. The educator may be ready to teach, but if learners are not ready to learn, little learning may transpire. Readiness is a complex functional state that depends primarily on learners' perceptions of how useful, meaningful, or worthwhile the material is to them. Educators may be able to enlighten, encourage, threaten, or sustain the need for learning, but readiness remains the individual learner's perogative.

Learning Is Social

As noted earlier, learning is an interactive and mutually shared responsibility that engages both learners and teachers. Other components in this interaction include the learning climate and the interactions among and between other learners. The climate for learning largely depends on the nature and attributes of the social relationship between instructors and learners.

If learning depends on the active participation of the learner, and, if this interaction forms the essence of the teaching-learning process, then any social interaction that promotes the learner's participation will enhance learning. An instructor's non-judgmental and democratic leadership style can facilitate learner participation by supporting the learner's right to disagree openly, to make mistakes, and to hold a different opinion. Authoritarian learning climates, characterized by a teacher's dogmatic, caustic, or belittling tone; rigid adherence to rules; critical, discounting, or defensive behavior, socially inhibit learner participation and discourage learning.

Educators can enhance the social elements of the teaching-learning process in numerous ways. Getting to know learners as individuals, engaging in frequent informal discussions, communicating clearly, critiquing constructively, and being available when needed are especially effective means to warm the social climate for learning. Maintaining and sharing enthusiasm for their interests, acting on learners' suggestions, being prompt, organized, and prepared for classes, providing adequate time for discussion and questions, listening intently, exercising patience, and ac-

cepting individual differences among learners will also be helpful. When this social interaction is managed effectively, the teacher and the learner become co-learners, each sharing and gaining insight from having encountered one another in an instructional setting.

Learning Is Influenced by the Learning Environment

Learning is influenced not only by the psychological climate of a learning situation but also by the physical environment. To foster active participation by learners, the educator needs to ensure that lighting and acoustics are adequate, that temperature control is comfortable for everyone, that projected media are clearly visible to the entire audience, that voices or tapes can be heard by all, and that seating arrangements and workspaces are sufficient and comfortable for learners. If formats such as group work or group discussions are used, participants need to be able to see and interact with each other easily.

Learning Proceeds Best When It Is Organized and Clearly Communicated

Regardless of the method selected to sequence instruction, educators need to enssure that smaller units of instruction are integrated into some meaningful whole so that learners are able to integrate the material with past, present, and future experiences. Learning unrelated bits of information outside their clinical context reduces the chance that learning will be retained or transferred to new situations. Depending on the subject matter and learners' backgrounds, the educator is free to select the organizing principle(s) that seems most appropriate and conducive to learning.

Good organization also requires that operational and support activities such as learning resources, instructional materials, and the physical setting are well planned and prepared ahead of time. Learners' time should not be wasted while media are readied, equipment is delivered, rooms are rearranged, or class locations are determined. Writing out a schedule of learning activities and preplanning for each day's sessions are important logistical aspects of the educator's responsibility.

Effective organization requires clear and unambiguous communication among all participants in the educational program. Learners, instructors, and all necessary support staff should understand the program's objectives, the subject matter to be addressed, the location and schedule of learning experiences, and when, where, and how learning will be evaluated. A clearly delineated schedule of classroom, laboratory, and clinical activities that is communicated to all participants can provide a more cohesive, orderly, and effective series of learning experiences.

A well-organized, lucid, and succinct presentation of

material can greatly assist learners in acquiring, integrating, and retaining instructional material. Less experienced educators might try-out their presentation by pilot testing it with peers or a representative group from their intended audience or by reviewing their organizational plan with more experienced counterparts. Even seasoned instructors need to solicit peer critique if they will be presenting new or particularly complex material.

Learning Is Facilitated by Positive and Immediate Feedback

Behaviorist theories of learning emphasize that positive and immediate reinforcement of a new behavior will tend to make that behavior recur. Positive reinforcement given shortly after learning leads to a lasting association between the learned behavior and its approval. In general, the closer the reinforcement occurs to the behavior itself, the greater its potential effect on influencing that behavior.

Positive learning reinforcement enables the learner to be successful in the learning experience by rewarding the desired, correct, or appropriate behavior. If learning is defined as a change in behavior, and, if the educator's responsibility is to foster these behavioral changes, then building reward systems into the learning situation will usually enhance learners' acquisition of the desired behavioral changes. The learner's feeling of success in the learning situation then constitutes a powerful motivating force for continuing the pursuit of learning as an enjoyable and self-satisfying endeavor.

Positive feedback can take many forms. Recognition, attention, approval, encouragement, and praise are extrinsic social rewards. Good grades, increased pay, career status or advancement are more tangible extrinsic reinforcers. Each of these is based on an appraisal of performance by others.

All learners have their own personal standards for self-appraisal of performance; the perception of success in learning, especially for adult learners, is as much or sometimes more determined by their own vs. others' evaluations of them. Some learners hold higher standards for their own performance than those who evaluate them; some hold similar or even lower standards. Educators and evaluators can assist in molding learners' perceptions of themselves by being sensitive to how learners seem to judge their own performance and by modifying the feedback given to learners so that they neither unduly over- nor underestimate that performance.

Instructors can improve their feedback to learners by being readily available, by providing an abundance of opportunities for success at learning, by offering approval freely and frequently, by communicating anticipated success in learning attempts, by exercising patience with slower learners, by evaluating constructively, and by being realistic in their expectations.

Retention and Transfer of Learning Can Be Facilitated

Retention of learning is facilitated by proximal recall and distributed practice. Proximal recall involves the review and reiteration of information shortly after it is initially presented. Distributed practice involves activities such as repetition or drill that are spread over a period of time rather than being provided all at once. Early review and summary combined with feedback on performance favors the solidification of new learning. Repetition without feedback has virtually no effect on learning. Spaced practice reinforces and refines previous learning, appreciably adding to its integration and retention.

Retention of learning is useful insofar as it enables the learner to transfer what has been learned to new situations. But before learning can be transferred, it must first be retained. As mentioned earlier, retention is enhanced when learning is meaningful and desired by the learner, when it is communicated in a systematic and comprehensible fashion, and when it is reviewed periodically.

Other factors that promote learning transfer include emphasizing principles and general concepts rather than minute details, providing adequate time for learners to integrate new material into their banks of experience, and providing for numerous applications of learning at increasingly more complex levels. For example, in teaching the skill of endotracheal suctioning, the educator should first review the principles (such as asepsis, oxygenation, effect of hypoxemia on hemoglobin saturation, cardiac and vagal responses to hypoxemia, and the like) involved with this skill. Following a review and discussion of these principles, the instructor should then demonstrate how to perform the skill. Learners should be provided with ample time to practice skill performance on mannequins, while the educator offers constructive feedback and reminds learners of the principles operating at various points in the procedure. Once the simulated performance is satisfactory, the same skill can be performed on real patients who have endotracheal tubes in place. Later, related and more complex skills such as nasotracheal suctioning of nonintubated patients, combining oropharyngeal with endotracheal suctioning, or suctioning patients with new tracheostomy tubes can be performed. Eventually the nurse might even demonstrate how to teach endotracheal suctioning to a patient's family so that they can provide this care following the patient's discharge. The wider the variety of experiences with the technique, the greater its transferability to each situation and the more proficient the learner will be in modifying and refining the skills needed in each situation.

Learning Is Creative

Learning is the sum of successively acquired behaviors. Learners engage in a continual process of integrating new learning with their past experience, and, in so doing, modify, delete, or add to what they previously knew. This process of integration results in a reorganization of understanding that is distinctively rewoven and reconstructed rather than merely representing an addition to what was previously known. The degree of significance and applicability of the learned material is highly specific to each learner; learning has different meanings for different people. For example, two critical care nurses may be learning endotracheal suctioning as part of their orientation. The nurse who will be working in the respiratory unit views suctioning as an absolutely essential clinical skill that will be needed on a daily basis; the nurse who will be working in the coronary care unit views suctioning as important but not as a skill that will be used often in daily practice. Thus the meaning and perceived importance of this skill can vary widely with different learners.

Learning Is Inferred Rather Than Observed

Learning is never directly observable. It must always be inferred on the basis of some visible behavioral change that can be measured by the learner's performance. Therefore, whenever evaluation of learning is necessary, the educator must remember that the evaluation process is, at best, only indirectly related to the learning process. Every instance of testing or evaluation, then, gives only one small behavioral reflection of whether learning has occurred. Evaluation represents a sample of what we expect a learner to be able to do following an educational program. These are important points to bear in mind when writing instructional outcomes and when designing evaluation tools for an educational program. In constructing both outcomes and evaluation criteria, educators need to be both highly selective and specific about what they require as the behavioral evidence of learning.

Learning Is Influenced by the Nature and Variability of the Learning Experience

Learning activities should be planned on the basis of the instructional outcomes, subject matter, and the learners' current knowledge and abilities. A logical correlation is needed between the method of instruction, the setting for instruction, and the learning outcomes. In general, classroom learning experiences are appropriate for didactic learning of content-oriented material, whereas laboratory and clinical settings are more appropriate for experiential learning of skill- and attitude-oriented material.

Once the nature of the instructional outcome has been determined, the educator is responsible for assigning that outcome to its most appropriate learning setting and for determining the teaching method(s) that will be employed. In this process, educators need not feel restricted in the kinds of learning experiences they select. Many types of learning are amenable to a variety of possible teaching methods. Novelty or variation in teaching methods is highly desirable, especially for extended programs. Persistent use of the same kind of learning experience inevitably induces boredom, the stifling of learner interest, and a diminished ability to profit from the learning activity. Novelty in teaching method not only stimulates and motivates learning, but exemplifies an openness toward making learning more enjoyable and introduces learners to new ways of participating in the teaching-learning process.

PRINCIPLES OF ADULT EDUCATION

Because the audience for nursing staff development programs consists of adults, educators need to tailor the teaching-learning process to accommodate the special needs of adult learners. Adult learners are not merely aging replicas of their juvenile counterparts. They are a distinct and qualitatively different group of learners who perceive and respond to the teaching-learning process differently than they did as children. As an adult educator, the staff development instructor has a responsibility to acknowledge these differences in planning, implementing, and evaluating learning experiences for adults.

It should be noted at the outset, however, that these characteristics are not universal among the adult population to the extent that every adult the educator encounters will exhibit them. Nor can it be said that all adults manifest these characteristics at all times. In different learning situations, individual adults may demonstrate varying degrees of these characteristics. Indeed, it has been asserted that the methodologies used in the education of children and those used in the education of adults differ more in degree rather than in kind.[16] Educators need to keep these considerations in mind as they review the principles of adult education.

The principles of adult education are founded on the distinguishing characteristics of adult learners. The following section describes some of these distinguishing characteristics and considers the implications of each trait for the educator.

Distinguishing Characteristics of Adult Learners: Implications for Educators*
Adults Are Heterogenous as Learners

Adults represent a heterogeneous group of learners who command the respect that is due to them as mature individuals.

*See references 11, 15, 27, 28, 30, 78, 83-84, 94, 96.

IMPLICATIONS FOR EDUCATORS

- Respect and encourage the unique perspective each adult brings to a learning situation; resist attempts to use the pressure of group conformity.
- Expect and encourage differences of opinion and interpretation; avoid being defensive or dogmatic.
- Involve learners in decision-making related to assessment of their needs and in planning, implementing, and evaluating programs.
- Avoid talking down to learners; minimize the use of unnecessary rules and policies.

Adults Have Multiple Responsibilities

Adult learners are often married and have responsibilities for children, spouses, homes, careers, and civic obligations. Adults place a high value on their time.

IMPLICATIONS FOR EDUCATORS

- Recognize adults' needs to assume comparable amounts of responsibility for their own learning and to be actively involved in decisions related to all phases of the teaching-learning process. Insofar as possible, provide opportunities for adults to determine what they need to learn, how they will best learn, when they are ready to learn, and whether their learning is successful.
- Respect the adult's time by not wasting it on irrelevant, repetitious, or ineffective learning experiences. Allow adults to plan their time by sharing with them course objectives, class schedules, and expectations as early as possible.
- Provide maximum flexibility in scheduling learning activities for times and locations that learners find most convenient.
- Start and stop learning experiences on time.
- When possible, provide alternative means for learning at home or at work so that learners' home and community commitments can be accommodated.
- Be sensitive to the fact that concurrent responsibilities of adult learners may affect their learning readiness and the quality of their participation in learning experiences. Financial, social, marital, and child care problems can interfere with the adult learner's performance.

Adults Have Numerous Life and Work Backgrounds

Adults enter learning situations with a large reservoir of life and work experiences. They value highly both their own experience and that of others.

IMPLICATIONS FOR EDUCATORS

- In some manner (formally via pretest or questionnaire or informally via asking questions) determine the background of knowledge, skills, attitudes, and past experiences of learners. Even in brief instructional situations, make an attempt to construct at least an overview of learners' backgrounds in relation to the program.
- Use your assessment of learners' past experiences and present capabilities in tailoring course content and activities to avoid coverage of areas already mastered, to incorporate those experiences in learning activities, and to concentrate instruction on areas of need.[108]
- Be overt in recognizing and valuing learners' knowledge and skills.
- Solicit and use learners' experiences by selecting teaching methods (such as group discussion, role playing, open seminars, patient care conferences) that are enriched by these experiences.
- Guide participants in the art of learning from their personal experiences; assist them with reflecting on the process and outcomes of their clinical experiences, with deriving principles learned, and with drawing generalizations to be used in the future.
- Emphasize transfer of experiential learning by relating how current learning influences an adult's past experiences and conclusions.

Adults May Be Less Flexible As Learners

Adult habits, attitudes, and perspectives formed over many years are more rigidly adhered to and more deeply imbedded than those of young learners. Adults may resist, challenge, discard, or discount ideas and approaches that differ significantly from what they are accustomed to or from what they have personally experienced.

IMPLICATIONS FOR EDUCATORS

- Be open-minded and adaptable in planning and conducting learning activities.
- Rather than being dogmatic in instruction, emphasize the many gray areas that exist in nursing practice, areas in which there is no one "right answer" or "right way" to manage a situation. Be candid and forthright in discussions.
- Attempt to help learners integrate new concepts, ideas, and approaches with their previous beliefs and practices. Avoid direct challenges to the validity of their ideas and habits. Try to develop open-mindedness in learners.
- Be mindful that ideas inconsistent or contrary to learners' perceptions may temporarily or transiently diminish your credibility as an educator. Don't expect adults to immediately accept alternative views. Give learners time to work through, consider, and reach their own conclusions.

Adults May Have Negative Past Learning Experiences

Many adults have had negative past experiences as learners that evoke feelings of inadequacy, fear of failure, and diminished self-confidence in learning situations.

IMPLICATIONS FOR EDUCATORS

- Provide frequent and generous positive reinforcement for learning.
- Avoid placing learners in situations where failure or feelings of inadequacy are probable.
- Assess readiness for learning and provide remedial instruction as necessary so that all learners are equally ready to proceed with instruction. Minimize the likelihood of large discrepancies among learners in their familiarity with content to be covered.
- Provide a learning environment and learning climate that are conducive to positive learning experiences:

    Informal and relaxed atmosphere

    Learners feel supported

    Non-judgmental interactions between instructors and learners

    Mutual trust and respect between instructors and learners

    Openness that accepts differences of opinion

    Learning activities that are realistic for learners

    Lack of ridicule, belittling remarks, censure, or embarrassment to learners

    Healthy sense of humor

- Convey confidence in learners' ability to acquire the necessary knowledge and skills.
- Coordinate the scheduling of learning activities so that instructional supports are provided when needed; provide sufficient resources for learning so that learners do not feel stranded when they need assistance.
- Ensure that comments concerning performance are constructive and helpful rather than demeaning.
- Clarify any misconceptions that others already "know everything."
- Be overt in demonstrating that the instructor is a co-learner with the participants in a learning situation. Cite instances when learners taught the instructor some lessons.
- If learners need to use instructional media, provide clear and full instructions on how to operate equipment and use study materials. Avoid making learners feel inadequate or dependent on instructors.

Adults Are Voluntary Learners

Adults are usually voluntary learners who engage in learning activities for a variety of personal and professional reasons.

IMPLICATIONS FOR EDUCATORS

- Take some time during the assessment process to determine the specific motivations of learners for participating in instruction. Determine how learners intend to use what they learn.
- Remember that adults' motives for participating in educational programs vary widely and are not likely to be uniform within a given class. Some adults may wish to update knowledge and skills, change jobs, advance their career, whereas others may just wish to take a break from work, change their environment, or do something different. Educators need to keep their expectations of adult learners realistic.
- Recognize that as voluntary learners, adults may "vote with their feet" when learning situations do not meet their needs. If learning activities bore, threaten, offend, or intimidate adults, they may walk out. Pay attention and respond to behavioral cues that suggest that learners' needs are not being met.

Adults Are Problem-Centered Learners

Adults are problem-centered learners who engage in learning activities with the intention of immediately applying what they learn to solve problems in their present roles and responsibilities. An adult's readiness for learning is highly dependent on the demands and problems that confront them daily. Problems that learners confront at work afford strong, self-sustaining, and highly motivating factors in the pursuit of learning.

IMPLICATIONS FOR EDUCATORS

- Manage adults' impatience in pursuit of learning by attempting to determine and meet their highest priority needs first.
- Focus instruction on concrete and immediate realities rather than on idealism or theory.
- Focus program content on the essentials that learners can apply immediately in their work assignments.
- Use a problem-centered approach to the subject matter, relating the usefulness of learning the material for managing current or anticipated clinical situations.
- Insofar as possible, sequence and time learning experiences to coincide with learners' present needs to know. Avoid attempts to teach everything they might eventually want to know; limit coverage to areas of greatest importance and clinical relevance.
- Before progressing to new content areas, verify that all issues and questions have been adequately addressed.

Adults Are Knowledgeable Learners

Adults work best with instructors who interact with them as knowledgeable colleagues, who help them learn, and who are subject to the same shortcomings as they are.

Adults can readily detect pretenses and facades in their instructors.

IMPLICATIONS FOR EDUCATORS[40,67]

- Be natural and unaffected in interactions with learners; avoid the "all-knowing expert" stereotype. Admit mistakes, areas of uncertainty, or lack of understanding.
- Convey a sincere and mutual respect for learners.
- Avoid approaches that suggest that "right answers" can always be supplied.
- Don't take yourself too seriously; be able to laugh at yourself.
- Make yourself available to learners when they need your support. Avoid an overbearing demeanor and resist taking over situations. Whenever possible, allow learners the freedom to experiment with solutions and learn from their mistakes.
- Be helpful, informative, clear, concise, and well-prepared; use realistic examples.

Most Adults Are Self-Directed in Their Learning

Adults need to be provided with opportunities to evaluate the effectiveness of instruction in relation to their own goals and expectations of the experience.

IMPLICATIONS FOR EDUCATORS

- In soliciting learners' evaluations, distinguish between individual and group learning needs addressed in the program to determine if both sets of needs are being met.
- Incorporate learners' evaluations as a primary tool for evaluating the program and for making modifications in future offerings.
- Use follow-up evaluations after the program to determine whether learners' clinical practice needs were met. Provide additional instructional support and supplementation if necessary.

- Remember that some adults are not self-directed in their learning activities and that some are self-directed in certain situations but not in others.[16] It is unrealistic for the educator to expect that all adults prefer to direct their own learning activities.

Adults of Different Ages Need Varying Degrees of Support in Learning

Some adult learners may be older and have a slower learning speed than their younger counterparts. Others may have visual or auditory deficits or require more frequent changes in position or activity. A physically comfortable environment is important to adult learners.

IMPLICATIONS FOR EDUCATORS

- Be sensitive to the pace at which learning activities proceed. Plan sufficient time for learners to acquire and integrate information before proceeding to subsequent activities. Verify that the pace of instruction is comfortable for learners.
- Provide a learning environment that is suitable for adults. Attend to details regarding comfortable seating arrangements, adequate ventilation and lighting, temperature and humidity control, good acoustics, and visibility of instructional aids.
- Confirm with the audience that media can be heard and viewed by everyone. Use a microphone if necessary.
- Plan for rest periods and breaks between learning experiences to minimize mental and physical fatigue on learners. When possible, cover more challenging areas early in the day and use interactive activities following lunch and later in the day.

COGNITIVE STYLE

Adults vary in the way they perceive, organize, and conceptually assimilate information from their environment.

TABLE 4.1 • DISTINGUISHING FEATURES OF FIELD-INDEPENDENT AND FIELD-DEPENDENT INDIVIDUALS*		
Feature	**Field-Independent**	**Field-Dependent**
General		
Perception of learning environment	Analytical (pays attention to details)	Global (pays attention to the whole context)
Standards used for decision-making	Internal	External
Stronger skills	Analytic	Interpersonal, social
Reliance	Self-reliant	Relies on others
Social		
Role in groups	Leader	Follower
Effect of peer pressure	Less affected by; less likely to conform	More affected by; likely to conform
Effect of others' evaluations, criticism	Relatively unaffected by	Likely to be affected by
Sensitivity to social cues	Relatively insensitive to	Sensitive to

*From references 39, 50, 68, 73, 74, 81, 100.

As a result, adults learn in different ways. The term *cognitive style* refers to an adult's predominant or distinctive way of structuring or processing information.

Cranton[27] describes cognitive style as an intellectual characteristic of a learner that reflects how the learner acquires, processes, stores, and uses information. One's cognitive style is established at an early age, is not readily altered, remains relatively stable through adulthood,[134] and represents a combination of traits or dimensions rather than a single, discrete feature.[27,28]

More than ten dimensions of cognitive style have been studied to date.[101] Of these, the dimension most widely acknowledged and most extensively researched is Witkin's notion of field independence/dependence (FID).[133,135] The foundational research on FID is derived from studies on human perception related to two areas: the ability to recognize one's body position (using body adjustment tests) and the ability to recognize a simple figure located within a complex design (using embedded figure tests). Findings from studies in this area reveal that individuals tend to be either field-independent or field-dependent in their perceptions of the environment.

Field-independent (FI) individuals use internal cues to orient themselves within their environment. They perceive their surroundings analytically and attend to the discrete parts that make up that complex environment. Field-dependent (FD) individuals, by contrast, use external cues to orient themselves. They perceive their environment globally, attending to the whole of their surroundings rather than to its component parts. FI and FD individuals also differ in relation to the effect of their social environment. In general, FI persons tend to remain relatively detached from their social surroundings, whereas FD individuals are strongly affected by it. Table 4.1 summarizes some of the general and social features that distinguish FI and FD individuals.

These bipolar attributes toward field-independence or field-dependence extend into learning situations as well. The same tendencies to use different cues (internal vs. external) and to perceive different aspects (parts vs. the whole) of one's surroundings persist in educational settings, where they serve to distinguish the cognitive styles of FI and FD learners. As can be seen from Table 4.2, differences in the cognitive styles of FI and FD learners suggest that the same teaching methods will not be equally effective for both types of learners. Learners who are field-independent will tend to favor formal instruction such as lectures or working alone on a self-directed basis at intellectual challenges that require use of their systematic analytical skills and that afford plenty of opportunity to apply scientific concepts and principles. Learners who are field-dependent will more likely favor informal group activities that require collaborative decision-making or highly structured and teacher-directed learning experiences.

Differences in cognitive style are important to acknowledge because they influence how a learner acquires, organ-

TABLE 4.2 • COGNITIVE STYLES OF FIELD-INDEPENDENT AND FIELD-DEPENDENT LEARNERS*		
Feature	**Field-Independent Cognitive Style**	**Field-Dependent Cognitive Style**
Type of learner	Abstract: derives concepts and principles to structure and organize learning	Concrete: needs assistance in organizing and structuring learning situations
Approach to learning	Analytic: can readily apply concepts and principles in ambiguous and complex situations	Global: context of overall situation limits ability to distinguish relevant details
Role as learner	Active participant	Passive observer
Orientation as a learner	Task-oriented	Group-oriented: cooperation, collaboration
Motivation for learning	Internal: meeting challenges, solving problems	External: social approval from peers, instructor
Autonomy as a learner	Self-directed, independent	Other-directed, dependent
Best learning environment	Quiet, solitary	Interactive, group
Favored teaching methods	Formal, didactic methods	Informal, group methods
	Lecture with opportunities to ask questions and apply learning	Group discussions, observation, demonstration, role playing
	Self-directed learning	Teacher-directed learning via preceptors, instructors, programmed instruction
	Experiential learning	
Feedback in learning	Primarily self-imposed; less influenced by grades and others' evaluations	Primarily dependent on external reinforcement such as grades, verbal and nonverbal appraisals of others
Ability to make decisions and solve problems in complex situations	Strong: enhanced by analytic and organizational skills	Weak: holistic perspective may obscure ability to detect subtle factors

*From references 39, 50, 68, 73, 74, 81, 100.

izes, and uses the information gained from instruction. There is no right or wrong or better cognitive style. Each reflects a different way of receiving, structuring, and processing information. No one style is best for all learning situations although one cognitive style may be more advantageous than another in a particular situation, for a particular type of content, or for a specific teaching method.

The cognitive styles of nursing students and practicing nurses have also been examined to a limited extent. These studies have noted that FI nursing students are more effective than FD students in the assessment[86,126] and evaluation phases of the nursing process;[79] and that FI students spend less time with their instructor and more time with their patients than FD students.[70,85] Jackson and Gosnell-Moses[73] assert that the findings of such studies suggest that the field-independent cognitive style would be most adaptive for critical care nursing practice because critical care nursing requires practitioners who can readily sort out complex clinical data, identify clinical problems, and evaluate the effects of interventions and therapies. In this environment, the analytic and self-directed skills of the FI critical care nurse might facilitate patient care, while the FD nurses' reliance on others for direction and decision-making might be problematic. Conversely, the FD nurse's interpersonal and social skills could enhance their ability to provide the psychosocial support for patients and families that FI nurses may neglect.

LEARNING STYLE PREFERENCES

In addition to having distinctive ways of receiving and processing instruction, individuals also have characteristic preferences for certain types of learning conditions. The collective term for these favored learning conditions is *learning style preference.*

Learning style preferences reflect how learners like to learn—that is, the manner in which they prefer to learn and the conditions in which they are most comfortable and receptive to learning. Learning style preferences reflect the various likes and dislikes learners have for particular instructional situations, conditions, and methods. Similar to cognitive style, one's learning style is not a single trait but represents a composite of many different attributes such as one's preferences for the sensory medium used in learning (visual, tactile, auditory, etc.), the social milieu (alone or in groups), the degree of desired instructor supervision (little or a great deal), and the desired degree of structure in the learning setting (unstructured or highly teacher-structured).

Unlike cognitive style, which tends to remain quite stable over time, one's learning style preference is more open to influence from a number of potential factors: environmental demands, current circumstances, personality type, new educational experiences, career demands, and the development of adaptive skills.[84] One or more of these influ-

ences can modify an individual's learning style preference. There is no one uniquely adult learning style.[16]

The development of inventories to measure learning style began in the 1960s.[127] Different workers in this area conceptualize learning styles and learning style preferences in different ways. Dunn and Dunn[35] organize learning styles in four categories according to a learner's preferences:

- Immediate environment: includes preferences related to
    Sound: silence vs. background sounds
        such as music
    Light: subdued vs. bright lighting
    Temperature: warm vs. cool
    Design: sitting at desk vs. lying on bed
- Social needs: includes preferences related to
    Learning alone vs. with others
    Learning with vs. without an instructor present
- Physical needs: includes preferences related to
    Sensory mode of learning
    Nourishment needs while learning
    Best time of day for learning
    Need for mobility while learning
- Emotional needs: includes preferences related to
    Learning under pressure vs. at a leisurely pace
    Persistence at learning tasks
    Responsibility toward learning
    Motivation for learning

Kolb's[84] "Learning Style Inventory" reflects an alternative notion of learning style. In Kolb's model,[85] learning style is the combined product of a learner's predominant mode(s) of learning (feeling, thinking, observing, doing) and a myriad of other features that together produce one of four types of learning styles: converger, diverger, assimilator, or accommodator. The characteristics of each of Kolb's learning styles are summarized in Table 4.3.

Renzulli and Smith's "Learning Styles Inventory" (as described by Ferrell),[47] Rezler's[110] "Learning Preference Inventory," Gregoric's "Gregoric Style Delineator,"[59] and the modified version of Hill's cognitive mapping technique (as described by Ehrhardt[41]), represent other conceptualizations of learning style.

A number of consistent findings related to learning style preferences among members of the health professions have now emerged. Rezler[111,112] found that a majority of students in allied health professions prefer concrete and teacher-structured learning situations. In 1983, Mays[92] likewise found that a majority of medical technology students prefer concrete and teacher-structured learning experiences. Studies by Garity[50] and Ostmoe et al.[99] found similar results for nursing students. Eagleton's[38] study on the learning preferences of practicing critical care nurses found comparable results. However, Eagleton found that among

TABLE 4.3 • KOLB'S FOUR LEARNING STYLES[6,61,85]				
Feature	**Converger**	**Diverger**	**Assimilator**	**Accommodator**
Modes of learning	Thinking and doing	Feeling and observing	Thinking and observing	Feeling and doing
Orientation to learning	Analytic and pragmatic	Emotional and imaginative	Theoretical and systematic	Emotional and intuitive
Likes learning via	Deductive reasoning; using general ideas, concepts, principles	Examining unique situations from many perspectives	Inductive reasoning and synthesis of observations	Trial-and-error, intuition, personal experience
Learning strengths	Practical application of ideas Solving specific problems	Generation of ideas Sensitivity to feelings Open-mindedness Creativity	Analysis of information into concise, logical form; creation of theoretical models; understanding vs. application	Learns by doing, likes challenges and projects, likes to experiment and take risks; adaptable, open-minded
Prefers to deal with	Things (tasks, problems)	People	Abstract ideas, information	People
Interests	Narrow, technical, physical sciences	Broad, cultural issues, social sciences	Understanding complexities, basic sciences	Doing things
Benefits most from	Learning situations where there is only one correct answer or solution	Discussion when many issues are involved or when ideas must be generated	Situations in which synthesis of information and logical analysis can be applied	Structured situations that need to be managed
Approach to learning	Pragmatic Likes to see results	Imaginative Likes to generate ideas	Scientific Likes to synthesize data	Risk-taker Likes to experiment
Most effective teaching strategies	Hands-on experiences Return demonstrations Clinical experiences Lectures followed by questions and practice Skills laboratories Workshops Simulations	Brainstorming Group discussions Small group work Role playing Seminars Drawing from past experiences	Lectures by experts with time for reflection and integration Self-instruction Reading Computer-assisted instruction Independent study	Learning from others Skills laboratories Computer-assisted instruction with feedback Case studies that require adaptations from routine care Preceptor-guided clinical experiences

critical care nurses, those who are CCRNs have a distinctive preference for self-directed or solitary pursuit of learning.

As with cognitive style, there is no one best learning style. Each represents an alternative way of learning that learners acquire and modify with experience. Each style is advantageous in particular instructional circumstances and represents the diversity of individual differences that exist among learners.

The value of acknowledging differences in learning style preference is similar to the value of acknowledging differences in a learner's cognitive style. If a learner's cognitive style and learning style preference can be identified, the educator is in a position to enhance the teaching-learning process by matching teaching strategies to accommodate the range and types of cognitive and learning styles found among learners.

The matching of cognitive and learning style with teaching methods is widely held to result in greater learning achievement, greater learner satisfaction with the learning experience, improved understanding, and better learning comprehension.* Habitual use of the same learning style, however—even if it is the learners' preferred style—can leave learners at a disadvantage when they must, of necessity, use some other learning style.[101] At times, divergers will need to acquire some of their learning through lectures just as convergers will at times need to learn by participating in group interactions; field-dependent learners will need to do some learning without the supervision and feedback of an instructor, just as field-independent learners will

*See references 6, 26, 33, 106, 127, 129.

at times need to learn by using observation. Educators, then, need to be sensitive to and aware of the diversity of cognitive and learning styles that exist among learners. They will want to use teaching strategies that both match those preferred by their students and also methods that vary from those preferred in order to broaden learner capabilities to gain instruction through more than just the predominant learning style. Both matching and mismatching of instructional methods are worthwhile.

TEACHING STYLE PREFERENCES

Just as learners have preferred styles of learning, teachers can be said to have preferred styles of teaching. An educator's *teaching style preference* describes his/her characteristic or customary way of providing instruction. One's preferred teaching style is expressed in the types of instructional activities that the educator typically employs.

Some educators prefer to teach in an informal, one-to-one relationship with learners in the clinical setting, whereas others may favor formal lectures to large audiences in a classroom setting. Some instructors perceive their role as providers of information, but others view their role as facilitators of learning. Some offer highly structured teaching through programmed instruction, while others prefer to merely stimulate learning by posing provocative discussion questions. Some like to employ multiple audiovisual aids and others prefer to teach by using their interpersonal or group process skills.

As with learning style preferences, instructors' teaching style preferences may be influenced by many factors. Some of these factors include their own cognitive style, their preferred learning style, the teaching methods that they received, the teaching methods that they have used, and the success they have experienced in using various teaching strategies. Educators may identify their cognitive and preferred learning styles using the same instruments that have been described for determining learning style. Educators who assimilate, structure, and process information in predictable ways may also share this information with learners in much the same style. If it is true that "we teach as we were taught," then many educators may be merely replicating the teaching methods they experienced as students because these methods are most familiar to them. The relative success (and failure) in using different teaching techniques may also shape the educator's repertoire of teaching strategies.

Educators need to have an awareness of their preferred teaching style for many of the same reasons that learners need to know their preferred learning style. Educators should be able to recognize when they are intentionally matching their teaching style to a segment of their audience's preferred learning style. Instructors also need to recognize the necessity of varying their teaching style so that they can effectively meet the needs of learners who have different learning styles. No one teaching style can possibly be effective for every learner or for every instructional situation. Some learning situations require the transmission of facts and principles, but others require teaching applications or group decision-making. Although a majority of nurses may prefer concrete, teacher-structured learning experiences, this is not true for all nurses and is not applicable for all learning situations (e.g., resolving ethical dilemmas or setting patient care priorities). As a result, educators need to acknowledge their preferred teaching style but must be able to offer an array of teaching strategies that meet the learning needs of all learners and that are appropriate for a variety of learning situations. Just as learners need to expand their repertoire of learning styles, educators must also extend their repertoire of teaching styles.

Unlike learning style preferences, which have received a considerable amount of discussion and research, teaching style preference has, thus far, received relatively little attention. Teaching style inventories have not proliferated in the literature and no standard means to quantify teaching style has yet appeared. At present, educators can best analyze their teaching style by introspection, reflection, and surveying their learners and peers.

The fundamental precepts on which the instructional process are based afford a foundation for all aspects of program implementation. The educators' understanding of the principles of teaching and learning and the principles of adult education, together with the recognition of cognitive style, learning, and teaching style preferences, establish a framework from which the educator can then plan and provide specific teaching strategies for the program.

TEACHING METHODS

FACTORS THAT INFLUENCE SELECTION OF A TEACHING METHOD

The teaching-learning process is interactive and consists of one or a series of planned instructional experiences. A *teaching method* specifies how the educator will interact with learners to bring about the desired instructional outcomes. Teaching methods are the means by which educational programs are implemented. They characterize the specific types of learning activities or educational experiences provided for learners.

Today's educator has an ever-expanding array of available teaching methods. Although much research has been done in relation to the efficacy of different teaching strategies, no one method has emerged as the "right" way to provide instruction and no single method has yet been identified that is consistently and universally superior to all other methods. For any given learning experience, a variety of teaching methods may be employed with comparable effectiveness. Teaching strategies may be used in their relatively pure form or may be modified or combined with other methods for various instructional purposes. As a general guideline, the most reliable indication that a teaching method is effective is whether it results in learners' attainment of the instructional outcomes for the program. This section describes a number of factors that the educator needs to consider in selecting among various teaching methods and offers some guidelines for each factor.

Instructional Outcomes To Be Attained

Remember that learning is evidenced as a change in the learner's behavior. The desired behavioral change may be a change in what the leaner knows (cognitive behavior), feels (affective behavior), or does (psychomotor behavior). The single most influential factor governing selection of a teaching method is the behavior specified in the instructional outcomes for the program. The teaching strategy selected should afford learners the opportunity to perform the same behavior that appears in the instructional outcome.

The instructional outcomes established for the program will determine both the domain of learning (cognitive, affective, psychomotor) as well as the taxonomic level within that domain. Some teaching methods are more appropriate for one domain of learning than for another. For example, consider the following three instructional outcomes:

- The nurse will be able to describe the initial management of head trauma patients.
- The nurse will be able to provide effective crisis intervention for the families of trauma patients.
- The nurse will demonstrate how to set up traction for a patient with Crutchfield tongs.

The first outcome represents a cognitive behavior and might be met through a lecture or discussion with the learner. The second outcome represents an affective behavior and might be provided by role playing. The third outcome represents a psychomotor behavior and might be provided by demonstration and practice. A lecture would not be appropriate for developing affective or psychomotor capabilities any more than role playing would be appropriate for a cognitive or psychomotor behavior.

The behaviors contained in the instructional outcomes also determine the taxonomic level of performance expected of the learner. Different teaching methods are appropriate for particular levels within each taxonomic domain. For example, consider the following three instructional outcomes:

- The nurse will be able to define the term *nitrogen balance.*
- The nurse will be able to correctly compute the nitrogen balance for three assigned postoperative patients.
- The nurse will be able to judge how a negative nitrogen balance modifies nursing management of a postoperative patient.

The first outcome requires a behavior (defining) at the lowest (knowledge) level of the cognitive domain. Instruction

for this behavior could be provided by simply providing the learner with relevant journal articles. The second outcome requires a behavior (computing) at a middle (application) level of the cognitive domain. Instruction for this behavior could be provided by some written exercises or a self-study module. The third outcome specifies a behavior (judging) at the highest (evaluation) level of the cognitive domain. Instruction for this outcome might be provided by making patient rounds with the preceptor and reviewing the charts of four or five patients. Both the domain of learning and the taxonomic level of the behavior contained in the instructional outcomes, then, have a bearing on which teaching method(s) are most appropriate to employ.

Guideline

The teaching method(s) selected should provide learners with practice in performing the behaviors specified in the instructional outcomes. Teaching strategies should afford experiences that match as closely as possible the type and level of performances dictated in the instructional outcomes.

Content Indicated in the Instructional Outcomes

The subject matter or content that appears in the instructional outcomes also influences the selection of teaching method. The breadth and scope of the content to be learned as well as its difficulty and complexity may suggest that one teaching strategy might be more appropriate than another for this content.

For example, nurses who work in postanesthesia recovery (PAR) may need limited capabilities in the area of cardiac monitoring. Your institution may only require that PAR nurses be able to recognize and intervene for lethal cardiac dysrhythmias. Nurses who work in a coronary care unit, by contrast, may need a commensurably greater capability in this area. Since the depth, scope, and complexity of instruction may vary widely between these two groups of staff, the number and types of teaching methodologies may also differ. The PAR nurses may be provided with a relatively brief lecture on lethal dysrhythmias followed by some workbook practice. The coronary care unit nurses, on the other hand, may require a series of lectures with case studies, a number of workshops to practice their interpretation skills, audiovisual simulations that afford feedback on their interventions, and considerable preceptor role modeling of dysrhythmia analysis and interpretation on the clinical unit.

Guideline

The teaching method(s) selected should relate directly to the depth, scope, and complexity of the content reflected in the instructional outcomes.

Agent of Instruction

Instructional methods can be broadly categorized into those that are controlled and provided by someone other than the learner and those that are controlled and provided by the learner. The former are referred to as *other-directed* methods and the latter are referred to as *self-directed* methods. Some institutions use exclusively other-directed teaching methods in which all instruction is provided and managed by one or more educators. Some institutions use primarily self-directed teaching methods in which learners are expected to pursue and manage their own learning and in which educators function only as resources to the learner. Other institutions use some combination of these two possible agents of instruction, whereby some segments of the program are teacher-directed and some segments are self-directed. The use of other- vs, self-directed methods can emanate from a philosophical or financial rationale. Philosophically, an institution that ascribes to strong beliefs in adult education may be particularly devoted to extensive use of self-directed learning techniques. At other times, the personnel or budgetary resources may make it impossible for a single educator to provide all of the staff development programs required at that agency; self-directed learning may then be included to relieve some of this labor-intensive burden.

Other-directed teaching methods include strategies such as lecture, role modeling, and demonstration of clinical skills. Self-directed methods may include independent study, self-learning modules, and some forms of computer-assisted instruction.

Guideline

The teaching method(s) selected should reflect both philosophical beliefs and operational realities related to the agent responsible for instruction.

Learning Setting

A traditional means for categorizing teaching methods is according to the instructional setting where they are most appropriately employed. The traditional instructional settings for nursing staff development are divided into classroom, laboratory, and clinical settings. The instructional setting, in turn, is dictated by the type of behavior contained in the instructional objective or outcome.

A group discussion concerning problems in patient management is not appropriately conducted at the patient's bedside any more than practice in how to admit a patient can reasonably be located in a classroom. The very nature of the learning experience usually dictates where it should properly be held. Once the instructional setting has been identified, a different array of teaching methods becomes available. The latter section of this chapter will detail the teaching strategies typically employed for each of these instructional settings.

Guideline

The teaching method(s) selected should be appropriate to the setting in which it will be employed.

Learner Characteristics

Learners' previous background of education and experience; their present knowledge, attitudes, and skills; their cognitive style and learning style preferences; their need to be actively involved in learning experiences, and their need for variation in instructional methods all influence the selection of teaching strategies. Learners with limited knowledge and experience in the areas addressed by the instructional outcomes may initially benefit by instruction, via lectures or assigned readings, that provides them with the knowledge base for those areas. More experienced staff would likely be bored by these techniques since they already possess knowledge of these fundamentals; that group of staff might benefit more by teaching methods such as case studies or simulations that require application of their knowledge base.

As adult learners, nurses need to be actively involved in learning experiences. Experiential teaching methods, such as written or computerized patient simulations, role playing, nursing rounds on the unit, workshops, or skills laboratory exercises, might be planned to maximize active participation.

The need to provide variation in teaching methods originates from three major sources: differences among learners in cognitive style, differences among learners in learning style preference, and the more generic need to avoid monotony in the means of instruction. The influence of cognitive style and learning style have been described earlier in this chapter. Using the same teaching method for virtually all learning experiences disregards the influence of the behavior and content included in instructional outcomes and ignores regard for individual differences among learners. In addition, any teaching method may become ineffective over time if it no longer continues to stimulate learning and the active involvement of learners.

Educators who fail to expand their repertoire of teaching strategies may not only stifle learners' interest in learning but diminish their own creativity, interest, and effectiveness in teaching. Freitas, Lantz, and Reed[48] explored the attributes of creative nurse educators. Their research identified the following seven techniques of creative teaching that:

- *Connect the learners' life experiences with the educational material.* Instruction is made "real" by providing opportunities for learners to experience the kinds of situations and problems that clinical nursing presents.

- *Include humor.* Teaching that incorporates humorous and light-hearted segments can relieve tension in the learning setting and maintain learner attention.
- *Use feeling-focused experiences.* Teaching methods such as guided fantasy (close your eyes and imagine that you are lying paralyzed in a cold hospital room) and role playing can heighten learners' sensitivities to the types of situations that many of their patients may experience. Rather than giving volumes of information about what these situations are like, the instructor can illustrate important points by acting them out with the learner.
- *Involve learners in the role of the patient.* Providing learners with the opportunity to experience first-hand what patients experience (e.g., having an IV started, being restrained) can afford learning more poignant than any lecture or textbook could offer.
- *Exhibit risk-taking behavior.* Educators can effectively and creatively address a number of process skills (e.g., resolving legal and ethical dilemmas, resolving family disagreements regarding organ donation, making case management decisions) where no one right answer exists by allowing learners to debate and reach consensus regarding these issues. Allow for uncertain outcomes and permit learners to make mistakes that won't harm patients.
- *Use teaching methods that match the material to be learned rather than the personality of the teacher.* Creative teachers adapt their teaching method to the subject matter rather than using the same method(s) they customarily use.
- *Present information dramatically.* Learning experiences that surprise, shock, or intellectually jolt learners can engage them more profoundly than merely providing information to be absorbed and assimilated.

Guideline

The teaching method(s) selected should reflect recognition of differences among learners' education and experience; their present knowledge, attitudes, and skills; their cognitive style and learning style preferences; their need to be actively involved in learning experiences; and their need for variation in instructional strategies.

Number of Learners

Some teaching methods such as computer-assisted instruction or self-learning packages are ideal for individualized, self-paced learning experiences. Other methods such as brainstorming, workshops, or clinical conferences are more suited for small groups. Still others such as lectures or seminars are teaching strategy alternatives available for large numbers of learners. Just as certain audiovisual media are appropriate for different size audiences, teaching methods need careful selection in relation to audience size.

Guideline

The teaching method(s) selected should reflect the number of learners who need instruction.

Available Resources

The resources available within the agency may affect the feasibility of using various teaching methods. In these days of austerity and diminished educational budgets, educators have a responsibility to use instructional resources judiciously when they consider the range of possible teaching strategies that may be used. These instructional resources include the following categories:

- Personnel (both prospective program faculty as well as support staff such as secretaries, audiovisual technicians, computer programmers, and the like)
- Physical facilities (number, type, and size of facilities; possible seating and room arrangements; spaces available for learning laboratories, computer-assisted instruction; workshop practice; amount and location of storage space)
- Equipment and supplies (audiovisual and instructional hardware, software, and aids)
- Time (amount of time available for development of instructional materials, for class preparation, and for learning new teaching skills or techniques)
- Financial (funds available for purchasing instructional programs, equipment, and supplies; fiscal budget for orientation, in-service, and continuing education programs; funds available for developing instructional materials in-house).

Guideline

The teaching method(s) selected should be within the resource capability of the agency. Insofar as possible, educators should employ teaching methods that can afford the greatest effectiveness at the greatest efficiency. When two or more teaching methods are equally effective in relation to attainment of learning outcomes, the more efficient method(s) should be used.

Educator's Familiarity and Expertise with Teaching Methods

Regardless of the purported efficacy of any particular teaching method, if the instructor is unfamiliar with the technique, is inexperienced or unskilled in using it, the potential value of that teaching strategy is negated. Even educators who would like to be more creative and diverse in the instructional techniques they employ will have varying levels of proficiency in using each technique. Time and graduated experience in practicing new teaching strategies will enhance the educator's range of instructional skills, but instructors have a responsibility to learners to use teaching methods they can employ with some predictable degree of effectiveness.

Guideline

While being open to both experimentation and the need for variation in teaching strategies, the teaching method(s) selected should be ones that the educator is skilled in using.

The following section describes a variety of teaching methods available for use in nursing staff development programs. These teaching methods can be differentiated into one of two broad categories based on who controls the variables in the teaching-learning process. *Other-directed teaching methods* are those in which someone other than the learner controls a majority of the elements in the instructional process. *Self-directed teaching methods* are those in which the learner controls a majority of these instructional variables. In both categories in the teaching-learning process the instructional variables include the following ten instructional elements:

- Identification of learning needs
- Determining the topic and purpose of the learning activity
- Establishing the objectives or expected outcomes
- Selecting appropriate learning experiences
- Incorporating human and material resources
- Determining the learning environment or setting
- Deciding the time and duration of learning
- Determining the pace of learning
- Establishing the methods of evaluation
- Documenting evidence that the outcomes have been achieved.[2]

OTHER-DIRECTED TEACHING METHODS

When someone other than the learner controls most of the elements in the instructional process, that "other" person is usually the educator. As a result, other-directed teaching methods may also be called *teacher-directed* or *instructor-directed* methods. In nursing staff development, the most commonly employed other-directed teaching methods can be further classified according to the setting where these methods are generally used. These settings include the classroom, the laboratory, and the clinical setting. The following section provides an overview of teaching methods used in each of these learning settings.

Classroom Teaching Methods

The classroom setting is usually the locus for learning related to instructional outcomes within the cognitive domain. This is distinguished from both the laboratory setting and the clinical setting where psychomotor and affective outcomes are more appropriately addressed.

When the classroom is used for teaching, the educator must be certain that the principles of both the teaching-learning process and those of adult education are employed. A commonly held view is that classroom teaching methods often involve instructors teaching while learners passively listen or take notes. In reality, classroom teaching can be very interactive if the educator incorporates the fundamental principles of instruction and adult education.

The range of available teaching methods for the classroom includes the classical lecture, various forms of group discussion, conferences, seminars, and brainstorming. In the section that follows, a variety of classroom teaching methods will be described, including their appropriate use, limitations, and guidelines for use.

Lecture*

The lecture is, by far, the most time- and tradition-honored teaching method. It remains the most commonly employed teaching strategy largely because of its long-standing familiarity to both educators and learners, its economy of time and space, and its efficiency in managing large learner-to-instructor ratios.

The lecture holds the unique distinction of being not only the most widely used but also the most frequently misused and abused form of instruction.[3] It can be a personable, effective, and highly efficient vehicle for conveying a large volume of information to a large number of learners. At its best, a lecture provides a personable means of sharing information in an organized, systematic, and informative manner. At its worst, a lecture anesthetizes audiences with litanies of facts, reiterates the known and the obvious, or confuses learners. When poorly used, the lecture can stifle learner feedback and response while transforming an audience into a sea of note-taking sponges.

If used with care, the lecture can be extremely efficient as a cost- and time-effective method of summarizing, updating, assimilating, and correlating large bodies of knowledge in a particular content area. When well organized and developed, it can disseminate the expertise and insight of a single instructor to an audience size limited only by seating capacity and the adequacy of acoustics.

APPROPRIATENESS FOR TEACHING   The lecture method is appropriately used for instructional outcomes situated at any level within the cognitive domain of learning although it is most often employed with the lower cognitive levels.[27] It can be used when the instructional outcomes center on

*See references 3, 7, 24, 45, 52, 122, 124.

learners' attaining cognitive abilities such as definition, re-call, identification, relation, synthesis, explanation, description, understanding, interrelation, generalization, and differentiation among complex concepts. Lectures can be used to provide learners with the factual data needed to prepare for affective and psychomotor learning by supplying them with opportunities for critical thinking and for solving the intellectual challenges involved with application of theories, concepts, and principles. Lectures can also be used to clarify intricate ideas, delineate important concepts, assimilate information from a multitude of diverse sources, understand complex and interrelated concepts, critique, motivate, stimulate budding interests in new areas, and resolve discrepant multidisciplinary perspectives on selected issues and problems.

Limitations Some limitations of the lecture include the following[7,74]:

- The speaker may employ an ineffective presentation style.
- The speaker may possess limited expertise in the content area.
- The speaker may use a level of instruction that is inappropriate for learners.
- Retention of learning may be limited if learners are not actively involved in the presentation. Estimates are that only 10% of what is heard is retained and that nearly 40% of lecture content may be forgotten within 20 minutes.
- It is not an effective method of instruction for learning within the psychomotor or affective domains. Although lectures may afford the intellectual groundwork for modifying attitudes or clinical practice, they are generally confined to altering behaviors within the cognitive domain.
- If no question and answer time is provided, individual learners may be denied the opportunity to ask questions or to request clarification of specific points.
- If the lecture is not complemented by one or more forms of interaction and exchange with learners, the principles of adult education are neglected.
- Adult learners may experience fatigue and boredom if lectures last too long or are not combined with more participative teaching methods.
- Formal lectures may foster learner dependence on the instructor and disappoint adult learners with more interactive and social learning styles.

Guidelines for Use In preparing a lecture, planning is of the utmost importance. Some useful guidelines for planning a lecture include the following:[3]

- Use the instructional outcomes and a literature review to formulate an outline of key points to be covered. Limit the outline to words and phrases to reduce the likelihood of "reading" the lecture.
- Be certain that the outline introduces and develops concepts in a clear, logical sequence based on previous learning and anticipated future learning needs; supplement the outline with concrete clinical examples and illustrations.
- Organize your presentation around some meaningful sequence (such as simple to complex, concrete to abstract). Plan the transitions to be used to progress through each segment of the content.
- Know your audience: what they already know relative to the topic, clinical experiences they have had or will encounter soon. Cover the topic at an instructional level appropriate for your audience's knowledge, skills, and experiences.
- Prepare three elements for the presentation: an introduction, the main body of content, and a closing summary.
- Introduce the lecture with the outcomes to be attained, key points to be discussed, issues to be addressed, questions to be answered, problems to be solved, and the like. If content is part of a continuing series, summarize previous coverage related to the topic. These measures will help to generate learner involvement and communicate the relevancy of the lecture content. Plan to alternate simple with more complex concepts and to illustrate application of principles and concepts by using clinical examples to which learners can relate.
- Allocate instructional time according to the importance and complexity of the content. Double-check that you have allotted adequate time for considering and integrating more difficult concepts. Use the margins of your lecture notes to mark the time required for covering certain sections. Avoid the tendency of attempting to teach "everything" about a topic in a limited amount of time.
- Anticipate questions, issues, and areas of misconception that may arise. Determine how you will respond to each of these.
- If unforeseen events could impinge on the amount of available instructional time, plan for this by highlighting the most important points to be covered. Should these time infringements occur, you will then have your coverage priorities already established. After some experience giving each lecture, make note of time allotment adjustments necessary for covering the topic.
- Distribute the class outline before the lecture so that learners will be able to more readily follow the presentation. A handout that includes an outline of all key points and copies of any complex diagrams, formulas, or calculations reduces the need for copious note-taking and enables learners to listen more attentively without fear of missing important elements in their notes.
- Plan to include audiovisuals to clarify and supplement the presentation and to provide information in a visual

medium. Learning retention is enhanced by using more than one teaching medium, and many principles and concepts can be more effectively communicated through visual explanations rather than just verbal ones.

- Have all support materials (handouts, outlines, worksheets, reading lists, etc.) available and all audiovisuals (software and hardware) readied well in advance of the lecture time. Ensure that all equipment is functioning properly and that replacement components such as slide projector bulbs are readily at hand.
- Plan for at least a 10-minute break after every 50 minutes of instruction.

The following guidelines can help the educator implement the lecture teaching method more effectively:

- Find a comfortable posture and location where you can be easily seen and heard.
- Exemplify enthusiasm for the material by using an energetic yet conversational tone of voice. Avoid being overly dramatic, affected, or listless. Vary the pitch, intensity, and rate of delivery throughout the presentation. If necessary, practice voice projection and modulation using an audiotape or videotape of practice teaching sessions.
- Use a microphone whenever learners may have difficulty hearing you. When in doubt, use the microphone; learners should not have to strain to hear a presentation.
- Use pauses to interrupt the steady flow of the presentation. Use the pause to offer intriguing thoughts to ponder, to raise issues or problems for discussion, to elicit learner reactions, to encourage challenges, to clarify or reiterate major points, or to request clinical examples from the audience. Make time during the presentation to validate that the content is meaningful and useful to learners.
- Emphasize immediate application of knowledge to clinical practice. Use transitions and pauses during the presentation to verify that learners know how to use and apply facts, principles, theories, and content to patient care. Don't expect learners to be able to integrate and apply new information; assist learners in this process. This might be accomplished by making rounds on the units where learners work to identify relevant patient situations they presently confront.
- Make yourself aware of any tendencies you may have to use habitual phrases ("you know") or distracting movements and gestures (continual pacing). Try to be natural and relaxed as you relate to learners. New instructors may find it helpful to have their first few presentations videotaped or observed by a peer to determine if their presentation style needs polishing.
- Develop your ability to recognize learners' nonverbal responses to instruction. Look for facial expressions and body language that indicate understanding and distinguish these from nonverbal cues that suggest confusion, bewilderment, boredom, or fatigue. Face learners as you present and scan their faces and behavior frequently. Validate their nonverbal reactions as readily as you would their questions or requests for clarification. For example, the educator might respond to a quizzical expression by asking, "Kate, did that point raise a question for you?"
- Confirm learners' comprehension of material by soliciting clinical examples of applications, by posing problems or issues related to the topic, asking followup questions, or interjecting discussion and critique.
- Conclude the presentation with a brief summary of the most important points and their clinical implications. Be sure to provide any clarifications or answers to remaining questions learners may have. Use review and reinforcement to help learners achieve a sense of intellectual completion and attainment of the instructional outcomes.

Group Discussion

Group discussion consists of a purposeful meeting of two or more individuals who collectively gather to share, deliberate, exchange, and/or critique perspectives regarding some specific issue, problem, situation, or topic of mutual concern. The climate for this exchange of ideas and opinions may be either formal or informal and requires some form of leadership to direct, focus, and summarize the discussion. This teaching method capitalizes on the aggregate knowledge, abilities, and experiences of group members who come together for the purpose of reaching some conclusion, consensus, or resolution of a problem.

APPROPRIATENESS FOR TEACHING Group discussion is appropriately used for teaching the following:

- How to formulate, organize, and coherently express one's perceptions and positions on issues and situations.
- The dynamics of group process and the collaborative management of problems.
- Problem-solving skills: how to identify, define, approach, reconsider, constructively critique, and differentially weigh various elements in the problem-solving process.
- Affective behaviors such as critical and analytical thinking about behaviors, consciousness-raising on relevant legal, ethical, and psychosocial issues.
- The skills required for effective communication and interpersonal or interdisciplinary relations.
- Effective and active listening to the views expressed by others, as well as tolerance for views that differ from one's own.
- Areas open to multiple interpretations, when hard data and concrete facts are less available for decision-making.

LIMITATIONS Some of the limitations of group discussion include the following[16,90]:

- If the group process elements are not managed effectively, group discussion may result in few learning outcomes.
- Some learners have an aversion to working in small groups because it requires considerably more effort of the learner than sitting and listening. Learners who prefer more passive roles in the learning process may find group discussions neither helpful nor enjoyable.
- Learners who prefer instructor-dominated learning experiences may resist this teaching method because they view it as an abdication of the educator's responsibility to provide them with instruction.
- Learners who prefer concrete and highly structured learning activities may be dissatisfied with group discussions because these experiences may not afford the degree of specificity and/or structure they seek.
- Learners who prefer self-directed and/or solitary learning experiences may resist situations in which they are forced to learn with others.

GUIDELINES FOR USE Group discussion can be an effective teaching technique when the following suggestions are incorporated:

- The instructor has a thorough working knowledge of group dynamics in learning situations.
- The discussion leader structures the activity by[90]

    Giving participants the purpose and rationale for the discussion session including both personal and professional reasons for the activity

    Identifying the issue or topic to be addressed

    Explaining the task to be accomplished (the product or outcomes sought) through discussion

    Providing clear and explicit instructions on how the discussion should proceed (including the size of each group, the composition of groups [e.g., homogenous groups of people who know one another or heterogeneous groups of strangers with different backgrounds], and the amount of time available for discussion)

    Allowing participants to organize themselves into groups based on the established criteria for group composition

    Explaining what is to be reported by each group following the discussion

    Facilitating exchange of information within each group by answering questions, resolving problems, and redirecting groups that have strayed from the focus of the discussion

    Posing thought-provoking questions or comments to stimulate discussion and interaction within the groups

    Providing a realistic means and adequate time for each group to report its determinations to all participants

    Providing a summary and closure of the discussion session and its findings.

- Learners are provided with clearly defined topics and objectives for discussion. The agenda may be communicated in advance of the discussion session so that participants may prepare for the session or it may be made known just prior to the discussion.
- Seating arrangements and acoustics facilitate conversation and exchange among participants.
- Group membership may be homogenous or heterogeneous, depending on the purpose of the discussion and characteristics of the total audience. Group members need to share a similar desire to accomplish the goals established for discussion.

Nursing Care Conference

When some particular aspect or problem related to an individual patient's nursing care arises, a nursing care conference may be convened to identify ways to manage that patient's care more effectively. Nursing care conferences are learning activities conducted as an ongoing part of that patient's care. In these conferences, nursing staff may learn from any of a number of sources: their peers, other staff such as clinical nurse specialists or nurse managers, literature reviews, and personal reflections on their experiences with this patient and other similar patients. The value of such learning experiences is the reality-based situation and the immediate applicability to nursing practice.

APPROPRIATENESS FOR TEACHING Nursing care conferences are appropriate learning vehicles when an individual staff nurse has seemingly exhausted their personal resources for managing a particular patient care situation and needs some input and assistance from other nursing staff to resolve or improve the situation. The initiating event for these conferences is typically some obstacle or problem that exists in providing nursing care to a specific patient, but it may also be just a desire to appraise the overall quality and effectiveness of nursing care for a particular patient. This type of teaching method is also useful for acquainting orientees with the types of nursing management situations they can expect to encounter.

LIMITATIONS Some limitations of the nursing care conference as a teaching strategy include the following:

- Staff nurses must have the insight to recognize situations that would benefit from this type of learning activity. All staff may not be equally adept at this process.
- Staff must feel that their identification of need for such a conference will generate interest and support from peers and managers rather than suggest that they are not able to manage patient care effectively. Managerial support is a necessary prerequisite.

GUIDELINES FOR USE Nursing care conferences can be effective teaching vehicles when the following guidelines are employed:

- Conferences may be scheduled or spontaneous, depending on the time available and the nature of the situation.
- The nurse assigned to that patient usually provides participants with an overview of the patient, the nursing care issue or problem, and the results of interventions provided to date. The nurse then specifies the nature of assistance that is requested (e.g., finding alternative ways to communicate with a neurologically impaired patient or finding a more efficient method of providing patient education).
- The decision regarding who will manage the conference should be made in advance. Leadership is usually vested in the nurse who presents the patient situation; other staff, clinical nurse specialists, or nurse managers can then be used as resources and consultants. The conference manager will need to clarify, validate, and summarize the opinions and suggestions offered during the conference.

Case Study

A case study presents a historical and chronological account of an actual patient situation that affords some lesson to be learned. The lesson is derived through an analysis of interventions and results as they actually happened. As the case is presented, learners are asked to use their problem-solving skills to answer specific questions related to the situation.[128] Case studies teach by example and the outcomes of real life events.

APPROPRIATENESS FOR TEACHING The case study is an appropriate teaching strategy when the complexity, novelty, or unique nature of a particular patient situation warrants more formal, comprehensive, and detailed consideration. The lessons derived from a case study may be positive or negative. Positive lessons might include how to provide nursing care for a patient with a rarely observed clinical problem, how to coordinate care of a complex patient situation, or how to provide patient education under severe time constraints. A case study can then be used to illustrate "what works." Negative lessons can also be beneficial learning experiences because they provide powerful exemplars of "what doesn't work." Examples of negative lessons might include analyzing particular cases to determine what nursing interventions are *not* effective in reducing nosocomial infections, which nursing measures *fail* to comfort and support a grieving family, or when is the *least effective* time to administer tube feedings. Trial-and-error learning and learning from mistakes are often precursors to discovering which nursing measures are more effective than others.

Case studies can be used either to introduce or to summarize a learning experience. Using the case as an introduction allows for intermittent return to the case throughout the presentation so that it affords a continuing reference point for nursing theory and practice. Using the case to summarize a learning experience provides learners with an opportunity to review, integrate, and apply what was learned to an actual patient situation. Case studies may also be used for formal or informal evaluation of learning.[128]

LIMITATIONS Some limitations of the case study include the following:

- Someone has to recognize patient situations that offer a lesson to be learned.
- Nursing staff need to be afforded the resources and support to develop and present the case study as a teaching vehicle. Administrative support and learning resources may not always be available to nursing staff.
- Learning the necessary skills (of reflective nursing practice, critical thinking, writing the details of a case study, leading and managing group discussion) take time to develop and refine.
- Nursing staff may be hesitant to openly discuss areas of mismanagement or inappropriate nursing interventions with their peers. An open and supportive administrative environment that recognizes the value of learning from mistakes is not always available to nursing staff.

GUIDELINES FOR USE Some suggested ways to implement the case study teaching method include the following:

- Educators can set the stage for nursing staff to identify patient situations appropriate for a case study by sharing brief anecdotes of lessons learned from various patients on that unit and by encouraging nursing staff to reflect on their practice in a similar manner.
- Once a case has been identified for study, the nurse (or group of nurses) who provided care for that patient generally assume responsibility for determining how the situation will be described and presented. Nurse educators can assist in the design phase by providing related articles and reference materials, by assisting with the summarization of relevant clinical data, by offering instructional expertise regarding how the case might best be presented and discussed, and by reviewing the principles of effective group discussion.
- When appropriate, the patient and/or the family and other healthcare professionals may be invited to participate in the discussion so that all perspectives in the situation are considered.
- Designated individuals need to provide leadership in managing the group, its deliberations, and its conclusions. A clear and concise synopsis of the group's findings need to be presented as the "lesson" learned from the case.

Case Method

The case method teaching strategy is similar to a case study, except that the "case" is usually not a real patient, but a representative composite or hypothetical patient situation that is constructed and then analyzed by learners to achieve specific instructional outcomes.[22,75,77] Although the "patient" is not real, the situation and circumstances depicted are true-to-life. The primary value of the case method of teaching is that it teaches problem-solving and critical thinking skills. The case method affords learners an opportunity to explore specific types of situations or problems, to analyze how these might have been prevented or how they might be managed, to apply theory to practice,[29] and to weigh possible outcomes and their ramifications.

Cases may be developed locally by the educator, be borrowed or adapted (with permission from the copyright holder) from cases described in publications within or outside of nursing, or may be purchased. The case itself is a comprehensive account of information relevant to the situation or problem to be analyzed. It needs to contain sufficient detail for learners to be able to fully understand the situation and the aspects targeted for discussion. Clinical cases would need to include all pertinent findings and laboratory data. Cases that focus on a situation such as violence in the emergency department (rather than on patient care) need to document all relevant information bearing on that situation that is available as a basis for decision-making. The content for the case is selected according to the instructional outcomes to be attained. No answers, outcomes, or leading questions are included.[77]

APPROPRIATENESS FOR TEACHING The case method is well suited as a teaching strategy when specific types of learning experiences are important but may not be available at the time desired. It is also useful for ensuring that certain types of clinical situations are experienced by all learners and that the desired instructional elements in the situation are all present. The case method can thus be used as an alternative and/or complementary teaching strategy to augment clinical experiences and to add a large dose of reality to the information provided in lectures.

Some additional uses of the case method include the following:

- It is particularly useful for teaching decision-making and problem-solving, to reinforce theory and principles, apply theory to practice, and test reality.
- It can be useful in transfer of learning from theory to reality, from familiar to unfamiliar situations, or from simple to complex circumstances.
- It is valuable as an adjunct for teaching moral reasoning, ethical[29] and legal decision-making, and affective instructional outcomes.
- It affords nurses an opportunity to sharpen their assessment skills, to differentiate and prioritize relevant clinical information, and to use critical thinking skills in arriving at appropriate decisions.[75]

- It enables the educator to structure learning experiences to cover certain types of health problems, patients of various ages, specific nursing diagnoses, various documentation methods, and to elicit highly specific learning behaviors.
- Well-designed cases can be used repeatedly with different groups of learners and for different instructional purposes.

LIMITATIONS Some potential limitations of the case method include the following:

- The case may include too much information so that learners are confused or uncertain regarding which information is pertinent.
- The case may be missing relevant data.
- The case may be presented in a disorganized manner.
- The discussion leader may not be effective in group process and group learning methods. The educator may lack the skills to guide learners in analyzing information, drawing conclusions, and making generalizations.[22]
- Developing cases and designing case materials can be time consuming.[29]
- Many of the cases available for adoption or adaptation may not be suitable for the specific instructional outcomes sought.
- The roles of both the educator and the learner are different from traditional classroom lectures. Passive students may resist or fear active participation, and educators may feel that they are less able to control the outcomes of instruction.
- The case method is most appropriate for field-independent learners who prefer analytic thinking and active group discussions. Learners with other types of learning style preferences may be threatened by this form of learning.[29]

GUIDELINES FOR USE Some guidelines for using the case method follow:

- Identify pertinent characteristics of the learners, including their knowledge, skills, attitudes, and clinical experience.
- Determine the instructional outcomes for the case. These should emphasize learning behaviors that can be attained in a classroom setting.
- Construct or select case materials that coincide with the desired outcomes. Content and details of the case need to be based on these outcomes. Remove all extraneous information and organize presentation of the case via some logical framework such as the chronological order of events.
- Determine the pertinent attributes of each character in the case scenario: their demographic, social, and economic traits, health problems, beliefs, and personality traits.
- Prepare discussion questions based on the instruc-

tional outcomes and details of the case. These questions should promote lively exchanges, stimulate multiple points of view on an issue, reinforce important points, and enable learners to summarize their learning.

- Whenever possible, prepare and distribute the case to learners in advance of instruction so that they can review this information and come prepared for discussion. If desired, concentrate learners' attention on selected aspects, key points, or questions that will represent the focus of discussion.
- When multiple cases will be considered, the educator may divide the class into small groups who each work on a different case. Each group then presents their analysis to the entire group.
- Open the discussion by highlighting the case and clarifying the focus of the discussion. Manage the discussion by keeping the dialogue moving, by ensuring that key points are not overlooked, by managing time appropriately, and by including the input of all participants. Group members can work as a team (vs. independently) to analyze the situation and arrive at solutions. The educator facilitates group exchange and outcomes but does not provide "answers" or indicate "correct" solutions.

Incident Process

The incident process is a group discussion technique that fosters development of skills in reasoned inquiry. As a teaching strategy, the incident process uses a single real-life situation (the incident) as a springboard to compel learners to solicit and analyze all relevant information before making decisions. The originators of the incident process, Paul and Faith Pigors,[102] believe that its greatest value is to help individuals learn how to generalize.

The discussion leader may be the educator or the group member who is most familiar with all aspects of the actual situation. The discussion leader presents a very brief description of the incident to the group either verbally or in writing. An example of an incident might be: *Mary Jackson is preparing Mr. Erickson for transfer to the operating room for open-heart surgery. Immediately after Mary administers Mr. Erickson's preoperative medication, Mr. Erickson states "I've changed my mind about this surgery. I don't want to go! I don't think I'm going to make it out of the operating room alive!" The operating team is awaiting Mr. Erickson's arrival.*

Once the incident has been presented, group members must uncover the facts bearing on the incident by soliciting further information from the discussion leader. After a period of fact-gathering and analysis, group members identify key factors influencing the incident and arrive at a decision. The discussion leader then determines the validity of that decision by comparing the group's decision-making outcome and process with the actual facts and decision reached in the real incident.

APPROPRIATENESS FOR TEACHING   The incident process is appropriate for teaching in following areas:

- Fundamentals of sound decision-making based on gathering and analysis of all pertinent facts
- Critical thinking processes
- Problem-solving skills related to nursing interventions: how to define problems, analyze situations, and find appropriate solutions[23]
- Using analytical approaches for nursing practice and management issues
- Reinforcing application of policies and procedures or standards of care and for identifying needed revisions in any of these documents
- Teaching learners how to distinguish among impressions, opinions, inferences, and facts
- Effective listening skills

LIMITATIONS   The potential limitations of the incident process revolve around the capability of the discussion leader. For the incident process to be used effectively, the discussion leader needs to be skilled in describing the substance of the incident cryptically, in offering only the information that group members solicit, in helping group members to define the problem or issue and the most relevant facts related to it, in selecting the most appropriate response, and in arriving at generalizations from the incident to similar situations. The leader also needs to describe the original incident in a manner that protects the anonymity of staff who were involved so as to avoid any possible embarrassment.

GUIDELINES FOR USE   Group participants do not need to prepare in advance for this teaching strategy. If group members are not familiar with the process, the instructor or group leader outlines how the incident process works and then presents the incident.

There are five discussion phases in the incident process[23]:

- *Study the incident.* Each participant reviews the incident and formulates questions designed to examine the situation more fully.
- *Get the facts.* Participants pose questions to the discussion leader who provides only the facts requested. As answers are provided, additional queries are raised in an attempt to determine what else needs to be known about the incident. The group decides when they have obtained all relevant facts bearing upon the incident.
- *Define the problem.* The group attempts to reach consensus on the nature of the issue that requires some action. If necessary, the discussion leader may be asked to supply more facts.
- *Determine appropriate action.* If the group is small, each member writes down a suggested action and its rationale. If the group is large, subgroups may work as teams to arrive at solutions and rationales. After

each solution is presented, the entire group attempts to reach consensus on the most appropriate action to take. The discussion leader then reveals what was actually decided in the incident and the outcomes of that decision.

- *Make generalizations.* Participants reflect on the incident in its entirety to identify principles and lessons learned in making the decision that could be applicable to other clinical situations.

Brainstorming

Brainstorming is a group idea-generating or problem-solving technique that aims at stimulating creative thinking. In a structured process, a group leader presents the problem to be worked on, solicits as many ideas and alternative solutions as participants can imagine, records all suggestions, and manages the time available. The idea-generating phase typically lasts from 60 to 90 minutes. Participants then form small groups to categorize each idea, appraise the relative effectiveness of each, and recommend the most promising solutions. Each group's deliberations are then shared and consensus regarding the best solution is then attempted.[57]

APPROPRIATENESS FOR TEACHING   Brainstorming is a useful instructional method when conventional approaches to clinical problem-solving have proven futile, when tried solutions are no longer effective, or when the problem or issue can not be solved by analytic or deductive means and more creative means are necessary.

LIMITATIONS   Brainstorming may not be effective if any of the following exist:

- If the problem described is ambiguous or vague
- If the meeting is scheduled at a time when participants are tired, stressed, or otherwise distracted
- If the time frame established for the session is not adhered to
- If the leader fails to enforce the procedural rules for brainstorming
- If suggestions offered cannot be heard by all participants

GUIDELINES FOR USE   Some suggested ways to implement brainstorming include the following:

- A week before the scheduled session, send a note to participants to suggest that they begin thinking about the problem.
- Schedule the meeting in the early part of the day when participants will be more alert and responsive. Establish a time limit and stick to it.
- Start the session with a warm-up that reviews the rules for brainstorming and relaxes participants with a practice exercise: "If you weren't working today, what could you be doing with your day?"

- Clarify the rules for brainstorming:
   Generate as many new and eclectic ideas as possible to solve the problem
   Quantity, novelty, and originality are desired
   Piggyback ideas
   Don't be afraid to suggest unusual or seemingly silly solutions
   No one is allowed to criticize or evaluate any ideas suggested
   Only one person can speak at a time
   All suggestions will be recorded for everyone to see
- After the real problem is presented, the leader controls and solicits participants' generation of ideas, clarifies their intent, records each so that everyone can see the list, and then manages the group consensus process.

Seminar

A seminar is a learner-directed guided discussion in which participants function as instructors or consultants in analyzing a selected problem. In a seminar, the discussion involves sharing of information, ideas, and opinions, and the exploration of relevant problems and questions.[31] Seminars require advanced preparation by group members so that they arrive at the seminar prepared to discuss, debate, exchange, and express their ideas and opinions related to the selected topic. The focus of a seminar should represent "a significant problem of current interest."[46] The ideal size of a seminar group is 10 to 15 members.[46]

APPROPRIATENESS FOR TEACHING   A seminar format is appropriate in providing the following types of learning experiences:

- Promoting active learner involvement in considering all aspects of a complex issue
- Providing learners with opportunities to assess, interpret, critique, describe, summarize, and apply ideas
- Providing first-hand experiences with group problem-solving
- Teaching related to affective and interpersonal issues.[31]
- Enhancing interactive skills, effective listening, verbal expression of ideas, and promoting critical thinking[89]

LIMITATIONS   Potential limitations of the seminar teaching method include the following:

- The topic selected for the seminar may not be appropriate for discussion; topics require some contrasting elements open to deliberation rather than admitting of a "right" or "correct" answer.
- Participants must come prepared if the seminar topic is to be thoughtfully considered.
- The seminar leader may fail to keep the discussion focused and meaningful.

- The seminar leader may dominate the discussion and inhibit participation by other learners.
- One or more participants may dominate the discussion.
- The group size may be too large or too small for effective discussion.

GUIDELINES FOR USE   Farley[46] recommends the following guidelines for using the seminar:

- Before the seminar, the educator needs to provide learners with instructional objectives, a list of recommended readings, and rules governing conduct of the seminar (coming prepared to present on the topic, keeping comments focused, no monopolizing of time, and respecting the opinions of others).
- During the seminar, the educator ensures an open and nonjudgemental climate for discussion among learners, keeps the exchange moving and focused toward its established outcomes, encourages participation by all learners, and refrains from providing answers, lectures, or direct contributions to the discussion.
- At the end of the seminar, the educator assists learners with summarizing the discussion outcomes and their implications for practice.

Laboratory Teaching Methods

In nursing, the term *laboratory* can be interpreted broadly to include all forms and settings for clinical experiences or more narrowly to imply a setting for learning that is wholly or partly a mock-up of the clinical setting. For the present discussion, a laboratory refers to a facility or process designed to provide learners with near real or simulated clinical experiences using the knowledge, equipment, materials, procedures, skills, or situations found in the actual clinical practice setting.

Laboratory learning experiences may be provided in locations far removed from the actual patient care area (e.g., in a skills lab in another building), in a nearby classroom, or in an unoccupied patient room on the clinical unit. The specific location of the laboratory is not important; what makes the setting a learning laboratory is the similarity the learning experience provides to the reality of the patient care area.

The purpose of the laboratory is to offer learners an opportunity for direct and supervised experiences in applying theory for problem-solving related to patient care; for developing, testing, and applying previously learned principles; and for hands-on practice of clinical skills. In the laboratory, learners are given an opportunity to confront and manage many of the realities they can expect to encounter in the normal course of daily nursing practice.

In contrast to the classroom setting which emphasizes instructional outcomes largely confined to the cognitive domain, the laboratory setting is used primarily for learning outcomes within the psychomotor and affective domains. In many instances, however, laboratory learning experiences also incorporate and/or reinforce cognitive areas of instruction.

The laboratory is intended to serve as a bridge between the knowledge acquired in the classroom and the refined application of that knowledge at the patient's bedside. Laboratory teaching methods comprise various means for simulating psychomotor, problem-solving, affective, and interpersonal skills and for interacting with the people, equipment, events, and experiences that exist in actual clinical situations.

Like classroom teaching methods, laboratory teaching methods bring together theoretical content and scientific principles that underlie clinical practice but provide these at a location removed from the actual patient care area. Thus laboratory teaching strategies are closer representations of reality than classroom teaching methods but are less realistic than real nursing practice.

In their intermediary position between the classroom and clinical unit, laboratory teaching methods offer a number of advantages over teaching in the clinical setting[62]:

- The laboratory setting provides learning experiences in a more controlled, consistent, and structured environment than that found in real patient care areas. This enables the provision of scheduled and specific learning experiences without the distractions, obstacles, and shifting circumstances so often present on the clinical unit.
- Laboratory learning can be provided with no hazard to patients, families, other staff, or learners themselves. Learners are then free to make mistakes or to make errors in judgment or execution without harmful consequences to themselves or others.
- It is easier for the educator to supervise and guide learning when learners are all in the same geographical area rather than dispersed throughout one or more patient care areas.
- More consistent learning experiences can be afforded to all learners when these activities can be structured and scheduled. The laboratory setting enables the provision of a comparable quality, quantity, breadth, and scope of instruction for all learners at whatever time is optimal for these learning activities. Structured learning can provide the types and variety of learning experiences necessary for the program.
- Rather than having a large group of learners all vying for similar types of patient assignments, laboratory learning experiences can be scheduled in a staggered manner to avoid congestion and competition for patients.
- The amount of time available for learning in the clinical area may be limited during an educational program. Rather than missing out on certain learning experiences, laboratory activities can be used to

supplement and complement classroom and clinical learning.

- The laboratory setting affords learners the opportunity to acquire, practice, and refine skills at their own pace and, usually, as often as they like.
- Learners can make mistakes without embarrassment, anxiety, or feelings of inadequacy or failure. Removal of these potentially negative episodes can make learning a more positive and satisfying experience for learners.
- Many of the formats for laboratory learning foster learner accountability and self-reliance since learners are able to determine when they will partake of laboratory experiences, how much practice they need, and when they will be evaluated.
- Learners who have an opportunity to acquire and develop some beginning proficiency in a laboratory learning experience may then be more skillful, self-confident, and poised in their clinical practice.

Laboratory experiences can serve as an adjunct to either classroom or clinical learning experiences. As in other learning settings, the instructor functions as a facilitator of learning. But in the laboratory setting, the learner's direct involvement in the learning process is notably and measurably increased. Depending on the nature of the learning format selected, direct instructor involvement in teaching may be moderate (such as demonstrating procedures), minimal (giving feedback on a learner's return demonstration), or absent (allowing learners to discover and correct their own mistakes).

When the laboratory is used as a learning setting, the following guidelines may be helpful:

- Insofar as possible, schedule laboratory experiences at times when they will best complement classroom and clinical learning experiences. This will assist in integration of learning.
- Be just as rigorous in defining learning outcomes for a laboratory session as in defining them for classroom instruction.
- Prepare learners by clearly stating the learning outcomes, the tasks or activities to be accomplished, and the criteria for successful performance. When appropriate and necessary, provide detailed instructions to learners on how to complete the required activities.
- Decide how laboratory experiences will be managed:
  What degree of direction will be provided to learners
  The extent to which learners will be allowed to make mistakes and find their own way through the learning activity
  When and how the educator will intervene in guiding learning
  How each laboratory learning experience will be integrated with classroom and clinical learning experiences

How the educator will facilitate transfer of learning from the laboratory to the clinical setting
Who will evaluate learner performance in the laboratory (self-, peer, or instructor evaluation)
What instrument (e.g., a performance checklist) will be used to evaluate learner performance in the laboratory

A variety of teaching methods may be used in the laboratory setting. These include three major categories: demonstration, learning laboratory, and simulation. Simulations may consist of physical simulations (models); simulated patients, simulation games, or role playing. The section that follows describes each of these laboratory teaching methods in the same manner as that used to describe the classroom teaching methods.

Demonstration

Demonstration is an enactment of a procedure or skill that exemplifies how it is to be performed. Although demonstrations are most often provided live, they may also be provided through instructional media such as a videotape program. Demonstration is most often used to teach technical psychomotor skills (e.g., how to perform endotracheal suctioning) but may also be used to teach procedural skills (such as how to admit a patient to the unit), or to teach affective or interpersonal skills (such as how to provide psychosocial support to a trauma victim's family or how to reconcile two conflicting physician orders). Live demonstration affords a multisensory method of instruction by simultaneously employing visual, auditory, tactile, and sometimes olfactory sensory paths: learners see how to do something; hear explanations of underlying facts, principles, and rationale; and obtain hands-on experience in using the materials normally used to perform the task.

There are four phases to a demonstration: the preparation phase, the instructive demonstration phase, the return demonstration, and the review phase. During the preparation phase, the educator assembles all necessary supplies and equipment, verifies that equipment is in working order, readies the room or patient care area, and prepares learners for the activity. Preparation of learners includes ensuring that they have the knowledge base necessary for understanding what will be demonstrated, why it is important, the underlying principles or theory involved, and the key points to observe. In the instructive demonstration phase, someone with expertise in the area to be demonstrated (e.g., the educator, a preceptor, clinical nurse specialist, or nurse manager) performs the procedure in a smooth, skilled, and successful manner.[31] Immediately following the demonstration, learners are afforded an opportunity to practice each aspect of the procedure, to manipulate and gain dexterity with the equipment and supplies, to obtain guidance and feedback on their performance from the instructor, and to begin developing some proficiency in the skill. During the review phase, the educator answers questions, clarifies any remaining areas of confusion, reiterates the purpose and steps in the procedure, and highlights major points of importance.

Oermann[98] offers a number of important considerations for using demonstration/return demonstration to teach psychomotor skills:

- Psychomotor skill development progresses from an inceptual phase when learners view the procedure and begins to develop a mental image of how it is performed through later stages when they practice the skill until their performance matches the mental image.
- Learning psychomotor skills requires that learners be given the opportunity to try out the skill repeatedly in order to refine their movements and achieve a smooth and coordinated performance.
- Learners who have a chance to perform parts of a skill and to manipulate related equipment may require less time to learn a new procedure.
- In acquiring a psychomotor skill, learners focus on the motor movements of the skill itself. Discussion of underlying principles, the rationale for how a skill is performed, and other cognitive aspects related to the skill should take place **before** the nurse practices the skill. Interjection of cognitive aspects during skill practice (e.g., asking the learner "what scientific principle was used in the step you just performed?") interfere with the learner's concentration on the motor aspects of performance.
- Supervision is necessary during the learner's beginning attempts at return demonstration because the accuracy and speed with which the learner performs the procedure can vary significantly from the desired performance. The learner needs time and practice to master the individual components of the motor activity and the correct sequence used to complete it. At this stage, the instructor should limit verbal feedback to the skill itself by offering verbal cues to guide the learner's performance, correcting errors in performance, and providing positive reinforcement.
- Subsequent practice sessions to refine motions and enhance speed and precision may be undertaken independently by the learner.
- Although the psychomotor aspects of the procedure will ultimately need to be integrated with its cognitive and affective components, clinical skill acquisition requires a segment of instruction that allows the learner to focus on developing smooth, coordinated, and precise movements that comprise the individual motor components of the skill.

A study by Gomez and Gomez[56] makes some useful distinctions between when psychomotor skills should be taught in a laboratory setting and when they should be taught in the patient care setting. Clinical skills that will be performed under environmental conditions that are sta-

ble and unchanging (called "closed skills") can be effectively taught in a laboratory setting. Examples of closed skills might include setting up a chest drainage system or documenting a patient's chart. Skills to be performed under environmental conditions that are unstable, changing, varied, and dynamic (called "open skills") are most effectively taught in the clinical setting where all of these environmental variables are confronted and dealt with by the nurse. The authors relate that most skills in nursing are open rather than closed skills. Examples of open skills are changing dressings, administering medications, or starting an intravenous line. Because of the limitations and variables, however, inherent in using the clinical setting as an instructional site, the laboratory setting can still be viewed as an intermediary site where the fundamentals and initial development of learners in procedures, skills, and use of equipment can be introduced. Beginning proficiency can be acquired in a stable environment before moving learners in a graduated fashion to the clinical setting where these skills are perfected and adapted to the realities that Gomez and Gomez mention.

APPROPRIATENESS FOR TEACHING   The demonstration method is appropriate for teaching how to perform procedures, operate and use biomedical equipment and supplies, carry out the sequential steps of a plan, apply principles and theories, and execute interpersonal and affective processes.

LIMITATIONS   Some limitations of demonstration as a teaching method include the following:

- The individual who provides the demonstration may overwhelm or intimidate learners.
- The size of the audience for a live demonstration is limited to the number of learners who can readily see and hear the demonstration. For some procedures and skills, this may be a very small group, adding to the time and costs involved.
- Videotaped demonstrations deprive learners of the opportunity to ask questions or to obtain clarifications regarding the procedure.
- The time available for demonstration and practice may be inadequate for learners to gain necessary facility and proficiency.
- The demonstration may proceed too rapidly for learners to follow and integrate.
- The actual equipment used in the clinical area may not be available for demonstration or practice of the skill.
- The actual performance of the skill in the clinical setting may require learners to modify and adapt what they learned in the laboratory setting.

GUIDELINES FOR USE   Guidelines for using this teaching method can be subdivided into the four phases of a demonstration:

- *Preparation phase.* Before the demonstration, the educator needs to do the following:
    Identify the instructional outcomes and related content to be covered
    Enumerate the key points, terms, and principles emphasized in the demonstration
    Assemble and pretest all equipment and materials to be used for the demonstration
    Mentally and physically rehearse all steps in the procedure
    Organize the sequence of steps so that all unnecessary details and steps are deleted
    Select a location where learners can readily hear and see the demonstration
    Create environmental conditions and use supplies and equipment that approximate as closely as possible those that the learner will encounter in the clinical setting
    Review the nature, purpose, and objectives for viewing the demonstration with an emphasis on key points and principles involved
    If possible, have learners prepare for a live demonstration by reading about the procedure and/or viewing taped demonstrations so they can begin forming a mental image of the skill(s)
- *Instructive demonstration.* During the actual demonstration, the educator needs to:
    Perform the demonstration in a smooth, organized, and sequential manner
    Proceed through the sequence of activities slowly enough for learners to grasp pertinent behaviors, quickly enough to sustain learners' attention, and frequently enough for learners to understand and integrate each step with the preceding and following steps
    Identify and describe the function of any equipment or materials that may be unfamiliar to learners
    Clearly specify all steps in the procedure, process, or skill
    Avoid references regarding what **not** to do
    Repeat the demonstration a number of times (entire or selected segments) for complex or lengthy procedures
- *Return demonstration.* Immediately following the demonstration, the educator needs to:
    Offer each learner an opportunity to practice the skill
    Provide adequate time, role models, and materials for learners to perform the required operations to attain beginning proficiency and meet the established outcomes
    Offer guidance, support, and feedback in a positive and constructive manner
- *Review.* At the close of the demonstration session, the educator needs to do the following:

Solicit questions and provide clarifications as necessary
Reiterate the purpose, procedure, and major points of emphasis
Where appropriate, clarify how incorrect performance of the procedure might adversely affect the patient
Allow learners an opportunity to evaluate the demonstration session either verbally or in writing.

Learning Laboratory

A learning laboratory (also known as a skills lab, clinical skills lab, competency lab) is a temporary or permanent instructional facility that offers learners hand-on experiences with one or more aspects of clinical practice. Learning labs are most commonly used to provide instruction in a wide variety of clinical procedures and skills but can also be used to teach principles related to physiology, pathophysiology, or pharmacology as well as the mechanism of action for various treatments and therapies.

Learning labs may be designed for self-directed or teacher-directed instruction. If the laboratory experience is designed for self-instruction, the educator will arrange and prepare all necessary learning resources and provide directions on how to use the lab so that learners can then proceed in a self-paced manner. If the laboratory activities will be led by an instructor, the educator will likely both organize and pace the activities. Some learning laboratories combine these two designs: the instructional resources are set up by the educator, who then returns to the laboratory at frequent intervals or whenever a learner requests assistance (by pager, beeper, or some other system).

The various components of a learning laboratory will depend on the specific purpose for the lab, but a few components will be necessary for virtually all labs:

- Some means (verbal or written) for introducing the laboratory experience to learners
- A list of the learning outcomes to be achieved
- A description of how the laboratory is organized (provided by posters, numbered skills stations, written directions, and the like)
- A means (verbal, written material, audiovisual programs) of providing instruction
- Some means for evaluating whether the instructional outcomes have been achieved (self-assessment, peer-assessment, written or performance assessments).

Learning laboratories enjoy widespread use in nursing staff development. Some of the advantages of this popular teaching method are[42,62,80]:

- *Realism.* Provides hands-on experience that affords active learner participation in performing essential clinical procedures and skills
- *Safety.* Provides experiential learning in a structured, protected, and virtually risk-free environment

- *Versatility.* Can be adapted to a wide range of clinical performance areas, including technical and clinical skills, operation of biomedical equipment, use of actual hospital supplies, and application of principles and knowledge that underlie clinical practice
- *Multisensory experience.* Enhances learning by affording visual, kinesthetic, auditory, and olfactory avenues of instruction
- *Self-paced learning.* Learners can determine when instruction occurs, what segments of the lab they need (or do not need) to use, how much and how often they will practice, and when they are ready to be evaluated
- *Relaxed style.* Affords a less anxiety-provoking means of learning clinical skills
- *Accessibility.* Can be made available 24 hours a day so that nursing staff on all shifts may participate
- *Self-directed approach.* Provides a means for staff to determine and meet their own learning needs in relation to specific areas, thereby fostering professional accountability
- *Efficiency.* Rather than instructors having to repeat instruction multiple times to reach all staff, labs can be set up and left in place over a period of days so that staff can use them whenever it is most convenient to do so
- *Cost-effectiveness.* Rather than the slow and expensive method of one-on-one teaching of clinical skills, laboratories enable a single educator to extend instruction to larger numbers of staff over a relatively brief period of time
- *Modularity.* Even very complex content and skills can be subdivided into small related units of instruction that can be more readily learned and practiced before needing to be fully integrated. These modules may then be learned separately at numbered stations or at designated areas in the laboratory.
- *Variety.* The unique features of each learning laboratory add some necessary variation to the teaching methods used in staff development programs.

APPROPRIATENESS FOR TEACHING   Learning laboratories may be used purely for instruction, for both instruction and evaluation, or purely for evaluation. As mentioned earlier, these labs can be designed to offer instruction in both cognitive and psychomotor areas but are more commonly used for the latter. They are most appropriately employed to supplement and complement (rather than to replace) other forms of instruction. For instruction in nursing practice areas, laboratories typically are employed for initial development and beginning proficiency in clinical skills and as a prelude to performing these skills in the clinical setting. They may be used for both new graduates as well as for experienced nurses.

Examples might include learning laboratories on various forms of monitoring (serum glucose, hemodynamic, cardiac, intracranial pressure), use of specialized pieces of equipment (intravenous infusion devices, ventilators, hy-

pothermia units, chest drainage systems), performance of procedures (insertion of a nasogastric tube, peritoneal and hemodialysis, endotracheal intubation, cardiac output determinations, chest physiotherapy), and the like.

Learning laboratories may also be used for evaluation of orientation, in-service, and continuing education programs. In addition, they may be one means by which the institution determines the clinical competence of nursing staff as part of their quality monitoring and accreditation programs.

LIMITATIONS   Some of the limitations inherent in learning laboratories include the following:

- *Availability of specialized equipment.* If certain pieces of equipment such as monitors or ventilators are not available in excess of patient needs, the lab may need to be disassembled to return equipment to the clinical area when needed for patient care
- *Portability and setup of biomedical equipment.* Some equipment (such as circoelectric beds or orthopedic traction is large, cumbersome, time-consuming to setup, and cannot readily be moved from patient care areas without potentially damaging it or making it inaccessible for immediate patient use. This generally requires that the lab be conducted in an empty patient room rather than moved to a distant classroom. Patient care demands might then dictate the need to disassemble, move, and reassemble the lab or to cancel it until the facilities and equipment are again available for an extended period.
- *Cost.* If materials or equipment need to be purchased to set up the laboratory in a realistic manner, the initial financial outlay can be considerable; if materials and supplies require frequent replacement, the annual cost can be high.
- *Time.* The initial design and preparation of resources for a learning laboratory can represent a significant investment of time for the educator. Although this investment is typically repaid afterward, the initial development time can be lengthy.
- *Lack of an instructor when needed.* If the lab is designed for self-study, learners may have no one to turn to if they need assistance. Although the educator may be summoned by beeper or page, the educator may not be able to leave the present location to come to the learner's assistance. Some learners may be frustrated by this situation and leave the laboratory. Others may hesitate to contact the educator if they believe that they should be able to complete the lab on their own.[42]

GUIDELINES FOR USE   Effective use of a learning laboratory requires two distinct phases: preparation and operation. During the *preparation* or design phase, the educator will need to accomplish each of the following:

- Determine the content area to be addressed in the laboratory experience. This may be accomplished by means of a needs assessment that identifies areas of practice that are appropriate for this type of learning experience.
- Formulate a list of instructional outcomes to be accomplished during the laboratory experience.
- Use the instructional outcomes to develop an outline of specific subtopics that warrant coverage within that content area. Limit content to that which is clinically relevant and essential for understanding and performing the skill or procedure correctly.
- Group the instructional outcomes (with their related content subtopics) into discrete units of instruction. This step enables the educator to modularize the laboratory into separate workstations or written modules.
- Once the laboratory experience content has been divided into units of instruction, decide the specific teaching devices to be used at each station. Background information might be provided by readings, notebooks containing summaries of important points, handouts, and diagrams. Procedures might be introduced by means of videotapes or a poster or flip chart that depicts each step. Practice and refinement of skills can be taught by using the actual equipment and supplies found in the clinical area with mannequins or other physical models. Evaluation can be provided by means of performance checklists, written tests (for cognitive areas), case studies to solve, or having learners videotape their own performance of the procedure.
- Prepare a set of instructions for introducing the laboratory experience to learners and for guiding them through each stage or station. Instructions need to be clear, brief but thorough, and well organized. If learners can challenge or bypass certain segments of the lab, this should be stated.
- Determine how the laboratory will be arranged to be a maximally effective learning experience. Decide how materials and stations will be displayed within the room, how each station will be set up and supplied, and how learners will progress from one station to another. Hodson[71] suggests that educators take photographs of how each station and the laboratory as a whole should be arranged so that maintenance, restocking, and assembly time are minimized and the consistency and quality of the experience are ensured. Diagrams of the room layout, placement of equipment and supplies, and location of instructional aids can be included with laminated photographs of how the final set up should appear.
- Arrange advertising of laboratory offerings to all pertinent members of the nursing staff. Offerings may be advertised in hospital newsletters, brochures, posters, staff meetings, and by other means. Prospective participants should be told the dates, times, and specific nature of the laboratory offerings.

During the *operation* phase of the learning laboratory, the educator will want to assure that each of the following are provided:

- *Accessibility.* Learners will need to be informed of when the lab will be available and who to contact if the laboratory site is locked or needs restocking, cleaning, or reorganization.
- *Supervision.* The educator needs to verify that learners are using and progressing through the laboratory experiences in the intended manner. This element is particularly important with newly designed laboratory experiences to be sure that learners are using materials appropriately and that the directions provided are clearly understood and followed.
- *Assistance.* An educator should always be immediately available to learners who may need instructional assistance in the lab. This may be accomplished through impromptu visits or by means of a beeper or paging system that can readily locate the educator. Even when a laboratory has been designed for self-instruction and directions are seemingly self-explanatory, it is best if educators avoid planning other activities that would significantly limit their availability to learners using the lab.
- *Support.* One or more educators need to visit the laboratory during hours of use to be certain that all learning resources are readied, that equipment is functioning properly, and to troubleshoot problems that may arise.
- *Evaluation.* Learners should be afforded an opportunity to critique the strengths and weaknesses of the laboratory activities. These evaluations might also include an opportunity to offer suggestions and to note any problems with materials, supplies, equipment, or arrangement of the lab that were encountered.

Simulation

Simulation teaching methods in nursing staff development attempt to replicate some or nearly all of the essential aspects of a clinical situation so that the situation may be more readily understood and managed when it occurs for real in the clinical practice setting. The more closely the processes and conditions of a simulation resemble the reality they are intended to represent, the greater the potential for transfer of learning to that situation.

Although no simulation ever equals confronting the real situation itself, simulations can be extremely useful in affording a controlled environment focused on the attainment of specific learning outcomes. Some of the other advantages of simulations are that they:*

*See references 43, 64, 76, 93, 103, 131.

- Can approximate the reality of a clinical situation more closely than classroom teaching methods
- Simplify reality by focusing only on the aspects intended for learning and by removing extraneous environmental factors that might interfere with learning
- Reduce the time required for learning by compressing into a single learning experience what might have taken days or weeks to obtain in the clinical setting
- May afford learning experiences that otherwise would not be available in the classroom or clinical settings
- Engage learners more directly and actively in the learning process than purely didactic or observational learning experiences
- Provide for novelty and variety in teaching methods
- Afford immediate feedback and reinforcement of learning
- Can be used without incurring the risk of adverse effects (of elements related to safety, comfort, privacy, learner inexperience) on patients
- Provide learners with the opportunity for self-paced learning and practicing of skills in a controlled setting and at times convenient to the learner
- Allow learners time to make mistakes and refine skills in an atmosphere free of danger, anxiety, censure, or embarrassment
- May enable the proficient nurse to attain learning outcomes in less time than by conventional classroom teaching methods
- Offer a means for teaching in the cognitive, affective, and psychomotor domains
- Use learner and instructor time more efficiently than in the clinical setting since an increased educator-to-learner ratio can be used
- Offer hands-on and socially engaging learning experiences for learners whose learning style preferences are in this category
- Provide an alternative learning setting if clinical facilities are crowded with too many students

Simulations are useful instructional devices for material that learners consider dry, for content that learners view as abstract or hard to relate to reality, and for applying theory to realistic practice situations. Simulations are also a preferred means for providing instruction when direct clinical experiences might be difficult or impossible to provide, when they could be dangerous or ethically troublesome, or when extraneous factors cannot be controlled to ensure an optimal learning experience.[55]

A number of different types of simulations can be used in nursing staff development programs. These can be broadly categorized into physical simulations, simulated patients, and simulation games.

PHYSICAL SIMULATIONS   Physical simulations consist of a wide array of devices for acquiring, practicing, and refining various clinical skills. Most nurses first encounter physical simulations when they meet the "Mrs. Chase" patient model in nursing school. Physical simulations include items such as the mannequins (head, upper torso, full body) used in the American Heart Association's Basic and Advanced Cardiac Life Support (BCLS, ACLS) teaching programs; adult, child, and infant intubation mannequins; training models for teaching tracheostomy care or for peripheral and central venipuncture; anatomical models for teaching physical assessment, for inserting various drainage devices such as nasogastric tubes or Foley catheters, or for applying dressings or ostomy drainage devices.

Appropriateness for Teaching   Physical simulations provide life-like, life-sized models for hands-on experiences in acquiring and mastering selected clinical skills. They are particularly appropriate for learning skills that require dexterity and coordination of complex refined motor movements. Learners are able to simultaneously see, feel, and manipulate materials and structures that closely resemble those they will encounter in the actual clinical setting. Their primary instructional value lies in the "hands-on" experiences they afford learners, particularly in the early stages of developing psychomotor skills. They can be use as a preliminary form of graduated instruction before learners are expected to demonstrate the procedures in the clinical setting.

Limitations   The major constraint of any physical simulation is the degree to which it may not closely approximate reality. Thus, if a mannequin or other model does not look, feel, or respond the way a typical patient would, its usefulness as an instructional device is diminished. If the model makes the customary procedure or skill too easy or too hard (compared to its usual degree of difficulty), the learning experience it affords will not be realistic.

Other limitations relate to the cost of simulation devices, their maintenance, and durability. Some devices, particularly those with computerized components, are very expensive. Others require a considerable amount of time and effort to maintain in working order, to keep clean, or to store properly. Others may require expensive repair or replacement at frequent intervals, increasing their "down time" and decreasing their availability to learners.

Guidelines for Use   Some guidelines for using physical simulations include the following:

- Be thoroughly familiar with each device used, its value and limitations, its idiosyncrasies and variations from real life
- Read and follow the manufacturer's instructions regarding maintenance, cleaning, disinfection, storage, and making minor repairs on the device
- Before using the model for instruction, be sure that learners understand the purpose of the learning experience, the instructional outcomes to be achieved,

how the model assists in achieving these outcomes, and how to properly use the model

- After learners have had an opportunity to observe how to use the device, describe the model's idiosyncrasies and variations from real life

SIMULATED PATIENTS As their name implies, simulated patients are individuals who pose as real-life patients. These individuals may be peers, other staff, or the educator. Simulated patients are assigned predetermined sets of symptoms, problems, personalities, histories (health, family, social), or illnesses for nurse learners to elicit, assess, and/or manage as they would in an actual patient care situation. Unlike physical simulations, these "patients" are real human beings rather than inanimate objects imbued with lifelike features.

Appropriateness for Teaching Simulated patients are used most often in teaching nursing assessment skills. They can be employed for teaching nurses how to obtain a health history or a history of the patient's present health problem(s), how to perform physical assessment techniques, how to arrive at pertinent nursing diagnoses and use these assessment findings to plan nursing care. Simulated patients can also be used to learn and practice a variety of noninvasive procedures such as how to record a 12-lead ECG, how to apply various types of dressings, or how to administer chest physiotherapy.[43]

Limitations The major limitation in using simulated patients for patient assessment is that these are usually healthy individuals. As a result, instructional experiences related to assessment will focus primarily on learning normal findings and normal variants rather than on detecting abnormal or pathologic findings. Limitations may also arise if the educator has failed to define the "patient" situation fully or if the "patient" enacts behaviors or responses that are different from those assigned or are inconsistent with those a typical patient would exhibit.

Guidelines for Use The guidelines for using simulated patients can be divided between those for the educator and those for the "patient":

- The instructor is responsible for deciding all necessary features of each "patient" and for communicating these to the prospective patient in a clear and concise manner. Guidelines need to include how the patient is to respond to certain questions or situations, what symptoms to demonstrate, what history to relate, and the like. The guidelines issued for demonstrating procedures might only include the suggestions to act naturally and react as they normally would to the situation.
- The individuals portraying "patients" must be sure that they understand their assignment before the in-

structional segment begins. In addition, they must be willing to be poked, probed, percussed, palpated, auscultated, and otherwise acted on as dictated by the learning outcomes. Persons selected to serve as patients need to offer natural, plausible, and spontaneous responses to learners.

SIMULATION GAMES Simulation games combine the usefulness of a simulated learning experience with the enjoyment of a game format. The simulation affords a safe, meaningful, and relatively controlled interaction among learners, while the game format fosters interest and motivation by providing a novel and fun way to learn.

Simulation games involve interactive activities among participants whose actions are governed and restricted by specified roles, contexts, constraints, rules, methods for differentiating winners from losers, and arbitrary, predetermined criteria for determining the end or winning of the game. Chance factors that relate to real-life unpredictable variables may be incorporated in games (by rolls of the dice, spins of a wheel, or game cards) to approximate their occurrence in reality. Taken collectively, the game elements comprise salient aspects of a situation that learners need to experience to heighten their understanding of some phenomenon. The more closely game elements resemble the reality they are intended to represent, the greater their validity and usefulness in transfer of learning to the clinical setting.

Games can be as simple in design as a scavenger hunt or a game of charades. A game may provide participants with an opportunity to lie in a bed with the monitoring and access lines usually imposed on their patients to see how they cope. More commonly, games are structured by having participants complete puzzles, card games, word games, or more sophisticated board games. Others are patterned after popular television game shows such as *Jeopardy,*[60,118,136] popular card games such as *Trivial Pursuit,*[44,65] or board games such as *Life*[117] or *Monopoly.*[120] Compilations that describe simulation games in the fields of education and training exist[58,72,121,137] as a resource for the nurse educator. In addition, Duke[34] has initiated development of a taxonomy of games and simulations to assist nurse educators in locating materials to match their learning objectives.

Because games typically require active learner participation and interaction and offer learners immediate feedback on their performance, they can afford learning experiences that are consistent with adult learning principles. Simulation games can be as effective and more enjoyable than more traditional methods of instruction in learners' acquisition of some cognitive and affective behaviors.

Appropriateness for Teaching Simulation games are generally used to supplement rather than to replace more traditional types of learning experiences. They can be used for teaching in all three domains of learning but are most often employed for cognitive and affective areas. Simulations can afford repetition, reinforcement, application to practice, and a multisensory mode of learning.[136] They may be used to introduce new content; to convey factual material in a more interesting way; to motivate learner interest in attending "mandatory" educational programs; to review or apply classroom learning; to predict clinical behaviors or evaluate learner knowledge or skills following classroom instruction; or to provide novelty and variety in teaching methods. Games are often used to teach highly abstract, intangible, or novel areas of learning. Intangible instructional outcomes include areas such as decision-making, interpersonal skills, work organization, communication, consciousness raising, or conflict resolution. Simulated patient management problems permit learners to make patient care or nursing management decisions and then experience the consequences of those decisions.[25,43]

Some criteria for determining if a game is a suitable instructional method are listed in Box 4.1.

Limitations   Some limitations inherent in simulation games include the following[60,114]:

- Although they may afford variety and enjoyment, games are not always the most effective method of instruction. Before using a game as a teaching device, the instructor needs to ensure that the purpose of the game is consistent with the instructional purpose and that the intended amount and nature of learning can, in fact, be achieved.
- Games may not be the most efficient vehicles for learning. Some games are very time consuming. The amount of time allocated to games needs to be carefully considered so that the game's entertainment value and its competitive elements do not outweigh its instructional value.
- Games will differ in the number of learners they allow or require. The number of players who simultaneously participate in the game may restrict its usefulness.

- When games require more than one player, there may be no mechanism for evaluating the performance of any single learner.
- Commercially available or already published games may not be suitable for a particular institution's needs. Many of these are not amenable to local tailoring or modification. Others may be too costly for purchase.
- If no game is available for meeting the instructional outcomes, the agency may need to design its own game. Nurse educators have described this process for various types of games.[60,118] Designing sophisticated simulation games can be time consuming and require expertise the educator may lack.
- Not all learners will enjoy using games or be able to readily relate their experiences to real-life situations.

Guidelines for Use   Some guidelines for using simulation games follow[76]:

- Before using a simulation game with learners, read the instructor's manual carefully. Determine your role during the exercise, identify any materials that will need to be prepared, and find out if any special equipment or seating arrangements will be needed. Determine whether any game materials will need replacement after each use.
- Pilot test the game with a group comparable to the intended audience before using it with learners. During the pilot test, practice how best to introduce the learning experience and see which rules tend to be most often violated. Decide what you will watch for, guard against, or admonish learners about. Tryout the game player's role to experience first hand the character, process, and various facets of the game. Try to identify potential pitfalls, problems, and learner responses so that these can be dealt with more effectively when the game is used with learners.
- Prepare learners to use the game by communicating

Box 4.1

CRITERIA FOR DETERMINING SUITABILITY OF THE GAME FORMAT

- The purpose and objectives of the game coincide with the purpose and objectives of instruction
- The physical facilities required by the game are available
- The required or optimal number of game players will be available
- The time required to complete the game coincides with the time available for instruction
- Resources exist to purchase, try out, and adapt a purchased game or design a locally prepared game
- Resources exist to supply replacement materials that the game requires
- The game requires only a limited amount of time for preparation and cleanup

From Gruending DL, Fenty D, Hogan T: Fun and games in nursing staff development, *J Cont Educ Nurs* 22:259, 1991, and Lewis DJ, Saydak SJ, Mierzwa IP et al: Gaming: a teaching strategy for adult learners, *J Cont Educ Nurs* 20:80, 1989.

the object of the game, its rules, roles, and sequence. Ensure that learners know how to start, proceed, and end the game. Keep the introduction as brief as possible. Check the instructor's manual to determine whether the instructional purpose of the game should be shared with learners in advance. For some games, divulging the instructional purpose undermines the effectiveness of the game.

- During the course of the game, listen to and observe learners' interactions and enforce game rules but avoid coaching, interceding directly, or giving feedback on learner behaviors. Keep the game going but limit your role to observing reactions and behaviors that will be considered after the game has ended.

- At the end of the game, allow sufficient time for a thorough debriefing. Allow learners time to reflect on their experiences. Then assist learners in sharing their feelings and impressions of the activity and its realism. Help learners to summarize the principles, concepts, and key points learned from the game. Help learners to extract the outcomes of their game experience and draw conclusions and implications for clinical practice. Be certain that the moral or lesson(s) derived from the game remain the focus of discussion rather than the details of the game itself.

Role Playing

Role playing is the spontaneous enactment of a true-to-life situation that involves human interaction. Use of this teaching technique typically involves identification of the purpose for the role play, assignment of specific roles to two or more participants, followed by a brief description of the situation to be portrayed. Role players then act and interact according to their assignments as if they were the actual persons in that situation. Once all relevant behaviors have been demonstrated, the play is terminated and the entire group reviews the events and their implications.

Unlike a drama, role playing has no written script; rather, the script or proceedings develop spontaneously by the actors. The actors in the play may be volunteers from the group of learners or, in some circumstances, may be the instructor. Although participants in the role playing are briefed regarding general attributes of their assigned role, their dialogue and behaviors proceed extemporaneously, based on their perceptions of how the person they are portraying would react and behave in that situation.

Role playing may focus on process skills from the past (problems nurses have encountered in communicating with physicians), on the present (how nursing staff approach families for organ donation), or the future (how one might tell the family that a patient had a terminal illness). The topic or issue selected for role playing may be selected by the educator, by the learners, by a consensus of both groups, or just spontaneously. Topics may also emerge spontaneously from other discussions. For example, a discussion regarding discharge planning might precipitate

role playing on resolving conflicting physician orders. When possible, learners may be asked to design their own role plays. This may help to make this technique more realistic, more clinically relevant, and more credible to learners.[87]

Role playing can be spontaneous or planned but is usually informal and untheatrical. Some educators refer to role playing as *reality practice,* a term that more directly suggests the focus on reality rather than play.[87]

Role playing affords learners an opportunity to put themselves in another's shoes, to view and respond to a situation through another's eyes and feelings. It is an instructional process that enables learners to participate in another's life experiences, to empathize and/or better understand the individual's situation, to reflect on their own opinions and feelings, and to generate confidence in managing specific types of difficult situations. When learners project themselves wholeheartedly into their roles, role playing can become rather intense. Acting out situations in this manner, however, is a form of protected projection because learners can "hide" behind the roles depicted while simultaneously evidencing the emotions and reactions they genuinely feel.[125]

APPROPRIATENESS FOR TEACHING   The purpose of role playing is to teach process skills or to develop attitudes rather than to convey factual content. Many of these skills involve management and interpersonal relations and include elements in the affective domain of learning. The primary value of this teaching technique is its ability to teach "soft skills" such as effective listening, communication, interviewing, and supporting patients and families. Role playing may be used to assist in teaching nurses how to elicit a patient's health history, to negotiate patient assignments or work schedules, to resolve conflicts, provide patient education, or counsel families of a terminally ill patient. It is most effective when dealing with topics and issues that involve values, emotions, controversy, and problem-solving.[125]

Role playing is a particularly useful device when learners need to try out new behaviors, to practice behaviors in order to make them habitual, to experience difficult situations from the viewpoints of others, and to test theories and suggested techniques in a realistic but safe environment.[87] It is also helpful for allowing learners to practice interpersonal skills where they need not be concerned about feeling awkward, uncertain, incompetent, flustered, or embarrassed over how they handle a given predicament.[54] Other uses for role playing include values clarification and developing sensitivity and empathy.

LIMITATIONS   One of the more common limitations of role playing is the adult learners' reluctance to use this teaching method. Some learners have had past negative experiences with this teaching technique and others may dislike any instructional method that forces them to perform in front of a group. In some instances, the educator may not be well versed in using the technique or in effectively managing its progress or conclusion. The discomfort may then be contagious with learners and result in an unsatisfactory learning experience for all.[123]

Some educators suggest that reticence to perform in front of a group can be overcome by assigning roles to everyone in the group and having them work in pairs rather than selecting just a few participants to perform at the front of the room. Use of role-playing pairs avoids the intimidating effects of spotlighting a small group of learners and also involves everyone more actively in the learning activity.[87]

GUIDELINES FOR USE   Some guidelines for the effective use of role playing include the following:

- Limit the topic for the role playing to some manageable component of a skill. Avoid attempts to teach the entire skill all at once.[54] For example, in teaching problem-solving skills, the educator might first have a role play that focuses on identification of the nature of the problem.
- Communicate the purpose of the session clearly to learners.
- Define the situational context for the role play clearly and succinctly. Keep the introduction simple and short.
- Cast the roles to optimize learning potential in the experience. Avoid casting extraneous roles and make sure that roles are distinct. The roles selected need to offer elements of conflict, ambiguity, or uncertainty that learners use to demonstrate the process skills intended.[87]
- Minimize learner discomfort and anxiety by establishing the scene and providing actors with a brief yet clear description of major role attributes they should exhibit. For example, "You are an acute MI patient who denies your diagnosis and demands to be discharged after 3 days in the CCU." Encourage players to act as they think that person would.
- Give players time to prepare themselves for their role.
- Limit the selection of role players to those who are willing to participate. Learners who feel uncomfortable or threatened will not likely be able to successfully become emotionally involved in their role to enact it effectively or credibly.
- Give specific written checkpoints to learners who are observing the role play. These observer sheets help to focus learners' attention on important aspects of the activity and assist in verifying that the instructional outcomes are attained. The observation sheet might include points to look for or questions they should be ready to answer during the discussion.[87]
- Guide learners so that they remain within their assigned roles.
- Monitor the interactions among participants for notable events and issues that should be highlighted later in the discussion period.
- Limit the enactment period to the time required to attain the objectives, usually not more than 10 to 15 minutes. The outcomes of a role play may consist of the solution to a problem, empathy for the individuals involved, or sensitivity to contrasting viewpoints on an issue. Within the available time frame, one or more of these outcomes or insights should have been attained. Whenever possible, allow the role play to conclude naturally.
- Use the discussion period following the role play to accomplish the following:
    Analyze what occurred (verbally and behaviorally), why and how it occurred, and the outcomes that resulted from these interactions
    Critique the players' actions rather than their acting.[123] Refer to players by their role name (rather than their real name) so that players will not feel that they are being evaluated
    Allow players to describe how they felt as they portrayed their assigned role
    Reinforce examples of effective ways to manage situations[123]
    Summarize and generalize the insights gained and their implications for nursing practice
    Elicit suggestions on how the role play could be improved
- When possible, allow learners to repeat the role play to practice and refine their skills. Reversing roles or selecting other players may be helpful.

Clinical Teaching Methods

Because nursing is a clinical practice discipline, the patient care setting represents the ultimate and most important location for teaching nursing practice. Indeed, all of the teaching methods discussed in this chapter are effective only to the extent that they eventually become evident in nurses' clinical practice. Knowledge of facts, concepts, principles, processes and skills without the attendant capability for applying these is, in a very pragmatic sense, of little value until this end is achieved.

Distinguishing Characteristics of the Clinical Setting

Unlike the classroom teaching setting, the clinical setting offers a less controllable, dependable, consistent, or structured learning environment. It is frequently less than the "ideal" that can be so readily presented in the classroom. Contrary to the secure and stable confines of the classroom, the clinical setting can be an anxiety provoking and volatile environment for learners.

The clinical setting is markedly less tolerant of mistakes, omissions, or errors in judgment than the laboratory setting. Clinical experiences may spotlight a learner's inadequacies and expose potential challenges that never surfaced without warning in the learning lab: bleeding patients, irate physicians, patients and families who do not speak English, itinerant support services, intimidating colleagues, and abruptly increased patient workloads. What the clinical setting **does** have to offer is the reality of nursing practice.

In some specialty areas of nursing (emergency department, critical care, operating room), the clinical setting is even more variable, frightening, and threatening to newcomers than many other clinical sites. Here, where acuity of illness, the weight and scope of professional responsibility, hectic pace, and limited margin for error are a way of life, the educator may find that it can be virtually impossible to "schedule" learners to encounter the right type of patients with the right nursing care needs at the specific times when learners are in that setting. Shortened hospital stays, combined with the unpredictability of a patient's clinical course, make it difficult to schedule particular types of learning experiences with any degree of confidence that they will actually be available at their scheduled times. As a result, nurse educators would do well to always make clinical teaching plans with the idea that they may need to be modified at the last moment or may need to be forsaken in favor of serendipitous learning opportunities. Fortunately, unforeseen events, emergencies, and unanticipated complications are often the most meaningful occasions for teaching in the clinical setting. In general, instruction in the clinical setting must be timely, flexible, and sensitive to the setting, individuals, patient care priorities, and events transpiring there.

Elements to Consider for Clinical Teaching

Teaching in the clinical setting is directed at assisting the learner to apply appropriate facts, concepts, and principles together with their affective and psychomotor components in providing direct patient care. To attain this end, implementation of clinical instruction needs to consider the following four elements:

- Instructional outcomes appropriate for the clinical area
- Teaching the nursing process in the clinical setting
- How nurses develop clinical expertise
- Intra- and interdepartmental cooperation

INSTRUCTIONAL OUTCOMES APPROPRIATE FOR THE CLINICAL AREA
As the educator reviews the instructional outcomes for the educational program and sorts those appropriate for the classroom and laboratory settings, the remaining outcomes should be those requiring some form of interaction with real patients. Outcomes for the clinical learning setting should refer to learner behaviors, such as applying and interrelating various principles, concepts, theories, and facts; displaying the affective traits important to effective

and compassionate nursing practice in a particular setting; and demonstrating the repertoire of patient care and technical skills requisite for competent nursing practice. Outcomes relevant to the clinical setting will require nurse-patient interactions and the integration of learning with the complexities and variables usually encountered in direct patient care.

TEACHING THE NURSING PROCESS IN THE CLINICAL SETTING
Ultimately, all applications of learning in the clinical setting are included within one of the five phases of the nursing process: assessment, diagnosis, planning, implementation, or evaluation. Putting each of these phases of the nursing process into operation in various clinical environments requires the same fundamental abilities but sometimes to differing degrees. For example, nurses who work in an emergency department or critical care unit need an expansive degree of preparation in the assessment phase of the nursing process and in the intervention phase of managing acute and potentially life-threatening patient problems. Nurses who work in pediatric units need to be particularly skilled in planning and implementing care that involves the entire family unit. Nurses who work in neonatal units must be highly skilled in the evaluation of objective patient parameters that reflect the effectiveness of nursing interventions because their patients are unable to provide subjective indicators for these appraisals. Nurses who work in ambulatory care settings need to be particularly skilled in planning and implementing patient education programs because their patient populations will be returning home immediately after receiving health services. In general, nurses being groomed to function effectively in today's hospitals need additional breadth and scope of instruction in each of the following areas:

I. *Assessment*
   A. A broad range and depth in clinical observation skills
   B. Greater proficiency in using a comprehensive, multisystem approach to patient assessment
   C. Facility in employing biomedical instrumentation as a major source for deriving the many parameters of a clinical database
II. *Diagnosis*
   A. Reaching accurate interpretations of a large, complex, dynamic, and highly interrelated database
   B. Appropriately characterizing patient care needs as nursing diagnoses that can be influenced by nursing practice so that these may be communicated to all members of the healthcare team
III. *Planning*
   A. Precision in summarizing expected patient outcomes to be attained
   B. Close correlation between identified patient care needs and planned nursing interventions

     C. Facility in organizing a complex patient assignment so that it reflects the priorities of care and amount of time available to provide care

     D. Formulating a plan of care that is individualized, succinctly and clearly communicated, and feasible in light of existing organizational constraints

     E. Refined skills in analytic and critical thinking to produce sound clinical judgments and rationales for planned interventions

IV. *Implementation*

     A. Highly skilled execution of a large repertoire of clinical skills and procedures

     B. Adroit capability to improvise, modify, and troubleshoot obstacles that arise in providing patient care

     C. Capability to respond quickly and appropriately in emergency situations

V. *Evaluation*

     A. Expertise in measuring the degree to which interventions have been effective in attaining the expected outcomes of patient care

     B. Skill in identification of modifications needed in a plan of care to improve patient outcomes

     C. Capability to succinctly summarize, appraise, anticipate, and communicate the patient's situation for planning discharge care and ensuring continuity of care

HOW NURSES DEVELOP CLINICAL EXPERTISE Professionals' knowledge about something (knowing *that*) and their knowledge of how to practice their profession (knowing *how*) reflect two different types of expertise. Cognitive psychologists refer to the former as theoretical (or declarative) knowledge and refer to the latter as practical (procedural or skilled) knowledge.[20] Theoretical expertise refers to one's knowledge about things. It includes our knowledge of facts, principles, concepts, theories, rules, and how these interrelate. By acquiring information about these areas and by integrating and understanding relationships among these phenomena, the professional is able to know *that*. Practical expertise, by contrast, refers to one's skill in knowing *how*—that is, how to perform in various situations. Unlike theoretical expertise, which can be developed by transmission of relevant information to a practitioner, procedural or skilled expertise can only be developed by the experience of practicing one's profession. Many aspects of a skilled practitioner's know-how, moreover, cannot be readily reduced into a list of facts and principles that explain how they know what they know.

Over the past decade, Benner[8] has studied the development of expertise in clinical nursing practice. A central thesis of her model is that clinical experience is requisite to the development of clinical expertise. Over time, a nurse develops clinical expertise by repeatedly encountering certain types of patient situations. Based on these experiences, the nurse develops sets of expectations about those situations and compares these expectations to previously believed notions. Through these experiences, nurses gradually refine their understanding and management of various patient situations and quickly recognize when what they encounter in clinical practice does or does not match those experienced-based expectations. At this level of functioning, the expert nurse possesses a rapid and highly astute perceptual grasp of clinical situations based on prior experience with similar situations.

Benner's model points out that clinical experience is not the equivalent of longevity, seniority, or the mere passage of time.[10] Unless nurses reflect on their clinical experiences, compare these encounters to previously held knowledge and beliefs, and modify their expectations and practice accordingly, their clinical encounters will not qualify as experience. As Benner describes this process, "expertise develops when the clinician tests and refines propositions, hypotheses, and principle-based expectations in actual practice situations."[8] Clinical situations that are not examined and compared with previous expectations in this manner do not qualify as experience and will not lead to practical expertise. Only when experience challenges, refines, or disconfirms previously held notions and expectations does it lead to the practical know-how of an expert practitioner.

Clinical expertise takes a combination of experience and time to develop. Benner's work adapts the Dreyfus model of skill acquisition[8] to describe how practical knowledge and experience develop over time. The Dreyfus model asserts that practitioners progress through five levels of proficiency in developing practice skills. These levels include:

- Novice
- Advanced beginner
- Competent
- Proficient
- Expert

These levels reflect changes that practitioners make in three general areas of skilled performance. The first is changing from reliance on abstract principles to the use of past concrete experiences in actual nursing practice as a basis for practice decisions. The second is a change from viewing clinical situations as a compilation of equally relevant bits of information to viewing them more as a complete whole in which only certain parts are relevant. The third is a change from functioning as a detached observer of clinical situations to functioning as an involved participant in that situation.[8]

The section below provides an overview of how Benner's model applies each of the five levels of proficiency to nursing. It includes a description of the attributes of each level as well as their implications for staff development.[8,9,10]

Novice Level

Attributes

- Might be a nursing student or a nurse who has just graduated
- Lacks depth and breadth of experience in patient care situations
- May be overwhelmed by the complexity of clinical situations
- Unable to recognize objective attributes that are relevant in different patient situations
- Unable to distinguish which tasks are most important, which clinical findings are most pertinent, or when an exception to a "rule" is required (unable to use discretionary judgment)

Implications for Staff Development

- Begin by teaching simple rules that apply to all patients on the unit
- Help learners to begin distinguishing clinical parameters that are relevant to the patient population on that unit
- Monitor novices to ensure that they understand which rules to follow and that they do not follow these rules blindly
- Remember that even experienced nurses (e.g., floats, agency nurses, nurses with clinical experience in other types of units) may respond like novices if they are unfamiliar with the patient population and nursing practices on the unit
- The most appropriate preceptor for novices is likely a nurse at the competent level

Advanced Beginner Level

Attributes

- Might be a newly graduated nurse with less than 1 year of nursing experience
- Has sufficient clinical experience to recognize many of the global aspects of clinical situations that are relevant to the patient population on that unit
- Demonstrates marginally acceptable clinical performance
- Functions on the basis of general guidelines and a beginning ability to discern meaningful patterns in clinical situations
- Unable to clearly and consistently distinguish the most important patient data in a given situation

Implications for Staff Development

- Assist these nurses to reflect on their experiences in order to identify aspects and attributes most relevant to nursing practice
- Assist them in formulating their own guidelines of action based on sets of relevant aspects and attributes from different patient care situations
- Monitor advanced beginners to be sure that important

patient needs and problems do not go unattended
- Help these nurses establish priorities of care based on sound clinical rationale
- Most appropriate preceptor would be a nurse at the competent level

Competent Level

Attributes

- Is usually a nurse with 2 to 3 years of clinical experience on that unit or with similar patients
- Views nursing interventions in terms of long-range goals or plans that are deliberately developed; these plans dictate what will represent the salient aspects of each clinical situation
- Able to manage and adapt nursing practice to many of the contingencies encountered

Implications for Staff Development

- Most staff development programs that are aimed at teaching standard procedures and routines are geared to this level of practice
- Competent nurses need practice (through simulations, games) in decision-making for complex clinical situations
- Provide practice in planning and coordinating multiple, complex patient care demands through life-like examples
- Provide opportunities in improving work organization and priority setting for patients with complex needs and problems
- Most appropriate preceptor would be nurses at the proficient or expert levels

Proficient Level

Attributes

- Usually is a nurse with 3 to 5 years of experience
- Perceive patient situations as wholes (rather than as unrelated bits of equally important information)
- Makes clinical decisions based on anticipation of typical events to expect in that situation
- Able to recognize clinical problems quickly and to modify interventions when events and patient data differ from what they expect
- Incorporate subtle nuances of situations (maxims) in decision-making
- Able to recognize patient problems before they are explicitly manifested as changes in vital signs or other measurable, objective parameters

Implications for Staff Development

- In educational programs, these learners will need to be provided with examples that include a clinical context that is realistic and credible; they will be frustrated by attempts to structure learning around rules and principles that the novice uses because the proficient nurse will inevitably be able to identify exceptions based on their experience

- Are best taught inductively, starting with a case study that incorporates levels of complexity and ambiguity similar to real clinical situations
- Solicit and incorporate the proficient nurse's own experiences and examples for determining the optimum way to manage particular patient situations
- Ask these nurses to cite cases when their interventions were successful in resolving patient problems and cases where their interventions were not successful; such reflections help to distinguish effective nursing practice
- Assist these nurses to identify situations that confused them, when their past experiences could not be drawn on to help manage the situation; discussion of these incidents with other proficient nurses may afford useful insights to use in the future
- Most appropriate preceptor would be a nurse at the expert level

Expert Level
Attributes
- Usually are nurses with over 5 years of experience in working with similar patients
- Able to intuitively grasp each clinical situation and immediately zero in on the salient aspects that warrant attention; no longer need to rely on analytic principles (rules, procedures, guidelines) to understand and manage patient care
- Able to intuitively recognize and resolve patient problems and situations based on the clinical context and similarity/dissimilarity to similar patients

Implications for Staff Development
- Assist these nurses in explicating critical incidents from their clinical practice that illustrate expertise or ineffective management of complex clinical situations
- Assist them in verbalizing the patient cues they responded to and how they knew about the existence of patient problems or complications before these became overtly manifested
- Work with groups of expert nurses to develop consensus regarding their observations and interventions in various patient care situations; help them to record these areas of consensus so that they can be shared with proficient nurses
- Other nurses might systematically observe how expert nurses practice to better identify their attributes
- Encourage expert nurses to collect and record paradigm cases and critical incidents that made a lasting impact in their clinical careers; encourage them to use these cases as illustrations when they teach nurses at other levels of clinical proficiency

INTRA- AND INTERDEPARTMENTAL COOPERATION Because so many categories of healthcare workers participate in the care of hospitalized patients, the educator must be able to work closely and collaboratively with each of these groups during the conduct of clinical educational programs to avoid interference and maintain continuity of patient care. Learning experiences in the clinical setting, therefore, need to be planned in conjunction with daily unit activities and coordinated with the work and priorities of other healthcare professionals.

Some guidelines for scheduling learning activities for the clinical setting include the following:

- Consult with the nurse manager or charge nurse to determine when events such as medical rounds, major procedures, or diagnostic testing are scheduled so that nursing staff development activities may be planned in conjunction with or around these events.
- Consult with the nurse manager or charge nurse to identify when other groups of learners are expected to be on the unit to avoid crowding the clinical area with learners.
- Consult with the nurse manager or charge nurse to determine the staffing pattern and coverage planned. Although nurse learners should not be scheduled to make up for staff shortages, their presence on the unit at various times may complement staffing and lend support to better patient care. Conversely, removing nurse learners from the unit at certain times may compromise patient care, so learner entry and exit times need careful attention.
- If staff nurses will be functioning as instructors or preceptors for learners, ascertain the number and availability of these staff before arriving on the unit with a group of learners.
- Before planning educational programs, consult with other professional groups and departments to become more familiar with their responsibilities, priorities, and willingness to assist in the program.
- Be certain that initial scheduling of clinical rotations includes orientation of learners to the physical layout and routines of the unit so that staff are not unnecessarily interrupted for questions in these areas.
- Work with the nurse manager or charge nurse to decide how patient assignments can be made to secure specific types of learning experiences. Attempt to reach agreement on each of the following points:
  - Who will be responsible for making assignments for learners
  - Whether dual assignments (such as preceptor and preceptee) will be used
  - How the accountability and responsibility for patient care will be shared if dual assignments are employed

How and when learners will be gradually weaned
from preceptors

What roles the educator and nurse manager/charge
nurse will have with respect to supervision of
learners

Since the turn of the century, nurses have learned to
become expert clinical practitioners primarily through an
apprenticeship form of on-the-job training, working with
and under more experienced counterparts. Although this
role-model system of teaching has endured today, other
methods of clinical instruction have emerged and will be
considered here. These include bedside nursing rounds
and the use of criterion-referenced performance checklists.
It should be noted at this point that many of the teaching
strategies already discussed for the classroom and clinical
settings are also employed in the clinical setting. These include the classroom teaching methods of group discussion,
nursing care conferences, case studies, and the incident
process as well as the laboratory method of demonstration.
In addition, learning laboratories are often set up in the
clinical area. The discussion that follows focuses on those
teaching methods for the clinical area that are more or less
unique to this setting.

Role Model

As mentioned previously, role modeling represents the
most time-honored method of clinical instruction for
nurses. A *role model* is an individual who exemplifies
through his/her behavior how a particular role is to be
enacted. The role model method of teaching is based on
expertise for its legitimacy and authority: whoever is most
expert and capable of effectively demonstrating that expertise should function as the role model for that aspect of
the nurse's instruction.

Most new nurses acquire and develop their clinical competence by observing and emulating other nurses who already possess expertise in nursing practice. These other
nurses may include the clinical nurse specialist, the nurse
manager or charge nurse, the staff development or unit
instructor, or other staff nurses. Although their positions
and titles may vary, they all have in common both experience and expertise in nursing practice. Their instructional
responsibility is to exemplify how that institution expects
a nurse to function in an assigned role.

At some institutions, the role model's function is vested
in a single individual, while, at other hospitals, it is a shared
responsibility among two or more of the categories of
nurses mentioned previously. When the role model is a
single individual that person is typically designated as a
preceptor.* When the role model function is shared, each
participant assumes responsibility for teaching various segments of that nurse's role.

APPROPRIATENESS FOR TEACHING Of all the components of
staff development, the role model method of teaching is
most appropriately used for orientation programs. The primary reason for this is that, unlike in-service and continuing education programs, orientation programs are role-spe-
cific. Who better could demonstrate that role than one who
has already achieved expertise through experience in that
role? The logical corollary here is that the best role model
for a newly employed nurse is an experienced colleague in
the same role. Thus experienced staff nurses serve as role
models for new staff nurses, experienced head nurses function as role models for new head nurses, and the like. Although role modeling is most commonly used for the orientation of new staff nurses, it may also be used for
orientation of new clinical specialists, charge nurses, nurse
managers, nurse administrators, nurse educators, or any
other category of nursing staff.

LIMITATIONS Although role modeling has served the nursing profession well for many decades, some inherent limitations of this teaching method exist. These include the
following:

- Having individuals designated as role models who do
  not possess sufficient clinical experience or expertise
  to demonstrate the role effectively
- Having individuals functioning as role models who do
  not wish to serve in this capacity
- If role modeling is provided by more than one individual, differences and inconsistencies in exemplifying
  the role may cause confusion and frustration to the
  new nurse
- Overuse of nurses as role models, leading to their
  burnout and diminished effectiveness. Role models
  may find it exhausting to have their performance con-
  tinuously scrutinized and to have responsibility for another nurse's development.
- Expert nurses are not always able to explain the details
  of how or why something is done in terms that a novice can understand

GUIDELINES FOR USE Some general guidelines for the use
of role models follows. Guidelines specific to the use of
preceptors for orientation of new staff nurses will be provided in Part III.

- Before individuals are selected to function as role
  models for other nurses, there needs to be some mechanism in place to ensure that these nurses possess the
  requisite experience and expertise to function in this
  capacity.
- Those who will serve as role models should be given
  clear guidelines on the scope and breadth of their responsibility to the new nurse.

---

*The use of preceptors will be covered in detail in the discussion of orientation programs in Part III.

- Those who serve as role models should be afforded preparation in the instructional aspects of their responsibilities: how to teach, evaluate, and work effectively with new staff members.
- Those who are willing to function as role models need to receive administrative and educational support in their role so that they may obtain assistance if problems arise that they are unable to resolve.
- Those who are willing to serve as role models need some relief from their regular staff responsibilities so that they are available to work with new nurses.
- Role models need to foster increased independence with the nurses they orient; weaning the new nurse from dependence on the role model is the natural form of closure in this process.
- If the responsibilities for role modeling of new staff nurses are shared among various categories of nursing personnel, some guidelines for dividing these responsibilities might be as follows:

  Staff nurses could be responsible for teaching patient care routines, unit policies, procedures and protocols; the physical layout of the unit and location of equipment and supplies; documentation; patient transfers, admissions, and discharges; and the role of the primary nurse

  Nurses managers might be responsible for teaching unit policies and procedures related to administrative and personnel areas, employment policies, expanded management functions such as charge nurse, team leader, assistant nurse manager, and the chain of command and communication.

  Clinical nurse specialists could be responsible for teaching clinical and role responsibilities that require greater expertise or more advanced preparation than staff nurses are able to afford; they may also function as a clinical resource person to the role model or unit instructor.

  Staff development instructors might provide expanded educational support for role models in suggesting additional or alternative ways to teach specific clinical or role responsibilities; act as an educational resource to the role model if problems arise in the teaching-learning process; or augment the role model's instruction with supplementary educational offerings such as readings, audiovisual programs, or one-on-one demonstrations; may also be responsible for monitoring the effectiveness of the role model–new nurse relationship.

Bedside Nursing Rounds

Bedside nursing rounds involve the presentation of patients and discussion of nursing care at the patient's bedside. Rounds may be conducted in a number of different ways but typically consist of a presentation of relevant information about the patient by the nurse assigned to that patient, focusing the discussion on selected aspects of the patient's situation, group discussion that involves patient assessment and interaction, followed by some form of followup discussion.

Before the days of primary nursing, computerized medical information systems and taped reports, the charge nurse or team leader might use bedside rounds to solicit pertinent information regarding each patient from the nurse assigned to that patient. This nurse-to-nurse personal communication system afforded not only a means for charge nurses to better know their patients but also provided a valuable learning opportunity and a means for monitoring and improving the quality and continuity of patient care.

The origin of bedside nursing rounds is most likely the traditional rounds conducted by the medical staff at major teaching hospitals. Although similar in many ways, bedside nursing rounds tend to be more holistic in scope, more inclusive of patient participation, and more directed at experienced staff rather than at students.

Some of the advantages offered by bedside nursing rounds include the following:

- Provide a more realistic, concrete, and clinically meaningful learning experience than either laboratory or classroom teaching methods
- Enable learners to refine their ability to establish and modify priorities of care based on real rather than hypothetical patient situations
- Afford an opportunity for learners to share clinical information, to learn from and support each other, and to employ group problem-solving methods in dealing with clinical problems and issues and in making clinical judgments
- Offer experiences in assessing and evaluating a wide range of normal variants and the presentations of abnormal findings as they actually exist
- Illustrate first-hand how to modify techniques, procedures, and other elements of nursing care based on real-life constraints and situations
- Provide learners with an opportunity to present clinical information in an organized and succinct manner

APPROPRIATENESS FOR TEACHING   Bedside nursing rounds can be used for any of the following[119]:

- To develop and refine patient assessment skills in systematic observation, palpation, percussion, and auscultation.
- To integrate laboratory, diagnostic, and other clinical assessments of the patient with the nurse's ongoing assessments
- To demonstrate how to involve the patient and family in the plan of care

- To demonstrate and stimulate constructive and supportive methods of peer review
- To teach and reinforce classroom and laboratory learning sessions
- To reinforce principles of normal physiology, pathophysiology, and patient responses to nursing interventions
- To expose a larger number of learners to learning experiences available on the unit
- To provide a forum for learners' self-appraisal of learning
- To foster self-directed learning that is immediately applicable to nursing practice
- To develop learners' ability to synthesize, organize, and cogently present a patient's situation for their peers' consideration
- To identify clinical cases that may be used for future classroom or laboratory learning sessions
- To demonstrate how quality monitoring and improvement are related to daily nursing practice on the unit

In addition, Benner and Wrubel[10] suggest that joint bedside rounds by nurses at various levels of clinical proficiency in the novice-to-expert continuum may be useful for clarifying how nurses at different proficiency levels describe and record patient assessments. Rounds can be employed to enable nurses at each level to better understand the differences between novices and experts in managing the clinical database into meaningful information that influences nursing practice.

LIMITATIONS Some of the limitations of bedside nursing rounds include the following:

- Groups of nurses making bedside rounds can make the unit too crowded for other healthcare workers
- The space-occupying nature of this teaching method limits the number of learners who can be accommodated at one time; all participants need to be able to see and hear the discussions
- Time constraints may limit the number of patients included
- May not be able to use this teaching method when patient needs for rest, quiet, or privacy exist
- May need to leave the bedside for discussions of certain sensitive patient problems or situations

GUIDELINES FOR USE Following are some guidelines for using bedside nursing rounds[119,130]:

- Determine the maximum number of learners who can participate in bedside rounds on that unit and how rounds will be conducted
- Check with nursing staff to verify that nursing rounds will not interfere with unit operation or patient care

- Use preestablished criteria and objectives to select patients who will be presented at rounds
- Meet with participants before starting to specify the purpose and objectives for rounds, what will be discussed and observed
- Offer directions to participants on how to present patients (e.g., providing a summary of their health history; significant clinical problems; findings of laboratory, diagnostic, and physical assessments; overview of medical therapy and all pertinent nursing management strategies with highlighting of areas related to objectives)
- Provide a mechanism for patient participation in rounds, when appropriate and feasible
- Whenever possible, elicit patients' willingness and ability to participate
- Be sensitive to criteria for terminating rounds: patient fatigue or deterioration in clinical status, unit emergencies and patient care priorities, attainment of objectives
- Conclude rounds with a followup conference for discussion of observations, findings, and implications for nursing practice

Bedside nursing rounds are intended to supplement and reinforce other types of learning experiences. Because they deliver instruction to the forefront of nursing practice, they are potentially a most meaningful and reality-based vehicle for clinical instruction. When planned for the bedside staff nurse, nursing rounds afford an enriching learning experience complemented by elements of quality improvement and a truly professional colleagueship in nursing practice.

Criterion-Referenced Performance Checklists

When an individual's performance is evaluated in relation to predetermined criteria, the form of evaluation used is called *criterion referenced*. A criterion-referenced performance checklist is a device that enumerates each requisite behavior required in the performance of some procedure or clinical skill. This device may be used for either evaluation of learning or for teaching how a procedure or skill is to be performed. Table 4.4 illustrates an example of a criterion-referenced performance checklist that is sufficiently detailed for use in teaching and learning the procedure.

The behaviors included in the checklist may be limited to only those considered critical or essential or may include both essential and nonessential behaviors. If the latter approach is used (as it is in Table 4-4), the behaviors considered "essential" for performance are typically marked with an asterisk (*) or some other device to distinguish them from nonessential behaviors. When the checklist is used for evaluation, learners are informed that all essential behaviors must be demonstrated before their performance

TABLE 4.4 • EXAMPLE OF A CRITERION-REFERENCED PERFORMANCE CHECKLIST

Recording a 12-Lead Electrocardiogram (ECG)

Instructions: The checklist that follows delineates the steps necessary to record a 12-lead ECG. You may use this form to learn, practice, or perform this procedure. Steps marked with an asterisk (*) must be included for the performance to be considered as satisfactory.

Step	Done	Not Done
1. Prepares patient and equipment		
Verifies patient's name	☐	☐
Introduces self and explains purpose and procedure to patient	☐	☐
Plugs in grounded single-channel ECG recorder	☐	☐
Turns power switch to "on"	☐	☐
Checks for adequate supply of paper; places new roll if necessary	☐	☐
Draws curtain around patient's bed	☐	☐
Places patient in supine 45° semi-Fowler's position	☐	☐
Exposes patient's distal limbs and chest	☐	☐
Performs skin preparation on chest and limbs*	☐	☐
Applies conductive material to electrodes*	☐	☐
Securely attaches electrodes to chest and limb locations*	☐	☐
Records patient's name and date on ECG record	☐	☐
2. Standardizes ECG for time and voltage		
Turns control knob to "run"	☐	☐
Centers stylus on ECG paper	☐	☐
Verifies that paper speed is 25 mm/second*	☐	☐
Turns lead selector switch to "STD"	☐	☐
Presses STD (1 mv) button and obtains 10 mm deflection*	☐	☐
Verifies that sensitivity switch is on "1"	☐	☐
Verifies that all waveforms are observable; if necessary, adjusts sensitivity to obtain observable waveforms*	☐	☐
3. Records six frontal plane leads		
Records at least 5 ECG cycles for each frontal plane lead*	☐	☐
4. Records six horizontal plane leads		
Applies chest electrodes in correct location*	☐	☐
V_1 4th ICS, RSB		
V_2 4th ICS, LSB		
V_3 midway between V_2 and V_4		
V_4 5th ICS, MCL		
V_5 5th ICS, AXL		
V_6 5th ICS, MAL		
Records at least five ECG cycles for each horizontal plane lead*	☐	☐
5. Concludes ECG recording		
Turns power switch to "off"	☐	☐
Unplugs ECG recorder	☐	☐
Detaches electrodes from patient	☐	☐
Removes all conductive material from patient's skin	☐	☐

will be considered acceptable. By reviewing the elements in the list, learners can become familiar with each step to be completed and practice the procedure with or without an instructor present.

Because the checklist specifies exactly what is expected in performance of the procedure, criterion-referenced lists can be used for self-instruction at whatever time is conve-nient for the learner. In addition to fostering principles of adult education, this teaching method may also reduce learners' performance anxiety and uncertainty regarding expectations of their performance. Use of these checklists also standardizes clinical practice on the unit and dimin-ishes the subjectivity involved with evaluation of staff per-formance.

APPROPRIATENESS FOR TEACHING Criterion-referenced performance checklists may be used for teaching technical psychomotor skills, proper use of equipment, clinical procedures, and unit routines and protocols. They may also be used for review and practice of many elements of physical assessment, monitoring procedures, documentation, and management of emergency situations. One of the benefits of such lists is that they can be attached to various pieces of equipment that new staff may need to use when no instructor is present. Thus the checklist in Table 4-4 might be permanently attached to an ECG machine in a patient unit where ECGs are not often performed; when staff on that unit need to record an ECG at 3 AM, they can use the checklist to review and complete the procedure rather than calling for assistance from the critical care staff or a nursing supervisor. Similar checklists might be attached to the resuscitation cart, a hypothermia machine, or other such equipment.

LIMITATIONS Some of the limitations of criterion-referenced performance checklists are that they may:

- Be somewhat tedious and time-consuming to develop
- Duplicate information that already exists in procedure manuals, manufacturer's operating manuals, and other reference materials
- Be left in place long after their updating is warranted
- Be less useful for procedures and patient interactions that require a significant amount of variability (e.g., abdominal dressings) or tailoring to individual patient situations (e.g., providing emotional support)

GUIDELINES FOR USE Some guidelines for developing and using criterion-referenced performance checklists follow:

- Draft a list of all the unit procedures and skills for which these checklists might be used; from this list, identify the priority ones to develop
- Designate different work teams to develop the elements for each separate checklist
- Decide whether the performance criteria will include all behaviors or only those considered essential to satisfactory performance
- For each procedure or skill, enumerate all necessary behavioral components in the order in which they should be executed
- If all behaviors will be included, reach consensus on which of the behaviors are to be designated as essential or critical and then distinguish these in the list by an asterisk or some other marking system
- Solicit staff and nurse manager input on the performance criteria developed and revise the criteria as necessary
- Attach the performance checklists to their appropriate

locations or include them in a reference notebook for the unit.

SELF-DIRECTED TEACHING METHODS

As mentioned earlier in this chapter, self-directed teaching methods refer to instruction in which the majority of learning elements are controlled by the learner. Although the name of this category of teaching methods seems to suggest that all forms of self-directed instruction are carried out by the learner completely independently of any instructor, this is not the case. On the contrary, self-directed learning often involves the assistance of others. The difference is that, despite this assistance, the learner retains control over the learning process.[14]

Recent efforts aimed at healthcare cost-containment and staffing shortages in nursing have precipitated widespread interest and use of self-directed instructional methods. But, as with any other form of instruction, self-directed learning has its advantages and disadvantages. Before describing some of the more commonly employed forms of self-directed learning (SDL), the educator needs to consider the relative benefits and limitations of this mode of instruction.

Advantages of Self-Directed Learning

Self-directed learning offers the following advantages*:

- *Consistency with principles of adult education.* The varied forms of SDL offer an appealing means of providing educational programs that actively involve learners, enable learners to meet their own learning needs as they perceive them while meeting program outcomes, provide immediate feedback and reinforcement of learning, and promote independence and accountability for learning. A recent survey of 150 registered nurses in British Columbia[105] found that 70% of these nurses preferred SDL over learning provided by educators. In addition, SDL programs afford continuity with numerous features of adult education. These features include learners' determination of each of the following:

  Time of instruction
  Duration of instruction
  Pace of instruction
  Amount of instruction
  Sequence of learning
  Learning style(s) used
  Learning needs addressed

- *Flexibility.* In relation to the number of learners who can be provided with instruction at one time, the ability to schedule learning experiences, and the number and types of learning strategies employed.

*See references 4, 19, 91, 109, 116, 132.

- *Variety.* In instructional methods.
- *Individuality.* In learners' ability to proceed with instruction based on their unique needs.
- *Convenience.* In the time, place, duration, and pace of instruction.
- *Adaptability.* In being able to accommodate learners who differ significantly from each other in their education, expertise, and experiences.
- *Accessibility.* In learners' ability to avail themselves of instruction without leaving their clinical unit, regardless of their shift, whenever staffing demands diminish on the unit, and whenever they wish to obtain review or repeated use
- *Portability.* In locating instructional programs at sites most convenient to learners (on or adjacent to the unit, at home, in learning resource center, library, etc); some programs are housed on mobile carts that can be placed on the nursing unit and moved to other units as the need exists.[132]
- *Applicability.* Can be tailored to meet the hospital's or unit's specific needs; can be designed to include hands-on simulated or real clinical practice or evaluation of learning.
- *Privacy.* Eliminate learners' concerns and anxiety over making mistakes or showing inadequacies in front of their peers or supervisors, in learning more slowly than others in a group, or in feeling discomfort in group learning situations.
- *Cost-effectiveness.* As a rule, self-directed instructional programs are far less expensive to provide than traditional classroom instruction and eliminate the costs (travel, lodging, meals, tuition) associated with sending learners to outside programs. SDL programs can also effect savings by reducing the amount of time that nurses have to be away from their units and reducing the need for supplemental staffing to cover patients while they are learning. From the educator's perspective, the time saved in providing instruction can be used for counseling learners, resolving learning problems, supervising or evaluating clinical performance, or ensuring application of learning to nursing practice. SDL may also relieve the boredom of repeating the same instruction multiple times throughout the year and reduce the cost per learner for instruction with small groups of learners. If a hospital needs to provide instruction to experienced nurses, SDL programs can decrease the time needed for instruction because learners can proceed more quickly than in a formal classroom course.

Disadvantages of Self-Directed Learning

Although proponents of self-directed learning tend to emphasize its many advantages, the educator needs to recognize some of the potential disadvantages of this mode of instruction[19,36,91,109]:

- *Low completion rates.* Some of the reasons for low completion rates with SDL offerings include learners not liking or accepting this form of instruction or lack of self-discipline and/or motivation to seek instructional resources or to persist in finishing the program.[5] In other instances, these offerings may not be well advertised or promoted, or users may not be given the administrative support needed to take advantage of the programs. Some institutions may thwart use of SDL programs because space is not allocated for storage and accessibility to users, because funds are not provided to duplicate enough copies of the program, or because audiovisual hardware needed in the program is not maintained or repaired in a timely fashion. Low completion rates may also be caused by a lack of educational support for users—if the educator is not immediately available to answer questions, troubleshoot problems, or help with applications, prospective users may falter in their efforts. At times, the program design is of poor quality because the topic area is too broad, too narrow, or lacks clinical relevance for learners.
- *Lack of interaction between learners and instructor.* SDL provides no opportunity for learners to ask questions, obtain clarifications, or have discussions regarding the application of content to practice.
- *Format may be too structured and visually uninteresting.* Learners may become bored using this form of learning because the program materials lack visual and structural appeal.
- *Program materials are time-consuming to design, develop, and pilot test.* Although providing SDL programs is very cost-efficient, developing and refining them may be quite costly for the educator, staff, and clerical personnel.
- *SDL is not a suitable method of instruction for all learners.* Learners who are highly field-dependent and those with learning style preferences for social interaction, group work, and structured relationships with teachers are not likely to find SDL appealing.
- *Some forms of SDL require storage space and monitoring of use.* SDL materials may have to be catalogued, stored, restocked, and managed by some staff member to ensure that materials are accounted for and available for use.
- *SDL is not appropriate for all topic areas.* SDL is most appropriately used for cognitive learning outcomes and as a preliminary step for psychomotor areas. It is less useful for learning in the affective domain.
- *Some SDL program materials need frequent updating and revision.* In order to keep SDL materials current and clinically relevant, they may need to be reviewed and revised on a regular basis.

Self-directed instruction exists in numerous forms. Two forms, mediated instruction and computer-assisted instruction, were discussed in Chapter 3. That chapter covered the rationale for each method of instruction and for selection criteria, guidelines for using, and the characteristics of each. The remaining forms of self-directed learning that will be considered in this chapter include programmed instruction, self-learning packages, and learning contracts.

Programmed Instruction[27]

Programmed instruction presents printed information in a series of small, sequential blocks (called *frames*). After a certain amount of information has been given, one or more questions based on that information are presented for the learner's response. The learner then compares his/her answer with the correct answer, which is typically provided either on the same page in a separate right-hand column adjacent to the question in that frame or on the next page.

Programmed instruction may be linear or branched. *Linear programmed instruction* presents content in a serial manner so that the learner reviews all frames in the program from beginning to end. *Branched programmed instruction* directs the learner to specific pages of the program, depending on answers to the questions posed. For example, if a learner selects the correct answer to a question, the program may direct the learner to skip the next few pages and advance more quickly through the instruction. If the learner selects an incorrect answer, the program may direct the learner to earlier or subsequent pages of the program for additional review, reinforcement, or clarification. Following this review or supplementation, the program would return the learner to the question so that the correct answer might then be selected.

Programmed instruction is usually provided in a self-contained written booklet format that includes a brief introduction, directions for using the program, a list of instructional outcomes, and the instructional content and self-assessment questions. In addition to the printed text, programmed instruction may also include graphic enhancements such as diagrams, photographs, charts, and tables.

Some examples of programmed instruction include the variety of programs offered for many years by the American Journal of Nursing Company on topics such as interpretation of acid-base disorders and twenty-two programs in the Patient Assessment Series on the management of anxiety, hostility, and conflict.

Appropriateness for Teaching

Learners who prefer highly structured learning experiences and those who prefer to work alone in a self-paced, self-directed manner will likely enjoy programmed instruction. This form of instruction is also appropriate for learners who like immediate feedback on their performance and the ability to evaluate their own learning.

Programmed instruction is most appropriate for teaching within the cognitive domain of learning, especially at the lower levels. Although the content may at times relate to affective and psychomotor learning outcomes, programmed instruction will tend to emphasize mostly the knowledge base that underlies these areas of practice, rather than affective or psychomotor skills or behaviors per se.

Limitations

The primary limitations of programmed instruction relate to its presentation format. Some learners find the highly structured and serial nature of this instruction tedious and time consuming to use. This is particularly true if the program requires more than 15 to 20 minutes to complete and/or if there is no means for challenging out of the material to be covered.

Nurses who prefer group or interactive learning experiences may dislike this mode of learning. At times, the instruction itself may be rather boring if it is devoid of any illustrations, if it contains few questions relative to the amount of information that must be read, and/or if it fails to provide sufficient practice to reinforce learning. Programmed instruction is also limited by its use of a single sensory (written) medium for learning. When programs must be developed locally, they can be time consuming (and, therefore, expensive) to develop, pilot test, revise, and finalize.

Guidelines for Use

The guidelines for using programmed instruction include the following:

- Determine which instructional outcomes are appropriate and amenable to this form of instruction.
- Decide whether programmed instruction can be provided via commercially available programs by reviewing the content, objectives, ease of use, and assessment questions contained in the program. Carefully critique these products to ensure that they are accurate, up to date, and targeted to the content and audience you intend.
- If commercially prepared programs are selected for use, order a sufficient quantity of these to ensure ready availability for the number of learners anticipated. Plan to order a few extra copies to replace booklets that may be lost or damaged over time.
- If commercial programs are not available or suitable for your purposes, develop local programs by:
    Identifying the instructional outcomes to be attained
    Writing a detailed and subordinated outline of all major points to be covered in the program
    Dividing the content into small segments of information that afford step-by-step progression through the content

Drafting the content into frames that include pertinent questions to review, reinforce, and evaluate learning

Aiming at a completion time of 15 to 20 minutes or less

Designing a pretest for learners to be able to challenge out of the program by demonstrating that they can already meet the instructional outcomes

Pilot testing the program with a group of learners who are comparable to those who will eventually use the program

Determining the validity and reliability of the pretest and assessment questions used in the program

Printing and storing a sufficient supply of copies for the number of anticipated learners

- Store programs so that they are immediately available to learners.
- Create a mechanism that facilitates use and return of program materials.
- Evaluate the effectiveness and efficiency of using programmed instruction in the staff development program.

Self-Learning Packages

Self-learning packages (SLPs)* are self-contained, self-paced units of instruction that include all elements a learner needs for independent study of a particular topic or concept. A wide variety of terms are used for this type of teaching methodology. Some of these terms include: *modularized instruction, self-directed learning modules, self-instructional modules, self-instructional packages, self-paced modules, self-instructional units, self-instructional packets,* and *independent study units.* Some authors use these terms to describe slightly different instructional methods, but much similarity exists among the various materials.

Self-learning packages offer a number of advantages to both prospective learners and to the nurse educator.† Some advantages of SLPs to learners include the following:

- SLPs enable learners to pursue their own learning interests at their own pace
- SLPs actively involve learners in the instructional process
- SLPs can be used at learners' desired time, location, and frequency
- SLPs enable learners to interrupt and resume learning if work demands arise
- SLPs are typically easy to use

- SLPs avoid any competition or pressure from peers in the learning process
- SLPs place responsibility for learning on the adult learner, who is free to exercise his/her self-direction in determining when, how, and for how long he/she will study
- SLPs enable learners to obtain instruction without having to leave their work area and without needing other staff to cover their patient assignments in their absence
- SLPs can be designed to provide a variety of learning activities and thus to accommodate a wide range of learning styles; learners can then select a package that matches their preferred ways of learning
- SLPs encourage initiative and responsibility among learners for pursuing their own learning as their needs and desires dictate
- SLPs provide variety in learning experiences

In addition to their benefits to users, SLPs offer a number of advantages to staff development instructors:

- SLPs free the instructor from the monotonous repetition of didactic presentations to many groups of nurses over time
- SLPs afford the educator with time out of the classroom to identify and solve learning problems, work with learners who need extra assistance, and help learners apply knowledge gains in the clinical setting
- SLPs can afford a means to bring a large group of nurses with different amounts of knowledge and experience to comparable levels of comprehension in relation to a specific topic area
- SLPs can help the educator make learning more accessible
- SLPs provide a means to initiate orientation programs whenever a new employee enters the unit, rather than having to wait until the next scheduled orientation program
- SLPs can be as effective and more efficient than traditional classroom teaching methods for motivated learners[12,17,95,115]
- SLPs afford consistency in the depth, scope, and quality of instructional content

Self-learning packages come with a wide variety of different presentation formats and component parts and may incorporate a multitude of forms of media. Although their contents may vary, most SLPs include the following components‡:

- Title
- Table of contents
- Purpose or overall goal
- Statement of prerequisites

---

*See references 21, 27, 31, 51, 53, 66, 97, 104.
†See references 21, 27, 53, 63, 66, 69, 95, 97, 104, 107, 114.
‡See references 1, 31, 51, 52, 66, 95, 116.

- List of instructional outcomes
- Directions for use
- List of learning activities
- Pretest
- Content
- Instructional aids
- Posttest
- Learner evaluation of SLP

The *title* of the SLP should be concise and descriptive of its content. The *table of contents* will be helpful to learners in orienting themselves to the SLP and in later locating specific information if it provides a list of all subtopics included in the package and their corresponding page numbers. The *purpose or overall goal* needs to provide the learner with a clear indication of the topic area covered.

A *statement of prerequisites* identifies the knowledge, skills, attitudes, and/or experiences that the learner should possess *before* attempting to complete the SLP. Prerequisites should be stated with sufficient clarity and detail so that learners will know at once whether they are able to complete the instructional package. In some instances, the prerequisites section may also include a description of resources available to the learner for meeting the prerequisites. For example, a SLP on infection control measures may have prerequisites that say, "Has read hospital policy and procedures entitled 'Infection Control' and 'Universal Precautions.' within the last month" and "Has observed the use of universal precautions in the emergency department." If the learner had not read these documents within that time frame, there might be directions on where to locate the policy and procedure book and find those documents. If the nurse had not observed the use of universal precautions, the package might relate how to make arrangements for this observational experience.

The *instructional outcomes* for the SLP need to be written in clear and specific behavioral terms. These outcomes inform the learner of the instructional intent of the SLP and make explicit what is expected of the learner. The *directions for use* should afford clear and concise explanations of each component in the package: what it consists of, where to find it, how to use it, and how best to proceed in completing the SLP.

The *learning activities* included in a SLP are summarized in a list so that learners know what they will encounter as they use the package. The learning experiences provided in the package may comprise a single set of activities that all users will employ or a variety of learning options that users may select among to complete the package. These activities may include any combination of the following learning strategies: reading certain pages of the package, reading a set of journal articles or book chapters, observing various patient care situations, viewing videotapes, listening to audio tapes, using supplies or equipment, contacting specific resource persons or services, completing written practice exercises, or taking various quizzes or written

tests. Some SLPs may also require that learners practice certain clinical behaviors or skills in a simulated or actual patient care setting.

The *pretest* should relate directly to the instructional outcomes for the SLP. A sufficient number of test items should be sampled for each outcome to ensure that the behaviors contained in the outcome are adequately verified in the learner's performance. The pretest may be used for any of three possible purposes: (1) to provide a baseline performance measure for later comparison with the posttest score, (2) to indicate to the learner which sections or subsections of the SLP they will need to complete, or (3) to enable the learner to challenge the SLP. If the pretest is used for comparison purposes, the educator may be interested in verifying that the SLP is effective in achieving its instructional goal by establishing the gain in scores between the pretest and posttest values. In this situation, the posttest may use the same test questions as the pretest or may use different but comparable questions to those used in the pretest (equivalent or parallel forms test). If the purpose of the pretest is to indicate which sections of the SLP the learner needs to complete, test items are usually coded to specific sections of the SLP and the answer key informs the learner which sections may be skipped or bypassed and/or which sections need to be completed. If the purpose of the pretest is to provide an opportunity for learners to challenge the SLP, the answer key typically indicates the "passing score" that must be achieved so that learners will know whether they need to complete the SLP or not. Pretests are often scored by the learner, but, when they are used for challenging the package, they may be scored by the instructor.

The *content* of the SLP consists of small segments of information with generous use of repetition. Throughout the SLP, the content is frequently interspersed with questions that review, reinforce, and apply learning. The answers to these self-assessment questions (also called self-checks) are typically provided for the learner on the page following the question or at the end of that section of information. These self-assessment items afford the learner immediate feedback on progress and performance.

The learning activities selected for use in the SLP will determine which *instructional aids* are included in the package. These instructional aids might include any of the following: readings, handouts, worksheets, written case studies, copies of policies or procedures, practice exercises, study questions, audiovisual media, computer software, supplies, equipment, scavenger hunt checklists, and a bibliography (suggested and/or required readings).

As mentioned previously, the *posttest* for the SLP may be the same or different from the pretest. As with the pretest, the written test items that comprise the posttest are closely linked with the instructional outcomes for the program. When psychomotor or affective areas are included in the SLP content, the posttest may also include required demonstrations of performance. These may be provided by instructor observation or through use of a videotaped performance that is submitted to the instructor for evaluation. If all outcomes were not attained, the learner may be directed to repeat one or more sections, complete an alternate learning activity, or secure assistance from the instructor.

Learners should always be given the opportunity to evaluate their experience in using the SLP. Forms for a *learner evaluation of SLP* may be provided with the package materials and be returned (with the pre- and posttests) to the instructor once the package has been finished.

Appropriateness for Teaching*

Self-learning packages are most often used to provide instruction within the cognitive domain of learning or to provide the knowledge base for affective or psychomotor areas of learning. They can be readily used for instruction at any level of the cognitive domain and may be incorporated into any component (orientation, in-service education, continuing education) of the staff development program.

Self-learning packages may be used to replace traditional classroom instruction, to review infrequently used practice areas, to provide supplemental or remedial instruction, to offer optional learning strategies to match preferred learning styles, to afford a means of gaining instruction when the learner cannot attend classroom presentations, to attain entry behaviors required for a current position or to meet the requirements for a more advanced position. SLPs may also be used to make a heterogeneous group of learners more comparable with respect to their background on a particular topic or to keep nurses on leave (maternity, disability, sick) abreast of changes in practice.

These packages are perhaps best employed when learners need to acquire basic facts, principles, concepts, or skills, to review hospital policies and procedures, or to gain some initial capabilities in using equipment.[51] Cranton[27] suggests that SLPs are especially useful in situations where learners have wide variations in their prior experience in a specific area or where their ability levels vary widely. Another area often selected for use of SLPs is in mandatory requirements for accreditation, such as CPR recertification, fire safety, and infection control. Other examples of areas where SLPs are often used include instruction in basic anatomy and physiology, pathophysiology, physical assessment skills, and various types of patient monitoring (e.g., ECG, arterial blood gas, neurological, and hemodynamic monitoring) where information remains relatively stable over time. When the self-learning package covers psychomotor skills, the addition of a laboratory and/or clinical component to instruction and evaluation is necessary so that the learner's actual skill performance can be demonstrated, observed, and evaluated.

Limitations

As with any other teaching method, self-learning packages do not provide a panacea for instruction. Some of the potential limitations or disadvantages of self-learning packages may be grouped into those related to learners and those related to the instructor[21,27,31,91,95]:

The possible limitations of SLPs in relation to the learner include the following:

- SLPs require that learners are highly motivated, persistent, and able and willing to work independently. Unless learners are willing to take the initiative and responsibility for managing their own learning experiences, the development or purchase of SLPs may be largely wasted effort.
- Learners may begin but not complete the SLP because of distractions, extended interruptions, or their own procrastination.
- Learners with preferences for group styles of learning and those who prefer to learn from an instructor may not respond favorably to SLPs.
- SLPs may be incompatible with learning styles that favor social interaction; such individuals may perceive this type of instruction as depersonalized and lonely.
- SLPs may not be effective if learners fail to use pretest results in planning instruction, if they attempt to complete the package with the least time and effort, or if they are dishonest (e.g., in pooling answers to the posttest with other learners) in using the assessment, feedback, and evaluation devices included in the package.
- SLPs may not be effective if the package is poorly designed, highly pedagogical, if its appraisal devices fail to correlate closely with instructional outcomes, or if these devices are not valid and reliable evaluation instruments.
- Commercially produced SLPs may not fully match the outcomes and content desired for instruction or may be inconsistent with nursing practice at that institution.
- If staff development programs use SLPs exclusively or for a majority of instruction, learners may lose interest in using this technique. The need for variation in instructional strategies cannot be neglected by using SLPs.

From the instructor's perspective, some limitations of SLPs include the following:

- Today's restricted staff development budgets may limit the funds available for purchasing commercially produced SLPs.
- Many SLPs need to be locally designed. The development (drafting, piloting, refining, retesting, etc.) of

---

*See references 21, 27, 31, 51, 97, 104.

SLPs can be a very time consuming and, therefore, very costly endeavor, particularly if the packages must be developed at the same time that instruction in those areas is delivered by traditional methods.

- Educators may not be granted the release time needed for development of SLPs.
- A self-learning package alone cannot be used to teach detailed and complex psychomotor skills; the SLP needs to be complemented with laboratory and/or clinical instruction and supervised practice and evaluation.
- SLPs do not fully free the educator to pursue other activities. SLPs require instructor time for storing, maintaining, replacing selected pages, monitoring learners' use of the packages, scoring (written, laboratory, and/or clinical) evaluation results, record keeping, reviewing and revising, managing learners' access to the programs, and troubleshooting audiovisual equipment or software problems.
- The educator(s) who are responsible for developing SLPs may lack the knowledge, skills, and experience to fulfill this responsibility. As a result, locally produced SLPs may be of marginal educational value and quality.
- Educators may find that frequent use of this teaching device brings them less personal satisfaction in their role owing to the loss of personal interaction with learners, loss of control over the learning process, or feelings of inadequacy regarding their ability to design effective SLPs.

Guidelines for Use

The following are some guidelines for developing and managing the use of self-learning packages*:

- *Select an appropriate topic.* The topic or concept chosen should be amenable to self-instruction and require about 20 to 30 minutes for learners to complete.
- *Define the overall purpose of the SLP.* The purpose of the SLP will need to be communicated to learners in the introductory information.
- *Identify the target audience.* Describe relevant characteristics of the audience such as their knowledge, skills, and clinical experiences in relation to the topic. The attributes of the users are important to recognize because they influence the level and depth of instruction provided in the SLP.
- *Write the instructional outcomes for the SLP.* These outcomes need to be written in clear behavioral and measurable terms. Outcomes should be attainable within the time frame established for the SLP.
- *Determine prerequisites for the SLP.* Identify any knowledge, skills, attitudes, and clinical experiences

that the learner should have before beginning the SLP. For learners who may not yet possess all of these entry requirements, the SLP might provide an enumeration of suggested resources (e.g., people to contact, articles or books to read, other SLPs to complete, clinical experiences to acquire) for obtaining these.

- *Develop an outline of content for the SLP.* The content needs to be selected based on its pertinence to meeting the instructional outcomes.
- *Designate appropriate learning activities.* These activities will assist learners in attaining the instructional outcomes established for the SLP. When possible, provide learners with several options so that they may select those learning activities that best coincide with their preferred learning style preferences. Learning activities need to include active learner participation and practice in performing the behaviors designated in the instructional outcomes. In the introductory section, these activities may simply be listed or organized under the outcome to which they pertain.
- *Obtain and/or design instructional aids.* Audiovisual or computer-assisted instructional programs, journal articles, books, handouts, charts, worksheets, supplies and equipment, and the like should be prepared to support and assist learners as they proceed in the learning activities selected for the SLP. Instructional aids can provide a variety of sensory resources and means for learning relevant content.
- *Tailor content to the intended audience.* Content may be tailored by using an instructional level appropriate for the target audience and the established prerequisites for the SLP.
- *Develop content that will be user friendly and interesting to learners.* In writing content for the SLP, use a writing style that is clear, direct, concise, and conversational in tone. Format and lay out the information so that it is easy to read and comprehend. Limit coverage to the essential points necessary for meeting the instructional outcomes. The SLP may also be perceived as less depersonalized if it incorporates some graphics, clip art, and occasional use of humor in its informal presentation of material.[12,66]
- *Arrange the content in a series of small, sequential units.* Segregating the content into brief paragraphs or frames may assist in keeping learners' attention focused on relevant aspects. These units of instruction need to include periodic questions that learners can use for self-assessment of their progress as well as for feedback and reinforcement of learning. The self-assessment questions should review and apply information just presented. Answers for these questions may be located on a subsequent page of the SLP. Include some repetition and summarization of content to review and reinforce learning.

*See references 13, 31, 66, 69, 95, 104, 116.

- *Decide whether the pretest and posttest instrument will use the same or different evaluation items.* For written tests, this decision relates to whether the same test questions will be used in both instances; for performance evaluations, the decision is whether the same or different behaviors will be required of learners in these two instances. Once this decision has been made, design the pre- and posttests for the SLP. These tests need to correlate directly with the instructional outcomes established for the program.

- *Determine the achievement level or passing score required for each evaluation tool.* Passing scores for completion of the SLP may be established according to the relative importance of the information. For example, a passing score of 80% might be used for a SLP related to identifying appropriate support services at that hospital, but a passing score of 95% might be used for a SLP on titrating vasoactive medications. In general, behavioral evaluations of clinical or laboratory performances use an achievement level of virtually 100% for all performance aspects considered critical or essential to acceptable performance.

- *Write an introduction to the SLP.* The introduction explains the relevance, usefulness, and components in the package. Include explanations on how to take, interpret, and act on results of the pretest.

- *Prepare a set of directions for use of the SLP.* Directions should be kept brief, clear, and straightforward so that learners can readily understand how to proceed through the package. When appropriate, include directions on how to secure and use audiovisual or computer hardware and software and any other supplies required in the learning activities. The directions may be most appropriately placed after the introduction to the SLP.

- *Pilot test the SLP.* Solicit comments and critique to validate the design, content, and evaluative elements of the package. Feedback needs to be secured from representatives of the target audience, from individuals with expertise in staff development, and from individuals with expertise in the content area addressed in the SLP. Request input regarding the accuracy, clarity, and sequencing of content, ease of use, clarity of directions as well as the amount of time required to complete the package.

- *Revise the SLP based on results of the pilot test.* Finalize the content, structure, format, and evaluation devices to be used in the SLP.

- *Design a form for learners to evaluate their experience using the SLP.* Areas that might be addressed on the form include learners' appraisals of the SLP's ease of use, clarity, relevance of content, learning activities offered, use of media, usefulness of evaluation devices, and time required for completion. Check to see if learners found the program boring, overwhelming, or distracting or whether it afforded them sufficient practice and reinforcement of learning.[81]

- *Package the SLP for maximal learner convenience.* The program needs to be packaged so that it is as self-contained as possible. All materials, supplies, and instructional aids may be placed in a cardboard box, file box, or—if larger equipment and many supplies are necessary—placed on a cart. Whenever possible, minimize learners' needs to secure SLP materials from other locations and sources.

- *Develop procedures for managing the use of SLPs.* These management responsibilities may include the following:

  Making arrangements for support services such as the audiovisual department and the library to store and provide access to materials

  Developing a system for documenting the results of written pretests and posttests as well as laboratory and/or clinical evaluations

  Monitoring the amount of time learners are using to complete each SLP

  Arranging for location and storage of SLPs in a place accessible to staff on all shifts

  Applying for continuing education unit (CEU) approval of the SLP, if this is desired, and developing a means to document crediting of CEUs to staff

  Duplicating or printing sufficient copies of the SLP for staff use

  Devising a mechanism for maintenance of the SLP over time. This may include replacing worn or damaged components; restocking additional handouts, worksheets, pretests, posttests, and supplies; and maintaining equipment on a regular basis.

  Reviewing, revising, and updating each SLP at defined intervals on an ongoing basis

  Introducing and orienting new and existing staff to the use of SLPs

  Making yourself readily available to staff when they use SLPs: being available to answer questions, resolve and troubleshoot problems, and monitor the effectiveness and efficiency of this teaching method.

Learning Contracts

Many forms of SDL are not mutually exclusive but use multiple avenues for learning. Learning contracts offer learners maximum flexibility in designing and directing their own learning plans.

A *contract* is a formal, binding agreement between two or more individuals or agencies to carry out certain activities within some specified period of time. Although most contracts are written, they may also be verbal. The terms of a contract specify what is to be accomplished, how it will be accomplished, the responsibilities of each party in the agreement, and when these obligations are to be fulfilled. If circumstances affect either party's subsequent ability to meet the terms agreed upon, the contract may be renegotiated.

A *learning contract* is a mutual agreement, usually written and signed, between an educator and a learner that describes the responsibilities of both in relation to the learner's achievement of certain specified learning outcomes. Learning contracts make explicit the terms of the learning plan: what instructional outcomes will be attained, how the learner and educator will participate in the learning process, what instructional resources will be used or made available, which learning activities will be undertaken, how learning will be evaluated, and when the learning experience will be completed.

The potential benefits of a learning contract are many.[37] One of the foremost benefits of a learning contract is its recognition of the adult learner's need to be actively involved in planning, conducting, and evaluating his/her own learning experiences. Learning contracts also afford a means to provide instructional strategies for adults whose learning style preferences tend toward being self-directed, self-paced, self-designed, solitary pursuits of individual learning interests. Adults who respond negatively to teacher-structured and teacher-dominated learning experiences will enjoy the opportunity to control and negotiate their own learning activities.

Learning contracts can vary in the degree of discretion the learner is given in the learning process. At one end of the continuum, learners determine the terms of the contract and the educator concurs with these; at the opposite end, the educator determines the terms of the contract and the learner agrees to these. In between these two extremes, the leaner and educator can mutually negotiate the terms of the contract and mutually agree to these commitments.

As a result of these varying potential arrangements dealing with learning contracts, the role of the educator also changes from the traditional role of direct provider of information to that of advisor, facilitator, resource person, mentor, and/or evaluator of learning. The instructor works with the learner to identify and clarify the intended learning outcomes, to select appropriate instructional activities, to tap instructional resources, to guide the learning process, to help learners resolve any impediments they encounter, and to evaluate the learning experience. A large part of the educator's role involves helping nurses learn how to learn on their own.

The elements in a learning contract may vary somewhat from one facility to another or when the purposes for using the contract differ but typically they resemble the sample provided in Figure 4.1. Most learning contracts, however, include the following elements:

- A general description of the learner's purpose or goal for engaging in the learning process

- An enumeration of the specific learning outcomes to be achieved. These outcomes need to be expressed in behavioral and measurable terms.
- A description of the learning activities and instructional resources that will be used to attain the learning outcomes.
- Identification of the division of mutual responsibilities of the learner and educator in the learning process. The obligations of both need to be specified and clearly distinguished so that each party understands its contribution in the instructional process.
- Specification of the evidence required for indicating attainment of each learning outcome. These evaluative criteria may also include a description of who will be responsible for performing these evaluations: the learner, the instructor, or some other individual(s).
- The time frame within which the terms of the contract are to be met.
- Signatures of the learner and the educator.

Appropriateness for Teaching

Learning contracts may be used for any of the three components of nursing staff development. They are perhaps most often used for orientation and continuing education programs but can be used for in-service offerings as well. In these programs, learning contracts are typically employed in conjunction with other more traditional teaching strategies rather than as a replacement for these. They may also be used to provide alternative, remedial, or supplementary instruction that complements the standard offerings of the staff development department.

When learning contracts are used in orientation programs, the learning outcomes are generally determined by the hospital's established requirements for orientation; however, learners may be given considerable latitude regarding which options they select for attaining those outcomes. This is particularly true for institutions that make multiple learning options (self-paced instruction, self-learning packages, audiovisual programs, computer-assisted instruction, and the like) available to staff. The outcomes for in-service programs are similarly held constant. For continuing education offerings, however, where the learner may be given wide discretion to pursue personal learning interests, the terms and conditions of a learning contract can be completely open to the learner's influence.

Limitations

Some limitations associated with the use of learning contracts include the following:

- Some learners may balk at the expectation that they will have to assume responsibility for planning their own learning experiences. Those whose learning styles prefer more traditional teacher-structured, passive

Learning Contract

Name: _____   Goal: _____

Date: _____   _____

LEARNING OUTCOMES	LEARNING ACTIVITIES	RESPONSIBILITIES LEARNER / EDUCATOR		EVALUATION CRITERIA	TARGET DATE

Signatures: _____   _____
                                Educator   Employee

Renegotiation date(s):

Figure 4.1 Learning contract.

learning may be particularly resistant to the use of this teaching strategy.

- Learners may be unfamiliar with the process of contracting for learning. These individuals may require some preliminary explanation of what a learning contract is and how the contracting process works.
- Learners may not be adept in fulfilling the terms of a learning contract. Those who lack self-direction and motivation for completing their commitments for learning may require guidance, support, and encouragement to persist in progressing toward their goals.
- Instructors may not be familiar or experienced in using this teaching strategy effectively and may find their altered role somewhat ill defined.
- Instructors may find that the use of learning contracts increases the time requirements for monitoring and managing the instructional process.
- Educators may resist giving up control over the teaching-learning process and find their facilitator role less satisfying and more difficult to organize.

Guidelines for Use

The following procedural steps may be helpful when learning contracts are used as a teaching device:

- Verify that the learner understands what a learning contract is and how the contract process operates
- Assist the learner in identifying the goal or purpose for instituting the learning contract
- Work with the learner to define the instructional outcomes to be achieved by the learning contract
- Develop a plan for instruction that includes the activities that the learner wishes to undertake, the instructional resources that will be made available, and the division of responsibilities for the learner and educator in this process
- Negotiate with the learner to establish a target date for attainment of each learning outcome
- Mutually determine the criteria that will be employed for evaluating attainment of each learning outcome
- Determine the conditions under which the terms of the contract can be renegotiated and the degree of latitude that exists
- Designate how and when the learner's progress toward achievement of the learning outcomes will be monitored
- Provide an opportunity for the learner to evaluate the learning contract experience

This chapter has described the general features of how nursing staff development programs are implemented: the principles that guide program implementation as well as the teaching methods employed in providing instruction. Chapter 5 addresses the common features involved in the last phase of the educational process, program evaluation.

REFERENCES

1. Abruzzese RA: *Nursing staff development,* St Louis, 1992, Mosby–Year Book.
2. Ad Hoc Committee on Nontraditional Study of Self-Directed Learning: *Self-directed continuing education in nursing,* Kansas City, MO, 1978, American Nurses Association.
3. Alspach JG: How to prepare a lecture presentation, *Focus Crit Care* 9(3):27, 1982.
4. Alspach JG: *The self-directed learning readiness of baccalaureate nursing students,* doctoral dissertation, College Park, 1991, University of Maryland.
5. Armstrong ML, Toebe DM, Watson MR: Strengthening the instructional role in self-directed learning activities, *J Cont Educ Nurs* 16: 75, 1985.
6. Arndt MJ, Underwood B: Learning style theory and patient education, *J Cont Educ Nurs* 21:28, 1990.
7. Ballard A: Getting started: instructional methods, *J Nurs Staff Develop* 7:42, 1991.
8. Benner P: *From novice to expert,* Menlo Park, CA, 1984, Addison-Wesley.
9. Benner P: From novice to expert, *Am J Nurs* 82:402, 1982.
10. Benner P, Wrubel J: Skilled clinical knowledge: the value of perceptual awareness, *Nurs Educ* 7(3):11, 1982.
11. Bennett NL: Theories of adult development for continuing education, *J Cont Educ Health Prof* 10:167, 1990.
12. Benschoter RA, Hays BJ, Jackson AJ et al: Adapting an established curriculum to the self-instructional format: rationale and process, *J Cont Educ Health Prof* 11(1):43, 1991.
13. Boss LAS: How to prepare self-instructional programs for critical care staff education, *Dimens Crit Care Nurs* 4:246, 1985.
14. Brookfield S: Self-directed adult learning: a critical paradigm, *Adult Educ Q* 35:59, 1984.
15. Brookfield S: *Understanding and facilitating adult learning,* San Francisco, 1986, Jossey-Bass.
16. Brookfield S: Why can't I get this right? Myths and realities in facilitating adult learning, *Adult Learning* 3(6):12, 1992.
17. Brooks B: Self-learning: an approach to cost-effective staff development, *J Cont Educ Nurs* 16:165, 1985.
18. Bruner J: *Towards a theory of instruction,* New York, 1968, Norton.
19. Bynum MM, Rosenblatt N: Self-study: boon or bust? *Training* 21(11):61, 1984.
20. Cervero RM: *Effective continuing education for professionals,* San Francisco, 1988, Jossey-Bass.
21. Cochenour C: Self-learning packages in staff development, *J Nurs Staff Develop* 8:123, 1992.
22. Cooper SS: Methods of teaching revisited: case method, *J Cont Educ Nurs* 12(5):32, 1981.
23. Cooper SS: Methods of teaching revisited: the incident process, *J Cont Educ Nurs* 12(6):22, 1981.
24. Cooper SS: Some teaching dos and dont's, *J Cont Educ Nurs* 20:140, 1989.
25. Crancer J, Maury-Hess S: Games: an alternative to pedagogical instruction, *J Nurs Educ* 19(3):45, 1980.
26. Cranston CM, McCort B: A learner analysis experiment: cognitive style versus learning style in undergraduate nursing education, *J Nurs Educ* 24:136, 1985.
27. Cranton P: *Planning instruction for adult learners,* Toronto, 1989, Wall & Thompson.
28. Cross KP: *Adults as learners: increasing participation and facilitating learning,* San Francisco, 1984, Jossey-Bass.
29. Dailey MA: Developing case studies, *Nurs Educ* 17(3):8, 1992.
30. Darkenwald GG, Merriam SB: *Adult education: foundations of practice,* New York, 1982, Harper & Row.
31. deTornyay R, Thompson MA: *Strategies for teaching nursing,* ed 3, New York, 1987, John Wiley.

32. Dewey J: *Democracy and education,* New York, 1916, Macmillan.
33. Draper DO, Young W: Continuing education for athletic trainers based on learning style research, *J Cont Educ Health Prof* 9:193, 1989.
34. Duke ES: A taxonomy of games and simulations for nursing education, *J Nurs Educ* 25:197, 1986.
35. Dunn R, Dunn K: How to diagnose learning styles, *Instructor* 87:123, 1977.
36. Dyche J: *Educational program development,* Calabasas, CA, 1982, Tri-Oak Education.
37. Eagleton B: Contract learning, *Focus Crit Care* 11(6):19, 1984.
38. Eagleton B: *Learning styles and locus of control of critical care nurses,* doctoral dissertation, Kansas City, 1984, Kansas State University.
39. Eagleton BB: The teaching-learning process. In Alspach JG, editor: *Instructor's resource manual for the AACN core curriculum for critical care nursing,* Philadelphia, 1992, WB Saunders.
40. Eason FR, Corbett RW: Effective teacher characteristics identified by adult learners in nursing, *J Cont Educ Nurs* 22:21, 1991.
41. Ehrhardt HB: Utilization of cognitive style in the clinical laboratory sciences, *Am J Med Technol* 49:569, 1983.
42. Espersen S, Barber C: Learning labs: critical care, *Dimens Crit Care Nurs* 5:117, 1986.
43. Evans ML: Simulations: their selection and use in developing nursing competencies, *J Nurs Staff Develop* 5:65, 1989.
44. Everson L, Kasuboski L: Creative teaching strategies for mandatory classes: team teaching with Trivial Pursuit, *J Nurs Staff Develop* 6:147, 1990.
45. Farley JK: Methods of teaching: the lecture, *Nurs Educ* 15(2):5, 1990.
46. Farley JK: The seminar, *Nurs Educ* 15(4):3, 1990.
47. Ferrell B: Attitudes toward learning styles and self-direction of ADN students, *J Nurs Educ* 17(2):19, 1978.
48. Freitas L, Lantz J, Reed R: The creative teacher, *Nurs Educ* 16(1):5, 1991.
49. Gagne RM: *The conditions of learning,* ed 3, New York, 1977, Holt, Rinehart & Winston.
50. Garity J: Learning styles: basis for creative teaching and learning, *Nurs Educ* 10(2):12, 1985.
51. Gaston C: Self-learning packages: another tool of educators, *Health-care Educ Dateline* August 3, 1990.
52. Geissler EM: Teaching the dynamics of effective oral presentations, *J Nurs Educ* 26:87, 1987.
53. Gentine M: Methods of teaching revisited: self-learning packages, *J Cont Educ Nurs* 11(3):57, 1980.
54. Georges JC: Why soft-skills training doesn't take, *Training* 25(4):42, 1988.
55. Gohring RJ: All in the game, *Discovery* 3:20, 1979.
56. Gomez GE, Gomez EA: Learning of psychomotor skills: laboratory versus patient care setting, *J Nurs Educ* 26(1):20, 1987.
57. Gordon J, Zemke R: The creativity jargon jungle, *Training* 23(5):30, 1986.
58. Greenblat C, Duke R: *Principles and practices of gaming-simulation,* Beverly Hills, CA, 1981, Sage Publications.
59. Gregoric AF: *An adult's guide to style,* Maynard, MA, 1982, Gabriel Systems, Inc.
60. Gruending DL, Fenty D, Hogan T: Fun and games in nursing staff development, *J Cont Educ Nurs* 22:259, 1991.
61. Haggard A: *Hospital orientation handbook,* Rockville, MD, 1984, Aspen Publishers.
62. Hallal JC, Welsh MD: Using the competency laboratory to learn psychomotor skills, *Nurs Educ* 9(1):34, 1984.
63. Hamilton L, Gregor F: Self-directed learning in a critical care nursing program, *J Cont Educ Nurs* 17:94, 1986.
64. Hanna DR: Using simulations to teach clinical nursing, *Nurs Educ* 16(2):28, 1991.
65. Hartsock JM, Lange RL: Trivia games: stimulating student learning, *Nurs Educ* 12(1):24, 1987.
66. Hast AS: Self-learning packages in critical care, *Crit Care Nurse* 7(2):110, 1987.
67. Heinrich KT, Gladstone C: Orientation programs for nurse-adult learners: fostering a sense of community, *Nurse Educ* 17(1):8, 1992.
68. Higgins MG: Learning style assessment: a new patient teaching tool? *J Nurs Staff Develop* 4:14, 1988.
69. Hinthorne R: Methods of teaching revisited: self-instructional modules, *J Cont Educ Nurs* 11(4):37, 1980.
70. Hodson K: Cognitive style and the behavioral differences of nursing students in the clinical setting, *J Nurs Educ* 24(2):58, 1985.
71. Hodson K: Photographs as organizational aids for the skill laboratory, *Nurs Educ* 10(3):28, 1985.
72. Horne RE, Cleaves A: *Guide to simulation/games for education and training,* ed 4, New York, 1980, Sage Publications.
73. Jackson BS, Gosnell-Moses D: Cognitive style: a guide for selecting teaching strategies for learners in critical care, *Crit Care Q* 7(1):18, 1984.
74. Jiricka MK, Knauss P, Malan SS et al, editors: *Critical care orientation: a guide to the process,* Newport Beach, CA, 1987, American Association of Critical Care Nurses.
75. Johnson J, Purvis J: Case studies: an alternative learning/teaching method in nursing, *J Nurs Educ* 26(3):118, 1987.
76. Joos IR: A teacher's guide for using games and simulations, *Nurs Educ* 9(3):25, 1984.
77. Kelly H: Case method training: what it is, how it works, *Training* 20(2):46, 1983.
78. Kidd JR: *How adults learn,* New York, 1973, Association Press.
79. Kissinger J, Munjas B: Predictors of student success, *Nurs Outlook* 30:53, 1984.
80. Kleinknecht MK, Hefferin EA: Maximizing nursing staff development: the learning laboratory, *J Nurs Staff Develop* 6:219, 1990.
81. Knopke HJ, Diekelmann NL: *Approaches to teaching in the health sciences,* Reading, MA, 1978, Addison-Wesley.
82. Knowles MS: *Andragogy in action,* San Francisco, 1984, Jossey-Bass.
83. Knowles MS: *The modern practice of adult education: from pedagogy to andragogy,* ed 2, New York, 1980, Cambridge.
84. Kolb DA: *Experiential learning: experience as the source of learning and development,* Englewood Cliffs, NJ, 1984, Prentice Hall.
85. Kolb DA: *Learning style inventory,* Boston, 1985, McBer & Company.
86. Kreider M: *An investigation of the relationship of perceptual field independence-dependence, the mode of representation used in instruction, and the ability to recognize signs of nutritional deficiency,* doctoral dissertation, College Park, 1976, University of Maryland.
87. Laird D, House RS: How to turn bystanders into role players, *Training* 21(4):41, 1984.
88. Lewis DJ, Saydak SJ, Mierzwa IP et al: Gaming: a teaching strategy for adult learners, *J Cont Educ Nurs* 20:80, 1989.
89. Lowenstein AJ, Bradshaw M: Seminar methods for RN to BSN students, *Nurs Educ* 14(5):27, 1989.
90. Margolis FH, Bell CR: How to break the news that you're breaking them into small groups, *Training* 22(3):81, 1985.
91. Mast ME, Van Atta MJ: Applying adult learning principles in instructional module design, *Nurs Educ* 11(1):35, 1986.
92. Mays B: An investigation of the cognitive styles of 76 associate degree medical laboratory technology students, *Am J Med Technol* 49:719, 1983.
93. McDonald GF: The simulation clinical laboratory, *Nurs Outlook* 35:290, 1987.
94. Mezirow J: A critical theory of learning and education, *Adult Educ* 32:3, 1981.
95. Miller PJ: Developing self-learning packages, *J Nurs Staff Develop* 5:73, 1989.
96. Nielsen BB: Applying andragogy in nursing continuing education, *J Cont Educ Nurs* 20:86, 1989.
97. O'Connor CT: Brief: evaluation of a modular method of cardiopulmonary resuscitation instruction, *J Cont Educ Nurs* 21:271, 1990.

98. Oermann MH: Psychomotor skill development, *J Cont Educ Nurs* 21:202, 1990.

99. Ostmoe P, VanHoozen H, Scheffel AL et al: Learning style preferences and selection of learning strategies: considerations and implications for nurse educators, *J Nurs Educ* 23:27, 1984.

100. Ostrow CL: The interaction of cognitive style, teaching methodology and cumulative GPA in baccalaureate nursing students, *J Cont Educ Nurs* 25:148, 1986.

101. Partridge R: Learning styles: a review of selected models, *J Nurs Educ* 22:243, 1983.

102. Pigors P, Pigors F: The incident process—a method of inquiry, *Nurs Outlook* 14(10):50, 1966.

103. Plunkett EJ, Olivieri RJ: A strategy for introducing diagnostic reasoning: hypothesis testing using a simulation approach, *Nurs Educ* 14(6):27, 1989.

104. Pritchett LA: Developing independent study units, *Dimens Crit Care Nurs* 2:371, 1983.

105. Prociuk JL: Self-directed learning and nursing orientation programs: are they compatible? *J Cont Educ Nurs* 21:252, 1990.

106. Puetz BE: *Continuing education in nursing,* Rockville, MD, 1987, Aspen Publishers.

107. Puetz BE: Responding to changing times: converting a seminar to self-study, *J Healthcare Educ Training* 4(3):18, 1990.

108. Raudonis BM: Adult education: its implications for baccalaureate nursing education, *J Nurs Educ* 26:164, 1987.

109. Resko D: Self-learning in critical care: a debate, *Dimens Crit Care Nurs* 10:230, 1991.

110. Rezler AG: *Learning preference inventory,* Chicago, 1974, University of Illinois Center for Educational Development.

111. Rezler A, French R: Preferences of students in six allied health professions, *J Allied Health* 4:20, 1975.

112. Rezler A, Rezmovic V: The learning preference inventory, *J Allied Health* 10:28, 1981.

113. Rogers C: *Freedom to learn,* Columbus, OH, 1969, Charles E. Merrill.

114. Rosenthal KA: Multimethod teaching modules, *Dimens Crit Care Nurs* 8:310, 1989.

115. Rufo KL: Effectiveness of self-instructional packages in staff development activities, *J Cont Educ Nurs* 16(3):80, 1985.

116. Schmidt KL, Fisher JC: Effective development and utilization of self-learning modules, *J Cont Educ Nurs* 23(2):54, 1992.

117. Schoessler M, Yount S, Marshall D et al: Brief: Safety First—a board game for safety education, *J Cont Educ Nurs* 22:263, 1991.

118. Sisson PM, Becker LM: Using games in nursing education, *J Nurs Staff Develop* 4:146, 1988.

119. Skurski V: Interactive clinical conferences: nursing rounds and education imagery, *J Nurs Educ* 24:166, 1985.

120. Sparber AG: Brief: putting fun into continuing education—creating a disaster medical board game, *J Cont Educ Nurs* 21:274, 1990.

121. Stadsklev R: *Handbook of simulation gaming in social education,* Birmingham, AL, 1979, University of Alabama Institute of Higher Education Research and Services.

122. Strader MK: Guidelines for a first lecture, *Nurs Educ* 12(1):34, 1987.

123. Surplus SH: Overcoming role-play resistance, *Training* 20(12):93, 1983.

124. Szarek E: 16 Ways to save time in the classroom, *Training* 20(5):67,10, 1983.

125. Thompson JF: *Using role playing in the classroom,* Bloomington, IN, 1978, Phi Delta Kappa Educational Foundation.

126. Utz SW: *A study of field-dependent/field-independent cognitive traits and the critical skills involved in decision making,* doctoral dissertation, 1979, University of Southern California, *Diss Abstracts Int* 40: 707A, 1981.

127. VanVoorhees C, Wolf FM, Gruppen LD et al: Learning styles and continuing medical education, *J Cont Educ Health Prof* 8: 257, 1988.

128. Yoder RE: Another look at case studies, *J Cont Educ Nurs* 21:276, 1990.

129. Ward LD: Warm fuzzies vs. hard facts: four styles of adult learning, *Training,* 20(11):31, 1983.

130. Werner-McCullough M, L'Orange C: Putting "oomph" into clinical conferences, *Nurs Educ* 10(6):33, 1985.

131. Whitis G: Simulation in teaching clinical nursing, *J Nurs Educ* 24: 161, 1985.

132. Williams J: The mobile educational crash cart: self-directed learning supplement that meets staff needs, *J Cont Educ Nurs* 17:59, 1986.

133. Witkin HA, Goodenough DR: *Cognitive styles: essence and origins of field independence and field dependence,* New York, 1982, International Universities Press.

134. Witkin HA, Goodenough DR, Carp SA: Stability of cognitive style from childhood to adulthood, *J Personal Soc Psychol* 7:291, 1967.

135. Witkin HA, Moore CA, Goodenough DR et al: Field-dependent and field-independent cognitive styles and their educational implications, *Rev Educ Res* 47:1(1), 1977.

136. Wolkenheim BJ: Games that teach: a practical approach, *J Nurs Staff Develop* 6(1):45, 1990.

137. Zuckerman D, Horne RE: *The guide to simulations/games for education and training,* Lexington, MA, 1973, Massachusetts Information Resources.

CHAPTER 5

Program Evaluation

As discussed in Chapter 1, the ultimate goal of nursing staff development is the provision of quality patient care. The evaluation phase of the educational process enables the educator to determine the extent to which this far-reaching goal has been attained.

DEFINITION OF EVALUATION

Evaluation is the process by which a judgment is made concerning the relative value of something. It is a process that considers the various components of an endeavor and then ascribes some qualitative assessment to each of those components. The aim of evaluation is not merely arriving at the value judgments but, rather, using these appraisals as a basis for subsequent decision-making about the endeavor.

For evaluation to be useful in decision-making related to educational programs, it must be fortified by an orderly, comprehensive, and educationally sound appraisal mechanism. Educational evaluations are helpful to the educator when they afford valid, dependable, timely, and meaningful information needed to make decisions about the program. Evaluation of a nursing staff development program provides value judgments about each major component of the program so that decisions can be made for improving each of these elements.

FUNCTIONS OF EVALUATION

The evaluation process can render numerous useful and important functions. Some of the potential functions of educational evaluation include its ability to do the following:

- Determine whether instructional outcomes were attained
- Motivate and positively reinforce learning
- Diagnose the nature and extent of learning problems
- Offer both positive and constructive feedback to learners
- Identify areas in need of remedial instruction
- Determine the effectiveness of various teaching methods
- Provide direction for subsequent program planning, development, and implementation
- Improve the effectiveness and/or efficiency of instruction
- Justify continuation, expansion, or discontinuation of specific offerings or courses
- Provide a mechanism for quality monitoring and improvement in educational offerings
- Enable the program to meet accreditation and continuing education unit approval requirements

To understand how these functions might be accomplished, the educator first needs to consider the full spectrum of what program evaluation encompasses.

OVERVIEW OF PROGRAM EVALUATION

The various elements of a nursing staff development program can be viewed as a dynamic system of interrelated parts that, individually and collectively, contribute to quality patient care. Using the terminology of systems theory, these components include the input, throughput, and output of the staff development program.[5] A comprehensive evaluation of the staff development program will enable the educator to make value judgments related to each of these components.

COMPONENTS OF PROGRAM EVALUATION

Input

The input to a nursing staff development program includes all elements existing prior to the instructional process that may influence the outcomes of instruction. These antecedents of instruction include both the educational and administrative contexts within which instruction will be provided. Some examples of **educational** input elements include the following:

- Stated beliefs and values: mission and philosophy of staff development
- Staff development program goals, objectives, and priorities
- Learner characteristics
- Faculty qualifications

Examples of **administrative** input elements include:

- Organizational structure for staff development
- Administrative policies and procedures related to staff development
- Available resources: staff, facilities, budget, time, and materials
- Internal and/or external marketing of program offerings

Although these elements are not subject to frequent change, each needs to be reviewed and critiqued at predetermined intervals to ensure that the environment they afford for the educational process contributes to the attainment of employee and agency needs and priorities.[2]

Throughput

The throughput of an educational program includes all facets of the process that delivers instruction to learners. In a nursing staff development program, this entails a series of transactions among educators, learners, and others that occurs throughout all four phases of the educational process.

In order to appraise throughput, the procedures, tools, and outcomes of each phase of the educational process need to be evaluated at regular intervals to determine their usefulness and effectiveness in the program. Some examples of throughput evaluation elements include the following:

- Scope and depth of learning needs assessment
- Changes in priorities among learning needs
- Clarity and accuracy in statement of instructional outcomes
- Appropriate selection and sequencing of content
- Allotment of instructional time
- Quality of instructional media
- Effectiveness of program faculty
- Efficiency of teaching methods
- Usefulness of evaluation tools[9,12,14]

Output

The output of a nursing staff development program includes all of the results or outcomes that are attributable to the program. These results encompass both intended and unintended outcomes.

The scope, cost, difficulty, frequency, and time frame of output evaluations may vary widely. Many educators reflect this diversity by distinguishing various levels of output evaluation.* A description of these evaluation levels follows.

LEVELS OF EVALUATION

Satisfaction

The lowest level of output appraisal evaluates learners' *satisfaction* with offerings in the program. This reaction form (or "happiness index") affords participants an opportunity to indicate the degree to which they were satisfied with elements such as the content, instructors, course materials, teaching methods, audiovisuals, facility, location, refreshments, and attainment of their personal objectives for attending the offering. Although they do not provide any indication of learning, satisfaction measures are easy to design, complete, and tabulate and afford a general indication of learners' overall contentment with the educational experience and learning environment. These are especially relevant features when working with adult learners; if adults perceive that their time and efforts were well spent in learning and that their personal and professional needs were met, their learning may be more effective and transfer more readily to the work setting. Simerly[41] offers numerous tips for designing tools to evaluate learner satisfaction.

Learning

The second level of output appraisal evaluates whether *learning* has occurred. Instead of merely soliciting learners' subjective opinions and reactions, this level of evaluation

---

*See references 1, 7, 16, 23-25, 27, 29.

seeks to objectively determine whether the instructional outcomes established for the program were attained. The elements included in this level of evaluation are changes in the learners' cognitive, affective, and/or psychomotor behavior.

Learning may be evaluated both before and after the instructional process or only following instruction. The former approach is used when the educator wishes to compare learners' entry and exit capabilities in relation to a specific educational offering. In staff development programs, the nature and extent of learning typically entails important aspects related to job performance. Evaluation of learning is a necessary facet of all nursing staff development programs.

Application

A third level of output appraisal evaluates learners' *application* of learning in the work setting. In a nursing staff development program, this level of evaluation seeks to determine whether learning acquired in classroom, laboratory, and clinical settings has been integrated and transferred over time to the nurse's daily practice in the clinical setting. Evidence of lasting changes in nursing practice that reflect integration of the acquired knowledge, attitudes, and skills are sought here. Until learning is transferred to the work setting, no changes or improvements in nursing practice or patient care can be made.[37] Because this level of educational evaluation examines outcomes in nursing practice, it may be integrated with the hospital's quality improvement program.

Impact

The highest level of output appraisal evaluates the *impact* of the educational program on the organization and its clients. In a nursing staff development program, impact evaluation seeks to determine whether the program has effected improvements in patient care or in various concerns of the healthcare agency. Appraisals at this level might include elements such as length of stay, incidence of complications, patient satisfaction, mortality rates, readmission rates, accreditation results, productivity, and the like. In general, impact evaluations extend appraisals beyond the boundaries of the educational program to its effects on the system as a whole.[49]

MODEL OF PROGRAM EVALUATION

Evaluation models are sometimes used to assist educators in designing and implementing the evaluation plan for an educational program. Figure 5.1 represents a program evaluation model that incorporates the elements discussed thus far as well as various features of other currently existing evaluation models.[1,29,34,40,43-46]

In viewing the four levels of output evaluation in this model, the educator should keep in mind that success at one level of output evaluation is no guarantee of success at the next higher level.[23] Even though learners might be thoroughly satisfied with all aspects of the program, written tests and learner demonstrations of skills may well reveal that little or no learning occurred as a result of the program.

In addition, educators need to remember that, as has been mentioned earlier, the scope, difficulty, cost, frequency, and timeframes of output evaluation vary significantly from one level to another. The *scope* of output evaluation increases progressively from the lowest to the highest levels of appraisal. This means that evaluations of learner satisfaction afford the most narrow and limited scope of appraisal while impact evaluation offers the most broad and far-reaching critique. In a similar manner, the *cost* and *difficulty* of evaluation rise with each successively higher level of evaluation. Designing, conducting, and tabulating satisfaction/reaction forms can be accomplished with a minimum expenditure of money, time, and effort by even novice educators; the design and validation of learning and application instruments requires considerably more time (and, therefore, cost) and expertise; development of impact evaluation tools and procedures may demand that outside consultants be paid to supplement local staff and resources. In part due to these factors, the *frequency* of output evaluation is *inversely* related to the level of evaluation. Although virtually all staff development programs include appraisal of learner satisfaction and most incorporate evaluation of learning, far fewer include evaluation of application and very few provide impact evaluation. In addition, the *timeframes* for these appraisals are quite different: satisfaction and learning evaluations are secured during or immediately following instruction. By contrast, evaluations of application are typically performed some weeks to months after instruction and impact evaluations may not be completed for months or years following the program. The short- vs. long-term appraisals are dictated by the nature of the evaluative information sought and when this information would be most readily available.

In summary, then, Figure 5.1 illustrates a comprehensive program evaluation model for nursing staff development. Input components need periodic appraisal at regular intervals, and throughput components require ongoing appraisals for each offering in the program as well as for the program as a whole. Output component evaluation should always include evaluation of satisfaction and learning levels and, as resources allow, incorporate periodic appraisals for application to practice and organizational impact.

The latter section of this chapter will describe the primary focus of evaluation for nursing staff development programs—the evaluation of learning. Many pertinent considerations for evaluation of application to nursing practice can be found in the discussions related to competency-

Program Evaluation Model

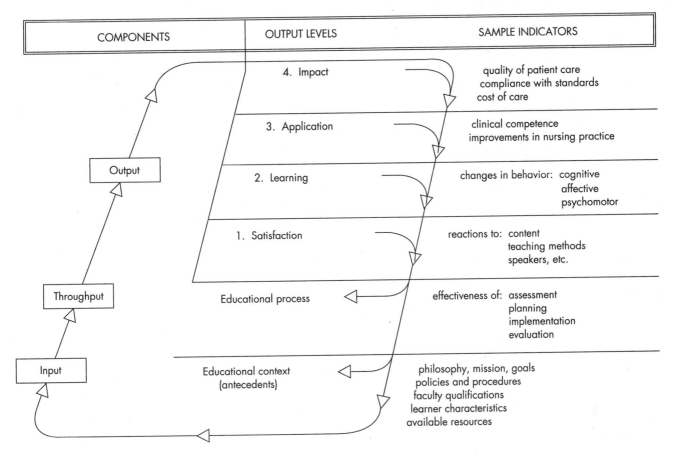

Figure 5.1   Program evaluation model.

based education in Chapter 6. Educators might also consider the extent to which salient aspects of evaluation for organizational impact could be incorporated within the staff development department's quality improvement process (covered in Chapter 8).

PARTICIPANTS IN THE EVALUATION PROCESS

Although educators may bear the greatest responsibility for evaluating nursing staff development programs, the evaluation phase of the educational process needs to be shared with many other individuals and groups. In general, everyone who is affected by any aspect of the program needs to be provided with an opportunity to participate in appraising that program so that their unique perspective is considered. From a practical point of view, the more inclusive and encompassing the evaluative input is, the more likely that the resulting conclusions and decisions will be accurate and complete.[4,38-39,42]

Obtaining an accurate appraisal of an educational program entails identification of individuals and groups who:

- Are in the best position to supply certain categories of information
- Have assisted in designing and planning the program
- Represent the learners in the program
- Represent the instructors for the program
- Represent the logistical, operational, staff, or financial support for the program
- Use the evaluative data for making decisions regarding past and future programming
- Will be directly or indirectly affected by the evaluations

The number of groups and individuals who participate in program evaluation and the exact composition of this group will depend on the scope and purposes established for the evaluation. Some suggested participants for the evaluation phase of nursing staff development programs include the groups listed in Box 5.1.

Box 5.1

PARTICIPANTS IN THE EVALUATION PROCESS

- Program director and educational staff
- Program participants: learners and their peers
- Program faculty: instructors, preceptors, clinical nurse specialists, and others as appropriate
- Staff nurses
- Administrators: unit, nursing department, hospital (when appropriate)
- Resource and support personnel:
  Clerical staff
  Professional staff (audiovisual, budgetary, public relations, marketing, human resource department, as appropriate)
- Advisory committee members (when appropriate)

TIMING OF EVALUATIONS

The optimal number, frequency, and occurrence of evaluations are determined primarily by the purpose for performing the appraisal and by the type of decisions and information sought. In general, evaluations should be performed as follows:

- Frequently enough to detect significant changes over time in the variables assessed
- At the times most likely to provide the information sought for necessary decisions
- In sufficient number to provide an adequate sampling of the outcomes established for the program
- With a sufficient variety of different methods to overcome the inherently limited validity, reliability, and scope of any one evaluation tool

Evaluations may be categorized into three major types on the basis of when they are performed. These three categories are preinstructional, formative, and summative evaluation.

PREINSTRUCTIONAL EVALUATION

Preinstructional evaluation is employed to measure learners' knowledge, attitudes, and/or skills before the provision of instruction. This category of evaluation is typically used either to determine if learners have the prerequisite knowledge, attitudes and skills necessary for instruction[27] or to establish a basis of comparison with evaluation(s) done following instruction. Although securing a baseline of learner capabilities is often helpful to verify learning that can rightfully be attributed to educational offerings, in many instances it may not be feasible because of limited access to learners, the cost and time involved, or other logistical constraints. An additional use of preinstructional evaluation occurs when challenge mechanisms are employed to determine whether learners can already meet the instructional outcomes of a particular program. If the evaluation reveals that some or all of these outcomes can be demonstrated, instruction in those areas can be bypassed.

FORMATIVE EVALUATION

Formative evaluation refers to appraisals that are conducted throughout the implementation phase of the educational process. The purpose of formative evaluation is to monitor the ongoing operational processes of teaching, learning, and related management and support activities in order to enhance the efficiency and/or effectiveness of these operations. Formative evaluations are usually dynamic and often informal, spontaneous and immediate in effect, sensitive to discrete incidents, and limited in the sphere of decisions they influence. The primary value of this type of evaluation is its ability to detect areas needing modification, revision, or improvement and to make necessary corrective adjustments that will resolve problems expeditiously before the program has been completed. To be most effective, formative evaluation should be a combination of systematically planned checkpoints together with informal mechanisms to continually monitor and minimize problems. The majority of formative evaluation data should be searched for rather than stumbled on.

Examples of formative evaluations include the following:

- Tests administered during a course to identify the areas or reasons for learning difficulties
- Periodic meetings with preceptors to determine their perception of how the new graduate orientation program is progressing
- Quizzes administered at the end of small subdivisions of the course to verify understanding before progressing to the next unit of study
- Self-assessments that learners complete to provide them with ongoing feedback on their progress and to uncover the need for remedial instruction or review

SUMMATIVE EVALUATION

In contrast to the ongoing focus of formative evaluation, *summative evaluation* has a terminal focus. Rather than concentrating on the unfolding educational process, summative evaluations examine the ultimate outcomes and final products of the program. In so doing, this type of evaluation affords a synopsis of the overall or net results of an educational program. Summative evaluations are directed at effecting improvements and necessary revisions in subsequent rather than current programming activities. The conclusions reached in these final judgments are usually more static and formal, more anticipated and thoroughly planned, less timely in their immediate effects on the program but more far-reaching in the decisions they influence. Because they incorporate data from numerous sources, summative evaluations generate the information needed to make major decisions regarding the program: whether it will be offered again, how much funding it will receive, which design elements will be modified and to what degree, which new procedures will be instituted, and the like.

Some examples of summative evaluation include the following:

- Comprehensive written or performance examinations aimed at determining successful completion of a course
- Certification or credentialing appraisals that determine whether a nurse may perform specific functions in an expanded role
- Questionnaires designed to solicit appraisals of a program from providers, learners, and support staff perspectives
- Budget reports that tabulate the cost-effectiveness of an educational offering

To direct the educational and administrative decision-making processes effectively, evaluations need to be incorporated into an organized schedule of assessments that coincide with the availability of useful information and the sequence of events being monitored. Neither formative nor summative evaluation alone is sufficient; each must be planned to complement the other if all phases of the program are to benefit maximally.

ELEMENTS OF EVALUATION

In the evaluation of nursing staff development programs, two primary elements are considered: effectiveness and efficiency. An educational program's *effectiveness* relates to whether the program achieves its intended instructional outcomes. An educational program's *efficiency* relates to the amount of resources that need to be expended to achieve those outcomes. Of these two elements, program effectiveness is more important: if an educational program fails to achieve the desired outcomes for which it was designed, its resource requirements are a somewhat moot is-

sue. In these days of budget reductions and staff downsizing, however, the necessity of maximizing program efficiency has gained increased importance.

Since program effectiveness is rooted in attainment of the instructional outcomes, the primary means of determining effectiveness is accomplished by evaluation of learning. Program efficiency, on the other hand, is determined by analysis and calculation of the resource costs of the program. Resource costs include expenditures for items such as staff salary and benefits, development and provision time, overhead, materials, clerical costs, instructional aids, and the like, which are incurred in relation to the program. The remainder of this chapter will be devoted to the evaluation of program effectiveness. Considerations related to program efficiency will be described in discussions on program budgets in Chapter 8.

EVALUATION OF LEARNING

In order to determine whether the cognitive, affective, and psychomotor outcomes sought for the educational offerings within a program were attained, the educator needs to be familiar with the steps involved in the evaluation process, the nomenclature used in educational measurement, and the benchmarks of educational measurement. Once these fundamentals are understood, the educator can then apply this information to evaluation of learning within each of the instructional domains.

STEPS IN THE EVALUATION PROCESS

There are four steps in the evaluation process: measurement, comparison, appraisal, and decision.

Measurement

Measurement determines the amount, extent, magnitude, capacity, or degree to which some characteristic or attribute is present in some object or person. A nurse, for example, may be interested in measuring a patient's body weight or blood pressure. Measurement is the core of evaluation because it provides the raw data necessary to make an informed appraisal. Measurement is a quantitative assessment that passes no judgment on the data collected.

Comparison

In order for a measurement to be amenable to interpretation, it must be viewed in relation to some common reference point that serves as a standard or criterion for *comparison*. In the second step of the evaluation process, measurements are compared to some agreed on standard of comparison that affords a meaningful context for appraising that measurement. For example, a measurement of body weight might result in the data "150." In order for nurses to interpret this data, they need to know whether the context or standard for comparison is pounds or kilograms. Measurement, then, incorporates observations with respect to some agreed on standard for that measurement (such as body weight measurements for drug dosage calculated in kilograms vs. pounds).

Appraisal

The third step in the evaluation process combines the first two steps and makes an *appraisal* of the measurement relative to the agreed on standard. For example, the measurement of 150 could be appraised as either "150 pounds" or as "70 kilograms." In this step the evaluator is interested in whether the measurement taken matches the selected standard for comparison: for this patient, what does 150 pounds or 70 kilograms imply?

Decision

The last step of the evaluation process involves making a *decision* regarding the appraisal reached in the preceding step. Unlike measurements, the decisions reached in this phase of evaluation constitute value judgments made on the data. Thus a nurse might decide that a patient's body weight of 70 kilograms represents an "ideal weight" for her adolescent male patient but is grossly underweight for a patient who normally weighs 95 kilograms and considerably overweight for a child. Although the measurement was the same, the nurse's decision regarding the suitability of that weight for different patient weight standards might vary considerably.

When the educator is interested in determining whether **cognitive** outcomes have been attained, *measurements* are typically derived by using the learner's responses to written test items (such as true/false items, multiple choice items, and the like). The learner's responses or answers to these test items are then *compared* to the correct or desired answers contained in the answer key for the test. The educator then *appraises* the learner's answer to determine if it matches the correct or desired answer and makes a *decision* regarding that appraisal (usually by giving the learner a designated number of points or credit for correct answers and deducting points or credit for incorrect or unacceptable answers).

The evaluation process works in a comparable way when the educator is interested in determining if **affective** or **psychomotor** outcomes have been attained. In these instances, *measurements* are usually derived by observations of the learner's performance in simulated or actual clinical situations. These samples of the learner's behavior are then *compared* to the desired or expected performance in that situation. These behavioral expectations might exist in the form of written performance criteria, unit procedures, protocols, or standards of nursing practice. Regardless of their form, they constitute the standard for comparison of the learner's behavior in that situation. The educator then *appraises* the learner's behavior to determine if it matches the desired performance and then makes a *decision* regarding the acceptability of that performance.

TERMS USED IN EDUCATIONAL MEASUREMENT

Educational measurement involves both the construction of one or more measuring devices and the provision of opportunities for learners to demonstrate that they have attained the learning outcomes established for that program. A measurement *method* is an overall approach, technique, or strategy for measuring learning. Cognitive learning outcomes are usually evaluated by the use of classroom evaluation methods, whereas affective or psychomotor outcomes are typically measured by simulation or clinical performance methods.

A measuring *instrument* or *test* refers to any means, tool, or device used to measure learning. A *test* may also be considered as a written or situational occurrence that provides one or more opportunities for the learner to demonstrate learning. Cognitive learning outcomes typically employ devices such as written case studies, worksheets, or other types of written tests to measure learning. A *written test* is composed of a number of written test items that may be structured in many different ways (such as statements, incomplete statements, questions, and the like). Affective and psychomotor outcomes, by contrast, are more often evaluated by means of one or more *performance tests* that specify behaviors the learner must demonstrate in a simulated or real clinical situation. Simulation devices such as role plays or clinical evaluation checklists serve as tools for these types of evaluation. The individual instances, questions, or entries that comprise the measuring instrument are called *test items*. These test items represent the behavioral samples or opportunities given to learners to demonstrate that they can meet the outcomes established for instruction.

BENCHMARKS OF EDUCATIONAL MEASUREMENT

If we hope to use the results of educational evaluation to make decisions regarding the instructional process and its outcomes, we need to have confidence that the information provided by our measuring instruments is accurate, dependable, and helpful. Since all measurement involves some degree of error, how does the educator determine the degree of confidence that can be ascribed to various measurement devices? How can the educator tell if the test scores or check marks obtained from educational measurements are truly sound indicators for making decisions? The three traits that serve as litmus tests for determining the legitimacy of a measurement tool are validity, reliability, and usefulness. Until the educator knows that the measuring device(s) being used are valid, reliable, and useful, they have no basis for confidence that measurements from that device can be used for sound decision-making.

Validity, reliability, and usefulness are the benchmarks of all educational measurement. Of this trio, validity is the most important attribute of an evaluation tool; without it, reliability and usefulness are virtually meaningless and decisions based on measurements from the tool are groundless. Ideally, all three attributes are maximally present in each evaluation device. In reality, each attribute is present to a greater or lesser degree, rather than being absolutely "there" or "not there." Because the educator needs to use these benchmarks to determine the quality of each evaluation instrument used in an educational program, it is worthwhile to examine each more closely.*

Validity

Validity may be defined as the degree to which an evaluation device measures what it is intended to measure. The validity of any testing instrument is always judged in reference to a specific purpose. If, for example, a 50-question written test is used to evaluate cognitive learning for a 1-week course on physical assessment and is also used to screen applicants for entry into an advanced medical-surgical nursing course, the validity of the test for measuring learning must be determined apart from its validity as a screening device. The same test may be highly valid for measuring a nurse's knowledge of physical assessment but have little or no validity as a screening device for the advanced medical-surgical nursing course. Multiple testing devices may be used for a single purpose or a single test may be used for multiple purposes. In each instance, validity must be determined for each testing device in relation to each evaluation purpose.

In its most basic form, validity refers to the degree to which the test situations or items elicit the behavior, content, and conditions called for in the instructional outcomes. If the test requirements or items are appropriate correlates of the instructional outcomes, the measurements should be valid indicators of whether those outcomes were attained. Conversely, if the evaluation instrument tests behaviors and content areas that are different from those that appear in the instructional outcomes, the scores or check marks produced have limited or no validity. For example, suppose that one outcome for an introductory medical-surgical nursing course was "Demonstrates the steps of crisis intervention with patient families." If this outcome were evaluated by a performance checklist that enumerated each of the essential steps of crisis intervention that the nurse would need to demonstrate, the check marks obtained would be valid indicators of that outcome. But if the only

means for evaluating this outcome were a written test item that required the nurse to list the steps of crisis intervention, the measurements obtained would tell the educator virtually nothing about that nurse's ability to execute those steps because *listing* and *demonstrating* the steps of crisis intervention are not the same behavior. In order for an educational measurement to be valid, the behavior and content area contained in the evaluation device should match those that appear in the instructional outcome.

There are four major types of validity. These include content validity, face validity, criterion-related validity, and construct validity.

Content Validity

Content validity refers to the degree to which the behaviors and content areas in the evaluation items are representative of the ones called for in the instructional outcomes. In assessing content validity, the educator or other content area expert(s) determines both the inclusiveness and the distribution of items in the evaluation tool (e.g., whether all of the behaviors called for in the instructional outcomes can be found somewhere in the tool and whether they are present in their appropriate proportion).

To appraise a measurement tool for content validity, it is necessary first to identify the behaviors and subject matter contained in the instructional outcomes. From the relative amount of instructional time (expressed as a percentage) allotted for each outcome, determine the weight that each outcome was given in the program. Then check that the evaluation tool requires demonstration of the *same* behavior related to the *same* content area as specified in each outcome. Finally, verify that the weight allotted in the evaluation device is comparable to that allotted for instructional time. To the extent that the distribution of items in the evaluation tool matches the distribution of items in the instructional outcomes, the tool has content validity; that is, it measures what it is intended to measure.

For most classroom tests, the appraisal of content validity is provided by a consensus of experts in the subject area. To the extent that evaluation items apportionately represent the instructional outcomes,† content validity is assured. Hospital-based nurse educators are likely to use content validity as their primary method for determining the overall validity of classroom, laboratory, and clinical evaluation tools.

Face Validity

A second type of validity, *face validity,* refers to whether a measuring instrument seems—from its superficial appear-

---

*Froman and Owen[21] describe an easy and enjoyable approach to learning about the concepts of validity and reliability.

†This apportionment is usually determined by using a test blueprint and table of specifications, both of which are covered later in this chapter.

ance—to represent the content areas and behaviors it is intended to represent. It differs from content validity in that the appraisal of face validity is largely superficial and random rather than comprehensive and systematic. Because this type of appraisal does not constitute a true measure of validity, it should be accorded limited legitimacy.

Criterion-Related Validity

Criterion-related validity refers to the degree to which an individual's performance on one measuring instrument correlates with present or future performance on another related instrument. As its name implies, criterion-related validity requires that the initial test results be compared with results on some valid criterion measure or standard related to the initial performance. If the second performance is a suitable and comparable measure of the first, then performance on the initial measure could be used to predict a learner's performance on the second measure.

Because criterion-related validity may involve the prediction of either another present performance or a future performance, the types of validity it provides are appropriately designated as concurrent or predictive.

Concurrent validity refers to the degree to which performance levels on one test correlate with performance levels on a second test taken at nearly the same time. For example, a staff development educator might be interested in determining the association between a staff nurse's score on the Basic Knowledge Assessment Tool (BKAT)[47] for critical care nursing and that nurse's score on the hospital's posttest for the "Fundamentals of Critical Care" course. If these tests were administered at more or less the same time, they could afford a measure of concurrent validity.

Predictive validity refers to the degree to which performance levels on one test correlate with performance levels on a second test taken in the future. For example, a consortium of local hospitals that offers a preparation course for certification in medical-surgical nursing might be interested in determining the association between participants' scores on the comprehensive examination taken at the completion of the preparation course with their scores on the actual ANA certification examination. If these two measurements correlate highly, then the results of the preparation test scores could be used to predict the participants' scores on the certification examination.

The term *correlation* has been used here a number of times in describing types of criterion-related validity. A correlation expresses the degree of relationship between two things. As a statistical index of relationship, correlations are determined by computing this relationship as a *correlation coefficient,* abbreviated as "r." The numerical value of a correlation coefficient (r) may range from -1.0 to $+1.0$.

If two sets of scores are directly related to one another so that one increases (or decreases) as the other set increases (or decreases), the sets of scores are said to have a

high degree of correlation. A high **positive** correlation has a correlation coefficient (r value) that approaches $+1.0$. If the two sets of scores had a perfect positive correlation, then as one set of scores increases (or decreases) by a given amount, the other would likewise increase (or decrease) by the same amount; scores on the two tests would tend to go up or down together. Lesser degrees of positive correlation (r values > 0.0, but $< +1.0$) indicate that this relationship is proportionately less than the maximum. Figure 5.2 shows

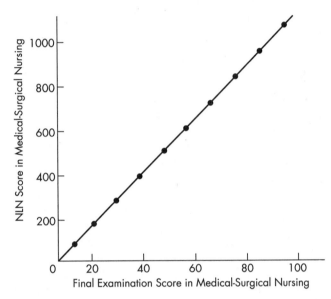

Figure 5.2   Perfect positive correlation. (r = +1.00).

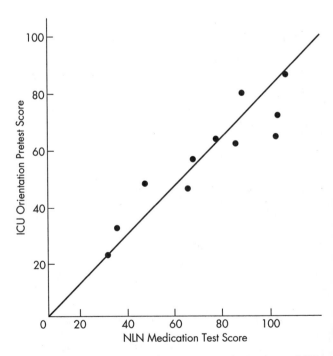

Figure 5.3   Lesser degree of positive correlation (r = +0.70).

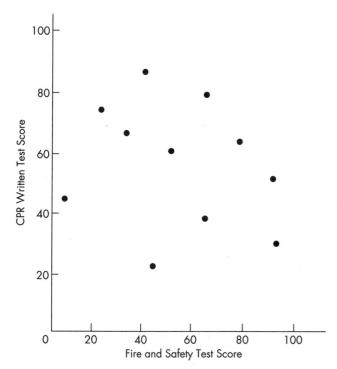

Figure 5.4 No correlation (r = 0.00).

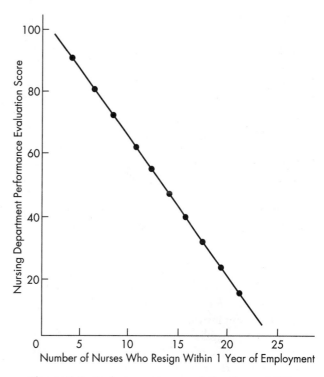

Figure 5.5 Perfect negative correlation (r = −1.00).

a graphic illustration (called a *scattergram*) of perfect positive correlation and Figure 5.3 illustrates a less than perfect positive correlation. If no relationship exists between two sets of scores, the value of r would be 0.00 (Figure 5.4), implying that no association exists between these two measurements.

Negative correlations afford equally important information. A high **negative** correlation has a correlation coefficient (r value) that approaches −1.0. If two sets of scores had a perfect negative correlation, then as one set of scores increases, the other set of scores decreases; the scores on the two tests are inversely related to each other. Figure 5.5 is a scattergram of a perfect negative correlation and Figure 5.6 shows a less than perfect negative correlation.*

Construct Validity

Construct validity is the third and least often used type of validity. Constructs are abstract, theoretical, or intangible qualities (such as anxiety, empathy, or leadership), which are assumed to be the basis for certain types of behavior. *Construct validity* refers to the degree to which specific constructs are represented in the measurement device. To the extent that these items appropriately and comprehensively measure the constructs, the results of measurement are explainable by the constructs included there.

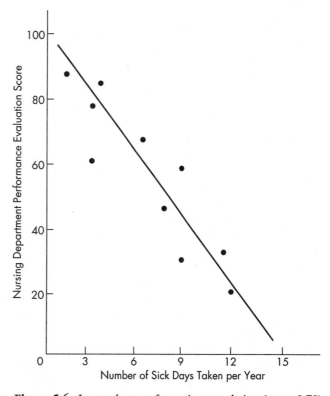

Figure 5.6 Lesser degree of negative correlation (r = −0.70).

*Calculating a correlation coefficient is beyond the scope of this book but may be found in any text on descriptive statistics.

Construct validity is most often employed with measures of affective behavior. If, for example, the educator were interested in assessing a nurse's "empathy" for the families of critically ill patients, the educator would need to determine what the constituents of empathy are and design an evaluation device to measure these. An obstacle in appraising construct validity arises because there are a limited number of available and valid tools with which to measure these qualities. Construct validity generally requires a substantial review of the literature and research findings related to the construct or its subcomponents. Calculation of construct validity may require that numerous correlations be made and demonstrated repeatedly among subcomponents to substantiate the proposed correlation.

Reliability

Reliability refers to the stability or consistency of measurements over time, the comparability of results between different measuring instruments or between different raters, the ability to generalize results from one situation to another, or the degree of consistency within a single test. In statistical terms, test reliability may be defined as the degree to which scores are free of measurement error.[3] Measurement error (i.e., errors in measurement owing to factors other than learning) can be caused by influences such as guessing, fatigue, test anxiety, item selection or the scoring procedure used in the test.[31]

If, for example, a nurse had reason to doubt that an arterial pressure monitoring system was working properly, the nurse might zero and calibrate the system and then take multiple readings over a specified period of time to see if the trend in readings remained comparable. The nurse might use another measuring device to cross-check the comparability of readings between invasive and noninvasive measurements of arterial pressure or the nurse might compare the readings obtained with those that another nurse obtains on the same device. Each of these comparability determinations represents a test for the reliability of a measuring instrument.

The degree of reliability of a specific measuring tool is expressed as an index (or coefficient) that ranges from 0.00 (no reliability) to 1.00 (maximal reliability). Many classroom tests aim for a reliability index between .50 and .70 or higher.[20]

Next to validity, reliability is the most important attribute of a measuring device. Reliability is an essential prerequisite for validity; a measuring device that has low reliability will not afford consistent findings and necessarily limits that tool's validity. The converse does not hold true, however; a measuring device may be reliable but not valid. If, for example, a central venous pressure (CVP) monitoring system always gave readings that were 10 cm H_2O below the patient's true CVP value, that consistent margin of error would represent a reliable but not a true measure of the patient's CVP. Even very high degrees of reliability, then, do not assure the validity of that measuring device.

Reliability, like validity, is always in reference to the purpose for which measurements are taken: a certain bed scale may be highly reliable for weighing adults, moderately reliable for weighing children, and not at all reliable for weighing infants or neonates.

As mentioned earlier, a number of methods can be used to determine reliability. One category focuses on administering or constructing an objectively scored measuring device, whereas another type focuses on subjectively scored measurements. Each method for determining reliability provides the educator with somewhat different information and implications regarding reliability. Therefore, in appraising how reliable a measuring instrument is, it is important to know which type of reliability is being considered. Methods for determining reliability that focus on test administration or construction include measures of stability, equivalence, and internal consistency.

Stability (Test-Retest) Reliability

One way of determining an instrument's reliability is to assess its temporal stability, the consistency of its measurements over time. *Stability reliability* refers to how repeatable the results of measurement are when the *same test* is administered to the *same persons* under the *same conditions* at two different times (T1 and T2) with no additional instruction intervening. Because the same test is given on both occasions, this type of reliability is also be called *test-retest reliability*. It is determined by calculating a correlation coefficient called a reliability coefficient.

The intervening time period between tests (the waiting period between T1 and T2) can vary from days to months or even years, depending on the purpose for retesting. For example, a nurse educator may be interested in determining the reliability of an evaluation tool for measuring staff nurses' understanding of the principles involved in managing diabetic emergencies after a 1-day course on this topic. To determine how reliable the evaluation tool is, the educator could test the same nurses at the end of the course and then again 2 weeks later. If the educator needed to provide long-term followup of the nurses to see how much of this information was retained, the second testing could be scheduled 6 months or 1 year following completion of the course.

Because the length of the intervening period between the test (T1) and retest (T2) vary, some potential problems arise that may influence the confidence with which reliability coefficients can be interpreted. Short intervening periods between T1 and T2 may produce falsely high reliability coefficients because the examinees can easily recall the test items and how they responded to them in T1 or because their familiarity with the test (T2) may reduce the test anxiety they experienced when they completed T1. Long intervening periods, on the other hand, allow many other variables to enter the test situation and possibly influence performance: the nurses may acquire a significant amount of additional learning, their ease or skill in test-taking may improve, their lives or work situations might change, or it may be difficult to replicate the conditions used for the initial testing. In general, test-retest reliability coefficients in the order of at least 0.4 are desirable for classroom tests.

Parallel (Equivalent, Alternative) Forms Reliability

A second method in this category attempts to verify reliability by computing the correlation between scores from two different tests that supposedly measure the same thing. Assuming the two test instruments measure the same behaviors and content area(s) under the same conditions, they should produce virtually the same results. This type of reliability is termed *parallel, equivalent,* or *alternate forms reliability.* Educators might be interested in determining parallel forms reliability in order to provide learners with different versions of the same test when offering a makeup test, appraising performance at a later date, or preventing cheating among learners seated close to one another.

When the educator is interested in determining equivalent forms reliability, both forms of the test are administered to the same individuals at a single test occasion. A reliability coefficient is then derived from a comparison of the results of each. The statistical device used to calculate this coefficient is called the Pearson Product Moment Correlation Coefficient. If T2 is truly an equivalent (parallel, alternate) form of T1, the results from each test should demonstrate a high degree of correlation with each other. Equivalent forms of the same test may also be administered with a specific intervening time period. Assuming that this intervening period is significant (i.e., more than just the time required to complete either test), the resulting correlations would indicate two types of reliability: equivalence and stability.

A problem encountered with equivalence reliability measures is that T2 is often not really equivalent to T1. Equivalence implies that each individual test item and the overall test has precisely the same range and scope of behaviors, content, difficulty, and discrimination as the other. Constructing a test instrument with this degree of precision can be a formidable task, even for experienced and knowledgeable educators. In reality, then, many alternate or parallel forms of the same test really are not interchangeable.

A second problem with using this reliability method is that it assumes the learners and test conditions remain unchanged. Even if T2 were administered directly after T1, the influence of test-taking skill, fatigue, and review of the content from the initial testing may be significant in determining the T2 scores and the correlation between the two sets of scores. The second testing situation might be in a small (vs. large) room that is dimly (vs. well) lighted where the test administrator gave scanty (vs. detailed) instructions on how to complete the test. Because these factors may affect reliability, they need to be taken into account when making interpretations of the results.

Internal Consistency Reliability

The third method of estimating reliability from an objectively scored device is called *internal consistency reliability.* This type of reliability considers the consistency of performance on items within the same test. It is a measure of the degree to which items intended to measure the same thing produce similar results.[14] Instead of administering the same test on two different occasions or constructing two comparable tests to be given at the same time, this method involves constructing a single test to be administered on a single occasion. Because it is economical of both instructor and examinee time, internal consistency reliability is the most commonly employed procedure for determining test reliability.

Constructing an instrument for estimating reliability by this method usually proceeds in one of two ways. The *split-half method* involves dividing the total test into two equivalent halves that measure the same thing. This can be accomplished by matching the items so that the second half of the test is an alternate form of the first half or so all evenly numbered items are matched with the odd numbered equivalents. Two separate scores are thus derived from this one test and compared with one another to estimate the degree of reliability between the scores. The split-half method computes reliability using a statistical device called the Spearman-Brown Prophecy Formula.

An alternate way to compute reliability is to compare the two scores from each test in terms of how many high vs. low scorers get the item correct and how much spread (vs. homogeneity) of scores was produced. This method uses a statistical device called the Kuder-Richardson Formula (KR20 or KR21). Readers are referred to Layton[31] for a detailed description of the formulas and procedures used in these calculations.

This second method for determining reliability is useful when scores or measurements must be derived from subjective judgments of raters who use some form of checklist or rating scale as the measuring device. Two different approaches are available to determine the reliability of this type of evaluation tool. The first approach calls for two or more evaluators to use the same device in rating the exact same performance. Videotape or equally good vantage points must be employed so that the performance being rated is, in reality, the same for both evaluators. The simultaneous ratings of the same performance are then compared with one another and provide for what is called *inter-rater reliability.*

A second way to estimate the reliability of subjectively scored measurements is to have the same rater observe the same performance (usually on some permanent record such as film) at two different times. Because the rater is the same in both instances and the performance being rated is the same, this is referred to as *intra-rater reliability.* Inter-rater reliability considers agreement between raters, whereas intra-rater reliability considers agreement by the same rater over time. In general, the greater the number of raters involved with estimating reliability, the more accurate will be the results of that estimate.

From the preceding section, it is clear that many factors may influence reliability and the overall implications of any given estimate of reliability.[31] When establishing acceptable reliability levels is a problem (i.e., when correlations are consistently less than 0.3), the educator may be able to attribute the problem to one or more of the following causes:

- Too few items in the test (restricts the number of behaviors and content areas represented)
- Some variation or error in test construction or administration
- Lack of objectivity in scoring
- Too many test items that are too difficult for learners
- Too few persons taking the test (a small sample size)
- Errors in calculating reliability
- Testing for an inherently unstable variable

Usefulness

The third benchmark of educational measurement is usefulness. The *usefulness* of an evaluation device refers to how feasible and practical it is to employ. Even if a measuring instrument is valid and reliable, if it is unwieldy to use, difficult to understand, or requires excessive resources (time, money, personnel, materials, support) to construct, administer, complete, score, or interpret, it is not very useful. Like validity and reliability, usefulness is also a matter of degree and must be viewed in relation to the other benchmarks of measurement. Unlike the other benchmarks, however, an instrument's usefulness is a more or less independent attribute, assessed with different criteria and on rather pragmatic and practical rather than statistical grounds.

How important are these three benchmark attributes of a measuring device? If a nurse were taking sequential blood pressures on a postoperative patient with a sphygmomanometer that did not work properly, the readings obtained would not be valid indicators of the patient's true arterial blood pressure. If that nurse used those (invalid) findings to titrate IV infusion rates and vasopressor administration, the patient might be seriously harmed. If the cuff gave accurate readings on some occasions and inaccurate ones at other times (i.e., was unreliable), the nurse would not know when titration of IVs or vasopressors should be made or not. If the patient had an upper body cast or had to be positioned so that use of the cuff was difficult and time-consuming (was not useful), the nurse might monitor the patient's arterial pressure less often than if an invasive arterial line was in place. Although these decisions are clinical rather than educational, they illustrate the importance of knowing that a measuring instrument is valid, reliable, and useful before one attempts to use its data to make important decisions.

EVALUATION OF LEARNING WITHIN THE COGNITIVE DOMAIN

There are two phases involved with evaluating learning in the cognitive domain: test construction and test item construction. The first phase involves designing the written test as a whole and the second phase involves developing the individual written test items.

Test Construction

The process for constructing a written test involves a total of seven steps. These steps are summarized in Box 5.2 and discussed in detail following.

Step 1: Identify the instructional outcomes to be evaluated. Since an educational program's effectiveness depends on learners attaining the instructional outcomes established for that program, the logical starting place for evaluation is with the instructional outcomes.

The instructional outcome statements are crucial to evaluation because they reveal both the specific **behavior** required of the learner and the **content area** to which that behavior must relate. In planning a test to measure learning, the educator must assure that the behaviors and content areas contained in the test instrument are the same behaviors and content areas specified in the instructional outcomes.

Box 5.2

STEPS IN CONSTRUCTING A WRITTEN TEST

1. Identify the instructional outcomes to be evaluated
2. Assign a relative weight to each outcome
3. Determine the amount of time available for testing
4. Decide on the type(s) of test item(s) to be used
5. Calculate the total number of test items that can be used in the time available for testing
6. Calculate the number of test items that should be allocated to each instructional outcome
7. Designate item numbers for the test

Step 2: Assign a relative weight to each outcome. In educational measurement, the term *relative weight* refers to the *evaluative weight* or emphasis that should be accorded to appraisal of a particular instructional outcome. An outcome's evaluative weight is a function of how important that outcome is within the program and is expressed as a percentage of the total test that relates to that individual outcome.

How does the educator apportion evaluative weights for each of the instructional outcomes in a staff development program? The answer is really rather straightforward: evaluative weights should be proportional to instructional weights. If you recall from Chapter 3 when we discussed allotment of instructional time, the educator needed to make some decisions regarding division of instructional time. The rationale for this decision was that, because the amount of teaching time is finite, it needs to be distributed in the most effective and efficient way possible according to its priority, complexity, and the amount of prerequisite subject matter that would need to be covered. As a general guideline, then, evaluative weight should be proportional to instructional weight. In practical terms, this means that if an instructional outcome was judged to be sufficiently important to receive 15% of the total amount of instructional time (i.e., its instructional weight was 15%), it should receive a comparable percentage of the total amount of evaluation (i.e., its evaluative weight should be 15% of the total test). Table 5.1 shows an example of how instructional and evaluative weights might be designated for a 2-week (80-hour) Coronary Care Unit (CCU) Course.

A few caveats related to assignment of evaluative weights are worth mentioning here. In calculating the percentages of evaluative weight for each instructional outcome, the educator will often find that the numerical values are not round numbers. If a certain outcome had an instructional weight of 8.5%, the educator will need to make a value judgment of whether that outcome will receive 8% or 9% as an evaluative weight. A second point is that the assignment of evaluative weights is not so much a matter of mathematical precision as it is one of attempting to strike a balance between instructional priority and evaluative priority. If a certain outcome had an instructional weight of 18%, it could conceivably have an evaluative weight of 15% or 20%, but not 8% or 28%. A third issue relates to the factors that influence instructional weight. Of the three major factors mentioned (priority, complexity, and the amount of prerequisite subject matter), the complexity and volume of subject matter usually affect teaching time more than they influence evaluation. Therefore the primary determinant for making decisions regarding assignment of evaluative weight is the priority or importance of that outcome for the program. The educator, as a result, should aim at allocating comparable amounts of instructional and evaluative weights, using the importance of each outcome to the program as the primary basis for decision-making.

Step 3: Determine the amount of time available for testing. In some types of tests, the educator is interested not only in measuring achievement but also in measuring the degree of achievement attained within a restricted time period. This type of test is called a *power test*. In a power

TABLE 5.1 • DISTRIBUTION OF INSTRUCTIONAL AND EVALUATIVE WEIGHTS FOR COGNITIVE BEHAVIORS			
80-HOUR CORONARY CARE COURSE			
❶			**❷**
Instructional Outcome	**Instructional Hours**	**Instructional Weight (%)**	**Evaluative Weight (%)**
Explain the clinical implications of abnormal physical assessment findings commonly encountered in the CCU patient	8	10	10
Distinguish normal from abnormal hemodynamic monitoring data from a series of written case studies	12	15	15
Recognize all common forms (sinus, atrial, junctional, and ventricular) of cardiac dysrhythmias and conduction defects	32	40	40
Describe the rationale for all major elements of nursing care for a patient with acute myocardial infarction	16	20	20
Specify the nursing care for patients in cardiogenic shock who require intraaortic balloon pump support	8	10	10
Identify the major nursing considerations in providing care to the patient with a temporary transvenous pacemaker	4	5	5
TOTALS:	80 hrs	100%	100%

test, one of the major variables affecting a learner's performance is the time available for testing.

The evaluation devices in a nursing staff development program are **not** intended to be power tests; that is, the educator does not want time to be a major influence on the learner's performance. What we want to evaluate for learning within the cognitive domain is what learners know about a certain subject area not what they know under the pressure of a tight time deadline. In order to avoid placing learners under a time constraint when they complete written tests, the educator needs to consider the time available for evaluation in planning the test. The amount of time planned for the test might be the same as for a regular class period or it might be longer or shorter. Whatever time frame is planned, it should be established at this point.

Step 4: Decide on the type(s) of test item(s) to be used. Many different types of written test items are available to the educator. These include *objective test items* that can be scored by anyone familiar with the scoring system or that can be machine scored and *subjective test items* that require a subjective appraisal by someone knowledgeable in the content area. Examples of objective test items include true-false, multiple-choice, short completion (fill-in-the-blank), and matching items. An essay question is an example of a subjective test item. Cranton[14] has designed a matrix of various types of test items that may be used for each cognitive level.

Educators need to make some preliminary decisions regarding the type of test item they intend to use because various types of items require different amounts of time to complete.[10] Some very general rules of thumb regarding the amount of time required for completing different types of written test items are provided in Table 5.2.

Step 5: Calculate the total number of test items that can be used in the time available for testing. Once the educator has estimated the total amount of time that will be available for testing and has decided on the type of test item to be used, calculating the number of items that can be used in

the time available is a matter of simple division. For example, if the total time available for testing is 45 minutes and the educator wishes to use complex multiple-choice items that would require approximately 1½ minutes per item to complete, the number of items that could be included in the test would be calculated as follows:

Total time for testing ÷ Time needed/item =
Number of items in test

For the example described previously, the calculation would appear as:

$$45 \text{ minutes} \div 1\tfrac{1}{2} \text{ minutes/item} = 30 \text{ items}$$

or, if conversion from minutes to seconds is easier, the calculation would be as follows:

$$2700 \text{ seconds} \div 90 \text{ seconds/item} = 30 \text{ items}$$

This calculation affords a good estimate of about how many test items of a specific type can reasonably be answered by learners in the time available for testing. After using the test a few times, the educator will be able to refine this figure up or down so that it reflects experience using the test and the needs of certain learner audiences.

The method for calculating the total number of test items described previously works quite well when the entire test employs only one type of test item. In other instances, however, the educator may wish to use two or more types of test items in the same test. This can also be accomplished quite readily by using the following guidelines:

- Decide the percentage of the total test that will use each specific type of test item (i.e., 60% of the test will use simple multiple-choice items, 20% will use complex true-false items, and 20% will use short essay items)
- Use the rules of thumb in Table 5.2 to estimate the amount of time each type of test item will require. These might be estimated as follows:
  Simple multiple-choice items = 45 sec/item
  Complex true-false items = 90 sec/item
  Short essay items = 4 min (240 sec /item)
- Calculate the subtotals for the time available for testing as indicated previously

These subtotals would be calculated as shown in Table 5.3. In that example, the total number of test items for a 1-hour test period is estimated to be 59. Remember that the educator would certainly be free to adjust this to 60 items in the test since mathematical precision is important but not absolute. What we are attempting to achieve here is balance between the instructional priorities and the evaluation priorities rather than rigorous arithmetic accuracy.

TABLE 5.2 • ESTIMATED TIMES REQUIRED TO COMPLETE VARIOUS TYPES OF TEST ITEMS	
Test Item	**Time per Item**
Simple true-false Simple multiple-choice Short completion	½ to 1 minute
Complex true-false (correct-false statements) Complex multiple-choice (select sets of options from a list) Short (5 to 10 elements) matching	1 to 2 minutes
Short (one paragraph) essay Long (10 to 15+ elements) matching	3 to 5 minutes

Percent of Test Using That Item	Subtotal Time for That Item (% times 3600 seconds)		Divided by Time/Item		Subtotal Number of Items
60	2160 seconds	÷	45 seconds/item	=	48 simple multiple-choice
20	720 seconds	÷	90 seconds/item	=	8 complex true-false
20	720 seconds	÷	240 seconds/item	=	3 short essay
100%	3600 seconds				59 test items

TABLE 5.3 • CALCULATION OF TEST ITEM DISTRIBUTION USING MULTIPLE TYPES OF TEST ITEMS*

*Assuming a total time for testing of 1 hour (3600 seconds).

Step 6: Calculate the number of test items that should be allocated to each instructional outcome. As Table 5.3 illustrates, once the educator has determined the total number of items to be used in the test, the number of items for each instructional outcome can be calculated by multiplying the evaluative weight for that outcome (stated as a percent of the total evaluative weight) times the total number of items in the test. For example, if a certain instructional outcome merited an evaluative weight of 20% in a test that included 50 total test items, the number of items that need to relate to that instructional outcome would be 20% of 50 items or 10 items.

In making these calculations, the product obtained is often not a whole number. For example, if the evaluative weight had been 15% rather than 20% for the 50-item test, the calculation would have resulted in a product of (15% times 50 items =) 7.5 items. As discussed in the caveats for determining evaluative weights, the educator simply makes a decision in these instances whether to round the number up or down, based on the importance of that outcome.

Step 7: Designate item numbers for the test. The last step in constructing a written test is a pragmatic one: deciding the order in which test items related to each instructional outcome will appear in the test. Some guidelines to consider here include the following:

- *Content that has an inherent sequencing order should follow this order in evaluation devices.* For example, items related to normal anatomy and physiology would usually precede items on pathophysiology and the latter would precede items related to nursing management. The rationale for this is comparable to the rationale for sequencing instructional content: it is easier for the learner to follow the material when the context is developed progressively.
- *Multiple items that relate to a similar content area should be grouped together.* For example, in a test on pulmonary disorders, all items related to adult respiratory distress syndrome could be grouped together and separated from items related to obstructive pulmonary disorders or those related to chest trauma. The reason for this guideline is that it minimizes the

learner's need to make cognitive shifts from one frame of reference to another. Intellectual shifts are time-consuming mental calisthenics that may detract from test performance.

- *When multiple types of test items are used, items of the same type should be grouped together.* If a test will include multiple-choice, true-false, essay, and matching items, each of these types of test items should, insofar as possible, be grouped together[10] so that the learner's approach for responding to the items does not continually need to change abruptly. Formulating a response to an essay item is, from the learner's perspective, quite different from formulating a response to a simple true-false or matching item. As in the case of items that address similar content areas, the aim here is to minimize the need for useless mental exercises that may adversely affect performance on the test.

Table 5.4 provides an illustration of all seven steps involved in constructing a written test, using the same instructional outcomes, instructional weights, and evaluative weights as those in Table 5.1. Following each of these steps will help to assure design of a valid evaluation device for both evaluation of learning and for making educational decisions. The product of test construction that appears in Table 5.4 is referred to as a test blueprint. A *test blueprint* is an evaluation plan that identifies the content (behaviors and subject matter) to be tested, the amount of time available for testing, the type and number of test items, and the distribution of items within the test. Test blueprints may be designed in a number of different ways.[31]

Another evaluative planning device derived from a test blueprint is sometimes employed in test construction. This device, known as a *table of specifications,* further distributes the test items allocated for each instructional outcome among the six cognitive levels. The rationale for using a table of specifications is to ensure that cognitive evaluation spans the full range of cognitive behaviors rather than being confined to only the lower levels of cognitive performance. As mentioned earlier in test item construction, testing at lower levels of cognitive behavior is a limitation of fill-in-the-blank, true-false, and matching items; the table of specifications attempts to minimize this potential limi-

TABLE 5.4 • SEVEN STEPS IN CONSTRUCTING A WRITTEN TEST: TEST BLUEPRINT

80-HOUR CORONARY CARE COURSE

❶ Instructional Outcome	Instructional Hours	Instructional Weight (%)	❷ Evaluative Weight (%)	❻ Number of Items	❼ Item Number
Explain the clinical implications of abnormal physical assessment findings commonly encountered in the CCU patient	8	10	10	3	01-03
Distinguish normal from abnormal hemodynamic monitoring data from a series of written case studies	12	15	15	4	04-07
Recognize all common forms (sinus, atrial, junctional, and ventricular) of cardiac dysrhythmias and conduction defects	32	40	40	12	08-19
Describe the rationale for all major elements of nursing care for a patient with acute myocardial infarction	16	20	20	6	20-25
Specify the nursing care for patients in cardiogenic shock who require intraaortic balloon pump support	8	10	10	3	26-28
Identify the major nursing considerations in providing care to the patient with a temporary transvenous pacemaker	4	5	5	2	29-30
TOTALS:	**80 hrs**	**100%**	**100%**	**30**	**01-30**

❸   Amount of time available for testing: 45 minutes
❹   Type of test item: complex multiple choice (90 seconds/item)
❺   Total number of test items that can be used:

total test time	divided by	time/item
45 minutes	÷	90 seconds/item
2700 seconds	÷	90 seconds/item = 30 items

tation by specifying that a certain number of items will test at the middle and upper taxonomy range.[15,19] Table 5.5 illustrates what a table of specifications might look like for the test blueprint in Table 5.4.

Once test construction and design of the test blueprint are completed, the construction of individual test items can begin.

Test Item Construction

The design of valid written test items requires that the educator be familiar with the features related to each type of test item. The section that follows provides an overview of the most commonly employed written test items, listing their appropriate uses, limitations, and guidelines for construction and use of each.

Essay Items

An essay item usually presents a problem or situation to which the examinee must formulate and organize a response. The required response may be limited to a few sentences or may extend over many pages, depending on the nature and focus of the information requested.

APPROPRIATE USES

- Measures complex cognitive behaviors such as the ability to organize, integrate, synthesize, differentiate, describe, and summarize
- Require learners to draw on past experience and breadth of knowledge, set priorities, use originality or creativity
- Elicits critical, logical, and analytical thinking and problem-solving

TABLE 5.5 • TABLE OF SPECIFICATIONS

80-HOUR CORONARY CARE COURSE

Instructional Outcome	Number of Items	Cognitive Level						
		Knowledge	Comprehension	Application	Analysis	Synthesis	Evaluation	
Explain the clinical implications of abnormal physical assessment findings commonly encountered in the CCU patient	3	0	1	0	1	1	0	
Distinguish normal from abnormal hemodynamic monitoring data from a series of written case studies	4	1	0	0	1	1	1	
Recognize all common forms (sinus, atrial, junctional, and ventricular) of cardiac dysrhythmias and conduction defects	12	1	1	2	2	3	3	
Describe the rationale for all major elements of nursing care for a patient with acute myocardial infarction	6	1	1	1	1	1	1	
Specify the nursing care for patients in cardiogenic shock who require intraaortic balloon pump support	3	1	0	1	0	0	1	
Identify the major nursing considerations in providing care to the patient with a temporary transvenous pacemaker	2	0	1	1	0	0	0	
TOTALS:	30	4	4	5	5	6	6	

- Measures learning related to affective and ethical areas, where more than one plausible approach is available

LIMITATIONS

- If posed as broad questions that require a long and complex response, the time required to answer may limit the number of outcomes that can be measured in a single test situation; limited sampling of outcomes reduces test validity
- May be too open-ended or ambiguous regarding the behavior and scope of content matter required in the response (e.g., "Describe the pathophysiology of asthma")
- If learners are given options regarding which or how many essay items they answer, all learners are not being evaluated on the same basis, thereby reducing both test validity and reliability
- Most forms of reliability testing (test-retest, equivalent forms, and the like) are difficult to achieve; inter-rater and intra-rater reliability are notoriously low
- Aspects of the response unrelated to learning (handwriting, grammar, punctuation, spelling, facility and quality of written expression, composition quality) may influence scoring of items
- Scoring can be a slow, time-consuming, and laborious task that requires coding of desired response(s)
- Scoring is fundamentally a subjective process that can lead to scorer bias

GUIDELINES FOR CONSTRUCTION AND USE

- Improve validity by increasing the number of behaviors sampled; rather than writing a few items that require long and complex responses, write a larger number of items requiring a brief, focused response
- Use verbs that restrict, clarify, and specify the behavior desired (e.g., contrast, summarize, outline, or list) rather than broad, ambiguous verbs (describe, discuss, explain)
- Present a clear and specific task to the learner that is not open to different interpretations[14]
- Verify that all behaviors in the instructional outcomes are covered in the essay item(s) and that learners will have sufficient time to respond to each item
- Include instructions to learners regarding the time available for completion, the point value of each item, and any restrictions or expectations regarding length and content of responses
- Develop a scoring guide for each item that identifies essential elements of the ideal response and the number of points allocated for each of these elements
- Score all responses to the same item before moving on to the next item so that consistency and uniformity in scoring are enhanced and scoring bias is minimized
- Randomly rearrange the order of papers before scor-

ing the next item so that papers at the bottom of the stack are not always subject to the potential effects of scorer fatigue

Short-Answer Completion (Fill-in-the-Blank) Items

Short answer or completion items may appear in one of two forms: as a direct question or as a sentence having one or more important words deleted. The direct question requires the learner to supply a word, a phrase, a few sentences, a number, or a symbol. The incomplete sentence usually requires the learner to supply only a word, a phrase, or a number that completes the statement correctly.

APPROPRIATE USES

- Evaluate cognitive performance at lower taxonomy levels
- Measure recall of facts, terms, symbols, definitions, functions, processes, and principles subject to limited interpretation
- Offer computational problems with few potentially correct answers
- Can be used to name numbered or lettered parts on an illustration, diagram, or model
- Offer ease of test construction and scoring
- Sample a large volume of information quickly
- Diminish the effect of guessing

LIMITATIONS

- Testing low levels of cognitive function (definition, recall, recognition), precipitates "lifting" words or phrases verbatim, and encourages rote memorization of bits of information
- Few content areas admit of only a single correct response
- Stems that lack sufficient information (e.g., "Arterial blood gases reflect _____") may confuse learners and cause scoring problems
- Ambiguous or imprecise wording of item leaves it open to multiple interpretations and scoring dilemmas[36]
- Problems in scoring may occur if responses are illegible, misspelled, or if they only approximate the desired response
- Content area expert must score items so that variants of desired responses can be fairly judged

GUIDELINES FOR CONSTRUCTION AND USE[26]

- Focus test items only on important areas
- Pose the statement or question so that only one possible response is correct or best
- When using incomplete statements, omit only the most significant words, phrases, or values[14]
- Include enough information (adequate stimulus) in the item for the learner to be able to respond (e.g., a completion item such as "Congestive heart failure

is _____ " does not afford the learner a sufficient amount of information to know how to direct and focus the response. A better wording might be "The nursing diagnosis most often associated with chronic congestive heart failure is _____)."

- For numerical or symbolic responses such as dosages, volumes, weights, or laboratory values, include the unit of measurement that is appropriate for the response (e.g., "A normal range of $PaCO_2$ is between _____ and _____ mm Hg)."
- Avoid grammatical cues by using both forms of indefinite articles such as "a/an"
- Locate blanks at the end of incomplete statements so that learners fully understand the information given before they must respond
- Keep the length of blanks uniform to avoid unwarranted cues
- Whenever possible, group similar forms of short answer or completion items together and provide explicit directions (e.g., "Provide one-word answers for each of the following ten questions" or "Use a brief phrase to correctly complete each of the following five statements.")
- Specify the scoring value of items and any special instructions (such as the need to show all computations in calculating a drug dosage)
- Devise a key of all acceptable responses for each item; review responses learners used to determine if any additional responses will be deemed acceptable
- Simplify the scoring process by either numbering each blank and providing a separate answer sheet or by using the right or left margins to list the completion entries that are printed alongside. An example of the latter is:

  _____ 1. The drug of choice for reversing narcotic effects is ⓵ .

TRUE-FALSE (ALTERNATE/FIXED RESPONSE) ITEMS

True-false items are declarative statements that learners must judge as either "true" or "false." Because responses to these items are limited to two options, they are also referred to as alternate, fixed response, or dichotomous items. Standard (simple) true-false items require only an indication of whether the item is true or false. Complex true-false items may additionally require the learner to cross out and/or correct the segment that is false.

APPROPRIATE USES

- Appraise knowledge and comprehension (cognitive taxonomy levels 1 and 2)
- Evaluate knowledge of facts that are categorically true or false
- Assess perceptions, misconceptions, fallacies, beliefs, and values
- Evaluate learners with limited verbal or writing capabilities
- Provide ease of construction and scoring (even by nonexperts, clerical staff, or computer)

LIMITATIONS

- Restricted in the number and types of instructional outcomes that can be appraised
- Restricted range of applicability because of the need for unequivocal facts; tendency to focus items on trivia and rote memorization
- May encourage guessing; standard format affords a 50% chance of guessing correctly
- Writing unequivocally true or false statements can be an onerous task because the truth or falsity of a statement is often contingent on a specific context, set of circumstances, or interpretation
- Qualifying statements intended to make the item less equivocal may give leading clues for the correct response

GUIDELINES FOR CONSTRUCTION AND USE

- Keep items brief, direct, and limited to a single idea
- Avoid determiners (*usually, often, in most cases, generally*) that cue the item as true (e.g., "Patients with acute myocardial infarction *often* have persisting substernal chest pain.")
- Avoid absolute determiners (*only, never, all, always*) that cue the item as false (e.g., "*All* patients with acute myocardial infarction have persisting substernal chest pain.")
- Avoid single or double negative statements that confuse the focus of truth or falsity (e.g., "*No* patients with acute myocardial infarction are *without* persisting substernal chest pain.")
- Avoid hiding the focus of the item in some inconspicuous feature such as a spelling error
- Reduce ambiguity and focus the learner's attention by underlining, CAPITALIZING, *italicizing*, or otherwise highlighting the focus of truth or falsity
- Reduce format cues by minimizing use of qualifying statements that make "true" statements longer than "false" statements
- Reduce guessing by having the examinee underline or correct the false segment of items
- Use random order for correct responses; avoid recognizable patterns in correct responses
- Use about (but not exactly) the same number of true and false statements
- To diminish problems in interpretation and scoring of responses, require learners to circle or check the words "true" or "false" rather than simply writing a letter "T" or "F" as a response. When learners are uncertain of the correct response, a handwritten "T" may assume features that make it difficult to distinguish from a handwritten "F."

Matching Items

A matching item consists of a series of problem items (called *stems* or *premises*) that are in some way associated with an accompanying series of possible responses or options. The separate series are arranged in a two-column format. The learner's task is to indicate which response or option corresponds to the item presented on the basis of some predetermined characteristic.

The problem items are typically numbered consecutively and arranged in the left-hand column. They may occur in the form of incomplete sentences, phrases, or words. All answers must be drawn from the same set of options.

APPROPRIATE USES

- Best for measuring knowledge (cognitive taxonomy level 1) of facts, associations, or relationships between two categories of words or phrases (such as associating anatomical structures with their functions, terms or concepts with their definition, drugs with their normal dosage, or poisons with their antidotes)
- Used primarily for evaluating a learner's ability to identify, recall, recognize, differentiate, or associate
- Can be used to match the names or functions of various parts with numbered or lettered diagrams
- Can be completed quickly by learners and scored quickly and easily by instructors[36]

LIMITATIONS

- Limited to evaluating the lower levels of cognitive function
- Item type is only appropriate when all responses are plausible alternatives for each premise
- Guessing may be a problem when some options can be readily discounted through the process of elimination
- Validity is impaired if each option can only be used once and the number of options is the same as the number of stems or premises; process of elimination can again become instrumental in determining responses

GUIDELINES FOR CONSTRUCTION AND USE

- Make each set within a column (both premises and responses) homogenous (i.e., related to similar content and phrased in a similar way) so that the basis for matching is clear and learners understand how the two columns relate to one another
- Plainly identify in headings over each column the commonality among entries in that column (e.g., the premise column might be headed as "Generic Name of Drug" and the response column could be headed as "Normal Maintenance Dosage Range." All entries under the "Generic Name of Drug" column would be the generic (not trade or brand) names of various drugs and all entries under the "Normal Maintenance Dosage Range" column would be the normal main-

tenance [not loading or resuscitative] dosages for different drugs)
- Reduce guessing and use of the process of elimination by providing more responses than there are items to match (premises) or permit responses to be used more than once
- Keep both column lists relatively short (greater than 5 but less than 15) and cryptic
- If either column has an inherent order, list its entries accordingly; otherwise, use alphabetical order (e.g., in the example, given previously, the column of generic names of drugs might be listed alphabetically and the dosages listed in ascending numerical order.)
- Place all entries for a column on the same page
- Ensure that designations for the entries within each column are readily distinguishable and employ different identification systems (e.g., each of the generic drug names could be listed alphabetically as entries A, B, C, D, and the like, whereas each of the possible dosages could be numbered as 1, 2, 3, 4. This will help to avoid the confusion of a single identification system where premise A matches with response A.)
- Give explicit directions that identify the basis for matching, whether responses can be used more than once, and whether any premises may require more than one response

Multiple-Choice Items

A multiple-choice item consists of a *stem* that formulates a problem or situation or asks a question and a series of alternative *options* that contain two elements: one element called a *distractor* that provide's plausible but incorrect or less desirable responses to the stem and another element called a *key* that designates the correct or best response to the question, problem, or situation posed (Table 5.6). Stems are formatted as either direct questions or as incomplete statements.

Multiple-choice items are sometimes distinguished according to the number of options they pose to learners. Most often, these items contain four options, but may, at other times, use three or five options. At least three options need to be used to avoid creating an alternate (either/or) item. More than five options, however, tends to create unwarranted complexity in reading and comprehension.

Multiple-choice items may be cast into a number different response formats, depending on the performance behaviors and content areas to be measured.[36] These formats include the correct response, best response, multiple response, negative response, and context-dependent response format.

The *correct response format* is used when the key is unequivocally correct and the distractors are indisputably incorrect. Its primary use is in measuring factual truisms and items of certainty.

The *best response format* is used when the key is clearly

TABLE 5.6 • TERMS USED TO DESCRIBE COMPONENTS OF MULTIPLE-CHOICE ITEMS

Component	Example
STEM	1. The percussion note normally heard over peripheral lung fields is _____
OPTIONS Distractors:	A. dullness B. tympany C. hyperresonance
Key:	D. resonance

and defensibly the most desirable or appropriate response among the alternatives offered, whereas the distractors are clearly less than optimal responses. Its primary use is in measuring areas having varying degrees of appropriateness or veracity, controversial issues and topics, or areas where certainty and fact are relative to circumstances or to complex, interrelated variables.

The *multiple response format* is used when the key includes more than a single option (multiple keys) or when multiple options are combined within a single key. Its primary use is in measuring more complex cognitive functions such as data interpretation and analysis, inferential and deductive reasoning, problem solving, and the determination of multiple causation or effect.

The *negative response format* is used when the key designates an option that is an exception, error, exclusion, anomaly, or other aberration that singles it out from the other options. Its primary use is for detecting errors or exceptions to general rules or procedures or for emphasizing contraindications and inappropriate ministrations.

The *context-dependent response format* is used when the key to a number of items is in part based on information provided in a picture, graphic, illustration, or narrative that accompanies or precedes the item series. It is primarily used for obtaining a more holistic and meaningful frame of reference for fuller consideration of more complex phenomena as they occur in a realistic situation.

Table 5.7 illustrates examples of each multiple-choice format. Other variations of these formats, such as combining two or more aspects of the response in a single option, are also possible.

APPROPRIATE USES

- Offers versatility, flexibility, and economy in measuring the full range of cognitive functions at any degree of difficulty[15]
- Appraises cognitive learning as well as or better than virtually any other written test item and often with greater effectiveness and efficiency
- Covers content to any desired breadth and scope
- Is reasonably easy to write, answer, score, and analyze

- Bypasses many of the logistical scoring problems (legibility of handwriting, ranges of skill in written expression, spelling, punctuation, variable degrees of accuracy, subjective scoring bias) that plague other types of items
- Scoring can be done by computer or by a person without expertise in the content area

LIMITATIONS[36]

- Best for written assessments of cognitive learning; less useful for assessing affective or psychomotor learning
- Reliance on recognition (vs. generation) of correct answer reflects lower level of cognitive performance tested
- Some content areas have few plausible distractors available
- Guessing can be a problem if distractors are inadequate in number, ineffective, inappropriate, or too close to readily discriminate among

GUIDELINES FOR CONSTRUCTION AND USE[10,11,35,48]

- Offer a stem that poses a clear, concise formulation of a problem admitting of only one correct or best response
- Develop a stem that contains all qualifying information relevant to the response and any words which would have to be repeated in each of the options
- Compose a stem so clearly that a knowledgeable learner can anticipate the correct answer before reading the options
- Avoid complexity, verbosity, jargon, and uncommon abbreviations in the item; use no more information in the stem than is necessary to elicit the correct response
- Use negative stems (e.g., "Each of the following is a clinical finding in CHF **except**" or "Which of the following is **not** an indication for oxygen therapy?") sparingly; if at all. Negative stems take longer to answer and may confuse learners or adversely affect test performance. When negative stems are used, the negative segment needs to be highlighted by <u>underlining</u>, CAPITALIZING, **boldfacing,** or *italicizing*
- Make each test item independent of all other items in the test. Check to be sure that the stem of one item does not reveal the correct response to some other item in the test. Verify that the correct or best response to the item does not depend on a correct response to another item
- Use different systems for designating the items and options (e.g., most multiple-choice items are numbered [1,2,3,4] and options are lettered with uppercase [A,B,C,D] or lowercase [a,b,c,d] letters)
- Avoid using terms that indicate extremes or absolutes (*never, only, every, always, all*). These words tend to cue the option as incorrect because few statements of this nature are true in every instance
- Avoid filler options (*all of the above, none of the above*)

	TABLE 5.7 • MULTIPLE-CHOICE ITEM RESPONSE FORMATS	
Response Format	**Use**	**Example**
Correct response	When the key is unequivocally correct	The mass movement of gases by bulk flow in and out of the pulmonary system is called _____. A. diffusion B. respiration C. ventilation D. osmosis
Best response	When the key is the most desirable or appropriate response	Patients should be suctioned for _____. A. as long as necessary every hour B. as long as necessary to clear the airway C. no longer than 30 seconds when scheduled D. no longer than 15 seconds when clinically indicated

Multiple response	When there are multiple key sets	The chief advantages of intermittent mandatory ventilation (IMV) over traditional methods of weaning are that IMV is _____.
		1. safer
		2. less physiologically demanding
		3. faster
		4. less burdensome for staff
		5. more readily accepted by patients
		  A. 1, 2, 4
		  B. 1, 2, 5
		  C. 2, 3, 5
		  D. 2 and 3 only

Multiple response	When there are multiple options within a single key	Weaning from mechanical ventilation should be discontinued immediately whenever there is any evidence of _____. A. hypertension, tachycardia, or anxiety B. hypertension, bradycardia, or diaphoresis • C. hypotension, tachycardia, or agitation D. hypotension, bradycardia, or ventricular dysrhythmias
Negative response	When the key designates an exception, anomaly, or aberration from general rules	When administering CPR, the victim's head would ***not*** be hyperextended if there were any possibility of _____. A. a fractured mandible B. an occipital fracture C. cervical spinal cord injury D. lumbar spinal cord injury
Context-dependent response	When the key is based on information contained in an accompanying illustration or narrative	On his fourth day of hospitalization for an acute MI, Mr. Casey experiences a sudden recurrence of chest pain that is positional and radiates to his left shoulder, fever of 102.6° F, and S-T segment elevation in nearly all 12 ECG leads. The most likely cause of this clinical picture is _____. A. extension of the original MI B. a new MI C. acute pericarditis D. pneumothorax

when other plausible options cannot be readily identified; fillers tend to cue the option as incorrect
- Make all options plausible but be sure that only one option (key) is best/correct
- Make all options grammatically consistent with the stem; options that lack this consistency may cue the option as incorrect
- Make all options homogenous in their context, terminology, part of speech, unit of measurement, frame of reference, and length

- If the options possess some inherent order (numerical, chronological, etc.), use ascending or descending order to list the options
- Limit the number of options to between 3 and 5, except when fewer options keeps all of them plausible
- Aim to keep the length of options comparable; avoid constructing keys so that they are usually the longest or shortest option
- Restrict the use of "none of the above" to computa-

tional or factual problems where the key is exactly correct

- Avoid overlapping numerical or narrative options so that more than one option could be correct (e.g., if option A was "10 to 20 mg/kg" and option B was "15 to 30 mg/kg" the two options would overlap one another)
- In a related series of items based on the same case study, be careful to avoid cueing answers to other items in the series
- Lay out the test so that various content areas and response formats are grouped together. Keep options on the same page as the stem to which they refer. Avoid crowding or varying the physical location of options on the pages of a test.[10]
- Give written directions regarding how responses should be recorded (separate answer sheet, circled, underlined, written in margin area)
- Once the key is defined for use in scoring, review the order of keys to be certain that no recognizable pattern of correct responses is evident (e.g., the key is usually option C or D or the key pattern of B-D-A-C repeats throughout the test)
- Keep a record of the references used to substantiate the key for each item so that any necessary verification can be readily located
- Provide learners with clear and concise directions for taking the test and for indicating their response to each item

The processes of test construction and test item construction described thus far generate a set of valid, reliable, and useful measurement devices that enable the educator to quantify cognitive learning. To derive evaluations from these measurements, the educator will need to compare these measurements to some reference point that affords a basis for making judgments about learning performance. The reference points available for making this comparison are considered in the section that follows.

Types of Evaluation

In educational evaluation, the reference point against which an individual's performance is compared may be either group performance or some specified criterion level of performance. The first type of evaluation is called norm-referenced evaluation and the second type is called criterion-referenced evaluation.

Norm-Referenced Evaluation

Norm-referenced evaluation is the more traditional type of evaluation. This type is used when the educator is interested in describing either an individual learner's performance in relation to group performance or when the educator simply wishes to describe the group's overall performance. The term *norm* refers to the entire group of learners who completed the test; in evaluation this group of individuals is considered as a peer (or "norm") group. The group itself establishes its own norm of performance that is distinct from that of the individuals who comprise the group.

Norm-referenced evaluation employs a relative scoring system because any one learner's performance is always interpreted in relation to the group's overall performance. The classic example of norm-referenced evaluation is grading on a curve. If an individual learner's test score was 68 out of a possible 100 points, that score of 68 might be equivalent to a grade of "A" if it was the highest score attained in the entire class. If virtually all members of that class scored higher than 68, however, that 68 might be equivalent to a letter grade of "F." If about half the class scored above 68 and the other half scored lower than 68, that score of 68 might be equivalent to a grade of "C." Other examples of norm-referenced evaluation include percentile scores (a percentile score of 68 indicates that 68% of the group scored lower than that learner's score) and quartile scores (a quartile score of 75 indicates that 75% of the group scored lower than that learner's score). Anyone who has taken a standardized achievement test such as the Scholastic Aptitude Test (SAT), Graduate Record Examination (GRE), or IQ test has been subject to norm-referenced evaluation. When competition, relative achievement, and/or differentiation among performance levels is needed, norm-referenced evaluation is the appropriate type to use.

Criterion-Referenced Evaluation

A second type of evaluation is used when the purpose of evaluation is to measure an individual learner's performance in relation to a predetermined set of behavioral criteria. In this type of evaluation, the educator is interested only in describing the performance of the individual learner without relating it to the performance of others. This type of evaluation is called *criterion-referenced evaluation*.

Criterion-referenced evaluation employs an absolute scoring system: either learners performed as described in the performance criteria or they did not. With written tests, learners either attained the established passing score (also called a cutoff score or cut score) or they did not. Likewise with clinical checklists, either learners performed as described by the performance criteria on the checklist or they did not. In either case, how the group as a whole performed is not relevant. One familiar example of criterion-referenced evaluation is the American Heart Association's Basic Cardiac Life Support course performance checklists for the various CPR scenarios (single rescuer, two-rescuer, obstructed airway, infant, and child resuscitation). Each of these scenarios has specific behavioral criteria that learners must demonstrate before they successfully complete the course. When individual performance in relation to a predetermined set of performance criteria is needed, criterion-referenced evaluation is the appropriate type to use.*

Educators may find that both types of evaluation are necessary at different times or for different purposes. The discussion that follows provides only an overview of norm-referenced evaluation methods because definitive aspects of this topic constitute discrete areas of study that are beyond the scope of this book. The purpose of acquainting readers with the fundamentals of educational evaluation is to familiarize them with evaluation's general features and encourage them to pursue these topics in greater detail as the need for educational evaluation warrants.

Description and Analysis of Group Performance

The concepts and techniques used in norm-referenced evaluation of cognitive learning are borrowed from the field of descriptive statistics. Its parent field, statistics, comprises all data analysis techniques applied to quantitative information derived from groups. The mathematical study of statistics is divided into two branches, descriptive and inferential. *Descriptive statistics* comprises techniques that enable one to summarize and characterize measurement data meaningfully and concisely. *Inferential statistics* includes analysis that enables one to validly infer or generalize measurement findings to other comparable groups or test situations. Because norm-referenced evaluation attempts to describe an individual's performance in relation to that of others, it requires that the educator first be able to describe group performance and then consider how the individual learner performed relative to the group as a whole.

Suppose you just administered a 60-item multiple-choice pretest to 20 nurse orientees (n = 20). After scoring all 20 tests, allotting one point (scoring unit) for each correct item out of 60 possible correct items, you reviewed the scores these nurses obtained and listed them as seen in Table 5.8. When the score data appear in that form, it is difficult to derive any clear indication of overall group performance on the test.

Some questions you might likely ask yourself at this point include the following:

- How could the data be organized so that it would be easier to recognize and describe group performance?
- Rather than considering each of these separate scores, how could I best summarize the overall performance of the group?
- Did everyone in the group do about the same or was there a lot of variation in individual performance on the test?

TABLE 5.8 • PRETEST SCORES OBTAINED BY 20 NURSE ORIENTEES	
Nurse	**Score**
A	34
B	59
C	39
D	58
E	42
F	41
G	57
H	45
I	54
J	45
K	52
L	46
M	52
N	47
O	52
P	47
Q	51
R	49
S	51
T	49

The sections that follow describe how to answer these questions.

Frequency Distribution

Consecutively listing each of the test scores (Table 5.8) does not offer much useful information to the educator who needs to evaluate these measurements. Because the scores are numerical values, it might be more helpful to arrange the scores in numerical order from the highest to the lowest attained score and to count the number of learners who obtained each score. The resulting tabulation (Table 5.9) is called a *frequency distribution*.

A frequency distribution is helpful as an initial device for counting the frequency of occurrences of any given score. Because the lowest score on the test was 34, the distribution does not need to include scores below this. But even after deleting these lower scores, the frequency distribution can be seen to offer only a limited ability to summarize the other scores adequately.

GROUPED FREQUENCY DISTRIBUTION   A further refinement of a frequency tabulation, which presents the data in a more succinct format, is achieved by tallying the scores according

*Criterion-referenced evaluation will be considered again later in the discussion related to competency-based orientation.

TABLE 5.9 • FREQUENCY DISTRIBUTION OF PRETEST SCORES OBTAINED BY 20 NURSE ORIENTEES	
X	**f**
60	
59	|
58	|
57	|
56	
55	
54	|
53	
52	| | |
51	| |
50	
49	| |
48	
47	| |
46	|
45	| |
44	
43	
42	|
41	|
40	
39	|
38	
37	
36	
35	
34	|
	n = 20

Legend: X = score obtained
 f = frequency of occurrence of that score
 n = total number of scores

TABLE 5.10 • GROUPED FREQUENCY DISTRIBUTION OF PRETEST SCORES OBTAINED BY 20 NURSE ORIENTEES (n = 20)	
Class Interval	**f**
56 to 60	3
51 to 55	6
46 to 50	5
41 to 45	4
36 to 40	1
31 to 35	1

TABLE 5.11 • GROUPED AND CUMULATIVE FREQUENCY DISTRIBUTIONS OF PRETEST SCORES OBTAINED BY 20 NURSE ORIENTEES (n = 20)			
Class Interval	**f**	**Cumulative f**	**Cumulative %**
56 to 60	3	20	100
51 to 55	6	17	85
46 to 50	5	11	55
41 to 45	4	6	30
36 to 40	1	2	15
31 to 35	1	1	5

to exclusive groups called *class intervals*. This provides a more visually convenient and economical form of frequency distribution that is referred to as a *grouped frequency distribution*.

As Table 5.10 illustrates, a grouped frequency distribution simply gathers groups of scores and determines the frequency of scores on the basis of these groups rather than on the basis of individual scores. Each group or class interval should be of equal size and should not overlap with adjacent groups.

CUMULATIVE FREQUENCY DISTRIBUTION   If the educator successively adds (accumulates) the number of frequencies within each class interval from lowest to highest, a *cumulative frequency distribution* is produced (Table 5.11). A cumulative frequency distribution enables the educator to consider the occurrences of each scoring interval in terms of the total number of persons who participated in providing the data (n = 20).

CUMULATIVE PERCENTAGES   A further extension of this process considers the cumulative frequencies in relation to the total number of individuals taking the test, expressed as a percentage. The far right column of Table 5.11 designates these *cumulative percentages,* obtained by simply dividing the cumulative frequency by the total number of frequencies (n = 20) and then multiplying by 100%. This provides helpful information relating to what percent of learners attained scores within each scoring or class interval. Just as the cumulative frequencies must total 20 (n), the cumulative percentages must total 100% (all 20 scores). Later discussion will show how these percentages can assist in deriving other features of group performance.

A frequency distribution is an extremely useful vehicle for succinctly organizing test data to see more readily where scores fell and how they were distributed. It visually indicates the highest, lowest, and all intermediate scores obtained, and reveals the scores and scoring intervals achieved most often or not at all.

Measures of Central Tendency

As helpful as frequency distributions are in summarizing a large number of test scores, they still involve a moderate amount of data manipulation and time to derive and provide limited information about group performance. In any testing situation where a large number of scores are produced, you could reasonably expect that a few individuals would score low, a few high, and most would earn scores somewhere between these two extremes. Your expectation is that scores would be distributed or spread out in a bell-shaped or normal distribution curve (Figure 5.7).

As the size of the group diminishes, the likelihood that scores will be distributed in this manner also diminishes. Even when group size is small, however, a majority of scores still tend to cluster around some central point and fewer scores will tend to exist toward peripheral areas on either side. This tendency of scores to pile up in the middle of a distribution of scores and thin out at the periphery enables the evaluator to locate one average, middle, or typical score that may be used to succinctly characterize the entire distribution and compare it with other distributions of scores. The determinations that represent these central or pivotal scores are called *measures of central tendency*.

There are three different measures of central tendency: the mean, median, and mode. Each refers to a different aspect of centrality, but all three can be used to characterize an entire distribution of scores.

MEAN   The *mean* refers to the average score of a group of scores. It is determined by finding the sum of all scores (Σ) and dividing this sum by the number of scores (n). If we added all 20 of the scores indicated in Table 5.8, the sum (Σ) would total 970. When 970 is then divided by the number of scores (n = 20), the average or mean score is 48.5.

The symbol abbreviation for a mean score is $\overline{X}$. Table 5.12 illustrates how to calculate a mean score.

The mean (also called an arithmetic mean) is the most widely used measure of central tendency because it considers the weight of each score and balances the total weight of the scores with how many scores contributed to that

TABLE 5.12 • CALCULATION OF A MEAN PRETEST SCORE	
Nurse	**Score**
A	34
B	59
C	39
D	58
E	42
F	41 $\overline{X} = \Sigma X \div n$
G	57
H	45 $\overline{X} = 970 \div 20$
I	54
J	45 $\overline{X} = 48.5$
K	52
L	46 where $\overline{X}$ = mean
M	52 Σ = the sum of
N	47 X = scores
O	52 n = total number of scores
P	47
Q	51
R	49
S	51
T	49
Σ = 970	

weight. As long as the scores follow a bell-shaped (normal) distribution, the mean is the single most valid representation of any set of scores. In general, the less symmetrical the distribution of the scores, the less valid the mean is for characterizing that set of scores.

Because the mean considers the relative weights of scores, it is susceptible to influence by any extreme score. An extremely high score will tend to deviate the mean upward, whereas an extremely low score will tend to shift the mean downward. Either way, the mean would then be a less valid and accurate characterization of all of the scores in that set. For example, suppose three groups of nurses took the same ECG test. All of the nurses in group I had about the same amount of experience in interpreting ECGs, but a single member in group II had many more years of experience in ECG interpretation, and a single member in group III had virtually no experience in ECG interpretation. The scores and means for each group are listed in Table 5.13.

As you can see, despite four of the five scores being identical across all groups, the extreme scores in group II (one extremely high score) and group III (one extremely low score) significantly alter the mean and make it a less accurate indicator of overall group performance. Barring these two instances (lack of a normal distribution curve or the presence of extreme scores), the mean remains the single best value to describe a distribution of scores.

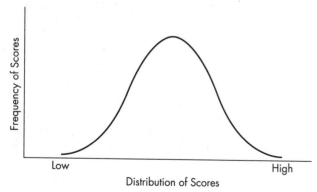

Figure 5.7   Normal distribution curve.

TABLE 5.13 • EFFECT OF EXTREME SCORES ON THE MEAN

	ECG Test Scores		
	Group I	Group II	Group III
	45	45	45
	51	51	51
	43	43	43
	44	44	44
	52	92	07
Sum of scores (Σ):	235	275	190
Mean (X̄):	47	55	38

MEDIAN   Whereas the mean indicates the *average* of a group of scores, the median indicates the *middle* in a distribution of scores. It can be variously defined as

- The score that divides the top half from the bottom half of scores
- The score that divides the distribution of scores into halves
- The score below which 50% of scores lie, or
- The score at the 50th percentile

With an uneven number (or odd number) of scores in the set, the median is the middle score; with an even number of scores, the median lies between the middle two scores.

To calculate a median, you must first rank order the scores: that is, list them from the highest to the lowest. Then you find the middle score in this rank order. For example, in the set of five scores listed in Table 5.13, the median in each set is the middle or third score (Table 5.14).

As you can see from this example, the median is nearly the same across all three groups of nurses who took the ECG test. Unlike the mean, the median is considerably less affected by the extreme scores in groups II and III. Because it is less influenced by extreme scores, the median is the preferred measure of central tendency for characterizing a set of scores that do not follow a normal distribution (bell-shaped curve) or that contain extreme scores. In general, the larger the size of the group being tested, the more likely

TABLE 5.14 • CALCULATION OF THE MEDIAN FOR AN ODD NUMBER OF SCORES (n = 5)

	Group I	Group II	Group III
	52	92	51
	51	51	45
Median:	45	45	44
	44	44	43
	43	43	07

the scores from that group will follow a normal distribution pattern. The smaller the size of the group (especially with groups of 30 or fewer learners), the less likely it is that scores will follow a normal distribution and the less useful the mean becomes to reflect central tendency. In this situation, the median will tend to provide a more accurate measure of central tendency than the mean.

The median is also the most valid summary statistic when rating scale categories are given numerical values such as when excellent = 5, very good = 4, good = 3, fair = 2, and poor = 1. When used in this manner, these numbers are not strictly arithmetic values, but numerical symbols that represent qualitative values.

In the ECG test example, the median is easy to calculate because there is an odd number of test scores; all the educator had to do was identify the middle or third of the five scores to find the median. In the earlier example of 20 nurse orientees, however, there is an even number (20) of test scores. Using the same scores for these orientees as appear in Table 5.12, the rank ordering of scores would appear as illustrated in Table 5.15. Because the two middle scores are both 49, the median is 49. If the two middle scores had been different numbers, the median would be the midpoint between them. For example, if the middle two numbers had been 49 and 48, the median would have been 48.5. If they had been 52 and 48, the median would have been 50.

MODE   The third measure of central tendency, the *mode,* represents the most *frequently* occurring score. The mode is the easiest of all measures of central tendency to determine because it only requires a visual scanning of frequencies (such as in Table 5.9) to identify the score attained most often. Whereas the mean represents the *average* score and the median represents the *middle* score, the mode represents the most *common* or typical score.

From the earlier example of 20 nurses (Table 5.9), it can be seen that the most commonly occurring score, the mode, is 52. The other example of three groups of nurses who took an ECG test contained no score that was obtained more than once within any of the groups. In this case, there is no mode. Other sets of scores could conceivably contain more than one score obtained with an equally high frequency. A distribution of scores, then, may contain no mode, a single mode, two modes (described as bimodal), three modes (trimodal), and so on.

Types of Distributions

In a perfectly symmetrical normal distribution of scores, all three measures of central tendency would fall on the same value (Figure 5.8, *A*). When scores predominate at either end of the distribution rather than in the middle, the distribution is said to be skewed. A *positively skewed distribution* (Figure 5.8, *B*) occurs when most scores are located

TABLE 5.15 • CALCULATION OF THE MEDIAN FOR AN EVEN NUMBER OF SCORES (n = 20)	
Median Score	**Scores**
	59
	58
	57
	54
	52
	52
	52
	51
	51
Median = 49	49
	49
	47
	47
	46
	45
	45
	42
	41
	39
	34

Measures of Variability

As you examine sets of test scores, you will find that they not only tend to cluster around some central value but that they also extend to varying degrees in either direction from that central point. In addition to central tendency, then, the other major feature to derive from a set of scores is the extent to which they spread, disperse, or vary from their central values. This is the property of *variability* or *dispersion*. Three measures of variability include range, interquartile range, and standard deviation.

RANGE   The easiest way to determine the spread of scores is by simply subtracting the lowest score from the highest score.* This procedure produces a measure called the *range* of scores. Range is the crudest but quickest measure of variability. In the example of the 20 nurse orientees, the highest score attained was 59 and the lowest score was 34, so the range was 59 minus 34, or 25.

The range of scores for the three groups of nurses who took the ECG test would be as follows:

Group I   52 − 43 = 9
Group II   92 − 43 = 49
Group III   51 − 7 = 44

Why are there such huge differences in the range for these groups? Remember that in these three sets of test results, Group I had no extreme scores, but both Groups II and III had one extreme score (Group II had one very high score of 92 and Group III had one very low score of 7). As a result, Group I's range of 9 indicates little variability or spread of scores within that group; Group II's range of 49 and Group III's range of 44 indicate a wide spread or variability among scores within those groups caused by a single extreme score.

Another problem with range that this example illustrates is its insensitivity to the actual proximity among scores. If you recall from Table 5-13, four of the five scores in each of the three groups were exactly the same. In cal-

toward the lower end of the distribution. With a positively skewed distribution of scores (also termed *skewed to the right*), the mean or average score is higher than both the median and mode scores. A *negatively skewed distribution* (Figure 5.8, *C*) exists when the majority of scores are located at the high end of the distribution. With a negatively skewed distribution of scores (also termed *skewed to the left*), the mean or average score is lower than both the median and mode scores. These findings underscore how the mean is vulnerable to influence by the presence of an asymmetrical distribution of scores.

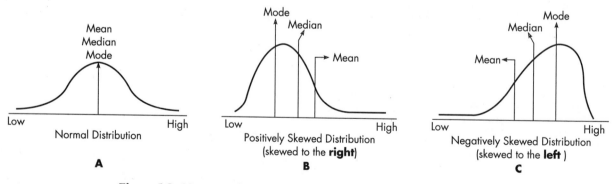

Figure 5.8 Measures of central tendency in normal and skewed distributions.

*When calculating the range for rating categories assigned numerical values (such as excellent = 5, very good = 4), the range is always *one less than* the difference between the highest and lowest number of categories.

culating the ranges for these three groups, the resulting drastic differences demonstrate that, were it not for the single extreme scores in two of the groups, the range for each of the three groups would have been quite small.

Although the range is easy and fast to calculate, its vulnerability to influence by extreme scores and its insensitivity to the true amount of actual dispersion among scores limit its usefulness and makes it a rather crude estimate of variability.

INTERQUARTILE RANGE   A second measure of variability of scores is the interquartile range. A quartile refers to a quarter or 25% of the distribution of scores. Every distribution contains four quartiles: the first 25% of scores represents the first quartile (called Q_1), the first 50% of scores represents the second quartile (called Q_2), the first 75% of scores represents the third quartile (Q_3), and all or 100% of scores represents the fourth quartile (Q_4).

One definition of the median was that it was the score at the 50th percentile. A percentile is a value that indicates the percent of a distribution that is equal to or below it. Thus, a score at the 50th percentile is the score value at which 50% of scores are located at or below it; it is the middle of a distribution of scores. After counting down (or up) half the total number of nurse orientee scores, you find that the score at the 50th percentile is 49 (Table 5.16). The *interquartile range* is determined by subtracting the score at the 25th percentile (Q_1) from the score at the 75th per-

centile (Q_3). In this example, the first quartile of scores (Q_1) falls at or below a score of 45 and the third quartile of scores (Q_3) falls at or below a score of 52. If Q_1 (45) is then subtracted from Q_3 (52), the interquartile range is calculated as 7.

This represents a very cursory description of how interquartile range is calculated and the values given here are primarily for purposes of illustration. Readers interested in calculating the true values for this measure are advised to consult a text on descriptive statistics.

STANDARD DEVIATION   A third measure of variability, the *standard deviation,* is the best and most widely used measure of dispersion. This measure is most suitably employed when scores follow a normal or bell-shaped distribution.

As a measure of variability, the standard deviation (abbreviated as "s") recognizes the mean of a set of scores as the measure of central tendency appropriate for a normal distribution and then considers how far each separate score deviates from the mean. By calculating each score's deviation from the mean, an average or standard deviation from the mean is identified to characterize how the scores are dispersed or spread around the mean.

Calculating a standard deviation is a relatively simple process but requires a fuller understanding than this brief description to perform it accurately. For raw data such as the 20 orientees' pretest scores, standard deviation is equal to the square root of the sum of squared deviations from the mean divided by the total number of scores. The formula for this would appear as follows:

$$s = \sqrt{\frac{\Sigma(X - \overline{X})^2}{n}}$$

Table 5.17 illustrates that the calculation of a standard deviation for the 20 nurse orientees' pretest scores is somewhat tedious but not really difficult. Computer software can greatly facilitate these calculations.

Knowing only the mean and standard deviation of a normally distributed set of scores, the educator can then describe the entire distribution of a set of scores and compare one group of scores with another. The details of how to accomplish this are beyond the scope of this text but can be found in any reference on descriptive statistics.

One of the values of knowing the standard deviation of a set of scores is that this information enables the educator to view scores on a normal distribution curve that contain the standard deviation about the mean of that set of scores. This constructs something called a *standard normal distribution curve* (Figure 5.9) that relates information such as the following:

- Of all scores in the distribution, 68.26% will fall within plus or minus 1 standard deviation from the mean (34.13% plus 1 standard deviation and 34.13% minus 1 standard deviation)

TABLE 5.16 • CALCULATING THE INTERQUARTILE RANGE

Interquartile Ranges	Scores
100th percentile (Q_4)	59
	58
	57
	54
	52
75th percentile (Q_3)	52
	52
	51
	51
	49
50th percentile (Q_2)	49
	47
	47
	46
	45
25th percentile (Q_1)	45
	42
	41
	39
	34

- Of all scores, 95.44% will fall within plus or minus 2 standard deviations from the mean (47.72% plus 2 standard deviations and 47.72% minus 2 standard deviations)
- Nearly all scores (greater than 99.7%) will fall within plus or minus 3 standard deviations from the mean

TABLE 5.17 • CALCULATION OF STANDARD DEVIATION FOR 20 NURSE ORIENTEE SCORES		
X	X − X̄	(X − X̄)²
59	10.5	110.25
58	9.5	90.25
57	8.5	72.25
54	5.5	30.25
52	3.5	12.25
52	3.5	12.25
52	3.5	12.25
51	2.5	6.25
51	2.5	6.25
49	0.5	0.25
49	0.5	0.25
47	−1.5	2.25
47	−1.5	2.25
46	−2.5	6.25
45	−3.5	12.25
45	−3.5	12.25
42	−6.5	42.25
41	−7.5	56.25
39	−9.5	90.25
34	−14.5	210.25
Σ = 970	Σ = 00.0	Σ = 787.00

$$\bar{X} = 48.5$$

$$s = \sqrt{\frac{\Sigma (X - \bar{X})^2}{n}}$$

$$s = 6.27$$

In the discussion of grading systems that follows the educator can see how the use of standard deviations also has a very practical value in the traditional methods of assigning grades to indicate relative achievement on written tests.

Grading Systems

Although staff development educators do not typically assign letter grades to learners' performance on written tests, understanding the procedure for determining grade assignments can be useful in understanding the entirety of the norm-referenced evaluation process and in viewing group performance on a given test.

A *grade* or mark is a symbol that represents an evaluation of performance in a condensed form. Grades may be derived and symbolized in various ways, depending on how that grade or mark will be used.

Traditional grading systems are norm-referenced in that the grades assigned are determined by comparing each learner's performance to that of others who completed the same test. Such grading systems use either numerical or letter symbols to represent the relative evaluation of a learner's performance.

Numerical grading systems assign grades as either absolute raw scores or percentages. Raw scores typically constitute the absolute number of points (scoring units) that a learner earned on the test. Percentages convert the portion of points earned into a percentage of points out of the total possible number of points that could be earned on the test.

Letter grading systems, using the traditional letter grades of A, B, C, D, F, are a bit more complicated to derive. They may incorporate one of three basic approaches to assignment of a letter grade:

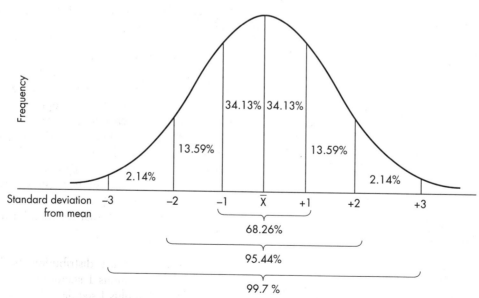

Figure 5.9 Standard normal distribution curve.

- **Direct conversion of a raw score or percentage to a letter grade.** For example, if scores were converted as follows for a 100-item test:

Score of 90 to 100	(90% to 100% correct)	= A
Score of 80 to 89	(80% to 89% correct)	= B
Score of 70 to 79	(70% to 79% correct)	= C
Score of 60 to 69	(60% to 69% correct)	= D
Score of less than 60	(00% to 59% correct)	= F

- **System of natural breaks.** This system may be used as a basis for assigning letter grades when a frequency distribution of grades reveals the absence of a normal distribution together with the presence of breaks of more than one consecutive score. These breaks create clusters of scores at well-demarcated levels. Visual inspection down such a frequency distribution will indicate whether the system of natural breaks will be appropriate for that set of scores (Table 5.18).

- **Standard letter grade system.** When a large number of scores (at least 30) fall into a pattern of normal distribution, letter grades may be assigned on the basis of the location of the numerical grade under the normal curve. This is the pure form of grading on a curve that is performed without adding or subtracting any factor that "corrects" the curve for grading purposes.

  In the pure form of this system, the mean test score

is used as the reference point for the middle range of a "C" grade. Ranges for the other letter grades are assigned according to the limits set by plus or minus 1, 2, or 3 standard deviations (SDs) from the mean:

A = +3 standard deviations from the mean
B = +2 standard deviations from the mean
C = ±1 standard deviation from the mean
D = −2 standard deviations from the mean
F = −3 standard deviations from the mean

Figure 5.10 illustrates an example of how this standard letter grade system would work for a 60-item test administered to 44 examinees when the mean score was 48.70 (out of a possible 60) and the standard deviation was 4.35. In addition to the full letter grades shown there, finer gradations for plus and minus letter grades could also be made if differentiation of a C^- from a C^+, for example, were desired.

When cognitive learning is assessed by means of a written test, the scores learners achieve are a function of both their cognitive performance (i.e., what they know) and test performance. *Test performance* refers to how effective the test items are as individual measuring devices. If test items are not well formulated, the test will be an inherently ineffective device for measuring learning. The following section describes how the educator can evaluate test performance.

Description and Analysis of Test Performance

Item analysis consists of a set of procedures for determining how well written test items function as measurement vehicles. It is used primarily with multiple-choice tests, but may also be employed for other types of items.[14,32] In item analysis, a norm-referenced approach is used to examine each test item in terms of how many and which learners marked it correctly or incorrectly.

Some of the benefits of performing item analysis are that this procedure may reveal unsuspected flaws and weaknesses in item construction, clarity, and form that may diminish the validity and usefulness of a test. This analysis also lays the groundwork for improved item writing and assists the educator in distinguishing between learning deficits and testing defects.

The primary rationale for subjecting a test to item analysis is to derive three pieces of information:

- How **difficult** the item was for a particular group of learners
- How well the items **discriminated** between more and less knowledgeable learners
- How effectively the **distractors** function within each item

These three considerations reflect the three major components of item analysis: item difficulty, item discrimination, and distractor effectiveness.

TABLE 5.18 • GRADE ASSIGNMENTS BASED ON SYSTEM OF NATURAL BREAKS

Score	f	Number of Scores	Grade
39	1	1	A
38	0	} natural break	
37	0		
36	0		
35	2		
34	1		
33	2		
32	1	6	B
31	0	} natural break	
30	0		
29	0		
28	2		
27	1		
26	1		
25	1	5	C
24	0	} natural break	
23	0		
22	0		
21	0		
20	2	2	D

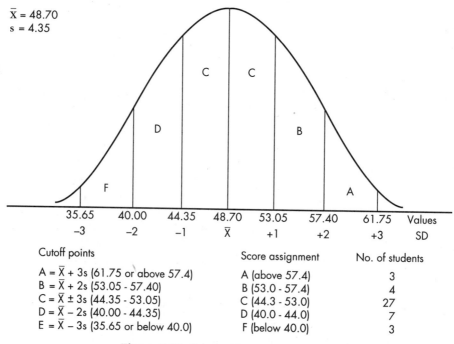

$\bar{X} = 48.70$
$s = 4.35$

Values	35.65	40.00	44.35	48.70	53.05	57.40	61.75
SD	−3	−2	−1	$\bar{X}$	+1	+2	+3

Cutoff points

A = $\bar{X}$ + 3s (61.75 or above 57.4)
B = $\bar{X}$ + 2s (53.05 - 57.40)
C = $\bar{X}$ ± 3s (44.35 - 53.05)
D = $\bar{X}$ – 2s (40.00 - 44.35)
E = $\bar{X}$ – 3s (35.65 or below 40.0)

Score assignment	No. of students
A (above 57.4)	3
B (53.0 - 57.4)	4
C (44.3 - 53.0)	27
D (40.0 - 44.0)	7
F (below 40.0)	3

Figure 5.10   Standard letter grade system.

Item Difficulty

Item difficulty is defined as the percentage of examinees who answer an item correctly. From this definition, it is obvious that a particular test item's difficulty is inversely proportional to the number of correct responses for that item; that is, as item difficulty increases, the percentage of correct responses to that item decreases, and vice versa.

Item difficulty may be determined by simply counting how many learners marked that item correctly and then dividing the number of correct responses by the total number of persons tested. If the result is left as a decimal proportion (of learners who answered the item correctly to the total number of learners tested), this figure is referred to as a *difficulty index*. If the result is converted into a percentage, it is called the *difficulty level* or *difficulty percentage*. Either term carries the same implications. A difficulty level may range from 0% (all learners answered the item incorrectly) to 100% (all learners answered the item correctly); a difficulty index may range from 0.0 (all learners answered the item incorrectly) to 1.0 (all learners answered the item correctly). Table 5.19 illustrates the calculation of item difficulty for a 10-item test taken by 30 nurses.

An earlier section discussed the notion of a skewed distribution. If a test had a large number of very difficult items, few learners would likely get them correct and most scores would accumulate at the low end of the distribution curve, producing a positively skewed distribution. If a test had a large number of very easy items, scores would tend to accumulate toward the high end of the distribution, producing a negatively skewed distribution.

TABLE 5.19 • CALCULATION OF ITEM DIFFICULTY (n = 30 EXAMINEES)

Item	Number of Correct Responses (n = 30)	Difficulty Index (correct ÷ n)	Item Difficulty (%)
1	18	0.600	60.0
2	15	0.500	50.0
3	11	0.367	36.7
4	14	0.467	46.7
5	14	0.467	46.7
6	13	0.433	43.3
7	15	0.500	50.0
8	11	0.367	36.7
9	8	0.267	26.7
10	10	0.333	33.3

When it is necessary or desirable to differentiate between high and low achievers (e.g., in competitive situations such as screening tests or tests for career advancement), having some moderately difficult items may be useful. In general, however, items that no one answers correctly (difficulty index 0.00) and items that everyone answers correctly (difficulty index 1.00) are not very helpful in differentiating among various levels of achievement. Most written tests, therefore, attempt to avoid these extremes and aim for an average difficulty range of 45% to 85% or 50% to 75%.[15,20,30] Items with this type of midrange difficulty level produce the highest test reliability.[31] Within each test, however, many educators aim at providing a distribution of items that includes easy, moderately difficult, and difficult items.[14,28]

The notion of item difficulty can be applied to either the test as a whole or to individual test items. In an objective test, a major influence on item difficulty is the number, content, and wording of the item's options. Because the likelihood of answering an item correctly is, to some extent, inversely proportional to the number of options available, the optimal difficulty level may be adjusted according to the possible influence of chance or guessing. The potential chance effect (the possibility that learners who lack the knowledge to answer the item could select the correct response simply by guessing) is inversely proportional to the number of options the learner must select among:

- Two-option items have a 50% chance effect
- Three-option items have a 33% chance effect
- Four-option items have a 25% chance effect

For example, in an alternate response (two-option) item such as a true-false question, chance alone gives the learner a 50% likelihood of answering the item correctly. As a result, the difficulty level for two-option items needs to be set at a higher level to compensate for the potentially heavy influence of chance in a correct response. Multiple-choice items with three or four options are much less potentially influenced by guessing or chance and could, as a result, have somewhat lower difficulty levels set for them. Overall, a test item should have a difficulty level established at some point between the chance effect and the maximum of 100%. For a four option multiple-choice item, the ideal difficulty index would be 62.5% or midway between the chance effect of 25% and no difficulty (100% correct).[20] Nunnally[33] recommends that the potential effect of guessing be factored in for various types of test items. He suggests a difficulty level of 60% to 95% for true-false items and 35% to 80% for four-option multiple-choice items.

As mentioned earlier, if an item is either very easy or very difficult, it does not allow for differentiating well between the better and less well-informed learner. If items are too easy, all learners will tend to perform well and the best learner will not be evident; if items are too difficult, all learners may perform poorly, including many of the best learners. The ability of an item to distinguish between well-informed and uninformed learners is the area of item analysis called *item discrimination*.

Item Discrimination

The *discrimination index* (level, power) is a statistical measure of an item's ability to distinguish between those who scored highest and those who scored lowest on the entire test. If an item discriminates well, the high scorers usually answer it correctly, whereas the low scorers usually answer it incorrectly. Knowing how well an item discriminates is

useful in supplementing instruction during test review and in indicating when improvement in item writing is necessary. In addition, the higher the average discrimination of test items, the higher test reliability will be.[31]

Discrimination levels are expressed as a ratio:

$$DL = \begin{array}{c} \text{Proportion of high} \\ \text{scorers answering} \\ \text{item correctly} \end{array} \quad to \quad \begin{array}{c} \text{Proportion of low} \\ \text{scorers answering} \\ \text{item incorrectly} \end{array}$$

Discrimination levels can range from a maximum of $+1.0$ (maximum or perfect discrimination) when all high scorers answer it correctly and all low scorers answer it incorrectly to 0.0 (no discrimination) to -1.0 (negative or reverse discrimination) when all high scorers answer it incorrectly and all low scorers answer it correctly. The more closely a discrimination level approaches a value of $+1.0$, the more effectively the item functions in differentiating between more and less knowledgeable learners and the less likely the item needs any revision. As positive discrimination values fall closer to 0.0, the less discriminating the item is and the more likely that item requires revision as a measuring device. Negative or 0.0 discrimination levels indicate that either the answer key is incorrect or that the item as written is ambiguous or structurally unsound. In either case, the item needs to be revised or deleted.

The optimal discrimination level, like the optimal difficulty level, falls within a moderate range because of the interrelatedness of these two item attributes. In general, the higher the discrimination index, the more effective the item is functioning. Most classroom tests using norm-referenced evaluation aim at a discrimination level between 0.35 and 0.60, or higher than 0.20.[15,17,20] With groups of 40 or fewer learners, a discrimination index of at least 0.20 may be used.[30] Items with higher discrimination levels are usually proportionately more difficult, whereas items with lesser discrimination levels are usually too easy. Highly discriminating items that are very difficult and less discriminating items that are very easy fail to provide the distribution or spread of scores sought in norm-referenced classroom testing.

Determining a discrimination level requires that the educator do the following:

- Identify the total number of examinees (n).
- Arrange the answer sheets or tests so that the highest score is the top paper and the lowest score is the bottom paper.
- Decide how the total number of examinees will be divided into distinct groups that constitute high, middle, and low scorer subgroups. Some options available here include the following:

    Dividing the total number of examinees into upper, middle, and lower thirds (this is particularly helpful with groups of 40 or fewer learners)

    Dividing the total number of examinees into an upper quarter, middle half, and lower quarter

Dividing the total number of examinees into an upper 27%, middle 46%, and lower 27%.[30] The smaller the fraction of people in the upper and lower groups, the more refined the discrimination analysis because the high and low scorers are increasingly more segregated from the mid-level performance group.

- From the fraction selected for the highest and lowest groups, pull the top and bottom of scores (33.3%, 27%, or 25%) and put the middle group aside, leaving separate stacks of papers with the highest and lowest scores.
- For each test item, separately tabulate how many of the high scorers answered it correctly and how many of the low scorers answered it correctly.
- Calculate the proportion of high scorers who answered it correctly from the total number of high scorers; do the same for the low scorers.
- Subtract the proportion of low scorers who answered it correctly from the proportion of high scorers who answered it correctly. The resulting net proportion is the discrimination level.

Table 5.20 illustrates how to calculate item discrimination for a 10-item test taken by 30 nurses. The top one-third (10) of scores constitutes the high scorer group and the lowest one-third of scores constitutes the low scorer group. Jenkins and Michael[28] describe how to perform item analysis by hand or computer.

Once item difficulty and discrimination are known, the item should be evaluated in light of each of these attributes to determine whether it is functioning effectively as written or needs revision. If subsequent revision of the item does not improve item performance, the educator should consider whether to discard or replace that item. Table 5.21 illustrates how the data from item analysis (see Tables 5.19 and 5.20) can be used as a basis for overall evaluation of a test item. In this process, the educator needs to keep in mind that other factors can influence item difficulty and discrimination: differences in learner characteristics, in teaching methods, test conditions, clerical errors in preparation of the test, or the physical formatting or layout of the test.[15]

In addition, it is important that the educator use item analysis results as an adjunct in decision-making about test items rather than as the sole criterion for these decisions. Although a difficulty index of .30 to .75 and a discrimination index greater than .30 may be ideal, these are not absolute cutoffs for acceptability of the item. For example, one item may be answered correctly by all learners (indicating 0.00 discrimination and difficulty of 1.00). The educator would not aim to have a large number of these items in a test, but a few easy items in a long test would be acceptable. Conversely, an item that has high discrimination

TABLE 5.20 • CALCULATION OF ITEM DISCRIMINATION FOR A 10-ITEM TEST TAKEN BY 30 NURSES (n = 30, SCORING GROUPS = HIGH, MIDDLE, AND LOW 33% OF SCORES)

Item	Group	Number of Correct Responses	Fraction of Correct Responses	Proportion of Correct Responses	Discrimination Index
1	H	10	$^{10}/_{10}$	1.00	
	L	8	$^{8}/_{10}$	0.80	0.20
2	H	9	$^{9}/_{10}$	0.90	
	L	6	$^{6}/_{10}$	0.60	0.30
3	H	7	$^{7}/_{10}$	0.70	
	L	4	$^{4}/_{10}$	0.40	0.30
4	H	7	$^{7}/_{10}$	0.70	
	L	7	$^{7}/_{10}$	0.70	0.00
5	H	10	$^{10}/_{10}$	1.00	
	L	4	$^{4}/_{10}$	0.40	0.60
6	H	8	$^{8}/_{10}$	0.80	
	L	5	$^{5}/_{10}$	0.50	0.30
7	H	10	$^{10}/_{10}$	1.00	
	L	5	$^{5}/_{10}$	0.50	0.50
8	H	9	$^{9}/_{10}$	0.90	
	L	2	$^{2}/_{10}$	0.20	0.70
9	H	6	$^{6}/_{10}$	0.60	
	L	2	$^{2}/_{10}$	0.20	0.40
10	H	8	$^{8}/_{10}$	0.80	
	L	2	$^{2}/_{10}$	0.20	0.60

Item	Item Difficulty	Item Discrimination	Item Evaluation
		TABLE 5.21 • ITEM EVALUATION FOR A 10-ITEM TEST TAKEN BY 30 NURSES	
1	0.60	0.20	Discriminates poorly. Difficulty falls within acceptable upper limits. Needs much improvement to retain it.
2	0.50	0.30	Discriminates only fairly well, but difficulty is very good. Revise and retain.
3	0.37	0.30	Too difficult at this level of discrimination. Revise to reduce difficulty; try rewording.
4	0.47	0.00	Fails to discriminate, although it has good difficulty. Will probably discard item.
5	0.47	0.60	Item difficulty and discrimination are very good. Retain as is.
6	0.43	0.30	Is too difficult for its discriminatory power. Revise to improve discriminatory level and retain.
7	0.50	0.50	Difficulty level is excellent, but discrimination could be improved. Modify slightly or retain as is.
8	0.37	0.70	Discriminates very well, although it is rather difficult; a challenger. Retain and locate at end of test.
9	0.27	0.40	Is much too difficult and discriminates only fairly well. Revise and reduce difficulty to retain.
10	0.33	0.60	Discriminates very well, but is too difficult. Try rewording to reduce difficulty level.

but was very difficult could also be retained since it tends to clearly segregate learners who know the content from those who do not. The major weaknesses the educator is attempting to isolate with item analysis are marginal or zero discrimination and reverse or negative discrimination. Weak items can then be improved for future use. When very small groups of learners are the norm, the educator may need to compile the results of a number of these groups to generate sufficient data for item analysis with greater precision. Regardless of the number of learners, item analysis can better assure the quality and effectiveness of classroom tests.

Effectiveness of Distractors

With multiple-choice items, item discrimination may be taken a step further to check how effective distractors are as plausible alternatives to the correct answer (key). Instead of merely indicating how many of the high and low scorers answered an item correctly, the specific options chosen (key or distractors) by members of the high and low scorer groups can be isolated and differentiated. Although this analysis is often overlooked,[28] distractor analysis assists in identifying the following:

- *Effective distractors* that are selected more often by low scorers than by high scorers
- *Ineffective distractors* that are selected more often by high scorers than by low scorers
- *Nonfunctioning distractors* that are not selected by either group

Table 5.22 illustrates how the effectiveness of an item's distractors may be determined, analyzed, and summarized.

EVALUATION OF LEARNING WITHIN THE AFFECTIVE DOMAIN

Affective behaviors embrace the expression of a complex variety of attitudes, beliefs, and values that incline individuals to respond toward specific situations or things in characteristic ways. The affective realm focuses not so much on the behavior displayed as it does on the disposition from which that behavior emanates. Evaluation of affective learning, however, must, of necessity, be inferred from overt behavioral evidence since the dispositions that generate those behaviors are not usually amenable to direct appraisal.

Special Considerations Related to the Affective Domain

Individuals acquire their beliefs and values through both experience and education. Instructional programs that include a practicum of some type may be able to influence learners' experiences to some degree. In addition, classroom and simulation experiences are often used to imbue learners with certain attitudes regarded as desirable, consistent, or appropriate for the professional roles that nurses undertake.[18]

Nursing has a substantial number of largely unwritten expectations for the deportment and demeanor of its prac-

		Options (*Indicates Key)				
Item	**Group**	**A**	**B**	**C**	**D**	**Evaluation of Distractors**
1	H	10*	0	0	0	All distractors functioning well.
	L	2	3	4	1	
2	H	1	1	8*	0	Option D not functioning at all; replace D.
	L	2	2	6	0	
3	H	3	1	2	4*	Options A and C are ineffective; need revision.
	L	1	3	0	6	Options A and D may be too close for even high scorers to distinguish between.
4	H	3	2*	2	3	Spread of high scorer responses indicates ambiguous or poorly constructed item; revise entirely or discard. Check accuracy of key.
	L	1	7	2	0	
5	H	1	1	7*	1	Distractors A and B are functioning effectively, but option D, less well.
	L	2	2	5	1	
6	H	5*	0	5	0	Option C is ineffective and may be too close to be distinguished from key.
	L	5	3	1	1	
7	H	0	0	1	9*	Options A and B are nonfunctional; replace.
	L	0	0	3	7	
8	H	2	6*	1	1	All distractors functioning at marginal level and fail to discriminate well between learners.
	L	2	6	1	1	
9	H	0	10*	0	0	All distractors functioning well.
	L	3	4	2	1	
10	H	0	0	7*	3	Option A is nonfunctional; replace it.
	L	0	4	6	0	Option D is ineffective; revise it.

TABLE 5.22 • Effectiveness and Evaluation of Distractors

titioners. Staff development educators often find themselves responsible for facilitating the acquisition, internalization, and expression of many of these expectations. Some of these expectations represent affective expressions related to patients such as caring, empathy, acceptance, respect, trust, confidentiality, sensitivity, and compassion. Some expectations relate to how nurses interact with others in performing their role: integrity, reliability, commitment, cooperation, sincerity, enthusiasm, initiative, and independence.

Challenges of Evaluating in the Affective Domain

Although certain dispositions and beliefs are clearly more therapeutic or desirable than others, the affective domain is fraught with many unique aspects that make teaching and evaluating this area truly challenging.[8] Some of the factors contributing to this situation are that affective behaviors are inherently:

- *Difficult to define precisely in behavioral terms.* Even when definitions are available for these abstract qualities, consensus on these definitions may not exist.

- *Difficult to measure because of their lack of precision and clarity in definition.* If an attribute cannot be clearly defined or if its expression is modified by an awareness of its being appraised, attempts to measure the attribute with any degree of reliability and validity are open to question. For example, if orientees know that their "cooperation with others" is being evaluated that day, human nature suggests that they may be especially cooperative in their working relationships then, perhaps more than they might usually be. We are, in many instances, limited in our knowledge of how to measure many affective behaviors. The number and types of valid instruments available for evaluating attitudes is quite limited in some areas and nonexistent in others.

- *Complex and difficult to isolate.* Apart from the context in which they occur, beliefs and attitudes have no independent focus that can serve as a basis for isolating them as discrete entities. For example, one cannot demonstrate "empathy" unless they are in a situation where this trait is called for and appropriate. In order for affective behaviors to be evaluated, learners must have an opportunity to experience a value-related issue or situation, examine their beliefs about that value, consider alternative courses of action and the consequences of each, and select the most appropriate course of action.

- *Inaccessible.* Learners are the only persons who can know what their true feelings and beliefs are. The behavior that a nurse demonstrates may arise out of genuine beliefs, out of what the nurse anticipates others expect, or even out of what is perceived as necessary behavior to successfully complete an educational program. Because educators must infer that overt behaviors correspond to a given set of convictions and because individual nurses may not be consciously aware of all the influences governing their behavior, inferences made concerning that behavior may be wholly inaccurate. Unlike other learning behaviors that are more or less directly attributable to specific causes, the genesis of affective behaviors may be less accurately inferred or even be inaccessible to direct inference. Each of us has experienced situations when our own behavior was misinterpreted by others; some nurses also express their beliefs and values in less overt ways that may make their affective basis for behavior difficult to detect much less characterize correctly.
- *Unstable.* Even if the measurement of affective behaviors were not problematic, the instability of these attributes makes them less than amenable to reliable measurement. Unlike cognitive or psychomotor behaviors, affective behaviors may not always be developed in a linear fashion and may change on the basis of a single life experience. For example, a nurse with many years of experience may not have genuinely felt or demonstrated much compassion toward patients who have attempted suicide. After providing nursing care to one of her friends who survived that experience, however, that nurse's compassion for similar patients might forever more be heightened.
- *Open to questions of propriety with respect to their assessment and evaluation.* Some educators are reluctant to judge the attitudes and value systems of others and are resistant to the notion that these can be mandated in time or degree by some educational program. The demonstration of a newly acquired attitude or belief cannot be programmed as readily as other types of learning nor scheduled for integration within specific time periods. This lag time between providing instruction in affective areas and demonstration of its acquisition is a particularly thorny problem. Because of many concerns such as these, affective outcomes are often clothed as concomitant or serendipitous components to more tangible and conventional aims of learning.

In spite of the fact that many of the more subtle aspects of human behavior are rather elusive and difficult to appraise objectively, the educator needs to make every attempt to appraise learning in the affective domain. As anyone who practices or receives the ministrations of nursing can attest, there is much more to being a capable nurse than merely knowing the science of nursing or performing its technical procedures. The art of nursing merits its due in evaluation too. Some of the methods that have been considered useful in evaluating affective learning are listed in Table 5.23.

EVALUATION OF LEARNING WITHIN THE PSYCHOMOTOR DOMAIN

Learning related to the psychomotor domain is traditionally evaluated in relation to the myriad of tasks, procedures, and skills that nurses must be able to perform in the clinical area. As opposed to tests that measure a learner's *knowledge about* an activity, skill, process, or procedure, psychomotor evaluation is intended to measure a learner's ability to actually perform that activity, skill, process, or procedure.

Challenges of Evaluating in the Psychomotor Domain

The evaluation of psychomotor behavior in nursing commonly presents a number of challenges to the educator. These challenges include the following:

- The number, range, and complexity of psychomotor behaviors required of nurses is considerable, especially in high-tech areas such as the operating room, emergency department, or critical care unit. This lays a heavy instructional and evaluational burden on both learners and educators.
- Operational definitions of what constitutes acceptable, correct, or satisfactory performance of psychomotor procedures may vary over time, from one agency to another, from one evaluator to another, and from one locality or region to another. The norms or standards by which these practices are judged tend to be based on those established by the individual agency. Although the use of local norms is often necessary, it creates the need for each institution to develop its own evaluation criteria rather than adopting or adapting criteria developed elsewhere. The time and expense required for developing these standards can be considerable.
- Performance tests typically require more time to design and are more difficult to use than cognitive tests.[26]
- The validity and reliability of evaluating psychomotor learning may be called into question because of the potential influence an observer's presence may have on learner performance. When they know that they are being observed and evaluated, learners may perform differently than they otherwise would.
- Scoring on tests of psychomotor performance may be

TABLE 5.23 • METHODS FOR EVALUATING AFFECTIVE LEARNING	
Method	**Comments**
Videotaping spontaneous performance	May be supplemented by self, peer, and/or instructor critique. Potential for bias in learners' behavior if they are aware that they are being videotaped.
Direct observation of performance	May be supplemented by a checklist or rating scale* to structure the observation,[8] detect trends in behavior, or search for behaviors such as responding judgmentally toward patients, cooperating with others, or labeling patients. Observations and impressions need to be verified and validated to be certain that they accurately reflect learner's belief systems.
Process recordings	Informal and serendipitous notes based on observations of nurse-patient interactions and interpersonal dynamics to detect patterns of values and beliefs demonstrated in various situations.
Simulations	Written, taped, or live enactments of specific true-to-life vignette situations to see how learners respond to the circumstances and variables presented. Discussion following the simulation can then uncover the beliefs, values, and attitudes elicited.
Patient care conferences	Selected patient situations may be used to highlight how various affective traits influence nursing care. For example, the situation of a newly diagnosed AIDS patient and a newly diagnosed cancer patient might be used to contrast how social mores and value systems affect the health care system's response to these two types of patients.
Role-playing	Role-playing can be designed to illustrate the influence of specific affective behaviors on nursing practice. Behavioral criteria with or without peer critique may be used to determine the manner in which desired behaviors are demonstrated.
Debate	Learners can be divided into groups to represent and contrast all sides of an issue or set of circumstances that revolve around the potential influence of certain affective behaviors. Following the exchange of viewpoints, some form of resolution and outcomes can be reached to afford guidance in nursing care.
Survey analysis	Established or newly designed survey instruments may be used to determine the range of values and attitudes related to sensitive or controversail issues and to afford a basis for discussion that reflects what learners believe about those issues.
Plan of care reviews	Some affective traits may be reflected by nursing interventions that appear in patients' plans of care. For example, nurses who are nonjudgmental in regard to patient values would plan interventions to meet patient needs even if they personally did not ascribe to them. Although a nurse might believe in the sanctity and preservation of life, the nurse would provide education and discharge care to assist a patient who preferred to be discharged rather than receive chemotherapy and surgery.

*See section on psychomotor evaluation instruments for construction of these tools.

more subject to bias than on objective tests of cognitive performance.

- Evaluations of psychomotor performance in the clinical area can seldom be fully controlled or standardized. In general, the closer the test situation approximates actual performance conditions, the greater the problems in minimizing the effects on uncontrolled situational variables.[26]
- The instructional outcomes related to psychomotor learning may lack clarity, organization, and specificity. When this is the case, both the learner and the educator may encounter difficulty in isolating what must be demonstrated for successful completion of these expectations.

Methods for Evaluating Psychomotor Learning

Each of the methods available for evaluating the psychomotor aspects of performance attempts to resolve one or more of the challenges mentioned previously. Although none is a panacea for evaluation in this area, some are more promising than others in circumventing these obstacles. In addition, educators may find that using a combination of evaluation methods affords more valid evaluation than using any single method alone.

Psychomotor evaluation may be conducted in either a simulated laboratory setting or in the clinical setting. The advantages and disadvantages of each of these settings for the instructional process have already been described (Chapter 4) and are equally applicable for the evaluation process.

As mentioned in Chapter 4, many of the methods used for teaching in the laboratory and clinical settings are also employed for evaluation. In many cases, the laboratory setting may be employed primarily for appraising the early development and initial tryout of psychomotor skills, for determining a learner's readiness for clinical evaluation, for performance of skills that cannot be readily provided in the clinical area, and for demonstration of skills that involve some potential element of harm to the patient. The clinical setting might then be reserved for validating the refined execution and modification of these skills under the constraints and variables typically present in the real world of nursing practice.

Some of the methods for evaluation of psychomotor learning are listed in Box 5.3. Of these, the most commonly employed method is observation. *Direct observation* involves the physical presence of an evaluator during a demonstrated performance. Although this may appear to be the most natural means of observation, educators must recognize that their presence interjects an unnatural element into the situation that may interfere with or artificially augment the learner's execution of a skill or procedure. Despite this recognized limitation, direct observation often represents the only feasible means to evaluate the totality of a complex clinical situation, especially when nonverbal communication and a multitude of subtle and highly specific variables exist in the situation. Many of these variables (such as the context or circumstances of the situation) may not be evident in a taped account of performance. Although it is time-consuming and open to bias, first-hand witnessing of performance may be the most reasonable and expedient way to measure psychomotor proficiency.

The technique of *indirect observation* entails the use of videotape, audiotape, or some other means to record and preserve observations for later review and appraisal. By providing a permanent and retrievable record of performance, learners and educators can both participate in the evaluation process as often as necessary or desired. Although indirect observation is less obtrusive and eliminates the potential bias that the observer's physical presence may cause, learners may also become preoccupied with being taped and fail to provide natural behaviors in that situation. Recordings are also limited in their failure to convey the emotional overlay of a nurse-patient interaction and in their restricted view (camera angle and distance, adequacy of

lighting and acoustics, microphone sensitivity) of the situation.

In order for observations and other methods of evaluating psychomotor learning to be valid and reliable in educational evaluation, they must be focused, systematically organized, and standardized. This is typically accomplished by the design and use of one or more tools or instruments to structure the measurement of psychomotor performance. These tools may also be used for appraisal of affective learning when the appraisal method involves observations of live or taped performance.

Psychomotor Evaluation Instruments

The design of psychomotor evaluation tools involves the same general procedures as those used in the design of cognitive evaluation tools: test construction and test item construction. But in place of the seven steps for constructing a written test, the educator follows the seven steps for constructing a performance evaluation tool. In place of test item construction, the educator develops the items or entries to be included in the performance evaluation tool.

Construction of Performance Evaluation Tools

To better ensure that psychomotor evaluation devices meet the same measurement benchmarks as those for written tests, the educator needs to employ a systematic and educationally sound procedure in designing these tools. The procedural steps listed in Box 5.4 will help the educator develop psychomotor evaluation instruments that are valid, reliable, and useful.

Step 1: Specify the instructional outcomes for psychomotor evaluation. After reviewing all of the instructional outcomes for each program offering, the educator sorts the outcomes into those appropriate for cognitive, affective, or psychomotor evaluation. If these outcomes are listed manually on some device such as index cards or sheets of paper,

---

Box 5.3

METHODS FOR EVALUATION OF PSYCHOMOTOR LEARNING

- Observation of performance
- Return demonstration
- Learning laboratory
- Training mannequins
- Simulated patients
- Simulated patient situations (such as ACLS Megacode stations)
- Role-playing
- Videotaped performance
- Review of written documentation such as plans of nursing care, discharge teaching plans, and the like
- Self-evaluation (typically used to a limited degree or used to augment instructor evaluations)

BOX 5.4

STEPS IN CONSTRUCTING PSYCHOMOTOR EVALUATION INSTRUMENTS

---

1. Specify the instructional outcomes for psychomotor evaluation
2. Determine the basis that will be used to judge learner performance
3. Design the evaluation tool
4. Develop the evaluation tool entries
5. Decide the setting(s) where psychomotor evaluation will be conducted
6. Pilot test the evaluation tool
7. Finalize the evaluation tool and its entries

---

the educator could sort the different domains for evaluation into three separate stacks. If the outcomes are included in a word processing file, the educator may just delete all outcomes that will not be evaluated by an appraisal of psychomotor performance.

During this process, the educator needs to carefully scrutinize the resulting list of psychomotor instructional outcomes to be certain that it is complete and accurate. Once this determination has been made, a second perusal can be made to verify that all outcomes are observable and measurable.

Step 2: Determine the basis that will be used to judge learner performance. The standard against which learner performance is measured may be in either of two categories: the degree of performance or the presence (vs. absence) of performance. The purpose of evaluation influences which of these two categories is the more appropriate. The former may be used more often for appraising affective areas, whereas the latter may be more suitable for evaluating psychomotor areas.

The *degree of performance* category includes evaluations that aim at appraising differences in learners' performance along some type of continuum. See Table 5.24 for examples.

The *presence of performance* category includes evaluations that aim at simply determining whether learners performed a particular behavior (or not). In this category of psychomotor evaluation, the degree of performance is not relevant; its presence or absence is the focus of appraisal. When this category of evaluation is used, it is important that all required behaviors be clearly enumerated so that the performance can be readily identified. With either category, the basis for evaluation represents the standard used to judge the learner's performance.

Step 3: Design the evaluation tool. If the purpose for evaluating psychomotor performance is to identify the degree of learner performance, the educator needs to design a rating scale to measure performance. If the purpose for evaluation is to determine whether certain behaviors are performed by the learner, the educator needs to devise a checklist to measure performance. The major features and formats for each type of evaluation device will be described in further detail later in this section.

Step 4: Develop the evaluation tool entries. The entries for rating scales and checklists are typically taken directly from the original list of instructional outcomes. This procedure assures the correlation necessary between intended instructional outcomes and evaluation items that is requisite for a valid evaluation instrument.

For many instructional outcomes, the detail and level of specificity contained in the wording of the outcome will be sufficient for use in the psychomotor evaluation tool. In other instances, the educator may find it necessary or helpful to add further detail or explanation in the evaluation entries to adequately cover all dimensions needing appraisal. For example, suppose the instructional outcome for an inservice education program was originally written as: "Demonstrates the staff nurse's responsibilities in the event of a fire alarm." This outcome may be expressed with sufficient clarity and specificity that no additional performance expectations are necessary for the evaluation process. By contrast, suppose that the outcome had been written as "Demonstrates the staff nurse's responsibilities in management of hospital emergencies." The educator might then distinguish separate entries on the evaluation form for management of a fire alarm, a disaster, cardiac arrest, and similar situations. Adequate detail needs to be provided so that the evaluator can readily distinguish among and between the performance behaviors, but unwarranted detail should be avoided.

Step 5: Decide the setting(s) where psychomotor evaluation will be conducted. As mentioned earlier, psychomotor evaluation may be provided as a simulated experience in the laboratory setting or as an actual experience in the clinical setting. When appraisal of specific psychomotor behaviors is targeted for evaluation in one setting rather than the other, the different evaluation settings need to be distinguished so that both learners and evaluators know where these activities should be completed. Some psychomotor behaviors may be evaluated in a single setting, while others may be evaluated in both settings; in other cases, the setting may be optional or left to the discretion of the instructor. Unless all behaviors will be appraised in the same setting, however, it is useful to distinguish this feature on the evaluation tool.

Though many hospitals have all psychomotor expecta-

Degree of Performance	Performance Continuum				
Frequency of performance	never	rarely	sometimes	usually	always
Dependency of performance	totally dependent	usually dependent	often dependent	minimally dependent	independent
Quality of performance	poor	fair	good	very good	excellent
Accuracy of performance	no errors	few errors	some errors	moderate errors	numerous errors
			or		
Consistency of performance	inconsistent		usually consistent		consistent
Assistance in performance	performs only with assistance		performs with some assistance		performs without assistance
Acceptability of performance	unacceptable		minimally acceptable		acceptable
Average of performance	below average		average		above average

TABLE 5.24 • DIFFERENCES IN LEARNERS' PERFORMANCE

tions enumerated on the same list, others find it helpful to use separate lists for laboratory and clinical setting evaluations. At times, this segregation by setting is used because different evaluators or different times are employed for different areas of evaluation. Individual preference and ease of use can help dictate this decision. The most important feature is to be sure that both learners and evaluators know where evaluations should occur.

Step 6: Pilot test the evaluation tool. Once the rating scale or checklist has been developed, it needs to be pilot tested to verify is validity, reliability, and usefulness. The validity of the tool can be verified by having users and clinical experts critique the scale or checklist entries for clarity, accuracy, correlation to instructional outcomes, timeliness, relevance, and inclusiveness. Inter-rater reliability can be determined by simultaneous ratings using live or videotaped performances; intra-rater reliability can be tested by having the same evaluator review multiple instances of a taped performance. Feedback from users regarding usefulness (ease of use, reading level, format, layout, and length) of the device can also be readily secured at this time.

Step 7: Finalize the evaluation tool and its entries. The findings from the pilot testing phase can be compiled and summarized to lend direction to changes that need to be made in the evaluation tool.

Construction of Performance Evaluation Tool Entries

As mentioned previously, psychomotor evaluation tools most often consist of either a rating scale or a checklist or, less often, anecdotal notes and self-evaluation devices. This discussion will focus primarily on the design of rating scales and checklists.

RATING SCALES A *rating scale* is a device used to record and evaluate observations. The dimension of behavior being rated constitutes some type of observable behavior such as a skill, procedure, task, or technique. Rating scales may also be used to evaluate expressions of affective traits such as attitudes or beliefs. Rating scales enable an observer to measure the degree to which a performance is evidenced.

Rating scales consist of two major parts: the behaviors to be evaluated and a scale for rating those behaviors. Once the behaviors to be evaluated have been determined, the educator needs to decide the type or format of scale to be used, the number of points along the scale, and whether one or more than one type of scale will be employed.

Rating Scale Formats All rating scales consist of a range of distinguishable, mutually exclusive (nonoverlapping), and equidistant degrees of behavioral performance arranged along a continuum. Though rating scales can employ anywhere from 3 to 20 scale points, most rating scales for evaluation of nurses' clinical performance employ a 5-point scale[6] Any of the performance attributes mentioned in step 2 may be used in this type of scale. All produce qualitative data that can be tabulated and summarized for evaluation.

In general, rating scales can be either narrative or numerical in their format. *Narrative rating scales* employ descriptive words, phrases, or paragraphs[13] to distinguish the relative degree of performance for a behavior. Examples of each of these are illustrated in Box 5.5.

Numerical rating scales may either designate numerical values for the points on a narrative scale (i.e., these convert a narrative to a numerical scale) or assign numerical values along a continuum anchored only at the endpoints by behavioral descriptions. Box 5.6 provides examples of each of these types of numerical rating scale.

Benefits and Advantages of Rating Scales Rating scales are relatively easy to construct and take little time to score and tabulate. Passing scores may consist of a preestablished narrative or numerical rating or a minimum requirement for each behavior in the list. By standardizing the focus of observations and facilitating their appraisal and recording, rating scales help to reduce the breadth of factors considered in the evaluation process, improve its accuracy, and diminish its reliance on the observer's memory of events. Because they employ a range of evaluation points, rating scales can be especially useful in monitoring the progress of learners over time as their performance advances along the continuum. In this regard, rating scales can be helpful in providing constructive feedback to learners about their relative learning achievements.

Limitations and Disadvantages of Rating Scales Some types of rating scales (particularly the paragraph narrative format) are tedious and time-consuming to design. Even with a well-designed scale, the ratings provided may be invalid or spurious if the evaluator has an aversion to assigning extreme scores, is unwilling to take the time necessary to observe and rate carefully, or has a vested interest in the outcome of the ratings.

Categories or points along the scale may not be mutually exclusive, leading to appraisals that actually overlap the available rating points. Qualitative scale categories (such as never-rarely-sometimes-usually-always) and normative category labels (such as excellent-very good-good-fair-poor) are virtually impossible to determine behaviorally in any objective manner.[6] The interpreted meaning of terms such as "average," "satisfactory," or "sometimes" can vary with each evaluator, making ratings unreliable and invalid.

Box 5.5

EXAMPLES OF NARRATIVE RATING SCALES

NARRATIVE RATING SCALE USING WORDS

Behavior to be evaluated	poor	fair	good	very good	excellent

NARRATIVE RATING SCALE USING PHRASES

Behavior to be evaluated	performs only with continuous assistance	performs with frequent assistance	performs with moderate assistance	performs with minimal assistance	performs with no assistance

NARRATIVE RATING SCALE USING PARAGRAPHS

Behavior to be evaluated	Patient assessments are never complete, accurate, or well documented. Never identifies all pertinent nursing diagnoses.	Patient assessments are rarely complete, accurate, or well documented. Rarely identifies all pertinent nursing diagnoses.	Patient assessments are sometimes complete, accurate, and well documented. At times identifies all pertinent nursing diagnoses.	Patient assessments are usually complete, accurate, and well documented. Usually identifies all pertinent nursing diagnoses.	Patient assessments are always complete, accurate, and well documented. Always identifies all pertinent nursing diagnoses.

Box 5.6					
EXAMPLES OF NUMERICAL RATING SCALES					

NUMERICAL RATING SCALE USING NUMBERED TERMS

Behavior to be evaluated	never (1)	rarely (2)	sometimes (3)	frequently (4)	always (5)

NUMERICAL RATING SCALE USING NUMBERED ENDPOINTS

Behavior to be evaluated	Requires continuous prompting and assistance from preceptor to perform (1)	(2)	(3)	(4)	Able to perform with no prompting or assistance from preceptor (5)

Descriptive categories regarding the learner's relative dependence on an instructor or preceptor may be of some interest in basic nursing education and nursing orientation programs[6] but do not represent the true focus of the instructional outcomes. Psychomotor outcomes all inherently assume that the nurse performs these procedures and processes independent of any form of prompting or assistance. In effect, then, a learner's need for assistance in performance is a more developmental consideration than the real emphasis of evaluation.

Because of these limitations and disadvantages, rating scales have limited usefulness in the evaluation of psychomotor learning in nursing staff development programs. They are, perhaps, more effectively and appropriately used for evaluation of affective learning outcomes and for appraising the input, throughput, and satisfaction level of output components of program evaluation.

CHECKLIST A *checklist,* as its name implies, is a recording device that lists behaviors to be performed and provides a place to check each behavior as it is observed. In order to be valid, reliable, and useful, the behaviors included in the checklist must be observable and measurable. Validity can be enhanced if the checklist entries are derived directly from the instructional outcomes for the program. Reliability may be augmented by stating the behaviors in clear and unambiguous terms that all evaluators will interpret in the same way. Usefulness can be improved by using a simple and straightforward recording system and form.

Checklists are similar to rating scales in that they are used to record and evaluate observations of learner performance. They differ from rating scales in that they require no judgment regarding the degree of performance but merely indicate whether a behavior was performed or not. Thus checklists use a dichotomous (either/or, pass/fail) system for making appraisals regarding learner performance.

Checklist Formats Checklists may be constructed in three basic formats. In its most rudimentary form, the checklist may only list the behavior to be performed. For example, a checklist entry may be written in this *summary format* as "Records a 12-lead ECG." A second format includes all component behaviors for performance of that skill, procedure, process, or technique. The component behaviors are typically enumerated in the order in which they are to be completed. An example of this *comprehensive format* is provided in Table 5.25. A third possible format restricts the behaviors included in the list to only those that are essential or critical to satisfactory performance. Table 5.26 illustrates the *critical behavior format* for a checklist.

The differences among these checklist formats are worthy of note. Although the summary format is easy and time-saving to construct, it affords no indication of the standards by which the evaluator is to judge the learner's performance. Lacking a standard to compare the observed performance against, there is no basis for the evaluator to determine whether the performance observed is acceptable (satisfactory, successful) or not.

At the other end of the format spectrum, the comprehensive format can be very laborious and time-consuming to construct. In addition, this format produces performance checklists that are lengthy; when a collection of comprehensive checklists is compiled, it can result in a document that resembles an encyclopedia more than an evaluation tool. Both the educator who would design these lists as well as the learner who would be subjected to them tend to recoil at their sheer bulk.

The critical behavior checklist format represents a useful compromise between the limitations of the summary

TABLE 5.25 • Comprehensive checklist format		
Records a 12-lead electrocardiogram		
Behavior	**Done**	**Not Done**
Prepares patient and equipment		
a. Verifies patients' name	☐	☐
b. Explains purpose and elements of procedure to patient	☐	☐
c. Plugs in grounded single-channel ECG recorder	☐	☐
d. Turns power switch to "on"	☐	☐
e. Checks for sufficient paper supply	☐	☐
f. Replaces paper roll if necessary	☐	☐
g. Draws curtain around patient's bed	☐	☐
h. Places patient in supine position at 45° semi-Fowler's	☐	☐
i. Exposes patient's distal limbs and chest	☐	☐
j. Prepares skin surfaces by cleansing with alcohol pad and mildly abrading friction	☐	☐
k. Applies conductive material to underside of electrode plates without allowing leakage	☐	☐
l. Attaches each electrode plate securely to its appropriate limb without straining or kinking cable wires	☐	☐
m. Records patient's name, date, and time on ECG paper	☐	☐
Standardizes ECG for time and voltage		
a. Turns control knob to "run"	☐	☐
b. Centers stylus on ECG paper	☐	☐
c. Sets paper speed to 25 mm/second	☐	☐
d. Turns lead selector switch to "STD"	☐	☐
e. Presses STD (1 mV) button	☐	☐
f. Produces of a 10-mm boxed deflection	☐	☐
g. Verifies sensitivity switch is "on"	☐	☐
h. Verifies that all waveforms are observable	☐	☐
i. If necessary, adjusts sensitivity to obtain observable waveforms	☐	☐
Records six frontal plane leads		
a. Records at least five ECG complex cycles for each frontal plane lead	☐	☐
b. Records frontal plane leads in the following order: I, II, III, aVR, aVL, aVF	☐	☐
c. Identifies each frontal plane lead by its respective code marking	☐	☐
Records six horizontal plane leads		
a. Turns control knob to "on"	☐	☐
b. Attaches small suction cup to chest lead cable	☐	☐
c. Applies electrode gel to each of six chest lead locations: V_1 = 4th ICS, RSB V_4 = 5th ICS, MCL V_2 = 4th ICS, LSB V_5 = same level as V_4, AAL V_3 = midway between V_2 and V_4 V_6 = same level as V_4, MAL	☐	☐
d. Applies suction cup to each V position	☐	☐
e. Turns lead selector to V position	☐	☐
f. Turns power switch to "run"	☐	☐
g. Records at least five ECG complexes for each horizontal plane lead	☐	☐
h. Records chest leads in standard order: V_1 through V_6	☐	☐
i. Identifies each horizontal plane lead by its respective code marking	☐	☐
Concludes ECG recording		
a. Turns power switch to "off"	☐	☐
b. Unplugs ECG recorder	☐	☐
c. Detaches electrodes from patient	☐	☐
d. Removes conductive material from patient's skin	☐	☐

TABLE 5.26 · CRITICAL BEHAVIOR CHECKLIST FORMAT

RECORDS A 12-LEAD ELECTROCARDIOGRAM

Behavior	Done	Not Done
Prepares patient and equipment		
a. Explains purpose and elements of procedure to patient	☐	☐
b. Turns power switch to "on"	☐	☐
c. Places patient in supine position at 45° semi-Fowler's	☐	☐
d. Prepares skin surfaces by cleansing with alcohol pad and mildly abrading friction	☐	☐
e. Applies conductive material to underside of electrode plates without allowing leakage	☐	☐
f. Attaches each electrode plate securely to its appropriate limb without straining or kinking cable wires	☐	☐
g. Records patient's name, date, and time on ECG paper	☐	☐
Standardizes ECG for time and voltage		
a. Sets paper speed to 25 mm/second	☐	☐
b. Presses STD (1 mV) button	☐	☐
c. Produces a 10-mm boxed deflection	☐	☐
d. If necessary, adjusts sensitivity to obtain observable waveforms	☐	☐
Records six frontal plane leads		
a. Records at least five ECG complex cycles for each frontal plane lead	☐	☐
b. Records frontal plane leads in the following order: I, II, III, aVR, aVL, aVF	☐	☐
Records six horizontal plane leads		
a. Applies electrode gel to each of six chest lead locations:	☐	☐
V_1 = 4th ICS, RSB V_4 = 5th ICS, MCL V_2 = 4th ICS, LSB V_5 = same level as V_4, AAL V_3 = midway between V_2 and V_4 V_6 = same level as V_4, MAL		
b. Records at least five ECG complexes for each horizontal plane lead	☐	☐
c. Records chest leads in standard order: V_1 through V_6	☐	☐
Concludes ECG recording		
a. Unplugs ECG recorder	☐	☐
b. Detaches electrodes from patient	☐	☐

and comprehensive formats. With the critical behavior format, the only behaviors listed are those that are essential to acceptable or desired performance in that area. Use of this format not only shortens the checklist, but, more importantly, recognizes two salient features of psychomotor performance: (1) that all behaviors in a procedure or skill are *not* equally important but that some are more important than others; and (2) that, although some behaviors could be executed in a number of alternative ways and still be acceptable, other behaviors must be executed in a specific manner for the performance to be acceptable. For example, with the procedure of recording a 12-lead ECG, it may be useful that the nurse "checks for sufficient paper supply," but even if the nurse neglected to do that, it would not necessarily detract from the quality and usefulness of the recording. But if the nurse neglects "to set the paper speed at 25 mm/second" or fails to standardize the voltage properly, the resulting ECG tracing could be interpreted incorrectly and cause unwarranted changes in the patient's med-

ical or nursing management. Other behaviors (such as recording the patient's name, date, and time) could be performed in many different ways and all of these would likely be acceptable. For all these reasons, the critical behavior checklist format is often preferred over both the summary and the comprehensive formats.

In constructing checklists, it is important to understand how the behavioral components of performance are generated because these constitute the standards against which the learner's performance will be judged acceptable or not. If an existing written document (e.g., written policies, procedures, standing orders, protocols) delineates how certain procedures are to be executed, the behaviors listed in that document can be directly applied or summarized for use in the checklist. If a particular performance area has no reference document to provide these behavioral components, the educator will need to develop the list of required behaviors. The following five steps can assist in this process[22]:

- *Secure the assistance of a nurse who might be considered a local "expert" in the performance area.* The expert might be identified by soliciting suggestions from nurse managers and nursing staff regarding the nurse whose practice in that area represents what all nurses should emulate. Then, ask that nurse to perform the procedure while the educator observes and records the performance (either in writing or on videotape). The desired performance attributes can then be listed as a rough draft of the behavior list with each entry indicating a single behavior.

- *Ask a few other nurses to perform the same procedure.* This step is helpful in identifying differences between the expert's performance and those of others to distinguish alternate but equally acceptable behavioral components and sequences of behavior from those that are considered essential. The educator then attempts to secure consensus among these nurses and the expert on which features of behavior are truly critical and which are not.

- *Pilot test the list of behaviors with one or more representatives of the prospective learner group.* This activity can help to determine if wording of the behaviors needs further clarification, simplification, or detail.

- *Note the types and frequency of errors in performance made by prospective learners.* Errors that commonly occur among learners will likely warrant reflection in the checklist to ensure they are not committed in the procedure performance.

- *Have those who assisted in developing the behavioral attributes of the performance use the checklist.* These nurses may be asked to enact the roles of both the learner and the evaluator to determine if the list of behaviors needs any additional refinements.

The steps described here represent a means of establishing a local standard for performance in a particular area. Use of this developmental process can help in assuring that the standards used in judging learner behaviors are as valid, reliable, and useful as those for which there are written standards of performance.

Benefits and Advantages of Checklists Checklists are helpful in overcoming many of the weaknesses of rating scales for evaluation of psychomotor performance. Because checklists use a dichotomous scoring system, the evaluator need not be concerned about appraising degrees of performance or avoiding extreme scale scores. Likewise, issues related to the equidistance between scale points and overlapping of categories are not encountered with the more straightforward, either/or evaluations used on checklists. Varying definitions of ambiguous terms such as "satisfactory" are less problematic with checklists because the behavioral attributes of what is satisfactory replace the ambiguous term. Thus scoring is easier, more direct, less subjective, and more valid and reliable.

In addition, checklists offer two other advantages for the educational process: () critical behavior checklists clarify and highlight all necessary and desired attributes of psychomotor performance so that both learners and evaluators can decipher the most important features of clinical performance, and (2) comprehensive checklists can be very useful as teaching devices for self-instruction. Learners can use these detailed lists of behaviors to learn, review, or practice procedures before being evaluated or whenever they wish to refresh their memory.

Limitations and Disadvantages of Checklists As mentioned earlier, the summary checklist format has very limited utility in psychomotor evaluation. Except for identifying the skill or procedure to be appraised, it affords no standards for judging the performance observed and, thus, precludes meeting the measurement benchmarks of validity, reliability, and usefulness.

The comprehensive and critical behavior checklists are time-consuming to design and refine, especially if the behavioral attributes must be developed "from scratch." The latter takes even more time and effort since essential vs. nonessential behaviors need to be clearly distinguished. For most areas of clinical nursing practice, however, the critical behavior checklist will repay this investment of time and effort many times over and give both learners and educators a useful, valid, and reliable means for evaluating psychomotor performance.

Anecdotal Records Although used less often in nursing staff development than in basic nursing education programs, anecdotal notes or records may be incorporated in psychomotor evaluations. *Anecdotal records* consist of brief narratives that describe observations of learner behaviors in a particular situation or instructor-learner interactions and their outcomes. These unstructured and informal notations may be used to help summarize or substantiate evaluation decisions, to indicate a learner's progress, to identify learning and/or performance problems, or to facilitate negotiations between the learner and instructor (e.g., in a learning contract). At times, these anecdotes include verbatim comments of learners or educators that occur during these exchanges.

The major disadvantages to using anecdotal records lies in their use and interpretation. Analysis of instructor comments, especially if there is a time lag since the recording, can be problematic for capturing the purpose and details of the account. Instructors may record them in a less than balanced manner, citing learner problems more often than their progress. Rather than recording facts and observations, educators may dilute the usefulness and validity of the records by interspersing their personal opinions and interpretations of events. If notes are not recorded immediately, the contents may suffer from faulty memory and recall of the events. A useful way to focus anecdotal records is by including a comments section on the psychomotor evaluation tool so that narrative notes can be targeted to specific behaviors. Alternately, an anecdotal record could be attached as a separate sheet to the evaluation tool so that both records are kept up-to-date.

SELF-EVALUATION DEVICES   Self-evaluation of one's psychomotor performance is an increasingly popular means of appraisal, especially at institutions where adult learning precepts are strongly held and applied. Such devices may be employed in a number of different ways.

Hospitals that use learning contracts for staff development programs may incorporate self-evaluations throughout the instructional process. Although educators or preceptors still must validate the nurse's performance, learners may be expected to critique themselves as a necessary component of the evaluation process much as they do for their regular performance evaluations. Agencies that use any form of self-instruction (written, audiovisual, computer-assisted) also typically include self-appraisals during the assessment and evaluation phases of instruction. In many of these self-instruction formats, formative and summative

self-evaluations are already included in the instructional materials. These evaluations may be employed in classroom, laboratory, or clinical settings.

Construction of self-evaluation tools follows the same guidelines as though these devices were to be administered by an instructor, preceptor, or staff development educator. Thus rating scales, checklists, anecdotal records, and the like for self-appraisals should be comparable to the instruments already described.

The primary value of using self-evaluation in nursing staff development is to actively involve nurses in the educational process. Since evaluation represents the litmus test for the effectiveness of instruction, learners must be afforded an opportunity to participate in this crucial phase.

This chapter on evaluation concludes the discussion of the educational process elements common to all staff development programs. The next chapter initiates coverage of educational considerations specific to orientation, inservice, and continuing education programs.

REFERENCES

1. Abruzzese RA: *Nursing staff development,* St Louis, 1992, CV Mosby.
2. Alspach JG, Bell J, Canobbio MM et al: *AACN education standards for critical care nursing,* St Louis, 1986, CV Mosby.
3. American Psychological Association: *Standards for educational and psychological testing,* Washington, DC, 1985, American Psychological Association.
4. Benjamin S: Evaluation principles for healthcare training institutions: the basics, *J Healthcare Educ Train* 7(1):7, 1992.
5. Bille DA: *Staff development: a systems approach,* Thorofare, NJ, 1982, Charles B. Slack.
6. Bondy KN: Criterion-referenced definitions for rating scales in clinical evaluation, *J Nurs Educ* 22:376, 1983.
7. Bowman B: Sins of omission, *Training* 24(5):45, 1987.
8. Bucher L: Evaluating the affective domain, *J Nurs Staff Develop* 7:234, 1991.
9. Caldwell RM, Marcel M: Evaluating trainers: in search of the perfect method, *Training* 22(1):52, 1985.
10. Cassidy VR: Test construction techniques, *J Nurs Staff Develop* 3:154, 1987.
11. Chenevey B: Constructing multiple-choice examinations: item writing, *J Cont Educ Nurs* 19:201, 1988.
12. Coleman EA, Thompson PJ: Faculty evaluation: the process and the tool, *Nurse Educ* 12(4):27, 1987.
13. Cottrell BH, Cox BH, Kelsey SJ et al: A clinical evaluation tool for nursing students based on the nursing process, *J Nurs Educ* 25:270, 1986.
14. Cranton P: *Planning instruction for adult learners,* Toronto, 1989, Wall & Thompson.
15. Demetrulias DAM, McCubbin LE: Constructing test questions for higher level thinking, *Nurse Educ* 7(5):13, 1982.
16. Dunn S, Thomas K: Surpassing the "smile sheet" approach to evaluation, *Training* 22(4):65, 1985.
17. Ebel RL: *Essentials of educational measurement,* ed 3, Englewood Cliffs, NJ, 1979, Prentice-Hall.
18. Ellis C: Incorporating the affective domain into staff development programs, *J Nurs Staff Develop* 9:127, 1993.
19. Farley JK: The multiple-choice test: developing the test blueprint, *Nurse Educ* 14(5):3, 1989.
20. Flynn MK, Reese JL: Development and evaluation of classroom tests: a practical application, *J Nurs Educ* 27(2):61, 1988.
21. Froman RD, Owen SV: Teaching reliability and validity: fun with classroom applications, *J Cont Educ Nurs* 22:88, 1991.
22. Geis GL: Checklisting, *J Instruct Develop* 7(1):2, 1984.
23. Gordon J: Measuring the "goodness" of training, *Training* 28(8):19, 1991.
24. Gordon J: Romancing the bottom line, *Training* 24(6):31, 1987.
25. Gosnell DJ: Evaluating continuing nursing education, *J Cont Educ Nurs* 15(1):9, 1984.
26. Gronlund NE: *Constructing achievement tests,* ed 3, Englewood Cliffs, NJ, 1982, Prentice-Hall.
27. Holzemer WL: Evaluation methods in continuing education, *J Cont Educ Nurs* 23:174, 1992.
28. Jenkins HM, Michael MM: Using and interpreting item analysis data, *Nurse Educ* 11(1):10, 1986.
29. Kirkpatrick D: *A practical guide for supervisory training and development,* ed 2, Reading, MA, 1983, Addison-Wesley.
30. Layton JM: Item analysis for teacher-made tests, *Nurse Educ* 10(4):27, 1985.
31. Layton JM: Validity and reliability of teacher-made tests, *J Nurs Staff Develop* 2:105, 1986.
32. Mehrens WA, Lehmann J: *Measurement and evaluation in education and psychology,* ed 3, New York, 1984, Holt, Rinehart, & Winston.
33. Nunnally J: *Educational measurement and evaluation,* New York, NY, 1972, McGraw-Hill.
34. Provus M: *Discrepancy evaluation,* Berkeley, CA, 1971, McCutchan.
35. Raymond M: *Guide to test item development,* Kansas City, MO, 1986, American Nurses Association.
36. Rosenberg MJ, Smitley W: Constructing tests that work, *Training* 20(9):41, 1983.
37. Rottet SM, Cervero RM: Clinical evaluation of a nursing orientation program, *J Nurs Staff Develop* 2:110, 1986.
38. Sarnecky MT: Program evaluation. Part 1: Four generations of theory, *Nurs Educ* 15(5):25, 1990.
39. Sarnecky MT: Program evaluation. Part 2: A responsive model proposal, *Nurs Educ* 15(65):7, 1990.

40. Scriven M: The methodology of evaluation. In Stake RE, ed: *Curriculum evaluation,* Chicago, 1967, Rand-McNally.

41. Simerly RG: *Planning and marketing conferences and workshops,* San Francisco, 1990, Jossey-Bass.

42. Sohn KS: Program evaluation in nursing, *Nurs Educ* 12(2):27, 1987.

43. Stake R: The countenance of educational evaluation, *Teachers College Record* 68:523, 1967.

44. Staropoli C, Waltz C: *Developing and evaluating educational programs for healthcare providers,* Philadelphia, 1978, FA Davis.

45. Stufflebeam DL, Foley W, Gephart W et al: *Educational evaluation and decision-making,* Philadelphia, 1971, FA Davis.

46. Tiessen JB: Comprehensive staff development evaluation: the need to combine models, *J Nurs Staff Develop* 3(1):9, 1987.

47. Toth JC: The basic knowledge assessment tool (BKAT)—validity and reliability: a national study of critical care nursing knowledge, *West J Nurs Res* 8:181, 1986.

48. Van Ort S, Hazzard ME: A guide for evaluation of test items, *Nurs Educ* 10(5):13, 1985.

49. Waddell DL: Differentiating impact evaluation from evaluation research: one perspective of implications for continuing nursing education, *J Cont Educ Nurs* 22:254, 1991.

Designing Staff Development Programs: A Competency-Based Approach

Nursing staff development programs may focus on any one of the three components of staff development: orientation, in-service education, or continuing education. In this unit, Chapter 6 will describe the design of nursing orientation programs and Chapter 7 will discuss the design of in-service and continuing education programs. The previous five chapters covered the elements common to constructing any nursing staff development program. Chapters in this unit will refer to these common elements and add considerations specific to each type of program.

CHAPTER 6

Orientation

The goal of an orientation program is to ensure that nursing staff are competent to fulfill the responsibilities and functions of their assigned position—that is, to ensure that nursing staff are capable of doing their job. Nursing staff may occupy any of a number of positions within the nursing department (e.g., staff nurse, charge nurse, nurse coordinator, nurse manager, clinical nurse specialist, associate director of nursing, and the like). Since the largest number of nursing positions are occupied by staff nurses, however, this chapter will use the staff nurse role as the frame of reference for describing the development of nursing orientation programs.

In contrast to the traditional approach to instruction used thus far, this unit will introduce the educator to the competency-based approach to designing instruction. *Competency-based education (CBE)* is an alternative approach to instruction that emphasizes a learner's ability to demonstrate integration of the knowledge, attitudes, and skills that are most important to a particular task, activity, or role. One of the primary distinctions between traditional and competency-based instruction is in the emphasis of the educational program: traditional instruction emphasizes what a learner should *know* by the end of an educational offering, while competency-based education emphasizes what a learner should be able *to do* to evidence competency for the task, activity, or role addressed in that program. Much of the rationale for employing a competency-based approach to a staff nurse orientation program is that CBE recognizes that the goal of this program is threefold: the orientee's demonstration of competence in the staff nurse role, tailoring instruction to that role, and offering emphasis on verification of clinical rather than purely cognitive performance.

If you recall from Chapter 2, the ANA defines orientation as the process by which new nursing staff members are acquainted with the philosophy, goals, policies, procedures, role expectations, physical facilities, and services of that agency.[14] Designing an instructional program to attain these ends follows the same procedure as for any other staff development program: needs assessment, program planning, implementation, and evaluation. This chapter will identify and emphasize features in each of these steps that merit special consideration for nursing orientation programs.

NEEDS ASSESSMENT

Educational needs related to orientation exist for all nursing staff when they enter the hospital as new employees or when they change roles at the institution. The latter might occur when an individual who had previously worked at a hospital as a nursing assistant obtains an associate degree in nursing and will now be working as a staff nurse.

While virtually all new employees are likely to need information related to the philosophy, goals, physical facilities and services available at that agency, their needs related to specific role expectations typically represent the major focus of the orientation program. The hospital's expectations for this role are usually summarized in the staff nurse position description. In practice, however, the agency's expectations for a staff nurse often derive from multiple sources rather than from this one source.

SOURCES FOR DETERMINING THE EDUCATIONAL NEEDS OF ORIENTEES

The sources used to identify the learning needs of orientees may include any of the primary, secondary, and combined sources of information described in Chapter 2. Of these, the sources of particular significance for an orientation program include a number of written documents as well as the perceptions of various members of the nursing staff.

Primary Sources
Written Documents

As mentioned in Chapter 2, the position description can be the single most important document for determining the educational needs of orientees. The position description usually provides an enumeration of organizational relationships related to that position, basic functions, necessary qualifications, and general work responsibilities of incumbents. However, because this document often comprises rather broad and generic descriptions of the agency's expectations for staff nurses, it may afford little more than a general framework with which to view the staff nurse role. If an orientation program must ensure that staff nurses are competent to perform their assigned responsibilities, then the specific components of what constitutes competent nursing practice in that role need to be enumerated in greater detail than the position description typically affords.

When a healthcare agency establishes standards of patient care and/or standards of nursing practice, these documents represent that agency's definition of how it expects nurses to function in relation to the care they provide and the practice they exemplify. The hospital's policies, procedures, protocols, and unit routines likewise represent defined sets of expectations for how a staff nurse functions, completes certain tasks or activities, and responds to specific situations in delivering patient care. Each of these documents implies that staff nurses are not entirely free to fulfill their responsibilities according to their individual opinions of how these are to be accomplished but according to the agency's written guidelines of how each of these are to be performed. Although the staff nurse is expected to exercise professional discretion in each of these situations, the hospital nonetheless uses these documents to communicate its expectations for many aspects of the staff nurse's role. Individually and collectively, these documents reflect the agency's expectations for those who occupy the staff nurse role.

Additional written documents important in this process are the accreditation standards of the Joint Commission on Accreditation of Healthcare Organization's (JCAHO's) *Accreditation Manual for Hospitals*[75] as well as requirements of the Occupational Safety and Healthcare Administration (OSHA). These agencies have requirements related to ongoing educational needs for instruction in areas related to infection control, fire safety, electrical safety, management of emergency situations, hazardous material and waste management, and cardiopulmonary resuscitation. These various safety areas are addressed for new employees at the time of their orientation program. In addition to these written documents, the hospital's requirements for a staff nurse are also partly determined from the expectations held by other members of the nursing department.

Nursing Staff

NURSE MANAGERS   The nurse manager of each patient care unit is administratively responsible for ensuring that all nursing staff on the unit are qualified and competent to perform their assigned duties. With this responsibility, nurse managers also have the final authority for determining the set of performance expectations that will apply to nursing staff on their unit. Nurse managers' perceptions of these expectations are, therefore, a pivotal element in the needs assessment process for staff nurse orientees.

The nurse manager's expectations for staff nurses are usually reflected in the criteria that make up the performance evaluation tool that the manager employs for ongoing appraisal of staff throughout the year. Although the nurse manager uses these criteria primarily for noninstructional purposes (such as decisions related to periodic quality monitoring, merit increases, and clinical ladder advancements), this set of managerial expectations for staff nurses reflects what the orientation program is directed toward achieving. At some institutions, the staff nurse performance appraisal criteria and position description mirror each other closely; at other institutions, they bear little overt resemblance to each other. The contents of both documents, therefore, need to be examined as part of the needs assessment process for orientation programs. In addition, if nurse managers have other expectations for their staff that are not included in either of these documents, these additional requirements need to be elicited.

PRECEPTORS AND/OR UNIT EDUCATORS   If the healthcare agency uses a preceptorship for the staff nurse orientation program, preceptors' perceptions (or those of unit educators or clinical nurse specialists who may serve as preceptors) of the educational needs of orientees to their unit merit special consideration. Preceptors' impressions from working with a diversity of orientees; from their experience in using the program's instructional materials, teaching methods, and evaluation devices; and from their observations and appraisals regarding development of the orientees' clinical proficiency during and after the program afford comprehensive and first-hand insights into the effectiveness of the orientation program and whether all relevant educational needs are identified and attained. Their unique perspective from working closely with orientees and with the orientation program makes their views regarding the learning needs of orientees particularly salient to the needs assessment.

ORIENTEES As adult learners, orientees should be afforded the opportunity to actively participate in identifying their own educational needs. However, rather than using an open-ended inquiry process to solicit these needs, the educator can help focus these responses by giving orientees a list of the unit's expectations of staff nurses and asking the orientees to indicate their learning needs relative to that list.

As mentioned in Chapter 2, nursing staff may vary in their ability to perform this self-appraisal, resulting in an over- or underestimation of their true educational needs. One reason for this variance may be attributable to the diversity in experience and capabilities that orientees possess as they enter a new work setting. Another possible reason may be that an experienced nurse is unwilling or hesitant to admit to areas where he/she lacks expertise.

As Figure 6.1 illustrates, a newly employed staff nurse's experience and capabilities to work in a particular unit can exist anywhere along a fairly broad continuum. Orientees who are registered nurses (RNs) can range from the newly graduated nurse who has no work experience in nursing to one who may have many years of experience working as a nursing assistant, nurse's aide, licensed practical/vocational nurse (LPN/LVN), or registered nurse. Newly graduated nurses may be recent baccalaureate program graduates who have prior experience working as RNs following their diploma or associate degree education. Others may have work experience in the RN role on one type of unit (e.g., a medical-surgical unit) but have no experience in providing care for the type of patients in their new unit (e.g., critically ill patients). The far end of this spectrum includes orientees with advanced degrees in nursing who have both considerable work experience as RNs and experience with the same type of patients as on their assigned unit.

When orientees are viewed in relation to a work experience spectrum such as this, it is obvious that the knowledge, attitudes, and skills they bring to their assigned unit may significantly influence the range and depth of their educational needs. The important point for educators is not to categorize an orientee but to recognize that diversity of capabilities may influence how well orientees will be able to accurately gauge their educational needs. Another feature likely to be influenced by an orientee's background is the number and type of educational needs that may be elicited: new graduates with limited or no experience in nursing are likely to identify a substantial number of learning needs, while their more knowledgeable, skilled, and experienced counterparts will likely have a more limited number and range of learning needs. In all cases, assessment of learning needs related to orientation requires validation of all required performance areas via direct observation of the orientee's actual clinical practice.

Despite anticipated differences in their entry characteristics, all orientees who will be functioning as staff nurses need to be assessed in relation to the ***same*** set of expectations for that role because, by the end of the orientation program, all of these orientees must have demonstrated that they are competent to function in the same role. When the agency's expectations for all staff nurses are the same, the assessment of their educational needs in relation to those expectations should also be the same. Unless a clinical ladder distinguishes different sets of expectations for different categories of staff nurses, all staff nurse orientees should be held responsible for attaining the same set of expectations. The individual differences that may be identified during the needs assessment are noted at this time and accommodated later during the planning and implementation phases of the educational process.

OTHER NURSING STAFF Although they may not work directly with orientees, other nursing staff on the unit can contribute to the needs assessment of orientees in at least three important ways. First, because the unit nurses are not personally involved with providing the orientation, their observations and appraisals of orientees may be more detached and less influenced by interpersonal factors than those of preceptors or unit educators. Secondly, as the orientation process progresses, unit staff will eventually be working with orientees and have opportunities to determine the existence or persistence of their learning needs.

A third avenue of unit staff participation in needs assessment arises when a competency-based approach is used for instructional design. When this approach is employed for orientation, the major source of information for identifying the educational needs of staff nurse orientees consists of nurses who are already competent in the staff nurse role on the unit where the orientee will be working. Competency-based orientation (CBO) programs, in effect, assume that the most valid and reliable sources of information related to the expectations of a competent staff nurse for a specific nursing unit are the individuals who are already competent in that role and setting. Although this group of "local experts" may also include nurse managers, preceptors, unit-based educators, and clinical nurse specialists, the remaining nursing staff who may not function as preceptors should be integrally involved in the determination and validation of orientee learning needs.

Secondary Sources

Other potential sources of information for the needs assessment of staff nurse orientees include healthcare professionals (such as dietitians, respiratory therapists, or clin-

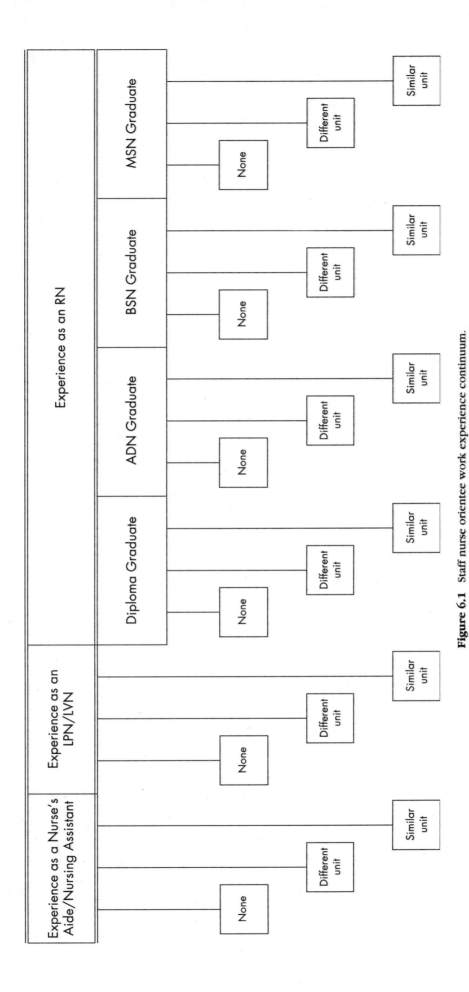

Figure 6.1 Staff nurse orientee work experience continuum.

ical pharmacologists) who may provide selected segments of the orientation program; physician members of the healthcare team; the professional literature related to the orientation of new employees; and the standards promulgated by various professional associations or service organizations.

The collaborative, interdisciplinary, and multidisciplinary nature of contemporary nursing practice requires ongoing communication among all healthcare professionals to achieve quality patient care. Orientation programs afford a logical forum to introduce new nursing staff to some of these professional groups, the services they offer, and how to work most effectively with them. The professional literature related to new employee orientation programs affords nurse educators with valuable perspectives from the fields of education, adult education, training, and human resource development to complement information gleaned from the literature of nursing education and staff development. Even fields as broad as psychology, sociology, and ethics offer useful insights related to issues on topics such as stress management, cultural diversity, and ethical dilemmas.

Many general and specialty nursing associations issue standards, guidelines, or core curricula that specify the capabilities and/or knowledge base necessary for nurses who function in those clinical areas. Examples of such standards include the American Nurses' Association (ANA) *Standards of Clinical Nursing Practice, Standards of Medical-Surgical Nursing Practice,* and *Standards of Cardiovascular Nursing Practice;* the American Association of Critical-Care Nurses (AACN) *Standards for Nursing Care of the Critically Ill* and *Outcome Standards for Nursing Care of the Critically Ill;* and the Association of Operating Room Nurses (AORN) *Standards of Perioperative Clinical Practice.* Examples of core curriculum texts include the AACN *Core Curriculum for Critical Care Nursing,* the AORN *Core Curriculum for the RN First Assistant,* the Association of Women's Health Obstetric and Neonatal Nursing (AWHONN) *Core Curriculum for Maternal-Newborn Nursing* and *Core Curriculum for Neonatal Intensive Care Nursing,* and the Emergency Nurses Assocation (ENA) *Emergency Nursing Core Curriculum.* Though these documents may not be adopted in their entirety, the requirements they establish should be reviewed for relevance and applicability to the orientation program under development.

Other worthwhile sources of information include the findings of quality monitoring and risk management activities. Either of these ongoing activities may identify deficiencies in nursing practice that are attributable to the need for instruction in certain areas of clinical performance. When trends in findings suggest the need for instruction, compliance with established standards and minimization or prevention of risks to patients, families, or staff may be enhanced among new employees if these needs are addressed during the orientation program.

Combined Sources

Some healthcare agencies prefer to determine educational needs for orientation by means of a task force or committee composed of representatives from all major input sources.[108] An orientation task force may convene only when the needs assessment warrants updating or revision, whereas an orientation committee may meet on an ongoing basis (e.g., quarterly or semiannually) to verify that needs addressed in the program are still current, complete, and accurate reflections of nursing practice. When a competency-based approach is in place, use of a task force or committee can be an effective and efficient means of determining educational needs, provided that a mechanism exists so that the nurse manager and entire nursing staff of each unit are provided with an opportunity to offer input and feedback to task force or committee proposals related to the orientation program for their unit.

METHODS FOR ASSESSING EDUCATIONAL NEEDS

Any of the direct or indirect methods for assessing educational needs reviewed in Chapter 2 may be employed to determine the educational needs of orientees. Thus the direct methods of interviews and questionnaires or the indirect methods of observation and review of written documents may be used alone or in combination with analysis of the staff nurse position description, review of the performance evaluation criteria, or written tests to determine what staff nurses need to perform their job in a competent manner.

When a competency-based approach is employed for orientation, the staff development educator works collaboratively with the nursing staff (preceptors, unit educators, other staff nurses, and clinical specialists) and the nurse manager of each unit to decide which of the available methods will be used for the learning needs assessment. The efficiency of the needs assessment process can be enhanced if all nursing units at that facility can reach consensus on the most appropriate methods to use. Because a competency-based orientation program emphasizes expectations related to *clinical* performance, methods that examine actual clinical performance (such as direct observation) tend to afford more useful assessment findings than would merely soliciting and/or summarizing staff opinions.

Some institutions assess the competency of newly hired staff nurses in a *clinical assessment center.*[127] These assessment centers afford a centralized location for determining the entry capabilities of new hires in simulated job situations. In the center, specially trained nurse educators assess the clinical skills of nursing staff in using the actual equipment and supplies found on their units and employ a variety of written (written simulations), audiovisual (audio tapes, videotapes, and games), and behavioral (role play) means to appraise clinical performance in areas such as problem-solving, decision-making, priority-setting, and care planning. Two limitations of the assessment center include the need to validate actual performance in the clinical setting and the costs associated with designing, equipping, and operating the center. Because start-up costs can range from $30,000 to $100,000, these centers are generally feasible only for larger (400+ beds) healthcare facilities.[41]

DISTINGUISHING BETWEEN EDUCATIONAL AND NONEDUCATIONAL NEEDS

Orientation programs seem especially vulnerable to including coverage of areas that do not represent true educational needs. Some content may endure in the program because it has existed there for many years, because the person(s) responsible for coordinating the needs assessment has remained in the same role for a prolonged period, because some quality assurance or incident report finding of some time ago (and long since resolved) has not been reexamined recently, or because the content represents "sacred territory" to one or more orientation instructors.

As discussed in Chapter 2, noneducational needs may also creep into staff development programs because a staff nurse performance problem exists and an educational remedy is being applied even though the deficient performance may not reflect a need for instruction. As with all staff development programs, the educator needs to work closely with the unit nursing staff and nurse manager to be certain that all the needs derived from the assessment process are truly educational in nature.

SETTING PRIORITIES AMONG EDUCATIONAL NEEDS

The four nursing education priorities (fatal, fundamental, frequent, and fixed) suggested in Chapter 2 need to be applied with great care for orientation programs. The more instructional resources are restricted, the more selective this priority setting process must be. The educator can use these four priority factors (the four Fs) to establish some general guidelines for deciding which of the educational needs proposed for the staff nurse orientation should and can be accommodated in this program. Some guidelines for such decisions are as follows:

- *All educational needs that relate to high-risk aspects of patient care (i.e., the **fatal** factor) merit the highest priority for inclusion in the orientation.* The rationale for this top priority is that if these needs (e.g., CPR procedures) are not addressed, the patient or staff might suffer grave harm or loss of life.
- *All educational needs that the nursing staff and managers deem as essential aspects of effective nursing practice on that unit (i.e., the **fundamental** factor) should be included in the orientation.* The working definition of "essential" needs to be restrictive so that coverage of "nice-to-know" performance areas can be deleted

to allow sufficient time and resources for coverage of "need-to-know" performance areas.
- *To be included in the orientation program, educational needs should represent an area of nursing practice that is often performed on that unit (i.e., the **frequency** factor).* In general, higher priority should be given to nursing practice areas that are performed on virtually a daily basis and a proportionately lesser degree of priority should be allocated to areas that are performed less often.
- *In general, only those learning needs that can realistically be attained during the time available for orientation should be included in the set of expectations for the orientation program.* Whenever the time available for orientation is limited or reduced, educators need to work together with the unit staff and nurse manager to trim the set of orientation expectations by deleting performance areas that cannot reasonably be completed within the maximum amount of time provided for the program. If, for example, a medical unit that has a 3-week orientation program only admits patients with upper gastrointestinal (UGI) bleeding once every 5 or 6 months, it is not very likely that an orientee will encounter this type of patient during the 3 weeks scheduled for orientation. Coverage of this area of practice within the orientation program, therefore, is less justifiable than coverage of the types of patients who are almost universally present on that unit. One way of identifying expectations that are subject to this consideration is by reviewing past orientation checklists to see which areas are most often incomplete at the end of the customary orientation time frame. Since it would be useful for the nurse to demonstrate the performance expectations for this patient population at some time, however, expectations in this group could be scheduled as part of that unit's ongoing in-service education offerings.
- *External accrediting agencies such as JCAHO may also impose requirements for staff orientation that represent priority areas of instruction and assessment.* Because these accreditation "mandatories" are imposed on the healthcare facility, they may be considered as **facility** priority factors. Because they must be provided during the orientation program, however, they may also be viewed as a variant of the **fixed** priority factors. In either case, they represent educational needs that must be accommodated at the time of staff orientation.
- *Performance expectations that do not fall under the guidelines for the fatal, fundamental, or frequency priority factors should be scrutinized very carefully before they are included in the orientation program.* Educators may need to remind unit staff and managers that orientation programs are not intended to prepare nurses for every possible situation they might encounter on that unit. Overwhelming orientees with large volumes

of instruction can result in diminished retention of learning since, by the time a nurse really needs to perform in that area, he/she may have long since forgotten what was taught during the orientation program. The nurse now assigned to a patient with active UGI bleeding may well feel a very pressing need to be able to competently care for this patient (i.e., the **fixed** factor). But if it has been 6 months since this area was covered in the orientation and no clinical experience in caring for these patients was available, it is not likely that much of what was learned during orientation will have been retained. As in the case of performance areas that occur infrequently, it would be more prudent to delete coverage of this area from the orientation program, make plans to cover it once every 4 to 6 months as an in-service offering, and designate a staff member (unit educator or clinical nurse specialist) to meet pressing educational needs related to that area when they arise.

Once the performance expectations for staff nurses that were identified in the needs assessment process are filtered through these priority factors, the expectations that remain should represent the following:

- A distillation of all of the various forms of expectations that the agency has for staff nurses put into a single list; this single compilation would reflect integration of all the separate expressions of these expectations: the staff nurse position description; performance evaluation tool criteria; existing standards, policies, procedures, and protocols; nurse manager, clinical nurse specialist, nursing staff, and recent orientees' suggestions; and relevant information secured from secondary sources both inside and outside the hospital
- A set of expectations for staff nurses that reflects the most salient and highest priority performance areas for competent nursing practice on that unit
- A set of expectations that can be completed in the time available for orientation

The next step is to summarize these expectations as instructional outcomes.

SUMMARIZING THE NEEDS ASSESSMENT AS INSTRUCTIONAL OUTCOMES

In contrast to the traditional approach to instruction that formulates instructional outcomes as part of the planning phase of the educational process, the competency-based approach to instruction specifies these outcomes during the assessment phase. The reason for this difference in timing is that traditional approaches to instruction typically employ a rather linear procedure wherein the instructor determines the knowledge, attitudes, and skills learners need

to know, composes program and instructional objectives to reflect those areas, provides the necessary instruction, and then evaluates the degree to which learning has occurred.

A competency-based approach to instruction uses a less linear process: during the assessment phase, learners (orientees) are assessed in relation to the performance outcomes for their role and clinical unit. Then, only those who are unable to demonstrate those performance expectations will undergo instruction and be reevaluated until the desired outcomes have been achieved. In effect, then, competency-based approaches to instruction link the needs assessment and evaluation phases of the educational process more closely: learners' needs are determined by appraising them in relation to the same set of expectations they will encounter during the evaluation phase of the orientation program.

A second way in which CBO programs differ from traditional orientation programs is in the expression of instructional outcomes. As Chapter 3 details, traditional approaches to education typically employ program and instructional objectives for this purpose. CBE programs, by contrast, express instructional outcomes by means of competency statements and performance criteria.

Competency statements describe a general or broad area of behavior/performance that is requisite for being competent in a particular role and work setting. For example, all hospital nurses need to be competent in the broad area of "planning nursing care." A competency statement for this area of behavior might be constructed as follows: "Develops a plan of nursing care based on a comprehensive assessment of patient data." Taken together, the competency statements identify all major areas or dimensions that relate to competency in a specific role and setting.

Performance criteria describe one or more specific behaviors that learners must demonstrate as evidence that they are competent in the area described by the competency statement. Performance criteria define the critical or essential behaviors that represent that competency. For example, before one is designated as competent to drive an automobile, that individual must perform each of the following essential behaviors: pass a written test on the rules of the road, pass a visual acuity examination, complete a driving test on a designated course or local roads, complete an application for a driver's license, and pay the required license fee. Only when all of these critical or essential behaviors have been achieved is one deemed competent to drive an automobile.

The process of drafting competency statements and performance criteria may proceed differently at various hospitals,[15] but typically it involves a collaborative effort among the nurse educator, nurse manager, clinical nurse specialists, and a number of nursing staff members from each unit. If only one clinical unit of the hospital is developing the CBO program, the nurse manager usually identifies which and how many members of the nursing staff will function on that unit's panel of experts to identify and draft the competency and performance criteria statements. The primary requirement for selection of this panel of experts is that each is already competent in the staff nurse role on that unit. For any one unit, only a small group of staff (perhaps two or three) need to be members of the panel. When multiple units are working on the program, however, each individual unit may have only one staff nurse serving as a representative for that unit and functioning as a liaison between the CBO task force and their home unit. Once all of the competency statements are drafted, the unit representative communicates these to the fellow staff and solicits their comments and critique as input to the task force. As each set of performance criteria are developed, the unit representatives again function as liaisons to secure feedback from their unit staff. Once both the competency statements and performance criteria are revised, unit representatives may coordinate pilot testing of the program on their unit to determine if any additional refinements are needed. A mechanism such as this minimizes the number of staff removed from the unit to work on the CBO task force, yet affords a means for all nursing staff to offer input and suggestions on the program. At each step in this process, the nurse manager or clinical nurse specialist supervises program development on his/her unit, while the educator facilitates the process to ensure development of a valid, reliable, and useful assessment tool* that is designed in accordance with the principles of CBE.

Writing Competency Statements

The set of expectations for staff nurses that has been developed thus far may be a long enumeration of expectations expressed in many different forms. These expectations might include orientation program objectives, performance evaluation criteria, position description elements, and the like. Some of these expectations may overlap, duplicate, or stand isolated from others in the list. Before one attempts to convert these expectations into competency statements, it is helpful at first to organize the list in some coherent way so that separate areas of competency for the staff nurse role can be more readily identified and distinguished from one another.

Some CBO work groups attempt to write competency statements without first deciding on an organizing theme or framework. This often generates a seemingly endless list of tasks, procedures, functions, duties, responsibilities, and the like, with no apparent order or endpoint. Use of an organizing framework to identify the areas of competency can, by contrast, afford much helpful direction in the competency writing process. In general, the approach(es) selected for organizing the competency areas will determine to a great extent how the competency is worded, the approximate number of competency areas that will be identified, and, at times, the logical starting and endpoints for drafting these statements.

There is no single, universally agreed on way in which the competency statements for a staff nurse orientation program must be organized and expressed. A number of alternative organizing frameworks are available, depending on how those involved with needs assessment prefer to view competency for the role.

For example, some hospitals may view nursing practice in relation to the nursing process. At those institutions, a "competent staff nurse" may be perceived as one who demonstrates proficiency in executing each of the five phases of the nursing process. Within the organizing framework of nursing process, then, five areas of competency would be identified, resulting in one competency statement for each phase of the nursing process (i.e., one competency statement each for the assessment, diagnosis, planning, implementation, and evaluation phases).

Another hospital might view nursing practice in relation to nursing diagnosis. At that facility, a "competent staff nurse" would be perceived as one who demonstrates all aspects of nursing care for patients with selected nursing diagnoses. Within this organizing framework, the unit could perform a retrospective care plan audit to identify the nursing diagnoses most frequently encountered on that unit (perhaps selecting the "15 most common" diagnoses) and then write one competency statement for each of these nursing diagnoses.

Nurses who work in the operating room might prefer to view nursing practice in relation to competency for three primary roles: the role of circulating nurse, the role of scrub nurse, and the role of first assistant. If this approach were used, three major competency areas would be identified, and, thus, three competency statements would be written. Nurses who work in an ambulatory care unit or surgical intensive care unit (ICU) might sort competency areas according to the most common types of surgical procedures performed.

Hospitals that ascribe to a particular nursing theory might view nursing in relation to the major tenets of that theory. As a result, competency areas could be organized around the different stages of adaptation for Roy's Adaptation Model or be organized around the most frequently encountered self-care deficits for Dorothea Orem's model.

The approach or framework selected for organizing and distinguishing areas of competency can be any one approach or a combination of approaches. For example, nurses who work in a mixed medical-surgical unit or medical-surgical ICU could organize competency areas according to body systems and then distinguish subcompetencies according to the patient's medical diagnosis, nursing di-

---

*See discussion of these benchmarks of measurement in Chapter 5.

agnoses, or phases of the nursing process. This combination of organizing approaches can be especially useful when patient populations, their healthcare problems, and nursing care requirements are diverse. Other healthcare institutions may use nursing practice standards or patient care standards to organize competency areas. Whichever organizing theme or combination of themes is selected, hospi-

tals typically find it easier to work within an organizing framework that they perceive as relevant to their patient population, meaningful to their view of nursing practice, and easy to use in distinguishing different areas of clinical competence.

As Table 6.1 illustrates, the organizing approach selected will also influence how the competency statement

TABLE 6.1 • SAMPLE ORGANIZING FRAMEWORKS FOR COMPETENCY STATEMENTS

Single Organizing Framework(s)	Estimated Number of Competency Areas	Example of Competency Statements
Nursing process	5 (1 per phase of the nursing process)	Develops a plan of nursing care based on identified patient needs (planning phase)
Nursing diagnosis	12 (1 for each of the 12 most commonly encountered nursing diagnoses)	Provides nursing care to patients with a potential fluid volume deficit
Roles of the staff nurse	2 (1 for each identified role)	Fulfills all major expectations for the scrub nurse role in the operating room
Patient's chief complaint	15 (1 for each of the 15 most frequently encountered chief complaints)	Demonstrates emergency department nursing management of patients with a chief complaint of "difficulty breathing"
Roy's Adaptation Model	4 (1 per adaptive mode in the model)	Promotes the patient's adaptation to physiologic needs anywhere along the health-illness continuum
Body systems	8 (1 per body system)	Administers nursing care for patients with neurologic health deficits
Medical therapies	20 (1 per frequently used therapy)	Manages nursing care of patients who require oxygen therapy

Combined Organizing Framework(s)	Estimated Number of Competency Areas	Example of Competency Statements
Medical diagnosis and nursing process	Depends on the number of medical diagnoses most commonly encountered on that unit	Provides nursing care for patients with diabetic ketoacidosis (DKA): • Obtains a comprehensive assessment of the DKA patient • Formulates a plan of care based on the needs of a patient with DKA • Intervenes effectively in managing the DKA patient's needs • Documents an evaluation of the effectiveness of nursing interventions for the patient with DKA
Body systems and nursing diagnosis	Depends on the number of body systems affected and nursing diagnoses most commonly encountered on that unit	Manages the healthcare needs of patients with renal dysfunction: • Manages patient needs related to fluid volume deficit • Manages patient needs related to fluid volume excess • Manages patient needs related to altered patterns of urinary elimination • Manages patient needs related to a potential for ineffective patient and family coping

may be worded. Although the specific wording of a competency statement will depend on the organizing approach(es) selected, all competency statements related to nursing practice define a broad yet distinguishable area of clinical competence and include behaviors that can be observed and measured.

Once all of the competency statements for staff nurses have been drafted, they should be shared with the nursing staff and nurse manager of that unit for suggestions and critique. The educator will want to elicit feedback to ensure that these statements include all major aspects of competency and that they describe the competency area clearly, fully, and behaviorally. This validation and consensus-building process is a necessary prerequisite to developing performance criteria for each competency statement.

Writing Performance Criteria

As mentioned earlier, performance criteria represent the behavioral evidence that learners must demonstrate to show that they are competent in the area described by the competency statement. In order for performance criteria to be effective and useful in judging an orientee's clinical practice, they need to do each of the following:

- Describe a behavior that the *orientee* must perform
- Describe behaviors that are *observable* and *measurable*
- Describe the behavior *fully, clearly,* and *unambiguously*
- Describe a *single* behavior
- Include a *basis* or *standard* for judging the behavior as acceptable (or not)
- Include only *essential* aspects of competent clinical performance
- Emphasize *clinical* rather than solely cognitive performance requirements

Performance criteria need to be written in terms of the learner (orientee) since it is the orientee's (rather than the instructor's or evaluator's) behavior that is being appraised. Since the preceptor must be able to see the orientee do something in order to appraise the behavior, performance criteria need to identify behaviors that are both observable (to see if the behavior is evidenced at all) and measurable (to determine if the nature or quality of behavior meets the specified requirements). Thus, behaviors such as *knows, understands,* or *appreciates* (see also those in Box 3.1, Chapter 3) are not appropriate for performance criteria because the observer can neither see nor measure those behaviors.

Performance criteria need to be stated as clearly and succinctly as possible so that both the orientee and the evaluator know what behaviors must be demonstrated. If the behavior is not sufficiently described (e.g., "administers medications"), both the orientee and the preceptor may have questions related to the expectations (which medications? which routes of administration? scheduled or prn

medications? unit-dose or calculated dosages?) and each may interpret the required behaviors differently. In addition, other preceptors or evaluators might interpret the required behaviors differently, creating concerns for the reliability of appraisals in these situations. In order to avoid or minimize ambiguity and uncertainty in both understanding and validating these behaviors, performance criteria need to be stated so that the required behaviors are understood and evaluated in a consistent manner from one orientee to another and from one evaluator to another.

Each performance criterion should consist of a single behavior in order to isolate that behavior for purposes of evaluation. If more than one behavior were included in the same criterion statement (e.g., "Auscultates and documents breath sounds"), the orientee might perform one behavior (auscultates) satisfactorily but not the other (documents), leaving the evaluator in a quandary over how to indicate this split decision.

Performance criteria need to include some basis for the evaluator to judge the behaviors as acceptable (satisfactory, correct, proper) or not. Just as a written test has an answer key to judge the learner's written response as "correct" or not, clinical performance evaluations must also include some standard for judging the clinical performance as "correct" or not. Performance standards serve as the reference point for the evaluator to make this decision. Many performance criteria include an implicit performance standard: that is, the performance criteria statement is worded so that it leaves virtually no room for differing interpretations. For example, the criterion statement "Completes preoperative teaching by 8:00 PM the night before the patient's surgery" represents a clear and unambiguous description of the behavior to be demonstrated with little or no room for misinterpretation or differing interpretations. Either the preop teaching was completed by that time or it was not. At other times, however, the performance standard may be less clear and warrant more detail to make it explicit. For example, if a performance criterion statement related that some procedure or function needed to be performed in a *satisfactory, acceptable, proper,* or *correct* manner, different preceptors might interpret these terms in different ways, leading to inconsistency in the assessment process and differing appraisals of the orientee's performance. As you may recall from discussion in Chapter 5 on the measurement benchmark of reliability, such inconsistencies diminish the confidence one can place in the results of these assessments and tend to invalidate the assessment process. Performance criteria such as these need to be made more explicit.

Performance standards may be made explicit by reference to some written document that specifies how a task or activity is to be performed. For example, the performance criterion might say *Admits patients as described in the nursing department's "Patient Admission Procedure."* Hospital or nursing department policies, procedures, unit protocols, or routines, nursing or patient care standards, and the like may all serve to define the expected standard of performance. At other times, however, there may be no written document that delineates how a particular competency area is to be evidenced. In this case, it is necessary to enumerate those expectations. For example, if there were no written documents that described what a competently performed patient admission consisted of, the unit or nursing department might either develop a procedure for this purpose or simply decide on the performance criteria for this competency area. This set of performance criteria might be drafted as appears in Box 6.1. Another institution might develop a totally different set of criteria for this competency area, depending on what the nursing department or unit required of its nursing staff.

When the performance standard refers to some written document, it is important that the contents of that document actually be used when that area is evaluated. In instances when it is not likely that the evaluator will actually retrieve the document and use it when observing and evaluating the orientee's performance, the performance standard may not really operate at all in judging the orientee's behavior. Another consideration is that lengthy documents, such as procedures, protocols, and unit routines, may contain a mixture of elements, some of which are essential to competent performance and others which are not. In order to keep criteria lists manageable in length and focused on the requirements for competency, performance criteria should be limited to only those aspects of performance that are truly essential to competency. Rather than repeating the entire procedure in the performance criteria, nonessential behaviors that may be performed in different ways or not

performed at all without compromising competency can be deleted and only those that are truly critical elements of competent performance can be retained. This process is analogous to creation of a critical behavior checklist (see Table 5.25) from a comprehensive performance checklist (see Table 5.24) as described in Chapter 5.

In traditional educational programs, a large majority of the behaviors required of learners are cognitive in nature. This means that the behaviors contained in the instructional objectives require learners to demonstrate that they **know** something. In CBE programs, greater emphasis is placed on learners' demonstration of competent job performance. That is, learners are required to demonstrate that they can **do** what their job requires of them. Performance criteria, therefore, typically employ clinical practice behaviors (e.g., *assesses, documents, provides, teaches*) rather than purely cognitive behaviors (e.g., *describes, explains, defines, relates*).

However, CBE programs recognize that there is always a cognitive component to competency; that is, before one can function in a competent manner, one must first know what it is he/she is to do in that situation. Where a traditional program often stops at verifying that the person *knows* what to do, CBE programs extend this appraisal by requiring the learner to actually *demonstrate* the performance. CBE programs, then, are described as performance-based because they require learners to apply their knowledge in actual practice rather than merely verify that this knowledge exists.

Although most behaviors in performance criteria require some form of clinical performance of the orientee, a

---

Box 6.1

SAMPLE SET OF PERFORMANCE CRITERIA

COMPETENCY STATEMENT
Demonstrates the procedure for admitting patients to the unit

PERFORMANCE CRITERIA
A. Obtains admission baseline data that include each of the following:
  1. Vital signs
  2. Height
  3. Weight
  4. Reason(s) for entering the hospital
  5. Allergies
  6. Current medications
  7. Nursing history
B. Completes a physical examination of the patient that includes all areas in the admission assessment form
C. Executes all admission orders
D. Completes the admission assessment form within 2 hours of the patient's arrival on the unit
E. Develops a patient care plan based on assessment data within 24 hours of the patient's admission

selected few cognitive behaviors are often included. Reasons for including cognitive performance criteria in a CBO program are the following:

- Ensures that the orientee is competent in areas that do not readily lend themselves to appraisal by clinical performance; examples might include knowing the actions, usual dosages, contraindications, and side effects of medications administered on the unit or understanding the clinical significance of an S_3 heart sound
- Includes coverage of essential areas of competency that occur infrequently. For example, this might include the ability of the orientee to recognize pacemaker malfunction, the clinical features of laryngospasm, or the symptoms of insulin shock

There is no required or usual number of performance criteria that need to be developed for a particular competency. The number of criteria should reflect the number of essential or critical elements necessary to demonstrate competent performance in that area—no more or less.

In summary, then, competency statements describe the broad areas of competence in which orientees will be assessed, and performance criteria represent the specific behaviors that orientees have to demonstrate to show that they are competent in those areas. The flexibility that CBE offers in how competency statements and performance criteria are organized and expressed is evident in the proliferation of CBO programs that have recently been published.

Information about competency-based orientation programs is now available for a wide variety of clinical areas: burn nursing,[19] cardiovascular nursing,[56,111,129] critical care,* emergency department nursing,[124] hemodialysis nursing,[130] operating room nursing,[123] orthopedic nursing,[48] pediatric nursing,[50] and psychiatric/mental health nursing,[18,60] to name a few. CBO programs have also been described for a variety of nursing roles such as preceptor,[11] staff nurse,[92,94,105] head nurse/nurse manager,[20,44,78,98] and clinical nurse specialist.[42,49] Additional examples of competency statements for staff nurses with their related sets of performance criteria are provided in Boxes 6.2 through 6.5.

VALIDATION OF EDUCATIONAL NEEDS

Before the set of performance criteria proposed for a particular competency area is used with orientees, it needs to be reviewed and critiqued by the nurse manager and nursing staff of each unit it pertains to. For example, performance criteria related to competency in hemodynamic monitoring should be reviewed by all nursing units that use this type of monitoring, while criteria related to care of the patient in traction might be reviewed only by the orthopedic and trauma units.

This validation process is helpful for ensuring that the performance criteria accurately reflect the behaviors most indicative of competency in that area and offer clear, measurable descriptions of those expectations. Revision and refinement of the performance criteria should continue until the widest possible degree of agreement is reached on the content and wording of the criteria. Although unanimity is not always possible, broad consensus on these inclusions and indicators of competent performance is necessary for a successful program.

In addition to establishing the validity of these performance criteria, attention should also be paid to ensuring the reliability of these criteria as assessment tools. Both intra-rater and inter-rater reliability can be determined, as described in Chapter 5. The former will verify that the same evaluator (preceptor) rates orientee performance in a consistent manner, and the latter verifies that different evaluators judge the same performance in a consistent manner. Videotaping or simultaneous observation of a few sample performance vignettes can afford the means to make judgments regarding both types of reliability.

VERIFICATION OF ORIENTEES' EDUCATIONAL NEEDS

Once the competency statements and performance criteria are finalized, they can be used to assess orientees' educational needs. In Chapter 2, an educational need was defined as the gap or difference between someone's present level of performance and the desired or necessary level of performance that can be satisfied through some type of instructional experience. For an orientation program, then, the last phase of the needs assessment process consists of verifying where gaps or discrepancies exist between the orientee's present performance capabilities and the performance expectations that have been identified in the competency statements and performance criteria for the role and work setting. Rather than assuming that all orientees have the same learning needs, CBE programs verify those needs by assessing orientees in relation to the competency statements and performance criteria that apply to their unit. Figure 6.2 (see p. 176) illustrates one example of how to construct a performance checklist for this purpose. The example uses the competency statement and performance criteria from Box 6-4.

Early in the orientation program, the preceptor can review these expectations with the orientees, have orientees demonstrate those performance criteria they are presently able to perform, and identify for orientees those compe-

*References 3, 7, 54, 69, 70, 72, 82, 88, 115, 126.

Box 6.2

COMPETENCY STATEMENT AND PERFORMANCE CRITERIA: EXAMPLE #1

ORGANIZING FRAMEWORK: BODY SYSTEMS

COMPETENCY STATEMENT:

Manages nursing care for patients with neurologic dysfunctions

PERFORMANCE CRITERIA:

A. Includes appraisal of each of the following parameters in documentation of patient assessment:
   1. History of neurologic disorders
   2. Recently ingested medications
   3. Orientation to
      a. Person
      b. Place
      c. Time
   4. Pupil characteristics
      a. Size
      b. Equality
      c. Reactivity to light
   5. Sensory deficits
   6. Motor deficits
   7. Level of consciousness
   8. Seizure activity
   9. Vital signs
      a. Blood pressure
      b. Pulse rate
      c. Temperature
      d. Respiratory rate
   10. Results of diagnostic studies
B. Notifies the attending physician STAT if signs of decreased cerebral perfusion exist
C. Within 8 hours of admission, develops a care plan that includes priority listing of patient health problems
D. Provides nursing interventions related to identified health problems as described in nursing department practice standards
E. Evaluates patient's response to each intervention provided
F. Documents all relevant aspects of nursing care in the patient record by the end of each shift

---

tency areas and performance criteria that remain to be achieved during the orientation program. The latter represent the focus of learning for the orientation program.

COLLABORATION WITH NURSING MANAGEMENT

CBO programs may be developed for a single nursing unit, a group of units within the same division, or all nursing units in the hospital. If CBO is new at that institution, it may be initially pilot-tested on one unit before being disseminated to other areas. Regardless of the scope of application selected, however, conversion from a traditional to a competency-based approach to orientation can entail a substantial amount of time and effort. In addition, because CBO program development requires the input and participation of nurse educators, managers,[47] clinical specialists,

preceptors, and other nursing staff, it must be accomplished through a collaborative effort. The organizational time, labor, and resources needed for this degree of collaboration makes the understanding, approval, and administrative support of nursing management imperative.

At many hospitals, it will be necessary for nurse educators to introduce the concept of CBE and its potential benefits to hospital and nursing administrators before their support can be expected. At times, it may be helpful to bring in a consultant to provide this background information and answer any questions that administrators might have regarding the efficacy and process used in CBO programs, the relationship of CBE to quality improvement and accreditation activities, to staff performance evaluations, clinical ladder criteria, and risk management initiatives.

Once concurrence on the potential benefits of CBE to

Box 6.3

COMPETENCY STATEMENT AND PERFORMANCE CRITERIA: EXAMPLE #2

ORGANIZING FRAMEWORK: ROLES OF THE NURSE

COMPETENCY STATEMENT

Fulfills all staff nurse responsibilities related to the role of patient educator.

PERFORMANCE CRITERIA

A. Determines patient/family readiness to learn about managing patient health problem(s)
B. Assists the patient/family in identifying specific health problem(s)
C. Provides patient/family with instruction that includes each of the following as appropriate:
  1. Pathophysiology of the disorder/problem
  2. Required medications
  3. Required therapies
  4. Lifestyle modifications (e.g., risk factors, diet, exercise, work)
  5. Potential complications
  6. Symptoms to report immediately, if any
D. Uses available instructional aids related to identified health problems and required care
E. Verifies that patient/family understand the instruction provided
F. Distributes written instructional materials for follow-up and postdischarge care
G. Documents the patient education process and its outcomes on the discharge plan of care

Box 6.4

COMPETENCY STATEMENT AND PERFORMANCE CRITERIA: EXAMPLE #3

ORGANIZING FRAMEWORK: MEDICAL THERAPIES

COMPETENCY STATEMENT

Provides nursing care for patients who require chest tubes

PERFORMANCE CRITERIA

A. Secures all equipment and supplies for chest tube insertion as listed in the written procedure
B. Sets up the chest tube drainage system as described in the manufacturer's directions
C. Prepares the patient for the procedure by describing events and effects on patient
D. Assists the physician with chest tube insertion by:
  1. Connecting chest tube(s) to the drainage system
  2. Taping all connections securely
  3. Applying an occlusive dressing to the chest tube site
E. Verifies the presence of a water seal in the drainage system
F. Sets the amount of suction as prescribed by the physician
G. Monitors each of the following according to unit protocol:
  1. Amount of drainage
  2. Characteristics of drainage
  3. Maintenance of water seal
  4. Presence of tracheal deviation
  5. Quality of bilateral breath sounds
H. On a mannequin, demonstrates how to manage each of the following situations:
  1. Patient transport
  2. Suspected air leak in pleural space
  3. Inadvertent chest tube removal
I. Changes dressing daily or as ordered according to written procedure
J. Documents nursing care considerations in plan of care

COMPETENCY Provides nursing care for patients who require chest tubes	COMPLETION		
PERFORMANCE CRITERIA	**DATE**	**SIGNATURE**	**COMMENTS**
1. Secures all equipment and supplies for chest tube insertion as listed in the written procedure			
2. Sets up the chest tube drainage system as described in the manufacturer's directions			
3. Prepares the patient for the procedure by describing events and effects on patient			
4. Assists the physician with chest tube insertion by: a) connecting chest tube(s) to the drainage system			
b) taping all connections securely			
c) applying an occlusive dressing to the chest tube site			
5. Verifies the presence of a water seal in the drainage system			
6. Sets the amount of suction as prescribed by the physician			
7. Monitors each of the following according to unit protocol: a) amount of drainage			
b) characteristics of drainage			
c) maintenance of water seal			
d) tracheal deviation			
e) quality of bilateral breath sounds			
8. On a mannequin, demonstrates how to manage each of the following situations: a) patient transport			
b) suspected air leak in pleural space			
c) inadvertent chest tube removal			
9. Changes dressing daily or as ordered according to written procedure			
10. Documents nursing care considerations in plan of care			

Figure 6.2   Sample CBO needs assessment checklist.

Box 6.5

COMPETENCY STATEMENT AND PERFORMANCE CRITERIA: EXAMPLE #4

ORGANIZING FRAMEWORK: NURSING DIAGNOSIS

COMPETENCY STATEMENT

Demonstrates nursing management of the patient with *decreased cardiac output* related to acute congestive heart failure.

PERFORMANCE CRITERIA

A. Assesses for each of the following signs and symptoms of decreased cardiac output at least hourly:
   1. Decreased systolic blood pressure
   2. Pulse < 60 or > 100 beats per minute
   3. Dyspnea
   4. Tachypnea
   5. Presence of S_3 and/or S_4 gallop
   6. Restlessness/agitation/anxiety
   7. Cool, cyanotic skin
   8. Urine output < 30 ml per hour
   9. Peripheral edema
B. Includes results of diagnostic tests in documentation of assessment findings
C. Places patient in position of maximal comfort for breathing
D. Administers all medications (including oxygen) as prescribed
E. Plans nursing care according to patient's response to interventions
F. Times nursing interventions to promote patient rest periods
G. Calculates intake and output by the end of shift
H. Documents all aspects of nursing care as listed in the unit protocol for patients in congestive heart failure

---

staff development is reached, the nurse educator collaborates with nurse managers regarding each of the following decisions:

- Who will coordinate development and pilot testing of the CBO program
- How many units will initially participate in conversion to CBO
- How many and which nursing staff will serve as unit representatives (that unit's panel of experts) for the CBO task force
- How many hours per week or month will be devoted as staff release time for program development
- What the target date is for the initial phase of program design and pilot-testing
- What the timetable is for dissemination of the CBO design to other units (if this is planned)

Since the nurse manager has final authority over the set of expectations that apply to staff nurses on that unit, nurse managers have a central role in all phases of the assessment process. Their support for the investment of staff time required for development of the program is essential for the success of this endeavor. In addition, their knowledge of the patient populations served on the unit, their awareness of the position description and performance evaluation tools used for staff nurses, and their responsibility for the competence of their staff underscore the necessity of the manager's active and ongoing participation in this process. Although nurse managers' understanding and support of CBO program development are required during all phases of the educational process, these elements are most crucial before and during the assessment phase, when resource demands for program development are maximal.

PROGRAM PLANNING

In a traditional approach to instruction, the planning phase consists of two major activities: specifying instructional outcomes and developing the curriculum. When a competency-based approach is used, however, the specification of instructional outcomes is accomplished during program assessment. As mentioned earlier in this chapter, the reason for this change is because the competency statements and performance criteria that constitute the instructional outcomes are used to assess the learner's entry capabilities and to determine the focus of the educational program that follows. For an orientation program, then, this mechanism enables knowledgeable and experienced orientees the possibility of challenging out of all areas of instruction if they can demonstrate that they are already competent in those areas. Both instructor and orientee time and resources can thereby be saved by avoiding teaching orientees content that they already know and skills that they already can perform to the hospital's expectations.

In both traditional and competency-based approaches to instruction, the process of curriculum development is quite comparable. When a CBE approach is employed, some curriculum development elements are modified, but each must be completed nonetheless. In addition to these customary aspects of curriculum development, orientation programs have some unique aspects that must be addressed. This section will review each of these considerations.

DEVELOPMENT OF THE CURRICULUM

As described in Chapter 3, traditional curriculum development includes the following activities: selecting instructional content, organizing and sequencing instruction, allotting instructional time, selecting appropriate media, and managing and supporting program faculty. Each of these activities is employed in orientation programs. In addition, planning for orientation programs also needs to include determining the level of the orientation, deciding on an appropriate orientation program format, and preparing and working with preceptors.

Selection of Instructional Content

Instructional content for an orientation program is determined in the same general two-step manner as content for any other type of educational activity. First, the educator reviews the instructional outcomes established for the program to identify the content area(s) reflected there. Second, the educator determines the prerequisite knowledge, attitudes, and skills that learners would need to have in order to attain those outcomes.

When a competency-based approach is used for the orientation program, two aspects of these steps differ. First, instead of deriving the necessary content from instructional objectives, the educator derives content from the competency statements and performance criteria. As Box 6.6 illustrates, this step requires that educators consider the performance criteria and ask themselves "If I am attempting to help an orientee meet that expectation [e.g., the expectation of *Determines patient/family readiness to learn about managing patient health problem(s)*], what content needs to be included in the instruction provided?" As the box suggests, relevant content might include definition of the term *readiness to learn,* identification of the many factors that may influence readiness to learn, and how one can estimate learning readiness.

The second way in which development of content coverage differs with a competency-based approach is that "content" includes providing orientees with an opportunity to actually practice using this information. As mentioned earlier, a major distinguishing feature of the competency-based approach to education is its emphasis on doing vs. just knowing. Because their job will require nurses to actually estimate a patient's readiness to learn, CBO programs go beyond merely verifying that the orientee knows what the term means, can identify factors that may influence learning readiness, and can describe the procedure for determining it. CBO programs extend these expectations by requiring learners to demonstrate that they can actually determine a patient's readiness to learn. This might first be done for practice as a simulation in a role-play scenario with other educators playing the role of patient and family members, but then this needs to be demonstrated by the orientee with actual patients and family members. Thus each of the content areas listed in Box 6.6 includes practice in demonstrating the area contained in the performance criteria. Where traditional orientation programs might only cover the cognitive components of competence, the content of CBO programs requires actual performance in a real-life situation (or in a simulation that is as close to "real" as possible).

If orientees have already been "checked off" after observation by the preceptor in any of these performance criteria during the assessment phase of orientation, the educator may delete the content related to that performance criteria from inclusion in that orientee's instruction. This type of challenge mechanism represents another feature often associated with CBE approaches to instruction.

Organizing and Sequencing the Curriculum

Organizing and sequencing the curriculum for an orientation program follows the same considerations and principles as described in Chapter 3. The order in which content is presented, the factors that may affect determination of the optimal sequencing pattern, and the general principles enumerated in Box 3.3 (Chapter 3) all apply to orientation programs.

In contrasting traditional with competency-based approaches to instruction, however, one important distinction emerges. In traditional approaches to education, the instructor typically makes all decisions regarding the order in which content is provided. In competency-based approaches, however, a concerted attempt is made to share this decision-making perogative with the learner. Insofar as possible, CBO programs provide some means for enabling the orientees to express their preferences regarding which competency areas and which performance criteria they learn about first, which they would like to cover next, and which they would prefer to address last. Although a number of organizational realities (such as classroom or laboratory space availability, the number of orientees being supported, shift rotation schedules, etc.) may place some constraints on this timetable, CBO programs try to accommodate the orientee's preferred order of instruction whenever possible. The educator may be able to assist orientees

---

Box 6.6

DERIVATION OF INSTRUCTIONAL CONTENT FOR A CBO PROGRAM

COMPETENCY STATEMENT

Fulfills all staff nurse responsibilities related to the role of patient educator.

PERFORMANCE CRITERIA

A. Determines patient/family readiness to learn about managing patient health problem(s)
B. Assists the patient/family in identifying specific health problem(s)
C. Provides patient/family with instruction that includes each of the following as appropriate:
   1. Pathophysiology of the disorder/problem
   2. Required medications
   3. Required therapies
   4. Lifestyle modifications (e.g., risk factors, diet, exercise, work)
   5. Potential complications
   6. Symptoms to report immediately, if any
D. Uses available instructional aids related to identified health problems and required care
E. Verifies that patient/family understand the instruction provided
F. Distributes written instructional materials for follow-up and postdischarge care
G. Documents the patient education process and its outcomes on the discharge plan of care

Role of the Nurse as Patient Educator

A. Readiness to learn
   1. Definition
   2. Factors that influence
   3. How to determine
   4. Practice in determining patient/family readiness to learn
B. Identification of health problem(s)
   1. Translating medical diagnoses into understandable "health problems"
   2. Health problems most often encountered on that unit
   3. Practice in assisting patients to identify their health problems
C. Providing health instruction
   1. For each common health problem identified, synopsis of its:
      a. Pathophysiology
      b. Usual medications
      c. Usual therapies
      d. Necessary lifestyle changes
      e. Potential complications
      f. Signs and symptoms to report immediately
   2. Practice in providing health instruction to patients and families on that unit
D. Use of instructional aids
   1. Rationale for using instructional aids
   2. Currently available instructional aids
   3. How to develop effective instructional aids
   4. Practice using instructional aids in patient/family education
E. Verification that instruction was effective
   1. Rationale for need to validate learning
   2. Techniques to verify that learning has occurred
   3. Practice in verifying effectiveness of instruction
F. Use of written instructional materials
   1. Purpose of written instructional materials
   2. Currently available instructional materials
   3. Practice in reviewing written instructional materials with patients and families
G. Documentation of patient education
   1. Rationale
   2. Unit requirements
   3. Practice in documentation of patient education process and outcomes

---

(especially inexperienced nurses such as new graduates) by suggesting organizing sequences that have been successful with others, but as much discretion as possible is given to the orientee.

Allotting Instructional Time

In contrast to traditional orientation programs where instructional time is the same for all orientees and determined according to the educator's appraisal of how much time each content area should receive, competency-based programs approach these decisions quite differently. Although CBO approaches still attend to all of the factors that may influence the allocation of instructional time (see Box 3.4, Chapter 3), CBO approaches tend to be more learner-controlled and less rigid about how much time is designated for each content area. In general, CBO programs allot instructional time according to how much time the learner needs to demonstrate the performance criteria: those who can meet some performance criteria on entry into that institution will not need to be provided with any instruction in those areas; those who need a minimal or moderate amount of instruction before they can meet the performance criteria will receive proportionate amounts of instruction. Instructional time, therefore, is based on the learner's needs rather than on the teacher's estimates and is flexible rather than fixed. As a result, the time required for CBO programs varies with the learner's needs and may be less predictable than with traditional orientation programs. While all orientees are subject to some maximal timeframe for completing orientation, some orientees may require more time and others will need much less time. The advantage of a CBO approach is that maximal amounts of instruction are only accorded to orientees who truly need more instruction rather than to all orientees regardless of need. With this approach, regularly scheduled blocks of instruction are replaced by flexibility in scheduling CBO learning experiences. Challenge mechanisms help to minimize or avoid the provision of unnecessary instruction for both orientees as well as educators and preceptors. The guiding principles for allocating instructional time in a CBO program are summarized in Box 6.7.

Selecting Instructional Media

When CBO programs incorporate instructional media, they do so in much the same way as is done for traditional orientation programs. If there is a difference in this aspect of curriculum development, it is that CBO programs use media more extensively than do traditional programs for a number of reasons. Because competency-based approaches to education are more flexible in relation to when and how learners learn, they foster use of instructional techniques that afford learners this type of flexibility. Since instructional media can be used when and where and for as long as and as often as learners desire, they are especially appropriate for educational programs that employ a competency-based approach. Although using instructional media is not required for the orientation program to be competency-based, media that facilitate self-directed learning are

often included in these programs to take advantage of flexibility in this area.

Distinguishing Among Levels of Orientation

The set of expectations that the hospital has for a newly hired staff nurse can be envisioned as existing at a number of levels. Some expectations such as those related to the general principles of fire safety and risk management apply to all hospital employees, not just those involved in patient care. Other expectations such as those related to documentation and CPR apply to all categories of nursing department personnel, not just to staff nurses. Other sets of expectations may apply to all staff nurses who work in related patient care areas such as maternal-child health units (labor and delivery, postpartum, newborn nursery, pediatrics), all of the medical-surgical areas, or all of the critical care units. Finally, some expectations of staff nurses apply only to the particular unit to which the nurse is assigned. As Figure 6.3 illustrates, then, four levels of orientation can be distinguished, based on the scope of applicability of various sets of expectations:

- Hospital
- Nursing department
- Nursing division
- Nursing unit

The expectations and learning needs addressed at the *hospital orientation* level apply to all employees and, thus, are universal in scope. The expectations and educational needs addressed at the *nursing department orientation* level apply to all members of the nursing service department: RNs, LPNs, nursing assistants, nurse's aides, and other ancillary staff, such as nursing technicians or orderlies who are considered members of the nursing department. Larger hospitals often cluster other sets of expectations according to different divisions within the nursing department. These *nursing division orientation* level programs encompass expectations and learning needs held in common by related

Box 6.7	
GUIDING PRINCIPLES FOR ALLOCATING INSTRUCTIONAL TIME IN A CBO PROGRAM	
Learner-centered	The primary determinants of time allocations are the orientee's needs and progress
Flexibility	Adjusting (increasing or decreasing) instructional time to the learner's needs
Efficiency	Only providing instruction to orientees who need it; only providing the amount of instruction that is warranted to meet established outcomes
Outcome-based	Helping orientees attain the performance criteria within the time limit for the program is the important element; the amount of time spent on learning in any one content area is less important
Performance-based	Sufficient time must be allotted for program outcomes based on actual job requirements to be achieved

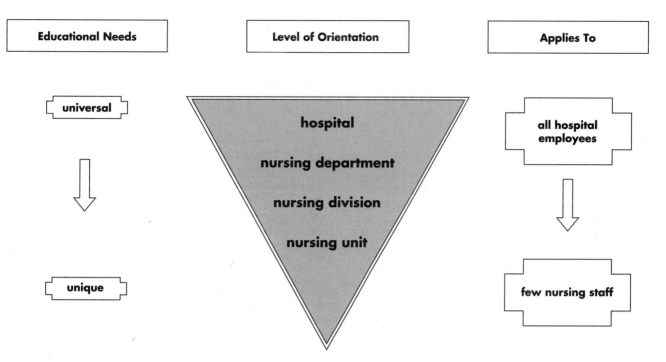

Figure 6.3   Orientation levels: scope of applicability.

units. For example, some competency areas and performance criteria will be shared by nurses who work in ambulatory surgery and those in postanesthesia recovery units; common areas will exist for staff nurses who work in coronary care and those who work in telemetry units; other areas will exist in common for nurses who work in any of the medical-surgical units. Finally, the *nursing unit orientation* level can be reserved for addressing only those expectations and educational needs that are unique to that unit.

The benefits of planning orientation programs at multiple levels are chiefly derived from enhanced efficiency. Rather than requiring each nursing unit to develop and provide its own curriculum to address all of the potential educational needs of its staff nurses, it is more cost-effective in time and labor to provide this instruction at its appropriate level of applicability. This type of cooperative planning avoids unnecessary duplication of both planning and provision efforts among the various nursing units.

As can be seen in Figure 6.3, the number of orientees who will need orientation decreases at each successive level of orientation from hospital to unit levels. To provide more efficient program planning, group teaching methods can be used when the number of orientees is large, whereas more individualized (one-on-one) teaching methods can be employed at the unit level, where the number of orientees is much smaller.

The organizational structure of the hospital and nursing department may, of course, modify the number of levels of orientation. Highly centralized organizational patterns with a human resource department (HRD) structure may only offer two levels of orientation: hospital and unit. Modified decentralized patterns with a nursing staff development department may offer three (hospital, nursing department, and unit) or all four levels of orientation. Fully decentralized structures may provide all orientation on the nursing unit. Although these organizational structures may influence the number of orientation levels, the most efficient planning and provision pattern, especially at larger hospitals, uses all four levels suggested.

When a competency-based approach is used for orientation, the only adjustment necessary is that the educational needs accommodated at each level relate to competencies and performance criteria rather than to instructional objectives. If CBO is to be used throughout the nursing department, each nursing unit drafts its own competency statements, preferably using the same organizing framework as other nursing units. Units then compare their competency statements to determine which competency areas they share in common with other units. Once these commonalities are identified, all units that have the same competency areas can work together to draft the performance criteria for that competency statement. Areas of commonalty among performance criteria are also acknowledged, with each unit having the freedom to add or modify performance criteria according to its own needs and requirements. In this manner, competency areas that are common throughout the nursing department can be grouped together, those common to multiple units within a division can be discerned, and those unique to a particular unit can be distinguished. When this process is used for other departments in the hospital, areas of commonalty across all departments can be revealed for coverage in the hospital orientation program.

The content covered at each level of orientation may vary somewhat at different hospitals but generally has many elements of similarity, especially at the hospital and nursing department levels. Hospital orientation programs for all employees often include the elements listed in Box 6.8. As can be seen from this list, the content of hospital orientation programs typically includes a combination of competencies related to work performance and communication of various other pieces of information to familiarize the employee with the institution. Box 6.9 lists some of the competency areas and information covered in nursing department orientation programs.

The content covered at the divisional level of orientation depends on the number and types of patient care units as well as on the manner in which these units are administratively arranged. In general, however, certain clusters of patient care units tend to share many competency areas in common with each other. Some of these clusters are enumerated in Box 6.10.

Once the orientation competencies have been identified and divided into appropriate levels for coverage, the educator will need to determine which format(s) will be most suitable at each level. As mentioned previously, large group formats are often used for hospital and nursing department levels of orientation and may, if the number of orientees is large, also be employed for divisional level orientation. The section that follows will describe program format options for the unit level of orientation.

Selecting an Orientation Program Format

The *format* of an educational program refers to its general organizational structure. Over the past three decades, a number of formats have evolved for hospital-based nursing orientation programs. These formats range from the apprentice-type and relatively unstructured coassignment and buddy system formats, to the more organized preceptorship and internship formats, to the learner-structured and learner-paced format. Although most of today's nursing orientation programs employ the preceptorship format,[5,6] it may be helpful to consider the features of alternative structures as well since many orientation programs combine the features of more than one format.

There is no one right or best format for an orientation program. Each format has advantages and disadvantages that need to be considered in relation to the particular circumstances that exist at each hospital. Virtually any format can be successful when the following conditions exist:

- All essential areas of performance are included in the outcomes
- The outcomes for the orientation are clearly specified
- Adequate resources are provided for instruction
- Orientees are afforded a support system
- The individuals who provide instruction are prepared for their role
- Administrative support exists for the program

Box 6.8

CONTENT AREAS IN HOSPITAL ORIENTATION PROGRAM

COMPETENCY AREAS

- Patient safety program
- Staff safety program: lifting, transferring, weighing patients
- Fire safety program
- Electrical safety program
- Hazardous material management program
- Infection control program
- Risk management guidelines
- Patient services: pastoral care, social service, dietary, occupational/physical therapy
- Compliance with universal precautions
- Hospital communication systems: telephone, computer, forms
- Disaster plan
- Patient rights
- Confidentiality of patient information
- Legal issues
- Ethical issues
- Quality monitoring and improvement program

HOSPITAL EMPLOYEE INFORMATION

- Welcome to agency
- Hospital mission, philosophy, goals
- Organizational chart
- Physical facilities: buildings, services, hospital floor plan
- Explanation of employee salary and benefit packages
- Employee health services
- Employee assistance and substance abuse programs
- Guest relations program
- Hospital security procedures, policies, ID badges
- Personnel policies, procedures, services, forms
- Staff development program offerings
- EEO policy

Box 6.9

CONTENT AREAS IN NURSING DEPARTMENT ORIENTATION PROGRAM

COMPETENCY AREAS

- Infection control policies, procedures
- Nursing procedures related to universal precautions
- CPR certification/recertification
- Nursing practice and patient care standards
- Nursing quality improvement program
- Departmental certification and credentialing programs
- Nursing responsibilities in fire, safety, and disaster management
- JCAHO accreditation requirements
- Patient advocacy: resolution of ethical and legal issues
- Patient classification system
- Patient care plans
- Patient education and discharge planning
- Documentation in patient record: mechanisms, forms, and procedures
- Medication administration policies, procedures, calculation test
- Multidisciplinary collaboration

NURSING STAFF INFORMATION

- Mission, philosophy, goals of nursing service department
- Nursing department organizational chart
- Nursing department policy and procedure manual
- Nursing department personnel policies and procedures
- Position description
- Patient populations served
- Work schedules and assignments
- Probationary period policies for nursing personnel
- Staff development services for nursing staff
- Performance evaluations
- Introduction to key nursing staff

Box 6.10

POSSIBLE GROUPINGS FOR DIVISION LEVEL ORIENTATION PROGRAM

MATERNAL-CHILD DIVISION
Neonatal ICU
Well baby nursery
Pediatric ICU
Pediatrics
Labor and delivery
Postpartum

SURGICAL DIVISION
Ambulatory surgery
Surgical clinics
Postanesthesia recovery
Operating room
General surgical units

MEDICAL DIVISION
All general medical units

CRITICAL CARE DIVISION
Medical ICU
Surgical ICU
Coronary care unit
Cardiac surgical unit
Telemetry unit
Emergency department

PSYCHIATRIC—MENTAL HEALTH DIVISION
Acute psychiatric inpatient unit
Psychiatric outpatient clinic
Substance abuse clinic

Features of Orientation Program Formats

At least six different formats have been developed for nursing orientation programs. These formats include: coassignment, buddy system, preceptorship, internship, self-directed, and the orientation unit. Each of these is described following.

COASSIGNMENT The *coassignment* orientation format involves the designation of one staff nurse per shift who shares a patient assignment with the orientee. The nurse coassigned with the orientee changes with every shift the orientee works. Coassignment is one of the oldest mechanisms for orienting new staff nurses. The advantages of this format include its simple design and management; minimal time and effort are required to provide the program, and virtually any staff nurse may be assigned to work with the orientee. In addition, some orientees enjoy the rotation of staff nurse instructors and learning their different approaches to nursing practice. Staff instructors benefit by not being burdened with instructional responsibilities for long periods of time. Some disadvantages of this format include a potential lack of continuity and quality in instruction, the potential for confusion in expectations if those assigned with the orientee practice differently from one another, the hit-or-miss nature of learning experiences, the duplication of staffing coverage required, a lack of ownership and accountability for helping the orientee develop, and a lack of overall coordination and supervision of the program. Some of these disadvantages are overcome by the buddy system format.

BUDDY SYSTEM   The *buddy system* format uses a limited number of experienced staff nurses who function as resource persons for orientees. The assigned "buddy" typically remains with the same orientee for a given period of time but might change with different patients or with shift and unit rotations. Buddies are not formally prepared for their role but function on the basis of their ability to model the staff nurse role on that unit. The advantages of the buddy system over coassignment include a greater continuity in the quality, style, and nature of instruction provided, more consistency in performance expectations, less duplication of staffing coverage, and an improved ability to monitor the overall progress of the orientee. Some disadvantages of the buddy system include its greater burden on staff who serve as buddies for longer periods of time and the lack of a stable one-to-one relationship in working with orientees. If the buddies change too often, there may be a lack of coordination, continuity, and supervision of orientees and failure to meet established outcomes. Because buddies receive no formal training for the involved instructional responsibilities, their skills as role models and instructors may be limited or weak and their expectations of orientees may not be realistic.

PRECEPTORSHIP   A *preceptorship* format is an organized instructional program in which staff nurses facilitate the development and socialization of newly hired nursing staff to the responsibilities of their position on their assigned unit. In this format, a *preceptor* is an experienced and competent staff nurse who has received formal training to function in this capacity and who serves as a clinical role model and resource person to the newly employed nurse (preceptee). In its classic form, the same preceptor remains with the same orientee/preceptee throughout the orientation program. Preceptors differ from buddies in that they are usually prepared for their role by some type of preceptor training program and, insofar as possible, work the same schedule as the orientee. Preceptors work closely with orientees on an ongoing basis to plan the orientation, monitor the orientee's progress, provide feedback on his/her performance, and help the new nurse feel welcomed and integrated into the unit and staff. The preceptor's judgment weighs heavily in the determination of when an orientee has completed orientation and is ready to function independently on the unit. The reported advantages of the preceptorship format are summarized in Box 6.11.

Box 6.11

ADVANTAGES OF THE PRECEPTORSHIP ORIENTATION FORMAT*

- Maintenance of a consistent role model in the 1:1 preceptor: orientee relationship
- Greater continuity in the quality and nature of instruction
- Improved knowledge and skill acquisition by orientees
- Smoother transition of the new graduate from student to staff nurse roles
- Enhanced socialization of new staff to the unit
- Orientees become more productive sooner
- Orientees learn nursing practice on that unit as it actually exists
- Increased retention and decreased turnover rates among new graduate nursing staff
- More cost effective
- Closer supervision and monitoring of orientees' performance based on mutual planning of goals, learning experiences, and weekly evaluation meetings
- Greater flexibility in modifying the content and duration of orientation to suit the orientee's individual needs
- Increased recruitment of new staff nurses
- More efficient use of staff development personnel to coordinate orientation of large numbers of orientees, troubleshoot problems, and support both orientee and preceptors
- Quality control over instruction via preceptor selection criteria and training
- Easier to adapt to meet the unique needs of smaller hospitals

*See references 9, 43, 57, 67, 86, 96, 125.

Giles and Moran[57] compared the buddy system and preceptorship formats for orientation and identified the following as advantages of the preceptorship format:

- Nurses oriented by preceptorship were more satisfied with their orientation than those oriented by the buddy system
- The orientation by preceptorship was more comprehensive, more standardized, better organized, better monitored, and progressed in a more logical sequence
- Preceptorship afforded better continuity in who oriented new staff and in what was covered
- The preceptorship orientation was more individualized and less stressful for the orientee
- There was greater accountability among those who provided orientation
- Although orientation by preceptorship lasted somewhat longer than with the buddy system, when the orientation was ended, the preceptorship orientees were more ready to assume their responsibilities than the buddy system orientees
- There was less turnover among new staff nurses

These authors concluded that the preceptorship method of orientation was both more effective and more efficient than the buddy system format.

Some disadvantages of the preceptorship format have also been reported. These are summarized in Box 6.12. Despite these possible disadvantages, preceptorships enjoy widespread use in nursing orientation programs. In a recent informal survey, 95% of 149 hospitals responding reported using preceptorship as the format for orienting critical care nurses.[5,6]

INTERNSHIP The nursing *internship* is somewhat of a hybrid educational program format that combines orientation with more extensive instruction. As conceived in the 1960s,[36] a nursing internship is a transitional educational

---

Box 6.12

DISADVANTAGES OF THE PRECEPTORSHIP ORIENTATION FORMAT*

- Transient or persistent staffing shortages may preclude consistency in the 1:1 preceptor:preceptee assignments
- Preceptors may not be relieved of their customary workload to allow them sufficient time with the orientee
- If preceptors are relieved of some of their customary workload, resentment may arise among other staff who have to carry heavier assignments to compensate
- Role conflict occurs if the preceptor also must function as charge nurse, team leader, or has more than one orientee to supervise
- If the hospital does not offer a training program to prepare preceptors for their role, individuals may function in this capacity without any consideration of their education, experience, or teaching ability
- Role of the preceptor can be demanding, stressful, and challenging, leading to stress, fatigue, and burnout among preceptors
- Lack of recognition or rewards for preceptors may lead to dissatisfaction
- Preceptors may find it difficult to relinquish direct care responsibilities and perceive precepting as less fulfilling than providing patient care
- Without peer support, preceptors' allegiance is divided between patient care demands and needs of the orientee
- Personality conflicts may arise between preceptors and orientees
- Differences in the educational preparation between preceptors and orientees may lead to differing perceptions, priorities, and frustrations
- Preceptors may be uncomfortable evaluating orientee performance, causing them to be too lenient or too harsh or to feel inadequate in this area
- Orientees who do not progress quickly may cause the preceptor stress and conflict
- The unit may not have a sufficient number of qualified preceptors, leading to burnout of the few available
- If precepting is mandatory or necessary for clinical advancement, it may be provided by nurses who do not enjoy this role or find it fulfilling, possibly leading to less than optimal performance
- Preceptors may feel pressured by other staff or nurse managers to designate marginally performing orientees as competent because of the need to fill staffing vacancies on the unit
- Orientees may rely on preceptors rather than on their own initiative to solve problems

*See references 5, 6, 9, 10, 57, 86, 102, 125, 143.

program for the orientation and development of newly graduated nurses.[8] Although some internships include interns who are not new graduates,[4] most internships are offered for that category of orientees. In contrast to medical internships that are provided by schools of medicine, most nursing internships are sponsored by hospitals rather than by schools of nursing.

Nursing internship programs are distinguished from traditional hospital orientations by their longer duration, more comprehensive curriculum, closer clinical supervision, more structured program of learning experiences, and more gradual and progressive development of the new graduate toward independent functioning in the staff nurse role.[8]

Nurse internship programs typically serve dual purposes. The educational purpose of an internship program has traditionally been to facilitate the new graduate's transition from the student to the staff nurse role. The organizational purpose of the internship program may include one or more of the following: increasing the supply of new nursing staff (recruitment), better preparing new graduates to function as staff nurses, and reducing the costs (turnover) associated with employment of new graduate nurses. In effect, then, hospital-sponsored nurse internship programs generally aim to serve their own needs as well as the special needs of newly graduated nurses. The characteristics of nursing internship programs have been reported in the nursing literature since the 1970s. A review of this literature reveals the characteristics listed in Table 6.2.

Internships have been described for many clinical areas of nursing.[87] These include internships for medical-surgical units,[17,27,36,106] critical care units,* pediatric units,[121] and surgical units.[55]

The potential advantages of internship programs may be divided into benefits to the intern, benefits to the hospital, and benefits to the unit nursing staff. The purported benefits of this format to nurse interns include the following†:

- Greater job satisfaction
- More self-confidence
- More self-sufficiency and independence in functioning
- More fully developed knowledge, attitudes, and clinical skills
- Better decision-making and leadership skills (such as priority setting and problem-solving)
- Smoother adjustment to the staff nurse role
- More time for rotation through different clinical unit(s)
- Better integration of classroom and clinical learning experiences

- Less pressure to quickly assume independent responsibilities as a staff nurse

The potential benefits of an internship to the hospital include improved recruitment and retention of new graduates and better patient care.* Internships are often credited as effective recruitment tools because new graduates perceive these programs as supportive and nurturing means of assisting them in making a smoother transition to the staff nurse role. The positive experience of nurses who enter the agency as interns often translates into lower attrition and turnover rates among the graduate nurse staff because internships tend to minimize the trauma of being a new graduate and having to experience the reality of nursing practice as well as assimilate the volumes of information and experience associated with most orientation programs. Nursing internships frequently include segments related to biculturalism, help new graduates through the stages of reality shock,[80] and are especially sensitive to the unique needs of new graduates. Nurses whose needs—educational, social, and developmental—are being met effectively will progress well and be ready to assume their full duties sooner than if one or more of these groups of needs is not being met.

In addition to the benefits that internships can afford to interns and the hospital, the unit nursing staff may also enjoy a number of positive benefits. Some that have been identified in the literature include the following†:

- Greater awareness and sensitivity to the needs of new graduates
- More realistic expectations for the new nurse
- Better rapport in working with new graduates
- Recognition of staff's knowledge, skills, and clinical expertise by the new graduates
- Improved staff morale related to the greater productivity of new graduates, fewer staff shortages, and lower turnover rates
- Renewed staff interest in continuing education

The potential disadvantages of nurse internships can also be viewed in relation to the hospital, the unit, and the intern. Because the associated costs of offering an internship program can be considerable, hospitals need to determine whether the returns on their investment are fully realized. Some related disadvantages in this context include the following‡:

- *Many of the qualitative outcomes for the internship are difficult to appraise.* Outcomes, such as increased self-confidence, job satisfaction, and smoother role ad-

*See references 2, 4, 23, 25, 30, 33, 63, 79, 89, 97, 117, 121, 133.
†See references 4, 17, 23, 28, 32, 52, 119, 122, 137.

*See references 4, 17, 23, 32, 52, 62, 77, 89, 117, 119, 122, 131.
†See references 4, 23, 32-33, 52, 137.
‡See references 8, 36, 37, 119, 122, 128.

	TABLE 6.2 • CHARACTERISTICS OF NURSE INTERNSHIP PROGRAMS*	
Characteristic	**Finding(s)**	**Comments**
Duration	Range from 1½ to 12 months Medical-surgical areas: 3 to 6 months Critical care areas: usually 6 months	Duration usually fixed, but some are variable; duration tends to be longer for specialty areas
Frequency	Range from 1 to 4 per year Usually 1 to 2 per year Critical care usually 1 per year	Many reports fail to mention frequency of offerings
Sponsor(s)	Usually a hospital	Occasionally a hospital cosponsors with a school of nursing[131,133] or a consortium of hospitals[137]
Funding	Hospital programs usually subsidized at the nursing unit or department level; less often, positions budgeted in staff development department	Most reports do not address this feature Programs offered by schools of nursing may be intern-subsidized via student tuition
Marketing	Usually by word of mouth, bulletins posted at schools of nursing, local newspaper advertising	Most reports do not mention
Enrollment	Ranges from 4 to 50 interns per program[119] Typically about 20 interns per program; fewer in critical care areas	Number of interns per program varies widely but is usually limited to enhance the learning experience
Intern compensation	Half provide full entry level (GN) salary and benefits; half offer reduced salary and benefits during program	Salary and benefits typically rise to full RN scale after RN license is obtained
Entry requirements	Graduation from an NLN accredited program, limited or no nursing experience, obtain RN license	Usually open to graduates of all three basic programs; less often, limited to only associate or baccalaureate degree graduates
Didactic emphasis	General orientation content Medical-surgical or specialty area orientation Reality shock/biculturalism	Emphasize policies, procedures, standards, documentation, medications
Clinical emphasis	Development of clinical skills Diversity of clinical experiences Progressive role development from staff nurse to manager	Patient care and refinement of technical skills; clinical rotations Varying role assignments.
Service commitment	Usually twice the length of internship program (e.g., 1 year service after a 6-month internship)	Not a legally binding contract
Cost	Depends on length of program, number of interns and instructors, salary and benefits of each, direct costs, and overhead	Rarely included in reports; the few estimates made are outdated and/or incomplete reflections of true costs

*See references 2, 4, 8, 17, 23, 25, 32, 36, 52, 79, 80, 87, 117, 119, 122.

justment, are largely derived from subjective verbal appraisals that are hard to substantiate. Many reports claim these outcomes but rarely measure them in any objective way.

- *A number of sought-after outcomes of internships cannot be determined until several years following the program.* Goals related to attrition, turnover, and quality of performance in the staff nurse role are long-term results that are not available for appraisal at completion of each internship program.
- *Attrition and turnover rates may not be lower following an internship program.* Problems in these areas that are attributable to some cause other than the preparation of new graduates are not likely to be positively affected by the internship program. If support for the program

is inadequate, attrition among both existing and intern nursing staff may actually increase. The former may leave if they are burdened with developing many interns without relief from their already heavy patient assignments. Interns may leave if they perceive that they were recruited more to fill staffing deficits than to participate in an educational offering.

- *Pressure may be exerted to retain interns whose performance is less than satisfactory.* Because of the sizable investments that hospitals make with an internship, program coordinators, preceptors, and staff may feel pressured to retain interns despite marginal or unsatisfactory performance in the program. This pressure may be especially strong towards the end of a long program. If no mechanism exists (or an existing mechanism is ignored) to release marginal performers, the program initially loses its quality control and, eventually, its reputation.

On units that participate in the internship program, potential disadvantages include the following[4,8,32,52,128]:

- *The internship may interfere with unit operations.* The addition of many new staff members, competition for certain patient assignments, and the need to both teach and provide patient care can lead to conflicts and disruptions in work flow. Extremes in staffing coverage may also occur: staffing ratios may be excessive when interns are on the units but deficient when interns leave for scheduled learning experiences. Friction, conflict, and split loyalties may then arise among both the regular staff and the intern group, leading to polarization between staff.
- *The internship may foster extended periods of dependence.* If the supportive and nurturing aspects of the internship are overly emphasized or unduly prolonged, interns may depend on their mentors much longer than is warranted or reasonable. A planned progression of weaning the interns toward greater independence in functioning can be incorporated in program planning to avoid this.
- *The internship may widen the education-service gap.* At times, the unit staff may perceive interns as privileged and pampered newcomers who "dump" their work loads on regular staff when they leave to attend classes. If this situation is not avoided (e.g., by the intern's preceptor taking the intern's patients), it sets up a classic we-they confrontation between the unit staff and interns. These circumstances may also arise if staff are not included in program planning and in determining ways to accommodate both patient care needs and interns' needs. Great effort, coordination, and communication must be exercised to ensure that unit staff are not misused or abused and that patient care is not compromised by efforts to provide the internship program. If such abuse occurs, unit staff will tend to resent rather than support the interns.
- *Roles and responsibilities of unit staff in relation to the interns may not be clear.* The boundaries of role responsibilities for providing instruction and patient care need to be clearly drawn so that loyalties towards patient care and the unit do not conflict with obligations to the interns.
- *Unit nursing staff may feel insecure about answering interns' questions.* Nursing staff who graduated many years earlier may not feel confident that they are well informed on "the latest" in nursing or may have fuzzy recall of specific points of physiology, pathophysiology, or some other area. An intern's explicit queries may then precipitate anxiety and insecurity among nursing staff. Making classes open and making readings and other assignments available to all staff can help to allay this staff concern.

Some potential disadvantages may also exist from the nurse intern's perspective. These include the following[8,52,133]:

- *The volume of instruction provided is overwhelming.* Especially when the internship lasts 3 to 6 months, the sheer amount of didactic and clinical instruction in the program may be beyond the intern's ability to assimilate and integrate. Rather than feeling nurtured and supported, interns may feel completely overwhelmed.
- *The internship may fail to deliver on its promises.* Interns may feel betrayed if they perceive that the program fails to live up to its advertising. Dubious organizational commitment to the program may be evidenced by an insufficient number of preceptors, preceptors who are not prepared to serve effectively in that role, poor program coordination, or a marginal quality of instruction.
- *The internship may be designed more for service than for education.* When an internship lasts for many months, crises and demanding situations may well arise that preclude the unit's ability to release a large portion of its staff to attend previously scheduled educational events. But when staffing needs run frequently in direct conflict with meeting interns' needs for instruction, it is easy for the interns to view this situation as sacrificing their instruction to meet unit staffing needs. If this situation arises often, interns may well look upon the internship as a "front" for filling staff vacancies. Rather than being glad to pitch in, interns may gradually develop resentment towards the hospital for using them in this manner. A related corollary to this situation exists when the interns' clinical instructors are continually unavailable to them because they are carrying heavy patient assignments and cannot leave their patients to assist the intern.

Despite these possible disadvantages, most internship programs reported in the literature indicate an abundance of positive outcomes for the hospital, the unit(s), and the interns. As a result, internship programs, despite their high costs, remain a popular means of recruiting and retaining new nurses.

SELF-DIRECTED FORMAT The *self-directed* orientation format requires that all outcomes for the program are clearly identified, orientees are provided with all necessary resources to achieve those outcomes, an identified time limit for completion of the orientation has been specified, and the orientee takes responsibility for completing the orientation under these conditions. Self-directed orientations are usually managed by means of a series of learning contracts, which are negotiated between the orientee and the preceptor at regular intervals. Although a few articles have reported on the use of this format as the primary means for orientation,[66,107,136] self-directed learning is more often integrated as a component of another orientation format. Rather than the orientation program being coordinated and managed by an educator or preceptor, the process and progress with the self-directed format is orientee-directed. In most cases, however, some amount of instruction is still provided by educators, preceptors, or other individuals.

The advantages of a self-directed format are its embodiment of adult education principles, its individualization and its flexibility,[74] its potential to accelerate completion of orientation for experienced nurses, and its potential for saving instructional time and, therefore, costs. Orientees are actively involved in each phase of the educational process and can pace and tailor the orientation to their individual needs and preferences.[116]

The potential disadvantages of a self-directed orientation format include the costs of program development and its limited usefulness for new graduates who may require and desire greater structure and personalized support in securing instruction. This would also not be an effective format for orientees whose learning styles are teacher-dependent or highly social. If resources and other supports are not readily available when and where orientees need these or if preceptors are not skilled at negotiating learning contracts, the format may not be successful.

ORIENTATION UNIT   One other orientation format occasionally mentioned in the literature is the orientation unit. An *orientation unit* centralizes the orientation process on one or more designated nursing units rather than requiring each nursing unit to orient its own new staff. On these designated units, orientation may be provided by the regular staff or by a group of orientation instructors; in either case, those who serve as instructors receive special training in that role. Because orientees on these units are not counted as staff, their instructors are always available to supervise and provide learning experiences. On completion of the expectations for orientation, the orientee transfers to the assigned unit of hire.

The purported advantages of an orientation unit are particularly noteworthy for new graduates and include consistency in the content and quality of instruction, provision of an environment where learning is emphasized and supported,[109] a decreased amount of instructional responsibility on all the remaining nursing units, a controlled working environment, and a progressive increase in the complexity and volume of clinical assignments.[40]

As Haggard[61] points out, however, there are some notable disadvantages to the orientation unit format that may account for its limited use. These disadvantages include the following:

- The orientation unit is an artificial environment that may be overly protective and unrealistic.

- The nursing staff on the orientation unit may grow weary and burn out from continually having the responsibility to provide instruction in addition to patient care.
- The time spent on such a unit only delays the orientees' familiarity and socialization with the staff of their assigned unit.
- Orientation units do not completely obviate the need for orientation to the unit of hire. Aspects of patient care unique to the assigned unit still need to be covered following the days spent on the orientation unit.

Decision on an Orientation Program Format

The decision as to which format is most appropriate for an orientation program rests on consideration of six major issues. These issues are:

- *The agency's philosophy of staff development.* As mentioned in Chapter 1, the nursing department's philosophical beliefs regarding the purpose of staff development, the nurse's responsibility for self-development, the role of the staff development department, and learning and adult education may significantly affect its selection of an orientation program format. For example, a hospital's deep commitment to fostering collegial relationships among nurses may lead it to adopt a buddy system format for orientation. By contrast, a hospital with abiding beliefs in the tenets of adult education and professional self-development might perceive that a self-directed format would be more consistent with these values.
- *The type of prospective orientees.* Hospitals that need or want to attract new graduate nurses would likely give serious consideration to using an internship format. By contrast, healthcare institutions whose orientees were primarily experienced nurses who required minimal educational support might select a coassignment or buddy system format.
- *The number of orientees to be processed at one time.* Orientation formats such as coassignment or the self-directed format can more readily accommodate relatively large numbers of orientees at one time. Others such as internships or orientation units, however, are considerably less accommodating of numerous learners at the same time. Because of this resource strain, internships and orientation units often need to limit the number of orientees who may participate at a given time to a relatively small number.
- *How comprehensive the educational needs are for orientation.* Unless supplemented by didactic instruction, some orientation formats such as the buddy system or coassignment may only cover the learning needs that happened to exist when orientees were on the unit. Because of its long duration, an internship can accommodate the largest breadth, depth, and vol-

ume of educational needs. In general, the ability of other formats to meet these needs depends on the length of time available and whether classroom and/or laboratory instruction supplements the orientees' clinical experiences.

- *How often the orientation program needs to be provided.* The frequency with which orientees enter the hospital may make one format more feasible than another. With some formats such as self-directed, coassignment, and the buddy system, orientees may enter the program at virtually any time. Other formats, such as internships, can only be offered a few times per year because of their extended duration.
- *The resources available for the orientation program.* The single most important resource for an orientation program is administrative support. With administrative support, other necessary resources (such as an adequate budget, a sufficient number of qualified instructional and clerical personnel, accessible and available teaching facilities, instructional aids and media, supplies and storage space, and adequate time to meet established outcomes) are likely to be afforded to the program. Even with managerial support within the department of nursing, organizational and fiscal constraints may impose challenges and obstacles to ensuring that these resources will be available on an enduring basis. As long as nursing administration continues to support the program, however, educators can at least be assured that the best possible matching of needs and resources will be achieved. In relation to resource expenditures, the self-directed and self-paced formats are usually the least costly, whereas internships are the most expensive. For orientations of comparable duration, those that use clinical instruction primarily or exclusively are less expensive than those that also include classroom instruction. In the clinical area, orientations that employ dual assignment of both orientees and preceptors to the same patient(s) are more costly than those that assign these individuals to different patients.

As mentioned earlier in this section, there is no one "best" format for an orientation program. The determination of what is best is relative to each hospital's circumstances, needs, and constraints. After weighing each of these six factors in light of those needs and constraints, the selection of the most appropriate program format (or combination of formats) should be more easily reached. Indeed, one of the reasons why the preceptorship format is so commonly employed for nurse orientation programs may be that this format is situated about midway on many of these factors. It is adaptable for any staff development philosophy, can be used for any type of orientee and for varying numbers of orientees, can meet a sizable number of educational needs, can be provided fairly often, and can be modified to variable resource availabilities.

When a competency-based approach is used for the ori-

entation program, any of these formats may be used to plan instruction. CBE offers program planners maximum flexibility in selection of a program format and imposes no restrictions on this feature.

MANAGING PROGRAM FACULTY

The faculty for an orientation program often includes both classroom and clinical instructors. At some hospitals, only clinical instructors are used for the unit level of orientation. Management of orientation faculty involves securing, developing, and supporting both types of instructors.

Classroom Faculty

Securing, developing, and supporting classroom faculty follows the guidelines provided in Chapter 3. Selection criteria for classroom instructors can be derived from the traits listed in Box 3.5. The development of classroom instructors follows the general approaches suggested for assisting faculty to prepare for and provide instruction, whereas support aspects follow Chapter 3's guidelines related to assisting faculty before, during, and after instruction. In relation to managing classroom instructors, then, orientation programs do not differ in any substantive way from any other category of staff development program. Because so many nursing orientation programs use the preceptorship format (or employ elements of it combined with other formats) and because so much of orientation occurs in the clinical setting, this section will focus on the management of clinical preceptors.

Clinical Faculty

For an orientation program, the educator's responsibilities for managing clinical preceptors comprise the same three major areas as for classroom faculty: securing, developing, and supporting preceptors.

Securing Preceptors

The selection criteria for clinical preceptors typically encompass four main areas: knowledge, attitudes, skills, and experience. Knowledge requirements usually emphasize clinical practice, attitude requirements emphasize social and work attitudes, skill requirements emphasize clinical and leadership abilities, and experience requirements emphasize familiarity with the staff nurse role. A summary of some of the selection criteria commonly used for preceptors in each of these areas is provided in Box 6.13. Although the list of selection criteria adopted by a hospital is typically much shorter than the lists in Box 6.13, the prerequisites enumerated are often implicit among whichever criteria are employed. For example, the selection criteria of "mature" may, in the minds of those who will designate new preceptors, include the related attitude attributes of "respectful," "collegial," "open-minded," and "realistic."

Box 6.13

SELECTION CRITERIA FOR PRECEPTORS

KNOWLEDGE	**ATTITUDES**	**SKILLS**
Documentation	Collegial	Clinical competence in patient care
Patient care	Committed to program	Communication
Policies, procedures	Constructive	Interpersonal relations
Practice standards	Desire to precept	Patient/family teaching
Unit routines	Empathetic	Technical procedures
	Flexible	Use of equipment
EXPERIENCE	Mature	Use of nursing process
	Open-minded	Use of resources
As staff nurse for ___ years	Patient	Leadership skills:
On that unit for ___ years	Realistic	Critical thinking
Satisfactory performance	Respectful	Decision-making
evaluations	Sincere	Delegation
Troubleshooting patient care	Supportive	Goal-setting
problems		Priority-setting
Modifying procedures to patient		Problem-solving
needs		Supervision
		Time management
		Work organization

Developing Preceptors

As mentioned in the earlier discussion related to orientation formats, one of the features that distinguishes preceptors from "buddies" or nurses coassigned with the orientee is that preceptors are prepared for their role by a formal instructional program, often called a *preceptor training program (PTP)*. The rationale for preceptor training programs is that functioning effectively as a preceptor requires *additional* knowledge, attitudes, skills, and experience beyond those required to function effectively as a staff nurse (Figure 6-4). Although serving as a role model of a staff nurse on that unit is an important part of good precepting, it is not inclusive of all that a preceptor must know or be able to do. PTPs concentrate primarily on those differences. In a competency-based framework, this implies that competence as a preceptor is more inclusive than competence as a staff nurse.

PRECEPTOR TRAINING PROGRAM Designing a preceptor training program involves four major considerations: the role of the preceptor, the content to be covered, the learning experiences to be provided, and the evaluation of participants.

Role of the Preceptor The preceptor's role consists of three components: (1) staff nurse role model, (2) socializer, and (3) educator.[11] Serving as a staff nurse role model on the assigned unit is the component most familiar and comfortable to staff who will serve as preceptors. The socializer component of the preceptor role involves helping the new employees feel welcomed and facilitating their integration into their peer group, their unit, and the hospital. These

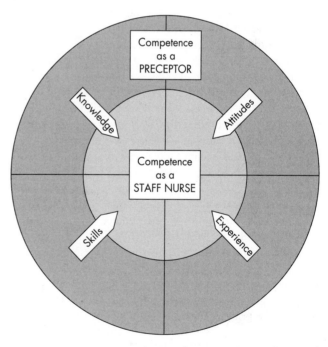

Figure 6.4 Relationship between staff nurse and preceptor competence.

responsibilities for socializing orientees are generally less familiar and less comfortable for the preceptor in comparison with their role model responsibilities.[9]

The educator component of the preceptor's role comprises four subsets of responsibilities that correlate with each phase of the educational process. These four responsibilities include assessment of the orientee's learning needs, planning learning activities, implementation of the teaching plan, and evaluation of orientee performance.[11] The educator component of the preceptor's role is usually the least familiar and least comfortable for preceptors.[9,138]

Program Content   Table 6.3 enumerates the content included in a preceptor training program that is organized around the three major components of the preceptor's role. If additional time is available for the program, other topic areas that might be considered include legal aspects of the preceptor's role and managing problems that may arise during the preceptorship program. The latter might include situations such as an orientee who is progressing too slowly or an orientee who depends on the preceptor for a prolonged time.

Learning Experiences   Because the nurses who participate in the PTP are adults, the learning experiences planned for this program should consist of highly interactive, adult teaching strategies.[11] Although one article describes the provision of a preceptor training program using solely self-instruction,[101] most published reports of this type of program employ a workshop to provide instruction.*

As Table 6.4 indicates, a wide variety of teaching strategies is employed in PTP workshops. An informal survey of 351 critical care preceptors[9] revealed that the most frequently employed learning experiences for this program included combined lecture/discussion (82% of PTPs), written handouts (77%), and role playing (52%). In addition to being interactive, the learning climate for these programs is often quite informal. A relaxed learning environment can not only enhance learning effectiveness but also help initiate feelings of camaraderie and support among members of the preceptor group.

Learner Evaluation   The evaluation of participants in a PTP needs to focus on their performance of elements considered essential to the preceptor role. Thus, rather than administering written tests to evaluate their knowledge about precepting, preceptor candidates are more appropriately afforded an opportunity to practice in each of the performance areas and to receive peer and educator critique as the primary means of evaluation.

COMPETENCY-BASED APPROACH TO PRECEPTOR TRAINING PROGRAMS   If a competency-based approach will be used to design the preceptor training program, the three components of the preceptor's role (staff nurse role model, socializer, and educator) may be adopted as competency areas with one competency statement written for each of these areas. For each competency statement, a set of performance criteria can then be drafted that specifies the ar-

TABLE 6.3 • PRECEPTOR TRAINING PROGRAM CONTENT AREAS*	
Program Segment	**Content Areas**
Introduction	Overview of preceptorship program
	Explanation of competency-based orientation
	Policies and procedures related to preceptorship
	Preceptor's position description
	Preceptor's support systems
Staff nurse role model	Role modeling process
	Differences between staff nurse and preceptor roles
	Responsibilities to orientee, patients, unit, nurse manager
	Practice as staff nurse role model
Socializer	Four stages of reality shock
	Biculturalism
	Healthcare team members
	Hospital support services
	Formal working relationships and rules
	Informal working relationships and rules
	Practice as socializer of new staff nurses
Educator	Assessment of learning needs:
	In relation to clinical instructional outcomes
	Setting priorities among learning needs
	Planning learning activities with the orientee:
	Developing a learning contract
	Negotiating learning contract terms
	Implementation of a learning plan with the orientee:
	Adult teaching methods
	Clinical teaching strategies
	How to teach clinical skills
	How to teach leadership skills
	Evaluation of the orientee's clinical performance:
	Providing feedback: positive, negative, constructive
	Practice using clinical evaluation tool(s)
	Practice in each phase of the educational process

*See references 9, 11, 38, 51, 67, 110, 125.

eas of performance considered as essential elements of competency for that area. Content for the PTP workshop as well as selection of appropriate learning experiences would proceed as described previously. Evaluation would then consist of verifying whether each participant had met the performance criteria established for each competency statement. Since a competency-based preceptor training program is already provided elsewhere,[11] it will not be described further here.

*See references 9, 11, 38, 51, 57, 92, 95, 99, 104, 110, 114, 125, 138, 143.

TABLE 6.4 • PRECEPTOR TRAINING PROGRAM TEACHING STRATEGIES*

Teaching Strategy	Examples of Applications
Assigned readings	Preparation for clinical experiences
Audiovisuals	Used in conjunction with instruction and discussions
Games	To identify principles of adult education, teaching, and learning
Group discussion	Phases of preceptor-orientee relationship
	Assisting orientees through each stage of reality shock
	Communication and feedback techniques
	Teaching skills
	Resources available for preceptor support
Handouts	Benner's novice-to-expert model
	Kramer's stages of reality shock
	Patient support services (names, telephone numbers)
Lecture/ discussion	Related to various content areas
Microteaching	Practice teaching clinical and leadership skills
	Live or videotaped practice with peer critique
Practice exercises	Using orientation checklists
	Teaching clinical and leadership skills
	Developing/negotiating learning contracts
	Counseling orientees
	Documenting orientee's progress
Reflection	How it feels to be "new"
	How it feels to be a new graduate
	How it feels to receive negative feedback
Role-playing	Giving orientees feedback on performance
	Managing conflicts, problems
Small group exercises	Pairs or triads practice each phase of educator role component
Written simulations	Case studies to practice leadership skills
Values clarification	Values of new graduates vs. experienced nurses
	Dealing with perspectives different from your own

*See references 11, 67, 92, 110, 114.

Supporting Preceptors

Support for preceptors needs to emanate from two sources: educational and administrative. In addition, preceptor support needs to be provided before, during, and after completion of each preceptorship program.

BEFORE THE PRECEPTORSHIP The best way for educators to support preceptors before their serving in this capacity is to provide prospective preceptors with an effective preceptor training program that prepares them for the duties and responsibilities that will be expected of them. In the PTP, preceptors should be afforded an opportunity not only to learn about but to experience and practice all major facets of their role.

Administrative support for preceptors before the preceptorship begins is required in two areas: financial support for the PTP and provision of a written position description for the preceptor role. Financial support for the PTP entails payment of salary and benefits to the educator who provides the program as well as to those who participate. In addition, financial support involves the cost of staffing coverage while preceptors are off their units. Some hospitals have found it more cost-effective to collaborate with other healthcare facilities in the area to regionalize the provision of preceptor preparation.[142] Preceptors need a written job description so that their duties, functions, and responsibilities and their obligations to the unit, to the orientee, and to patients, as well as their reporting mechanisms and relationships to others involved with orientation, are clarified.

Preceptors can also be supported before the preceptorship by nurse managers who share with them information about the orientee with whom they will be working. For example, the nurse manager might share the orientee's resumé and interview findings to give the preceptor a full and clear picture of the orientee's previous work history and clinical experiences, reasons for selecting that hospital as an employer, and personal and professional goals. If the orientee has already completed a self-assessment related to the performance expectations for staff nurses on a specific unit, this information could also be shared so that the preceptor may gain a clearer impression of the orientee's potential strengths and weaknesses. The nurse manager might also relate any other personal impressions that were gained from interviewing the orientee.

DURING THE PRECEPTORSHIP Staff development needs to maintain close contact with preceptors during the preceptorship to answer any questions that may arise, to troubleshoot any problems related to instruction, and to monitor the effectiveness and progress of the program. Since preceptor training programs are typically of limited duration (1 to 2 days or about 8 hours), they cannot realistically cover the entire scope of phenomena a preceptor might encounter. As a result, preceptors may require additional assistance in identifying or implementing strategies to perform any of their three role components. One may need help in supporting the orientee through the stages of reality shock, another may need guidance in selecting some audiovisual aids, and one may need additional suggestions on how to teach clinical skills. This type of immediate support should be readily available to preceptors on an ongoing basis and should be no more than a telephone or beeper call away. In addition, the educator may offer preceptors a set of guidelines consisting of suggested "do's and don'ts" while precepting (Box 6.14).

The nurse manager of each unit can support preceptors in numerous ways. A summary of this support is provided in Box 6.15. Obviously, from this enumeration, the nurse manager's support of the preceptor is of central importance to the success of any preceptorship program.

After the Preceptorship   Continued educational support for preceptors may exist in one or two forms: continuing education programs at more advanced levels of instruction and ongoing support groups. Some hospitals recognize the preceptors' persisting learning needs by offering both basic and advanced preceptor training programs.[103] The former concentrates on fundamentals necessary to function as a preceptor, and the latter concentrates on extensions of these. For example, all preceptors at a particular hospital may have regularly scheduled programs that cover more advanced topics such as:

- Matching teaching styles with orientee cognitive styles
- Matching teaching styles with orientee learning styles
- Matching preceptor and orientee personality styles[29]
- Adjusting teaching strategies for each level in Benner's novice-to-expert model[21]
- Managing conflict in the preceptor-orientee working relationship
- Solving orientee learning problems
- Developing creative clinical teaching strategies
- Handling interpersonal problems with preceptorships

A second form of continued educational support is the provision of ongoing preceptor support groups. In these groups, preceptors from all clinical areas may meet jointly on a monthly, quarterly, or semiannual basis to obtain assistance from educators, administrators, or others (clinical nurse specialists or psychiatric liaison nurses) to informally share their experiences; discuss problems, issues, and successes related to precepting; offer suggestions; and exchange points of view with each another. These regularly scheduled meetings can be instructive as well as highly satisfying in affording preceptors the organizational support they need to remain motivated and effective in their role.[95,118] The group may also be able to offer input into hospital policies, procedures, and the position description for preceptors.

Box 6.14

Preceptor Do's and Don'ts

Do

- Put yourself in the orientee's shoes; remember what it was like to be new
- Relate to the orientee as a colleague
- Get to know the orientee as an individual
- Elicit the orientee's perceived strengths and weaknesses
- Determine the orientee's preferences regarding the order and type of learning experiences
- Make every effort to help the orientee feel welcomed and accepted
- Respect the orientee's views, feelings, and values
- Prepare orientees for learning experiences and then proceed gradually at their pace
- Maintain the orientee's trust and confidence
- Offer feedback immediately after performance and at regularly scheduled times
- Be available when the orientee needs you
- Allow orientees to make and learn from mistakes (as long as patients are not harmed)
- Listen and learn from orientees
- Maintain your composure even during stressful situations when it would be easier to do it yourself
- Use learning contract terms to manage timely completion of the orientation program
- Keep your sense of humor and use it often to keep things in perspective
- Be generous in providing praise, support, and encouragement
- Be constructive and gentle with critiques
- Activate your educational and administrative support systems whenever necessary

Don't

- Relate to orientees as if they were student nurses
- Intimidate or be intimidated by orientees
- Overwhelm orientees with details
- Overwhelm orientees with situations beyond their capabilities to manage
- Do for orientees, except in emergencies
- Criticize the hospital, management, or other staff
- Over- or underestimate an orientee's abilities; verify these
- Assume that experienced orientees need little support or instruction
- Be unrealistic regarding expectations of orientees
- Embarrass the orientee in front of patients, family, or other staff
- Make the orientee feel unduly pressured or hurried
- Discourage questions from orientees
- Hesitate to give constructive criticisms of orientees' performance
- Use negative feedback to correct orientee performance
- Keep orientees in the dark regarding their performance and progress
- Hesitate to use your support systems
- Forget how important you are to the success of the orientation program

---

Box 6.15

NURSE MANAGER SUPPORT FOR PRECEPTORS DURING THE PRECEPTORSHIP
PROGRAM

- Ensure that staffing is adequate to enable preceptors to provide instruction to their orientee
- Schedule entry of new staff only when preceptor is available
- Ensure that preceptors are relieved of some of their normal work load so they will be available when orientees need their assistance
- Ensure that preceptors are not assigned other responsibilities (charge nurse, team leader, committees) that preclude their availability to orientees
- Plan patient assignments carefully to ensure the best possible matching of preceptors with orientees
- Encourage other staff to support preceptors on their unit
- Provide a sufficient amount of time for preceptors to help orientees complete orientation requirements
- Provide teaching aids (such as reference books, journals, self-study programs, audiovisual programs)
- Keep informed about how the preceptor-orientee relationship is working
- Allow time away from patient care for the preceptor to meet with and counsel the orientee
- Match the work schedules of preceptors and orientees
- Use the preceptor's appraisal of the orientee's progress as a primary means for determining completion of orientation
- Provide incentives for precepting orientees

Ongoing administrative support for preceptors is necessary in a number of areas. Paid release time for attendance at continuing education or support group meetings reflects recognition of preceptors' needs for continued professional development. Because precepting can be a stressful and exhausting activity, staff nurses who serve in this capacity need some intermittent relief from these additional responsibilities to avoid burnout,[59] fatigue, and diminished effectiveness. Assignment of preceptors, therefore, should include planned intervals during which the nurse may return to regular patient care duties and renew working relationships with peers. At times, the nurse manager may also provide temporary relief from the preceptor role by assigning an alternate or secondary preceptor to the orientee for a few days if some problem for the primary preceptor (such as a sick child at home) arises or if the preceptor just needs a break from the additional clinical burden. Nurse managers may also need to work with the educator to resolve any significant problems that may develop during the orientation process between the orientee and the preceptor.

Another avenue of administrative support for preceptors is the provision of some means of recognizing and rewarding preceptors for the added services they provide to the hospital. Although healthcare institutions depend on and derive much benefit from the time, efforts, and expertise of nurse preceptors, many give little or no overt recognition to reward preceptors for those contributions. A recent informal survey of nurse preceptors in critical care revealed that among the 351 nurses who participated in the survey, 62% received no rewards, incentives, or recognition for serving as preceptors.[10]

Some of the recognitions and rewards that might be afforded to preceptors are identified in Box 6.16. Incentives such as these acknowledge the contributions that preceptors make to the hospital and reflect organizational commitment to the preceptorship program as well as to those whose role is most instrumental in its success. Administrative support for preceptors is embodied in the "Preceptor's Bill of Rights" enumerated in Box 6.17.

PREPARING INSTRUCTIONAL SCHEDULES

Class schedules are most likely to be used at both the hospital and nursing department levels of orientation because instructional content and its presentation and evaluation at these levels are virtually universal for all learners and because larger groups of participants usually need to be accommodated. Instructors at both hospital and nursing department levels of orientation often need to manage the timing and use of faculty from multiple hospital departments and need to reserve facilities large enough for the anticipated audience well in advance to ensure that these facilities are available when new staff arrive at the hospital. Institutions that have a divisional level of orientation may also follow an established schedule if resources would be strained by the format(s) selected for the program. Program schedules are least likely to be employed at the unit level of orientation where maximal flexibility and individualization of the learning process are desired.

Box 6.16

POSSIBLE REWARDS/INCENTIVES FOR PRECEPTORS*

MONETARY
Base pay increase
Preceptor pay differential

EDUCATIONAL
Increased tuition assistance
Paid attendance at continuing education programs
Additional educational leave
Nursing reference book of choice

CAREER
Clinical ladder advancement

SOCIAL
Recognition at staff meetings
Luncheons, teas, dinners in preceptors' honor

OTHER
Letter of commendation in personnel file
Certificate of appreciation
Special name tag
Honorary title
Scheduling preference
Reduced floating assignments
Picture and recognition article in hospital newspaper

*Modified from references 10, 67, 86.

Box 6.17

THE PRECEPTOR'S BILL OF RIGHTS

PRECEPTORS HAVE A RIGHT TO:
1. A clear definition of their role
2. A clearly stated set of expectations for their performance
3. A clear delineation of their responsibilities to the preceptee
4. A clear distinction of their responsibilities in relation to others who are involved in the orientation process
5. A clear enumeration of all expected outcomes for the staff nurse orientation program
6. Valid and reliable evaluation tools to appraise preceptee performance
7. The resources necessary to fulfill their role responsibilities
8. Continuing and responsive support systems for fulfillment of their role responsibilities
9. Adequate preparation for integration of the preceptor role
10. Adequate training in the knowledge, skills, and attitudes necessary to fulfill their role responsibilities

From Alspach JG: The preceptor's bill of rights, *Crit Care Nurse* 7(1):1, 1987.

When a competency-based approach is used for orientation, every attempt is made to allow the orientee to determine the order in which learning experiences will occur. If a preceptorship format is selected for the orientation program, planning of learning experiences is negotiated between the orientee and preceptor with maximal consideration for the orientee's preferences.

New graduate orientees will often appreciate some guidance from their preceptor on how to best proceed with learning activities, but more experienced nurse orientees may have definite opinions in this regard. Whenever possible, competency-based orientation programs recognize and respond to these preferences so that orientees can schedule their own order of learning activities.

PROGRAM IMPLEMENTATION

The implementation phase of an orientation program proceeds as an outgrowth of the planning phase. Once all elements of the curriculum have been planned and faculty have been selected and prepared for their responsibilities, the orientation program may commence.

If you recall from Chapter 4, program implementation

is guided along its course by various sets of fundamental principles that reflect how teachers and learners interact most effectively. Thus the incorporation and application of the principles of teaching and learning and principles of adult education should be readily apparent in the implementation of an orientation program. In addition, the interactions between instructors and orientees can often be maximized when the principles related to cognitive styles, learning style preferences, and teaching style preferences are acknowledged and applied. The next section of this chapter will address these two areas. Following this, the selection of teaching methods for orientation programs will be considered, and special considerations for implementing both preceptorships and orientation programs for selected groups of orientees will be addressed.

GUIDING PRINCIPLES

Chapter 4 described each of the guiding principles related to teaching, learning, and adult education in some detail and explained their implications for nurse educators. The sections that follow provide the educator with some examples of how those principles might be incorporated and applied in a nursing orientation program.

Principles of Teaching and Learning

Chapter 4 identified 14 principles of teaching and learning that afford the educator direction for program implementation. Box 6.18 lists some ways in which each of these principles might be employed in implementing a nursing orientation program.

Principles of Adult Education

The ten principles of adult education described in Chapter 4 need to be made operational when an orientation program is implemented. Box 6.19 offers some examples of how the educator might apply each of the adult education principles in an orientation program.

Principles Related to Instructional Styles

The three sets of principles related to instructional styles (cognitive style, learning style preferences, and teaching style preferences) can be very useful to the educator during the implementation phase of an orientation program in at least three ways: (1) they remind the educator of important differences that may exist among orientees, (2) they represent a means to diagnose learning problems that may arise during the orientation process, and (3) they offer direction on ways to manage and resolve obstacles to effective instruction. Taken together, these three sets of considerations enable the educator and preceptor to better ensure that the process of orientation proceeds smoothly and effectively to its established ends.

Cognitive Styles

As you will recall from Chapter 4, cognitive style refers to an individual's customary or predominant way of acquiring, perceiving, organizing, and using information. Field-independent (FI) learners tend to acquire learning analytically by assimilating details into overall principles and concepts. FI orientees, therefore, will generally prefer hands-on approaches to learning that afford them an opportunity to learn theories, principles, and concepts by experimenting with these firsthand and on their own. FI orientees can be a fiercely self-directed group; they prefer to figure things out for themselves and on their own schedule. They won't appreciate an instructor hovering over their shoulder or anyone rushing them through a learning experience. Because they tend to prefer solitary and self-directed activities, FI orientees may resist or withdraw from group learning experiences that require collaboration and extensive interactions for consensus. FI orientees can also be expected to enjoy learning the details of technical tasks and procedures related to patient care.

Field-dependent (FD) orientees, by contrast, may get lost in the steps and details of procedures and encounter greater difficulty in reaching conclusions that require analysis of large volumes of clinical assessment data. These orientees tend to approach learning via its global or "big picture" features and experience difficulty recalling specifics. Because FD orientees are very sociable, holistic, and context-oriented, they may be more sensitive and therapeutic with families and more attentive to the psychosocial, ethical, and discharge-oriented aspects of patient care than their FI colleagues. FD orientees are often more passive as learners, prefer group teaching methods with lots of discussion, and feel more secure if their preceptor remains at their side. In extreme cases, FI orientees may tend to focus almost exclusively on patients' physiologic needs and the procedures and tasks that need to be accomplished, whereas FD orientees may get so involved with holistic aspects of care that the technical requirements never get completed by the end of their shift. FI orientees may tend to be independent prematurely, while FD orientees may be difficult to wean from their preceptors. If the educator and preceptor can recognize the differences between these two types of learners, potential pitfalls can be avoided or remedied quickly.

Learning Style Preferences

Learning style refers to one's preferred way of learning. It includes preferences related to a wide array of attributes: sensory route (seeing, listening, doing, etc.), instructor guidance (little or a lot), social aspects (individual vs. group work), degree of structure (highly structured or relatively unstructured), environmental noise (silence or music), time of day (morning vs. night person), and the like.

As discussed in Chapter 4, a number of different learning style preference tools are available for identifying one's

---

Box 6.18

APPLICATION OF TEACHING-LEARNING PRINCIPLES IN AN ORIENTATION PROGRAM

Learning is a self-activity of the learner

- At the commencement of orientation, have each orientee complete a self-assessment of their learning needs in relation to the expected outcomes for the orientation program
- Incorporate self-learning packages for instruction
- Manage the orientation program via learning contract terms established by the orientee

Learning is intentional

- Suggest that all orientees keep a pocket notebook to jot down questions or problems they experience as learning needs during their clinical time on the units so these can be used to focus their learning efforts with the preceptor
- Ask orientees to distinguish their personal goals for each week of the orientation
- Make every effort to achieve personal goals of orientee above and beyond the expectations for the orientation program

Learning is an active and interactive process

- Engage orientees in every phase of the educational process by having them take responsibility for developing the terms in their learning contracts
- Use teaching methods that involve active learner participation: interactive videodisc for learning history-taking, practice labs and mannequins for clinical skills, role plays for developing leadership skills, hands-on use of equipment and supplies, etc.
- Minimize the extensive or exclusive use of passive teaching methods such as reading or listening to audio tapes

Learning is a unitary process

- Create a learning environment for the orientee that minimizes stress and maximizes opportunities for success
- Plan patient assignments for orientees that are appropriate for their experience and ability to manage
- When an orientee's progress wanes, determine whether health or personal/family problems at home are affecting performance

Learning is influenced by the motivation of the learner

- Ask orientees why they decided to work at your hospital and on your unit, what their short- and long-term career goals are
- Before providing instruction to orientees who are new graduates, point out why instruction is important and how it will be useful in patient care
- Ask orientees to keep a record of any situations that make them feel unsure, inadequate, or uncomfortable so that these may be used to focus learning
- At the start of each clinical day, find out what the orientee most wants to accomplish that day

Learning is influenced by the readiness of the learner

- Use the orientee's self-evaluation to estimate readiness for learning various segments in the orientation program
- Verify your learning readiness estimate with the orientee before proceeding to plan learning experiences
- Heighten the orientee's learning readiness by posing thought-provoking questions or situations that the orientee needs to resolve
- Solicit the orientee's perceptions of what he/she feels ready to learn next, and monitor clinical performance for any areas where learning needs become apparent

Learning is social

- Relate to orientees as a trusted and supportive colleague whom they can depend on
- Maintain a sense of humor and enthusiasm for precepting
- Make every effort to help the orientee feel accepted and welcomed on the unit
- Early in the preceptorship, get to know the orientee as an individual; use breaks and meal times to relate to the orientee as a person

---

learning style. Some healthcare agencies have orientees complete one of these tools at the beginning of orientation to determine their learning style preference and then use this information for planning and providing subsequent instruction. Hospitals that use substantial amounts of self-directed learning in their orientation program and that offer a variety of learning options to orientees can maximize their responsiveness to this important feature of program implementation. On the other hand, healthcare agencies that employ self-directed learning more sparingly and/or that have fewer learning options to offer may find that their responsiveness to this aspect of learning is largely limited to two major areas: (1) implementing instruction that incorporates a wide variety of different types of learning ac-

tivities (reaching the widest possible range of learning style preferences and exposing orientees to new learning experiences) and (2) using their understanding of learning style preferences primarily for identifying and solving specific learning problems with individual orientees. An example of the latter might exist at a hospital that uses the Kolb Learning Style Inventory described in Chapter 4. In this situation, the preceptor, who has a "converger" learning style, teaches in much the same way that she prefers to learn: by "diving right in" to actual clinical situations that are encountered on the unit and requiring the orientee to perform at that moment. The orientee, who has an "assimilator" learning style, feels terrorized by these situations and dreads every day of the preceptorship. As an assimi-

Box 6.18

APPLICATION OF TEACHING-LEARNING PRINCIPLES IN AN ORIENTATION PROGRAM—cont'd

Learning is influenced by the learning environment

- In classroom settings, verify that all orientees can see and hear the instructor and any audiovisuals used; arrange room seating to facilitate communication with orientees; create an open and accepting climate for questions and solution of problems
- In laboratory settings, assure the orientees that it is all right to make mistakes in the lab and to practice as much as necessary to refine their skills
- In the clinical setting, minimize distractions (other staff, conversations, extraneous noise or equipment) that may interfere with learning; use a calm and relaxed manner for teaching; put the orientee at ease and provide instruction or practice that respects the orientee's status in front of patients, families, and other staff

Learning proceeds best when it is organized and clearly communicated

- With inexperienced nurses, learning in the clinical setting may be facilitated by first organizing it around gradually gaining proficiency in daily routines so that the overall patient care process can be mastered
- Remember that as adult learners, orientees will find it helpful if learning experiences can be organized around patient care problems, issues, and challenges they will encounter
- As a general rule, orientees can learn more effectively if a few general principles rather than a profusion of details can be used to explain phenomena; excessive amounts of information can easily overwhelm and confuse the novice nurse

Learning is facilitated by positive and immediate feedback

- Plan each day to include some experiences of success for the orientee in order to capitalize on the huge motivational value of success
- Even when you need to correct an orientee's faulty performance, do so in a supportive and constructive manner that clarifies rather than criticizes
- Meet frequently with the orientee to offer feedback on performance; avoid "dropping a bomb" long after or at the end of an extended period of subpar performance

Retention and transfer of learning can be facilitated

- Plan at least a brief period each day to meet with the orientee to review the day's experiences and what was learned
- Plan patient assignments for the orientee that build on and extend prior clinical experiences; identify and reinforce how nursing care was similar or dissimilar for each case

- Assist the orientee with integrating and applying classroom and laboratory learning experiences to the clinical setting by comparing and contrasting the "ideal" with the "real"
- When time allows, gradually relocate the learning setting from classroom (for theory, facts, principles) to laboratory (for familiarization and practice) to the clinical area (for refinement)

Learning is creative

- Teach orientees how to reflect on patient care experiences as a source of professional growth and development
- At specific intervals during the orientation program (weekly or monthly, depending on duration), ask orientees how their experiences have shaped their impressions and understanding

Learning is inferred rather than observed

- Remind new graduates that the way orientation differs from nursing school is in its emphasis on clinical performance rather than classroom performance
- Even with experienced orientees, never assume that prior experience equates with current competence; it is always necessary to validate the orientee's clinical performance to ensure that it matches your agency's expectations
- When using newly developed or recently revised evaluation tools, be sure that problems with orientee evaluations are not attributable to some weakness or fault in the evaluation tool or evaluation procedure

Learning is influenced by the nature and variability of the learning experience

- When planning learning activities for an orientation program, avoid prolonged classroom lecture sessions; even if blocks of classroom time are necessary, vary the type of learning experiences and teaching methods to maintain learner interest
- Whenever possible, allow orientees time in a protected area to gradually develop proficiency in clinical skills and use of equipment
- Provide orientees with an opportunity to give feedback on how effective different types of learning activities were

lator, the orientee would much prefer to read some articles or watch a video about the procedure first, then practice it on her own to understand it more fully, and then, when she was ready, perform the procedure on an actual patient. If one knew beforehand that this preceptor and orientee had contrasting learning style preferences, their mismatching could have been averted or, when problems such as these arose, they could be managed by pairing the orientee with a preceptor who has a similar learning style preference. Another possibility is that the educator who identifies

---

Box 6.19

APPLICATION OF ADULT EDUCATION PRINCIPLES IN AN ORIENTATION PROGRAM

Adults represent a heterogeneous group of learners who command the respect that is due to them as mature individuals

- Although the hospital and nursing department levels of orientation may, of necessity, relate to large numbers of orientees as more-or-less homogenous groups, plan ways to get to know orientees as individuals at the division and unit levels of orientation
- Always relate to orientees as adults rather than as students
- Enlist the assistance of more experienced orientees in teaching their less experienced colleagues

Adult learners often have multiple responsibilities for children, spouses, homes, career, and civic obligation; adults place a high value on their time

- Determine the demographic profile of your orientees
- Minimize the use of rigid time schedules for learning experiences if these often interfere with completion of orientation programs
- Consider the increased use of self-paced and self-directed learning methods that orientees can use at the time, place, and frequency they prefer
- Design challenge mechanisms that enable orientees to complete orientation expeditiously; don't waste their time by requiring them to endure learning experiences they do not need

Adults enter learning situations with a large reservoir of life and work experiences; they value highly both their own experiences and that of others

- Design learning activities based on case studies developed from orientees' actual experiences in patient care

- With new graduate orientees, have them draw upon past life or student experiences for comparison with their present work experiences
- Tap the past nursing experience of more seasoned orientees in group discussion, patient care conferences, and other types of learning activities

Adults may be less flexible as learners

- Expect orientees (especially experienced nurses) to question or challenge you or your institution's procedures and practices when these differ from their own
- Expect orientees to initially resist teaching methods that are unfamiliar to them
- For orientees who may seem very resistant about trying new types of learning experiences, try to give them special attention, support, and as much discretion as possible.

Many adults have had negative past experiences as learners that evoke feelings of inadequacy, fear of failure, and diminished self-confidence in learning situations

- Avoid the use of unannounced evaluations such as written or verbal quizzes during orientation programs; these may make orientees feel like students again
- Give orientees patient assignments that are within their present capabilities to manage; increase the difficulty of assignments as gradually as possible
- Inject as much fun and games into classroom and laboratory learning experiences as possible
- Be there when orientees need your assistance or reassurance
- Prime orientees for success by preparing them for their responsibilities in any given situation

---

the source of this incompatibility could suggest to the preceptor that his/her teaching style be modified to be sensitive to the preferences of orientees who are the assimilator type of learners. In either case, an appreciation of the notion of differences in learning style preferences among orientees and preceptors can be very helpful in maintaining and enhancing the effectiveness of the preceptor-orientee relationship.

Teaching Style Preferences

An instructor's preferred or customary way of teaching is, as has been mentioned, heavily influenced by his/her past experiences as a learner and by his/her own cognitive and learning style preferences. During the implementation of an orientation program, the most important considerations related to teaching style include the need to:

- Be cognizant of your usual ways of providing instruction to orientees

- Distinguish situations when your teaching style seems to be effective for most orientees and other situations where it seems less effective (e.g., hands-on learning may be very effective for teaching technical or procedural skills but may not be effective for teaching managerial skills or crisis intervention)
- Ascertain your orientee's learning style preference and cognitive style (inquire or look for behavioral clues if your hospital does not use published instruments)
- Determine, when you encounter teaching-learning problems during the orientation program, whether these could be attributable to a mismatching of teaching and learning styles; if so, either modify your teaching style to better match the orientee or secure the assistance of an alternate preceptor (even temporarily) to better match the orientee's learning style preference

The concept of matching teaching and learning styles offers much intuitive appeal, whether it is employed for matching preceptors and orientees or for recognizing and

Box 6.19

APPLICATION OF ADULT EDUCATION PRINCIPLES IN AN ORIENTATION PROGRAM—cont'd

Adults are usually voluntary learners who engage in learning activities for a variety of personal and professional reasons

- Minimize the "mandatories" in orientation programs by requiring only those learning activities that the orientee truly needs
- Ask orientees what their career goals are
- If orientees appear to find ways to avoid participating in certain types of learning experiences, determine whether this is attributable to legitimate reasons or represents a behavioral message that some problem exists with that learning activity

Adults are problem-centered learners who engage in learning activities with the intention of immediately applying what they learn to solve problems in their present roles and responsibilities

- If at all possible, allow orientees time to experience selected clinical situations before providing instruction in those areas
- Allow time for orientees to identify and get help solving problems they perceive as important and pressing
- If orientees are unable to appreciate the relevance of some areas of instruction, precede teaching by raising questions and issues that highlight problem areas

Adults work best with instructors who relate to them as knowledgeable colleagues, who help them learn, and who are subject to the same shortcomings as they are

- Be yourself and have a sense of humor when working with orientees
- Admit mistakes and share stories about some of these with orientees
- Place as much trust and confidence in orientees' judgment and actions as possible and convey this as often as possible

Most adults are self-directed in their learning

- Give orientees as much freedom as possible to manage their own orientation
- Using learning contracts, help more dependent orientees learn how to gradually assume more responsibility for their own learning
- Plan tentative time frames for orientees to progressively "wean" themselves from preceptor assistance and support

Some adult learners may be older and have a slower learning speed than their younger counterparts

- Be sure that the demographic profile of orientees includes identification of second career nurses and those beyond traditional new graduate age
- Incorporate at least some self-directed learning methods so learners can pace their own learning activities
- Avoid scheduling extended learning periods at the end of work days when orientees may be tired
- As a general rule, learning a few important things well is preferable to learning many things poorly

---

solving problems that may arise in their working relationship. Carroll[29] extends this application to the more enveloping notion of matching preceptor and orientee personality styles with much the same result. Although perfect and complete matches of preceptors and orientees are not often feasible or perhaps always desirable, the premise underlying this matchup has great validity and usefulness for orientation programs because of the pivotal nature of this relationship to the success of the orientation endeavor.

TEACHING METHODS

The teaching methods used in an orientation program can include any of those described in Chapter 4. The exact nature and number of methods used can be made on the basis of the eight factors that influence selection of teaching methods for any staff development program. The educator may also find it useful to experiment with at least one new teaching method for each orientation program to test its acceptance and effectiveness.

When a competency-based approach is used for the orientation program, a few overriding considerations need to be made. These considerations include the following:

- A CBO approach does not prescribe what teaching methods must be used; educators may employ any instructional strategy that is appropriate for the learning to be attained
- Because CBO approaches primarily emphasize outcomes related to clinical rather than cognitive performance, they typically employ relatively less emphasis on teaching methods aimed at information giving
- Although competency-based orientations have limited reliance on lectures, they do not preclude their use when large groups of orientees need to be provided

with the facts and principles that underlie clinical practice

- Because CBO programs emphasize clinical performance outcomes, they typically include greater use of laboratory and clinical teaching methods that enable orientees to practice and perfect clinical performance
- Because CBO programs reveal outcome expectations and do not mandate how learners must acquire instruction, they enable educators to incorporate as much self-directed teaching as resources permit
- Because CBO approaches do not require all orientees to use the same teaching methods, a variety of learning options may be made available to orientees
- Because CBO approaches make use of challenge mechanisms, some orientees may be able to complete orientation with little or no instruction
- When a CBO approach is used, educators need to review these points with preceptors during the preceptor training program

Beyond these considerations, the selection and employment of teaching methods during implementation of an orientation program is the same as for any other type of staff development program. Since preceptors will bear a substantial amount of the instructional responsibility in an orientation program, the educator needs to ensure that the preceptor training program prepares preceptors for their teaching responsibilities and that educators remain available to preceptors throughout the preceptorship to provide ongoing support and assistance. Continuing education programs for preceptors might include additional practice in using various teaching methods and introducing preceptors to new teaching methods for future use.

IMPLEMENTING PRECEPTORSHIPS: ROLES AND RESPONSIBILITIES

At smaller hospitals preceptors may be vested with virtually all responsibility for orienting the new nurse. At larger institutions, however, a number of nursing staff members may share this function with the preceptor. When the responsibility of orienting the new staff nurse is shared, it may be helpful to distinguish who is responsible for which aspects of orientation so that each individual understands the scope of responsibility and misunderstandings and potential conflicts are avoided. Table 6.5 outlines one way that these responsibilities might be divided.

TAILORING ORIENTATION PROGRAMS

As mentioned earlier in this chapter, staff nurse orientees may make up a very heterogeneous group of learners. At least five subgroups may be identifiable among the orientees and warrant special considerations when staff nurse orientation programs are implemented. Two of these subgroups consist of orientees from opposite ends of the staff

nurse experience continuum—that is, newly graduated nurses with no nursing experience and orientees with considerable staff nursing experience. Other subgroups that merit special attention include nurses being cross-trained (oriented to work on a unit with patients different from those on their customary unit), agency nurses, and nurses from foreign countries. The discussion that follows will present some considerations for each of these special subgroups of orientees.

New Graduate Nurses

At least three areas should be considered in relation to the orientation of newly graduated nurses. These include the new graduate nurse's (GN's) socialization, development of role identity, and development of clinical practice skills.

Socialization

In the earlier discussion related to preceptor training programs, one of the responsibilities identified for preceptors was to help the orientee feel welcomed and accepted as a member of the unit and department nursing staff, as a member of the healthcare team, and as an employee of the healthcare institution. In addition to introducing the new graduate to coworkers, the orientation program can facilitate the GN's entry into each of these social work groups by explaining both the formal and informal mechanisms of communication and operation, by revealing formal as well as informal working relationships, and by fostering an atmosphere of camaraderie and team work. Socialization of the new graduate also encompasses supporting and respecting the GN's abilities, recognizing the GN's progress, and enhancing the GN's self-confidence as a contributor to the healthcare team. Rather than feeling like outsiders or stumbling ex-students, new graduates can then experience a true sense of belonging among their peers. Needs for belonging can easily be overlooked in the torrent of new knowledge and skills the GN must acquire. Sometimes it is useful to remember that in Maslow's hierarchy of human needs,[90] only physiologic and safety needs are more important to meet than the need for belonging.

Development of Staff Nurse Role Identity

The plight of the new graduate nurse's need to develop role identity has been, perhaps, most clearly articulated in Kramer's work[80] on reality shock in nursing. In examining the reasons why nurses leave their profession, Kramer explored the cultural and professional conflicts that arise when the value system developed by the student nurse while in school conflicts with the value system that exists among nurses and other healthcare workers in the hospital bureaucracy. The transition from the identity of the student role to that of the staff nurse role depends on successful passage of the GN through the four phases of reality shock

TABLE 6.5 • DIVISION OF RESPONSIBILITY FOR UNIT ORIENTATION

Program Phase	Orientee	Preceptor	Nurse Manager	Nurse Educator	Clinical Specialist
Assessment	Completes all employment application forms Completes self-assessment related to outcomes of CBO program Relates strengths, weaknesses, short- and long-term career goals Meets with preceptor to identify educational needs Works with preceptor to determine priority of learning needs	Reviews information about orientee's past experience and self-assessment related to the CBO program Estimates orientee's current capabilities as a staff nurse Meets with the orientee to confirm strengths, weakness, and educational needs Assists orientee in developing initial learning contract based on priority of learning needs and orientee's preferred order of accomplishment Completes initial assessment of orientee's learning needs using direct observation of clinical performance Provides ongoing assessment of learning needs yet to be attained Documents learning needs assessment of orientee	Interviews and hires new nursing staff Determines work history and nursing experience Has interviewee complete self-assessment related to CBO outcomes Reviews all employment application information and self-assessment; verifies references Communicates relevant information about new hires to preceptor, educator, and clinical nurse specialist (CNS) Collaborates with above staff in making preceptor assignment Assigns preceptor to orientee based on best possible matching with orientee needs	Reviews information about the orientee's past experience and self-assessment related to the CBO program Administers any style inventories (if applicable) and communicates results to nurse manager Administers written tests and communicates results to nurse manager Collaborates with nurse manager in preceptor assignment Explains general plan for orientation to preceptor and orientee: expectations, time frames, staff involved, support systems available, use of learning contracts Monitors quality and effectiveness of learning needs assessment phase Lends support to the preceptor as requested or required	If unit-based, may review information on new nursing staff and participate in decision on preceptor assignment May be asked to provide selected aspects in clinical assessment of orientee and/or to verify selected areas of learning needs assessment Observes orientee's performance and shares observations with preceptor and/or nurse manager, as appropriate Lends clinical practice support to preceptor and educator related to assessment of orientee's needs
Planning	Identifies preferred order in which learning needs are to be attained Relates preferences among available instructional options Works with preceptor to develop initial and ongoing learning contracts to meet all outcomes of the CBO within the time frames specified	Meets with orientee initially to describe use of learning contracts Establishes a time frame (e.g., weekly) for planning or updating/revising learning contracts so that all outcomes are attained within an established time limit Works with orientee to mutually plan how outcomes for CBO will be achieved Counsels orientee	Supervises and keeps up to date on learning plan developed for orientee Reviews learning contracts on a regular basis to determine orientee progress Schedules orientee and preceptor to the same working hours Provides adequate time and resources for the CBO program	May assist orientee and/or preceptor in designing effective learning contract terms Reviews learning contracts on a regular basis to determine their educational soundness, feasibility, and appropriateness Communicates to the orientee instructional options currently available Assists the orientee and/or preceptor with any problems of an	Notifies preceptor of clinical situations that represent good learning opportunities for the orientee Collaborates with nurse manager and educator to schedule unit events so that orientees may avail themselves of learning experiences that arise on the unit Assists the orientee and/or preceptor with any clinical practice problems that may

Continued.

TABLE 6.5 • DIVISION OF RESPONSIBILITY FOR UNIT ORIENTATION—cont'd

Program Phase	Orientee	Preceptor	Nurse Manager	Nurse Educator	Clinical Specialist
		on need to adjust learning plan, when warranted Plans appropriate learning activities with orientee		educational nature that may arise in planning learning activities	arise in planning learning activities
Implementation	Attains all outcomes established for the CBO program according to the terms specified in the learning contracts Completes all learning activities required for achieving the CBO outcomes Seeks preceptor guidance commensurate with capabilities Gradually assumes increasing independence in staff nurse role	Functions as a role model and resource person Assists orientee's social integration into the unit and staff Provides clinical instruction in all areas not covered by the educator or CNS Applies principles of teaching, learning, and adult education in instruction Modifies instruction to meet orientee needs and/or to resolve learning problems Seeks assistance from nurse manager, educator, or CNS as warranted Communicates any perceived problems in relationship with orientee to the nurse manager Documents the orientee's attainment of CBO outcomes	Makes (or delegates) patient assignments that facilitate orientee meeting CBO outcomes Supervises effectiveness and progress of program completion Seeks feedback from orientee and preceptor regarding preceptorship Communicates problems with instructional support to educator Monitors effects of preceptorship on other staff and unit operations Provides resources and other forms of administrative support If circumstances warrant, schedules a second preceptor to temporarily provide support to the orientee	Provides instructional support as requested or warranted Makes instructional aids and materials accessible and available Monitors ongoing effectiveness and progress of each preceptor-orientee pair Communicates frequently with orientee and preceptor regarding their needs for support with any educational aspect of the program Communicates need for administrative support to the nurse manager Communicates need for clinical practice support to the CNS	May be asked to provide instruction in selected aspects of the program Provides clinical practice support to preceptor or educator Collaborates with nurse manager to support preceptorship among other unit staff and to minimize the program's disruptions to unit activities
Evaluation	Informs preceptor of when they are ready to be evaluated on specific competency areas Completes all necessary evaluations within the time frame specified for the program Evaluates own progress in relation to short-term	Uses established performance criteria to evaluate orientee's attainment of CBO outcomes Provides critique in a constructive and supportive manner Seeks assistance in evaluating orientee from nurse manager, educator, or	Keeps apprised of evaluation results on an ongoing basis Incorporates own observations and input from other staff nurses into appraisal of orientee Determines if orientation needs to be extended; if so,	Assists preceptor in evaluation of orientee's performance as requested Incorporates own observations on orientee performance and effectiveness of preceptor-orientee relationship into evaluations	May be asked to provide orientee evaluation in selected program areas Communicates own observation of orientee performance and input from other staff nurses to preceptor, nurse manager, and educator

			Nurse	**Nurse**	**Clinical**
Program Phase	**Orientee**	**Preceptor**	**Manager**	**Educator**	**Specialist**

TABLE 6.5 · DIVISION OF RESPONSIBILITY FOR UNIT ORIENTATION—cont'd

Program Phase	Orientee	Preceptor	Nurse Manager	Nurse Educator	Clinical Specialist
	goals and future needs for continuing education Provides an evaluation of the preceptor Completes an evaluation of the orientation program	CNS when appropriate Provides daily feedback and ongoing evaluation to orientee regarding performance Documents evaluations of orientee on all required forms Completes an evaluation of the preceptorship program	for how long; solicits assistance from educator and CNS as needed After consultation with preceptor and educator, decides when orientation has been completed Informs orientee when orientation is complete Evaluates the adequacy of administrative support for the orientation program; makes recommendations regarding future programs	Participates in decisions regarding extension of orientation program and meeting any educational problems that arise Monitors the validity, reliability, and usefulness of evaluation tools Evaluates the preceptor's performance Evaluates the overall effectiveness and efficiency of the orientation program; proposes revisions as indicated	May participate in decisions regarding extension of orientation and in resolving problems that may exist Reviews performance criteria used in evaluation to verify relevance and accuracy; communicates any concerns or suggestions to the nurse manager and educator

described in Table 6.6. If this transition in role identity from student to staff nurse is not effectively achieved, new graduates may become so disenchanted and disappointed with the reality of nursing that they may leave not only their employer but also their profession.

Orientation programs for new graduates must acknowledge and respond to the special needs of GNs for converting from the student to the staff nurse role identity.[26] Hospitals that employ more extensive orientation formats for GNs, such as internships, typically include concepts related to reality shock in the curriculum. Other agencies may provide this support as a separate offering (e.g., in a biculturalism training program) after or in the latter portion of the GN orientation program. If this support is provided separately, it is often scheduled some weeks to months following the start of employment so that the GN has already passed the honeymoon period and has begun to encounter elements of the shock stage. The rationale for this delay is that GNs will be able to relate to the concepts of reality shock and biculturalism more effectively if they have already experienced these conflicts between their expectations and the reality of nursing practice and have begun attempts to resolve these in their own minds. Specific suggestions on how to assist new graduates through each phase of reality shock are described elsewhere[11] and need to be included in the preceptor training program so that all preceptors who work with GNs are familiar with them.

Development of Clinical Practice Skills

Two major considerations need to be kept in mind in relation to the development of clinical practice skills in new graduates. The first consideration focuses on the entry capabilities of the new graduate, and the second focuses on the strategies used to develop those capabilities.

ENTRY CAPABILITIES The GN with no nursing experience may be a graduate of any one of three basic nursing education programs: diploma, associate degree, or baccalaureate degree. These programs differ not only in their duration (2 to 4 years) but in their curriculum, in the types and numbers of learning experiences provided, and in the criteria established for successful program completion. As a result, the clinical capabilities of graduates from these programs may vary widely.

While all programs cover traditional clinical areas, such as medical-surgical care, maternal-child health, psychiatric mental health, and community health, some programs may afford limited (observational) or no learning experiences in specialty and subspecialty areas such as critical care,[13,30,71] operating room, or labor and delivery.[35] Some provide an extensive coverage of clinical skills but confine these to execution in the simulated setting of a learning laboratory rather than to performance with real patients. Other programs cover clinical practice expectations in a very general way with skill and procedure training limited to serendip-

TABLE 6.6 · KRAMER'S PHASES OF REALITY SHOCK	
Phase	**Description**
Honeymoon	New graduate nurse (GN) perceives work setting and coworkers in a positive and perhaps overly glowing light. GN focuses on developing mastery in skills and unit routines and on becoming acquainted with the organization and its staff
Shock	New graduates experience weaknesses, obstacles, and practices in the work setting and among coworkers that are inconsistent with their expectations and goals, resulting in anger, frustration, and disillusionment
Recovery	GN is able to perceive the realities of the work setting with a more balanced view of positive and negative aspects; GN gains a sense of perspective regarding expectations of real nursing practice
Resolution	GN resolves the perceived conflict between school and work values either by rejecting one set of values or the other, or (ideally) by integrating the positive aspects of each set of values into one set that is realistic for the work setting; the term *biculturalism* refers to this blending of school and work value systems.

From Kramer M: *Reality shock: why nurses leave nursing,* St. Louis, 1974, CV Mosby.

itous opportunities the student may encounter. Some afford students preparation in beginning acquisition of leadership and management skills, while others are devoted almost exclusively to direct patient care experiences. Because of the differences among basic nursing education programs, graduates enter hospital orientation programs with a wide divergence of clinical practice capabilities. These differences among GN orientees exist in addition to the differences described earlier in the staff nurse experience continuum. As a result, those who plan and provide orientation programs for new graduates need to bear in mind that even among GNs who have no prior experience in nursing, there can be significant differences in the clinical practice capabilities they bring to their first work site and significant differences in their readiness for practice in specialty areas of nursing. These differences among GNs can be accommodated more readily during the implementation phase if the orientation program enables the new graduate to demonstrate current capabilities and thereby challenge out of unnecessary instruction. In addition to conserving instructional resources, challenge mechanisms also allow the GN to experience success and progress sooner, enhancing self-confidence and socialization as a contributing member of the nursing staff. Traditional orientation programs that require all GNs to undergo instruction (whether they need it or not) preclude these events

and may needlessly delay the GN's development and contribution to patient care.

STRATEGIES TO DEVELOP CLINICAL PRACTICE SKILLS   Benner's novice-to-expert model[21] provides a useful framework for understanding the unique ways in which new nurses acquire and develop clinical practice skills. Using the Dreyfus model of skill acquisition as a basis for her model, Benner's first two stages of skill acquisition (novice and advanced beginner) distinguish how nurses begin this process.

Novice nurses have no background of experience with the clinical situation they encounter. As a result, novices must learn and follow a fairly rigid set of rules and attributes to function safely in that situation. *Rules* may include the principles and theories learned in school, in textbooks, and from instructors, as well as the policies and procedures taught in the hospital. *Attributes,* on the other hand, are context-free features that are measurable and objective and can be explained and learned without exposure to a real patient situation. For example, the novice can be taught to take and record vital signs, height, weight, and allergies for every patient admitted to the unit. In situations where the GN truly has no prior exposure, then, the preceptor needs to provide instruction that conveys these general rules and attributes so that these elements can be acquired as a basis for further skill development. Criticism of GNs for being very task-oriented, then, may be unjustified: novices are merely focused on the objective, measurable parameters of patient care that must be acquired before their clinical capabilities can progress to higher levels. Until these concrete aspects of care are mastered, the novice will be unable to view or respond to the wider array of variables and needs that patients may exhibit. Novices approach clinical situations and focus immediately on parts rather than wholes. Until they master the technical details of patient care, novices are unable to perceive more holistic features. Thus acquisition of general rules and attributes can gradually progress from concrete task execution (*Before giving a patient digitalis, always take the patient's apical pulse for a full 60 seconds*) to more complex rule systems (*If the apical pulse is less than 60 beats/minute, hold the digitalis and notify the physician. If the apical pulse is less than 50 beats/minute, check the patient for signs of inadequate tissue perfusion and digitalis toxicity and record a 12-lead ECG.*)

The rule-governed practice that typifies the novice nurse has limited usefulness and flexibility because rules do not tell novices which of the tasks to be completed are most important and do not indicate when an exception to the rule is warranted. As a result, novice nurses' lack of experience leaves them ill prepared for organizing their work loads based on relevance of patient care needs, for setting and modifying priorities of care, or for executing care that differs in some way from established procedures. Their lack of clinical experience precludes their ability to make appropriate judgments, to reach appropriate decisions, and to distinguish necessary alternatives in care. Without the benefit of prior experience in the situation, the novice lacks the context necessary for direction of behavior and is unable to exercise discretionary judgment.

Nurses who are *advanced beginners* can demonstrate marginally acceptable clinical performance. Advanced beginners have had a sufficient number of similar clinical experiences to enable them to master the rules and attributes of these situations and to derive from these recurrent meaningful components that are now integrated into their practice. In contrast to the measurable and context-free attributes that the novice depends on, advanced beginners draw on recurrent components (called *aspects*) to afford them direction. For example, after admitting 10 or 12 patients to the unit, the nurse eventually learns about the questions that patients frequently ask on admission, how different patients look at admission, how families react to the admission process, and patient needs that commonly exist at this time. Although some of these aspects could be made explicit to orientees (by the preceptor's suggestion to look for them), aspects are recognized and acted on primarily on the basis of the nurse's previous experience with patients in similar situations. These more global features of the patient situation enable the nurse to gradually perceive and act on more than merely the discrete tasks to be performed. Advanced beginners are distinguished from novices chiefly by their having some clinical experiences to draw on and by their ability to recognize salient aspects of a clinical situation.

Although one might anticipate that GNs would be classified as novices in Benner's model, this is not the case. As Benner[21] points out, "In this book, novice should not be attributed to the newly graduated nurse because, in most cases, the newly graduated nurse will perform at the advanced beginner level." Benner's point reinforces the notion that even limited clinical experiences as a student nurse afford some context for patient care experiences. Only when the GN is in a truly and totally unfamiliar clinical area (possibly in the operating room or emergency department) would the GN be considered a novice. Otherwise, GNs are more likely to be functioning at the advanced beginner level for the majority of their orientation experiences.

Some implications that can be derived from Benner's work include the following:

- Early in the GN's orientation, the preceptor should validate that the GN knows the rules and attributes that govern patient assignments and provide any instruction and reinforcement indicated. (*For example, it is necessary to verify that the GN's admission assessment data include all areas stipulated in the unit's admission procedure [rule verification]. Look for evidence that the GN recognizes the need to assess other features relevant to certain types of patients: does the GN simply record that the patient takes insulin daily or does he/she also determine what the daily dose is and whether the patient received the morning dose of insulin prior to admission.*)

- Avoid or minimize reference to exceptions to rules until the GN demonstrates mastery of the general rules (operating concepts, principles, theories, and procedures). Until general rules are learned, the new nurse is likely to find exceptions more confusing than helpful.

- Assist GNs in formulating *guidelines* for practice that integrate as many aspects and attributes as possible. (*For example, help the GN formulate the following guidelines for when trauma patients are admitted: complete a detailed patient assessment first, search for indications of any injuries that may have been overlooked, stabilize the patient, and then anticipate that the family will need information and support when they arrive.*)

- Spend at least a few minutes with GNs at the end of each orientation day to help them reflect on their experiences so that they can learn to recognize salient *aspects* of various patient care situations. (*For example, how did the admission of a postoperative trauma patient differ from admission of a patient scheduled for elective surgery?*)

- Help both novices and advanced beginner GNs distinguish the relative importance of the various attributes and aspects for different types of patient situations. (*For example, on a surgical unit it might be relevant to ask the orientee how important age, prior medical history, and surgical procedure are to the incidence of postoperative complications.*)

- Work with the GN to develop capabilities to:
  Establish and readjust priorities of care as patient needs change
  Organize time and work load based on patient care priorities
  Modify rules and procedures when patient situations warrant
  Manage an ever-widening array of patient and family care needs toward more holistic practice

- While the previously discussed skills are being developed, closely supervise the GN's nursing care to ensure that important patient needs are being attended, that priorities of care are recognized, and that more holistic aspects of care (e.g., psychosocial needs, family support, or patient education) are not neglected.

- Have realistic expectations of the GN. Early in their orientation, *expect* the GNs to be preoccupied with the details of their own assignment, expect them to be fairly blind to other events on the unit, expect their practice to be more task-oriented than holistic, expect them to be slow and unsure of themselves, and expect them to know only one way of doing things.

- The best preceptor for the novice or advanced beginner is likely to be a nurse at the next higher (competent) level of practice rather than a nurse at the fourth (proficient) or fifth (expert) levels. The reason for Benner's assertion here is that nurses at the proficient and expert levels of practice process and respond to patient situations in a materially and qualitatively different way than the novice or advanced beginner does. Nurses at those uppermost levels may not be able to fully or clearly explicate how they derive their assessments, plan their care, or evaluate its effectiveness in language the novice or beginner can relate to and learn from. By contrast, a nurse closer to the novice or advanced beginner's skill level may be able to sort out and communicate these areas more clearly.

Some hospitals have recognized the progression of skill development necessary for new graduates and have instituted distinguishable levels of clinical performance for the GN orientation program.[93] Even if your hospital does not make these distinctions explicit, it is necessary that nursing staff on units that employ new graduates and those who function as preceptors for GNs understand how nursing practice skills are developed and have realistic expectations for these special orientees.

It should be noted that Benner's use of the term *competent* to denote the third of five stages in skill development differs from the use of this term in competency-based education. In CBE, a competent nurse is one who is able to demonstrate that he/she can perform assigned functions. Benner's competent stage of skill development refers to the nurse who has 2 to 3 years of nursing experience with the same or similar types of patients and who consciously plans and provides patient care in relation to long-range goals. This plan dictates which attributes and aspects of the situation the nurse considers most important. This conscious, deliberate planning helps the competent nurse achieve greater organization and efficiency in patient care than the novice or advanced beginner. Competent nurses are aware that they have mastered the basics and can effectively manage many of the contingencies associated with real nursing practice.

Within Benner's framework, then, orientation programs would aim at ensuring that all GNs have progressed from the novice to the advanced beginner level for patient situations that staff nurses will encounter daily on their assigned unit. Since attainment of the competent stage of Benner's model may require a few **years** of experience, it does not represent a feasible goal for the GN orientation program. Hospitals that incorporate elements of Benner's model and also adopt a competency-based approach to staff development need to be sure that they recognize the distinctly different ways in which the term *competent* is employed in each case.

Experienced Nurses

Just as new graduates with no nursing experience represent one end of the staff nurse orientation experience spectrum, newly hired staff *with* nursing experience represent the opposite end of this spectrum. Although groups of new graduates will share many attributes in common with each other, they may, as described in the previous section, also differ substantially from one another regarding the extent of their entry knowledge base and clinical skills. This potential for heterogeneity is even greater in relation to the pool of experienced nurses who may enter hospital orientation programs.

The experience that a nurse brings to a new employer needs to be viewed with a broad perspective that includes its duration, nature, range, quality, and effects. "Experienced nurses" may have anywhere from 1 to 20 or more years of nursing experience. The nature of their clinical experience may be with the same, similar, or different patient populations than the one(s) they will be working with in their new job. Their range of experience may be narrow or broad, depending on the nature and complexity of patient problems they have managed, the acuity vs. chronicity of patient health problems, the scope of their prior job descriptions, and the number of different types of patient populations they have worked with. The quality of their nursing experience may also vary from high-quality experiences gained in state-of-the-art healthcare facilities with exemplary standards of patient care to many years of work at institutions with lesser levels of scientific and quality-oriented control. Some nurses develop and mature in expertise throughout their careers, whereas others seem to stagnate at marginally acceptable performance levels. Knowing that a staff nurse orientee has nursing experience, therefore, should prompt more queries than conclusions regarding what that experience represents.

How can the educator recognize and respond to the special needs of experienced staff nurse orientees? This may be most readily accomplished by contrasting these experienced nurses with their inexperienced GN counterparts. As Table 6.7 shows, the differences between GN and experienced staff nurse orientees suggest certain implications for the educator to consider in working with experienced nurses. Foremost among these considerations are the following:

- Respecting experienced nurses' knowledge, skills, and abilities
- Recognizing the anxiety and insecurity that experienced nurses may feel when placed in the learner role
- Being sensitive to experienced nurses' perceived need to have to prove themselves to a new group of peers and staff
- Facilitating the experienced nurses' full participation as members of the nursing staff in as short a time as possible

An additional set of considerations for orienting experienced nurses can be derived from Benner's novice-to-expert model. In that model, a nurse with more than 2 years of experience could be functioning at any of the three top stages in skill acquisition: the competent, proficient, or expert stage.

Nurses at the *competent* level typically have at least 2 or 3 years of experience working with the same or similar patients. Competent nurses* view their interventions in relation to long-range goals or plans that they consciously construct for the patient. These plans then dictate which attributes and aspects of the patient's situation are most relevant and which can be ignored. The nurse's plan for the patient is based on deliberate, abstract, analytic deliberations of the patient's current and future needs. Benner[21] suggests that competent nurses benefit most from decision-making games and simulations that afford practice in planning and coordinating multiple, complex patient care demands.

Nurses functioning at the *proficient* stage perceive and respond to clinical situations as wholes rather than in terms of specific aspects or attributes. Experience over 3 to 5 years has taught the proficient nurse the typical events to expect in certain situations and how plans can be modified in response to these events. The clinical picture presents itself holistically to the nurse rather than being derived through analytic deliberations. This holistic understanding of a clinical situation not only improves the efficiency of decision-making but also enables the proficient nurse to recognize when the anticipated clinical picture is not present—that is, when one or more elements of the "normal" set of events are missing. Proficient nurses use maxims to guide their performance. *Maxims* are nuances of a situation that provide direction to the nurse in deciding which aspects of the situation are relevant. Maxims vary with each situation and are derived from experience. An example of a maxim might be the nurse's suspicion that a patient could be having an allergic reaction to a drug; the patient's vital signs, color, and respiratory pattern might still be within normal limits, yet *something* about their appearance and behavior suggests that the patient may be experiencing the early stages of anaphylaxis.

Benner relates that proficient nurses are best taught inductively by case studies where their ability to grasp the totality of a clinical situation is solicited and challenged. Case studies could be offered for orientees to respond to, or orientees could be asked to relate a clinical situation where they felt their interventions were particularly effective or ineffective. Discussion could then center around the process of sorting out relevant and irrelevant data to arrive at the most appropriate intervention. If educators or preceptors attempt to use context-free rules or general principles with proficient nurses, these orientees will become frustrated and readily identify exceptions to these general rules. Proficient nurses are recognizable by their frequent response that "it all depends on the situation."

Nurses at the *expert* level no longer rely on analytic principles (rules, guidelines, or maxims) to understand clinical situations and guide their actions but have an intuitive grasp of the situation that focuses on salient elements immediately. The process used by expert nurses is, unfortunately, difficult to articulate because it does not lend itself to explicit, analytic steps that can be distinguished and enumerated. Expert nurses are often unable to relate how they arrived at their assessments or decided on their interventions; they just knew these were correct for that patient. Providing instruction for and learning from expert nurses requires attention to their descriptions of how they perceived the circumstances and the effectiveness of their nursing actions within that context.

It should be kept in mind that Benner's stages of clinical skill development are not static and irreversible; nurses tend to remain at their attained level of performance as long as the clinical situations and patient populations they encounter are familiar to them. When faced with novel or unfamiliar situations (such as a medical diagnosis or drug unfamiliar to them or a new procedure or piece of equipment to use), nurses will tend to regress in that situation to the more analytic and procedural, rule- and principle-based functioning of novice or advanced beginner nurses.

One admonition is also worth mentioning in relation to orientees with nursing experience: regardless of the amount and presumed quality of a new hire's nursing experience, no newly hired staff nurses should ever be "grandfathered" through the orientation process—that is, be exempted from having to demonstrate that they can meet the expectations for the orientation program based on their prior experience. Grandfathering selected orientees erases all quality control over the orientation program and may be fraught with innumerable erroneous and unfounded assumptions regarding how well that prior experience has prepared the nurse for current job responsibilities. An additional consideration here is that such grandfathering also represents a breach in compliance with the Joint Commission on Accreditation of Healthcare Organization's (JCAHO's) requirements for verification of the clinical competency of all nursing staff on entry into employment. Just as with the basic premises of competency-based education, educators need to be mindful that competency cannot be assumed; competency must be demonstrated, verified, and documented. An orientee's experience in nursing may also have been in a different role

---

*Please refer to preceding discussion regarding differences between Benner's use of the term *competent* and its use in competency-based education.

TABLE 6.7 • CONSIDERATIONS FOR WORKING WITH EXPERIENCED STAFF NURSE ORIENTEES

Attribute	GN with *No* Nursing Experience	RN with Nursing Experience	Implications for Working with Experienced Nurse Orientees
Self-perception	New; limited knowledge and skills; have much to learn	Mature; knowledgeable and skilled; already know and can do a great deal	Respect the knowledge and skills the orientees bring: • Recognize their abilities and expertise • Inquire about how they are accustomed to doing things and whether policies and procedures differ from those they have used • Resolve weak areas in performance as expeditiously as possible • Encourage suggestions and questions from orientees • Individualize orientation as much as possible via learning contracts • Use challenge mechanisms to decrease unnecessary instruction
Willingness to admit lack of knowledge or skill	Usually comfortable doing so	May hesitate to admit limitations because of concern that this will result in lack of respect for their experience	Enable the orientee to "save face" by observing practice rather than asking direct questions regarding abilities Avoid attempts to impress the orientee with your expertise or that of others; orientee may be intimidated by new peers Be careful to avoid blatant or subtle criticism of orientee's former employer(s) or previous clinical practices
Openness to learning	Typically very receptive	May resist changing established habits and practices	Maintain openness to orientee's comments and suggestions Explain rationale for local practices without becoming defensive Anticipate being challenged if hospital policies, procedures, and standards differ substantively from what orientee believes to be better
Time since graduation	Brief: weeks to months	Years to decades	Minimize use of extended classroom teaching sessions: avoid making orientee feel like a "student" in learning situations
Study habits	Accustomed to reading, studying, completing assignments	May not have continued these habits since graduation	Try to plan time during orientation for reading and other assignments to be completed so that study habits can be reestablished
Experience writing goals and objectives	Accustomed to writing personal goals and objectives for learning experiences	May be unfamiliar or out of practice with this skill	Explain purpose of these activities in relation to learning contracts; provide ample opportunities to practice in simulated situations; offer feedback to orientee on these areas when learning contracts are drafted
Test-taking skills	Sharp; well-honed	May not have undergone testing since school; often view all forms of evaluation as threatening and potentially embarrassing	Use self-assessments with instructor feedback during instruction and/or self-learning packages that include self-evaluations of performance; describe completion of clinical checklists as means to verify attainment of performance criteria rather than as testing instruments; reassure orientee that remedial instruction and retesting are available

Attribute	**GN with *No* Nursing Experience**	**RN with Nursing Experience**	**Implications for Working With Experienced Nurse Orientees**
Theory vs. practice capabilities	Theory base up-to-date and exceeds clinical practice skills	Despite confidence in clinical skills, may fear knowledge base is outdated and incomplete	Provide reference materials, readings, and study guides to support augmentation of knowledge base according to orientee's needs; cover principles, theory, and rationale for clinical practice more as reminders to enhance nursing effectiveness than as facts to be memorized
Deference to instructors	Will likely defer to expertise of instructors and not question their authority or accuracy	Likely to challenge instructor or content taught if instruction does not coincide with own beliefs or experience	Past experience as a full-fledged and autonomous staff nurse is better acknowledged if instructors/preceptor relate to orientee as colleague; make every effort to listen and respond constructively to questions or issues the orientee raises regarding what is taught; direct orientees to mechanisms that exist to improve and update policies, procedures, and standards if they have suggestions to offer
Age	Tend to be younger	Tend to be older	Keep expectations regarding enthusiasm for learning realistic
Family responsibilities	Usually limited to self	May be considerable	Respect the orientee's time and stature as a staff member
Financial responsibilities	Usually limited	May be considerable and pressing	Financial needs may pressure orientee to complete orientation program as soon as possible so that off-shift differentials and progression up the clinical ladder become available; make every effort to assist orientee in this process

TABLE 6.7 • CONSIDERATIONS FOR WORKING WITH EXPERIENCED STAFF NURSE ORIENTEES—cont'd

(e.g., a newly graduated RN may have had experience as an LPN). Because a number of significant differences in responsibilities exist between the LPN and RN roles, the orientation of RNs who previously worked as LPNs must ensure that the former LPN can now demonstrate the capabilities required of the new role as an RN.[31]

Cross-Trained Nurses

Cross-training consists of a planned educational program to prepare individuals to work in an area different from their customary work area. In nursing staff development, cross-training programs are designed to prepare nurses to function in a safe and effective manner on a nursing unit or with patient population(s) that differ from those the nurse is accustomed to and experienced with. In relation to competency-based education, cross-training involves provision of an instructional program that ensures the nurse is competent to function in the new nursing unit.

Cross-training differs from orientation by its more restricted scope and depth in content coverage and outcome expectations. Because cross-trained nurses work in units other than their customary unit only on a periodic basis, they are not usually prepared to the same depth and scope

of responsibilities as nurses who work on that unit full-time. Cross-training differs from *floating*, which is typically only a transitory and sporadic change of work assignment to a different unit that is not preceded by any planned preparation for the assignment. Cross-trained nurses' reassignment is anticipated rather than sudden and is preceded by a structured instructional preparation. Cross-training also can be distinguished from *retraining*, which consists of a full and complete reorientation to a new work area for a permanent change in work assignment.[81]

The potential benefits of cross-training may accrue to both the hospital and the nurse who will be cross-trained. For the hospital, cross-training offers the following potential benefits[53,64,65,76,95]:

- Flexibility to adjust staffing to fluctuations in patient census, patient acuity, and other unit demands
- Greater efficiency and productivity in use of existing staff
- Reduced incidence of staffing shortages
- Expanded range of job skills among participating staff nurses
- Greater teamwork and collaboration between hospital units

- Maintenance of quality patient care when using other than regular unit staff
- Reduced need for use of expensive agency nurses

For the nurse who is cross-trained, the potential benefits include the following[53,65,76,95]:

- Opportunities for professional growth and development in new clinical practice areas
- Potential for career advancement with expanded knowledge and skills
- Potential for increased salary if differential paid
- New relationships with colleagues from other nursing units
- Opportunities for mutual learning and sharing of expertise among nurses from different hospital units
- Decreased vulnerability to mandatory released time if staffing demands on home unit decrease

Although many hospital cross-training programs have been instituted to meet variable staffing demands or to initiate changes in nursing care delivery systems (e.g., with the conversion to case management), the Joint Commission on Accreditation of Healthcare Organization's (JCAHO's) requirements for cross-training programs have also been instrumental in encouraging healthcare institutions to consider the development of these programs. Thus cross-training programs may evolve either because the hospital needs or wishes to use the program to enhance staffing efficiency, productivity, or delivery or because the hospital seeks compliance with JCAHO accreditation requirements. In this regard, it may be useful to review a few points related to current JCAHO accreditation requirements for cross-training.

JCAHO nursing care standards state that "If a nursing staff member is assigned to more than one type of nursing unit or patient, the staff member is competent to provide nursing care to patients in each unit and/or to each type of patient." Another standard indicates that "Adequate and timely orientation and cross-training are provided, as needed."[75] Some related considerations include the following:

- The JCAHO does **not** require that every nurse is competent to provide nursing care to every patient in the hospital
- The JCAHO does **not** require cross-training every time nurses are temporarily reassigned to a nursing unit different from their home unit
- The JCAHO does **not** require cross-training if an RN who *is* competent on that unit is immediately available to supervise and assist the nurse who is new to the unit

- The JCAHO does **not** require cross-training if the scope of responsibility for nurses new to the unit is restricted to those elements of nursing care they have already been deemed competent to perform
- But when a nurse is expected to **routinely*** or **frequently*** provide nursing care that requires knowledge and skills for which that nurse has not been deemed competent *and,* if a competent RN is not immediately available to assist that nurse, then the new nurse must be provided with cross-training prior to giving patient care

The "bottom line" relative to JCAHO's requirements for cross-training is quality assurance: nursing staff cannot be assigned to work in areas or to care for patients until their competency to do so has been demonstrated.

When cross-training is either desirable or necessary, then, the process used for program development is analogous to that used for any other orientation program and includes each of the following elements: determination of goals and outcomes, assessment of learning needs, planning of instruction, implementing the instructional plan, and evaluating instruction and the program as a whole.

The analysis of cross-training goals and outcomes includes identification of which nursing units need additional nursing staff and how many nurses need to be cross-trained for those units. These preliminary issues are best determined as a collaborative effort among nurse managers, educators, and staff. Some of the decisions that need to be made at this point include the following:

- *The number of units nurses will be cross-trained for.* Will cross-training be limited to a single unit or more than one unit?
- *The scope of the cross-trained nurse's responsibility.* Will cross-trained nurses be expected to function independently at the same level as the regular nursing staff of that unit or will they have a somewhat dependent role with some restrictions placed on the type of assignments and responsibilities they are given?
- *The crossing of nursing divisions.* Will cross-training occur only between units with similar patient populations (between two ambulatory surgery clinics or between the labor and delivery unit and the postpartum unit) or will it include crossovers to different patient populations (between the postpartum unit and the newborn nursery or between a medical and a surgical unit)?
- *The crossing of patient acuity levels.* Will cross-training occur only between units with comparable levels of patient acuity (among all critical care units) or will it include crossovers with units having different patient acuity levels (between the neonatal ICU and the new-

---

*Current JCAHO accreditation standards do not define the terms *routinely* or *frequently.* Each hospital defines these terms for its own use.

born nursery or between the coronary care unit and the cardiac telemetry unit)?

- *The direction of cross-training.* Will cross-training occur up an acuity level (from a stepdown ICU to the acute ICU), down an acuity level (from the coronary care unit to the telemetry unit), or in both directions?

The decisions made regarding each of these elements will form the basis for all program components that follow.

The assessment of learning needs for nurses to be cross-trained will be based on a comparison of their current areas of competence and the additional areas of competence needed to function effectively and safely on the new unit. The more the patient populations and acuity levels on the new unit resemble those on the nurse's customary unit, the fewer and less extensive the educational needs will be in the cross-training program. Conversely, the more the new unit differs from the nurse's home unit with respect to patient populations and acuity levels, the greater will be the scope of learning that the cross-training program will need to provide. Sorting out these similarities and differences is the primary task in needs assessment. Competency areas and performance criteria that are the same for both units do not need to be repeated in cross-training; only differences between the two units that fall within the scope of the cross-trained nurse's responsibilities need to be covered.

The instruction planned for cross-training programs builds on the instruction already provided in the orientation program. In hospitals that use a competency-based approach to orientation, planning is facilitated by the ease with which competency areas and performance criteria can be readily compared between the two units and areas unique to the new unit can be readily discerned. Once the competency areas and/or performance criteria yet to be attained are distinguished, planning for the cross-training program focuses solely on differences between the two units.

In general, the content and learning experiences for cross-training programs concentrate on several distinct areas where differences may exist between the home and new units: patient population (ages, medical diagnoses, and nursing diagnoses), patient acuity (clinical and laboratory parameters monitored, treatments administered, and procedures used), medications, documentation (procedures, forms, and charting systems such as POMR vs. SOAP), and nursing delivery systems (primary vs. team vs. case management).

The specific teaching strategies and instructors (preceptors) used for implementing a cross-training program may be the same as those customarily used in the orientation program. Cross-training programs generally attempt to provide instruction as efficiently as possible. Didactic instruction that is prerequisite for working on the new unit may be provided as self-instruction (self-learning packages; videotapes; copies of relevant policies, procedures, and

protocols; and readings) so that the nurse can secure this learning when time is available without leaving the home unit.[65] Clinical instruction on the new unit can then be scheduled with unit preceptors at mutually convenient times. The amount and time required for clinical instruction will be functions of the degree of similarity between the nurse's customary responsibilities and those expected on the new unit. Cross-training that remains within the same nursing division typically minimizes the time and amount of clinical instruction necessary. Cross-training down one acuity level may only require 1 or 2 clinical days for demonstration of competency, whereas cross-training up an acuity level may demand 3 to 5 clinical days before all performance criteria are attained.

The evaluation processes and tools used for cross-training are derived from those (the same or an abridged version if the scope of responsibilities is limited in some way) used in the unit's orientation program. As a general rule, when cross-trained nurses are expected to function at a level comparable to that of the regular nursing staff, the performance criteria used in clinical evaluation are the same as those in the regular orientation program. When cross-trained nurses are held accountable to the same performance criteria as any other staff nurse on that unit, this ensures that quality patient care is maintained whenever cross-trained nurses provide patient care.

An additional consideration for the cross-training program is development of a mechanism that guarantees that the knowledge and skills gained from the initial cross-training effort are maintained over time and are updated periodically. This may be accomplished by establishing a minimum number of days (per month, per quarter, or per year) that nurses must work on the new unit to maintain their expertise and by requiring periodic reassignment to that unit to meet these requirements if staffing needs alone do not warrant this. Other hospitals institute annual updating sessions for such nursing staff.[64]

A successful and effective cross-training program requires a considerable amount of cooperation and collaboration among nurse managers, nurse educators, preceptors, and nursing staff. Administrative support is a necessary ingredient throughout this process. Nursing management can be particularly useful in coordinating the development of job descriptions for cross-trained nurses that specify the limits of their responsibilities, by developing policies and procedures for the cross-training mechanism as well as its competency monitoring and documentation, and by disseminating this information to all participating staff.

Agency Nurses

Two phenomena have combined over the past few decades to accelerate and expand development of independent agencies that provide supplemental nursing staff for hospitals. These phenomena include (1) the persistence of periodic shortages of nursing staff in some areas of the United

States and (2) nurses' growing interest and need for acquiring greater autonomy, flexibility, control, financial independence, and satisfaction with their careers, working environment, and work schedules.[73] Nurses who work for independent staffing services may be referred to as *agency nurses, registry nurses, temporary supplemental nurses,* or *independent contract nurses.* Hospitals that rely on such supplemental nursing staff confront three major issues: (1) ensuring that the nurses are competent to provide quality patient care, (2) orienting the nurses in an effective yet efficient manner, and (3) evaluating the quality of care provided.

Ensuring the Competency of Agency Nurses

In the past, hospitals in dire straits to cover acute and pressing staffing shortages depended largely on an outside agency to screen and ensure the competency of their employees. Except for verifying that the agency nurse had a current license to practice nursing in that state, few quality controls were used. The current Joint Commission on Accreditation of Healthcare Organization (JCAHO) accreditation standards[75] specify that the **hospital** now bears the responsibility for verifying both the licensing and the competency of these nurses. Nursing care standards specify that "Documented evidence of licensure and current clinical competence in assigned patient care responsibilities are reviewed and approved by the hospital before nursing personnel from an outside source(s) engage in patient care activities."

The JCAHO requirements notwithstanding, concerns for patient safety and the quality and continuity of nursing care provide ample rationale for hospitals to verify rather than assume that independently contracted nursing staff are capable of providing safe and effective patient care for the duration of their assignment at that hospital.

Although the responsibility for verification of the clinical competency of agency nurses rests with the hospital, the burden of developing and maintaining this competency may be borne by the contracted nurse or the agency service or be shared with the hospital. The growing number of supplemental staffing organizations has created enough competition among providers so that agencies can both require demonstration of competency in nursing practice as a prerequisite for hiring eligibility and can offer inservice and continuing education programs for maintaining competence as part of their benefit package to attract nurses to and retain nurses at that agency. The only time a hospital might become involved in developing the basic competency of agency nurses would be if their demands for this service were high and their resources for securing supplemental staff were very limited. Under these circumstances, the costs in time and labor required for this effort might be a reasonable investment for the hospital. In most circumstances, however, hospitals should be able to expect the contracted nurse and that nurse's agency employer to assume these costs.

However, when the outside agency provides the documentation that verifies the clinical competency of its nurses, hospitals have a responsibility to compare the agency's requirements against their own position descriptions, policies, and procedures, to determine whether the agency's scope, depth, and nature of "competency" are comparable and to identify and resolve any discrepancies that may exist. Both general areas of competency and the performance criteria used to appraise competence need to be examined to ensure that the agency's validation of a nurse's practice is acceptable to and consistent with the hospital's requirements.

In addition to these considerations, hospitals may develop and employ other screening devices as adjuncts to the hiring of individual agency nurses. Leidy[84] describes development of a preemployment screening test (on administration of medications, intravenous therapy, and blood products) given to contract nurses who worked at the hospital infrequently or for short durations. Different versions of the test were constructed for RNs and LPNs, and an additional section (on dysrhythmias, pressure monitoring, and advanced assessment) was added for critical care nurses. Failure to pass the test after two attempts prohibits the agency nurse from administering medications or IV therapy but does not necessarily preclude employment.

Orienting Agency Nurses

The JCAHO accreditation requirements related to orientation stipulate that "The organization provides an individual who is new to the organization . . . with an orientation of sufficient scope and duration to inform the individual about his/her responsibilities and how to fulfill them within the organization or department/service." In the scoring guidelines for this standard, the Joint Commission further clarifies that "Whether done by the hospital or the off-site agency, the hospital is responsible for assuring that each individual from an off-site agency who is permitted by the hospital to provide nursing care to patients has completed an adequate and timely orientation to the hospital." The hospital is also required to document the agency nurse's completion of orientation. The "adequacy" of this orientation relates to the expectations and job description for the agency nurse: the agency nurse's responsibilities could be a less inclusive or a virtually exact version of that used for regular full-time hospital nurses. Hospitals are free to modify the scope of the agency nurse's responsibilities as they deem appropriate. The "timely" nature of the orientation relates to its provision prior to that nurse's engagement in patient care activities.

Because the use of agency nurses is very costly and the duration of their temporary employment may be very brief (a few days, weeks, or months), an overriding concern for hospitals in orienting independent contractors is limiting the costs of the orientation program. Since the "time is money" adage holds true here, hospitals need to find ways to provide all necessary orientation instruction at the least possible cost. Because the costs of orientation are chiefly a function of the time, labor, and salaries to be paid to provide the program, orientation programs for agency nurses are typically provided over a brief duration, by as few staff as possible, and are usually limited to essential content only.

The content considered essential usually includes the topics listed in Box 6.20. Hospitals may add or delete content but usually cover only selected policies and procedures that are directly related to the unit(s) on which the nurse will work and areas that are needed to meet JCAHO requirements.

The duration of agency nurse orientation programs is variable. Bertucci[22] described a 4-day orientation for agency nurses, whereas Leidy's[84] program consisted of only 4 hours of hospital-provided instruction. In other institutions, the agency may provide videotaped "introductions" to key personnel, videotaped "tours" of the facility to which the nurse will be assigned, and videotaped explanations of personnel policies, as well as a set of pertinent hospital and nursing department policies and procedures. If agency nurses are responsible for reviewing this information prior to their arrival at the facility, it can save the hospital time and money involved in providing this information on site.

The teaching methods selected for the agency nurse orientation program can have a direct impact on program duration. Leidy's[84] 4-hour program also required orientees to complete independent study of a prepared information manual and to use learning contracts to indicate their agreement to review the information prior to the 4-hour class. The class provided an opportunity for highlighting the information reviewed in the manual and evaluating return demonstration performance of selected skill areas. Excluding program development and materials, the cost of orientation per agency nurse was $110, a substantial savings compared to the cost of orienting regular nursing staff.

The 4-day program described by Bertucci[22] consisted of 1 full day of personnel orientation and processing and 3 days reviewing nursing department policies and procedures via lectures, videotapes, and demonstrations. The latter included an 8-hour self-study package of core orientation material and testing in medications, safety, and infection control procedures as well as medication instruction and testing via computer-assisted instruction. Unit preceptors then work with agency nurses for the first 2 days of their unit assignment.

Bliss and Alsdorf[24] describe another cost-effective option for providing orientation for agency nurses in which a consortium of hospitals developed a 5-hour course that covered general features for the JCAHO safety areas (infection control, universal precautions, chemical safety, electrical safety, and fire safety). The hospitals reached consensus on the behavioral objectives, content outlines, and

---

Box 6.20

CONTENT OF AGENCY NURSE ORIENTATION PROGRAMS*

LOCATION OF EMERGENCY AND ROUTINE EQUIPMENT AND SUPPLIES

HOSPITAL POLICIES, PROCEDURES, PROTOCOLS, AND UNIT ROUTINES RELATED TO:

Patient admission, transfer, and discharge

Medication administration
- NLN medication administration test (passing score)
- Medication administration system and hours
- Commonly administered medications, narcotics
- Administration of blood and blood products
- Needle disposal
- Dosage calculation and titration
- Transcription of written, verbal, and STAT orders

IV therapy
- Venipuncture
- Venous access devices
- Parenteral nutrition
- Glucose monitoring

CPR and resuscitation

Documentation
- Manual vs. computerized records
- Forms, methods, formats (SOAP, POMR, etc.)
- Patient care plans

Nursing care delivery system (primary nursing, team, case management, etc.)

Safety programs
- Fire safety
- Electrical safety
- Hazardous waste handling and disposal
- Infection control
- Universal precautions
- Lifting and positioning patients

"Do Not Resuscitate" orders

*From Bertucci RC: *J Nurse Staff Develop* 4(1):34, 1988, and Bliss JB, Alsdorf P: *J Cont Educ Nurs* 23(2):60, 1992.

TABLE 6.8 • CULTURAL CONTRASTS: THE UNITED STATES AND OTHER COUNTRIES*		
Cultural Attribute	**United States**	**Other Countries**
Communication style	Direct; open; democratic; assertive to peers and authority figures; express opinions freely; ask questions; direct eye contact; emphasizes verbal language	May be indirect; passive; submissive and subtle, especially towards authority figures; desire to protect others' feelings may lead to circumlocution or evasive responses; may consider direct communication and eye contact as offensive, harsh, and rude; much communication is nonverbal
Time orientation	Very time conscious; deadline-oriented; requires being on time; rushed; hurried; impatient; important to accomplish tasks within specified time	Time may be less important than other (family) responsibilities; tardiness or absences may occur for seemingly trivial reasons
Life priorities	Setting priorities is important; work is a consuming, driving force; work/career may take precedence over home and family	Family and relationships may take precedence over virtually all other obligations
Work attitudes	Results-oriented; competitive; highly organized; accustomed to giving directions; work for recognition of individual performance; respect for boss needs to be earned; expected to make suggestions and report problems; expected to make decisions; professionals would be offended by telling them every step to take	Team oriented; collaborative; follow directions given; work for group recognition; implicit respect for persons in authority; defer decisions and problem identification to those in positions of authority; even individuals in highly skilled positions may prefer explicit and detailed directions for work
Social orientation	Highly individualistic; value being self-directed, self-made, independent of others' assistance; prefer to do things on their own; competitive; both accomplishments and mistakes are attributable to individuals; nepotism disdained; want to be treated and recognized as individuals	May be highly group-oriented; value social ties, group harmony, cooperation; singling out individuals for praise or criticism may cause discomfort and social alienation; use family ties for many aspects of work; prefer to be treated and recognized as members of social groups
Political system	Democratic; freedom to express opinions; egalitarian	Range from dictatorships, coups, to socialist or democratic; freedom of expression may be limited
Economic system	Capitalistic; individual enterprises; private ownership of property; competitive	Variable; may be unaccustomed to private enterprise or have limited ownership of property
Family structures	Fewer have traditional structures of two parents with children; many nontraditional variations exist	Traditional family structures may predominate; strong family and community ties could have pervasive influence on life and work
Authority figures	Prefer authority figures at work to treat subordinates as peers as much as possible and to have a sense of humor; those in positions of authority may de-emphasize status to reduce gulf between themselves and workers; traditional deference to authority waning	May expect authority figures to be serious in demeanor and to demonstrate good manners, maintain distance from workers; authority figures may not be questioned, challenged, or interrupted out of respect for their status; status of others always noted
Religious beliefs	Variable; range from none to traditional	Traditional; often deep-rooted and strong
Emotional expression	Generally try to suppress strong emotions in work settings; adults expected to control strong emotional expressions; expressions may be interpreted as signs of immaturity	Feelings and emotions may be valued and expressions of these encouraged
Response to kidding, joking	Teasing usually viewed as playful and sign of friendship, amiability	May be interpreted as offensive, rude, deprecating, especially if by authority figure

TABLE 6.8 • CULTURAL CONTRASTS: THE UNITED STATES AND OTHER COUNTRIES*—cont'd		
Cultural Attribute	**United States**	**Other Countries**
Response to personal questions	Generally considered friendly; sign of interest in getting to know someone	May be considered intrusive and cause discomfort
Response to criticism	Expect feedback on performance; tell it like it is; give criticism as warranted but only to individual it pertains to; accept it if presented in constructive and objective manner	May cause loss of dignity, loss of face, especially if directed at an individual
Response to praise	Praise is a strong positive motivator; feel honored to be singled out for individual recognition of achievement	Being singled out for praise may cause embarrassment within the group, loss of face, and diminished sense of affiliation
Healthcare system	Capitalistic; private; available to those who can pay; expensive; high technology; cutting edge; aggressive care of elderly and dying may be fraught with legal and ethical issues; nurses perform many technical procedures; documentation systems may be highly structured and detailed with numerous abbreviations and acronyms; many ancillary and support staff; family involvement may be limited to education related to postdischarge care	May be highly centralized and socialized or rudimentary at village level; if fully socialized, is available to all without charge; less technologic; more traditional/folk medicine used; supportive care of elderly and dying; physicians perform most technical procedures; documentation primarily via unstructured narrative notes with few abbreviations and their own local medical jargon; no ancillary staff may exist; family often provides personal hygiene care and remains with patient in hospital
Basic nursing education	Three programs, lasting 2 to 4 years; most offered at colleges and universities; theory emphasized over clinical practice time, especially with longer programs; curriculum includes consumer rights notions of patient rights, patient advocacy, patient education; increased amounts of self-directed instruction included in curriculum; expected to know limits and to ask questions if something is not understood; respect for instructors is earned	Length and location of programs vary; Philippines emphasizes 4-year BSN; Great Britain and Ireland offer mostly hospital-based diploma programs; Sweden offers 20 ways to become an RN; programs emphasize clinical experiences over theory; issues related to consumer orientation may not exist; learning experiences are highly structured and teacher-directed; asking questions or indicating lack of understanding are avoided since these may imply that teaching was not effective; implicit respect for instructors as persons of high status and honor
Role of nursing	Wide scope of practice; function with independence and collaboration with other healthcare professionals; legal and ethical accountability for practice; documentation receives much attention and requires much paperwork; expected to function in cost-effective manner; patient has right to participate in own care; legally bound to question/clarify physician orders in certain instances; highly stylized nursing care delivery systems; in high-tech areas, nurses perform many complex technical procedures	Often have somewhat restricted scope of practice; role is more dependent, passive, and submissive, especially to physicians; accountable primarily for completing medical orders; documentation often anecdotal and limited in volume; cost of care not usually a nursing consideration; patients should not be burdened with providing their own care; may not question medical orders out of respect for physician's status; team nursing often used; physicians perform most technical procedures

*Modified from references 1, 16, 34, 61, 68, 83, 135, 141.

evaluation tools for the course and then transferred responsibility for providing the course to a local community college. All agency nurses who wish to work at any of the participating hospitals have to show their certificate of successful course completion before they can receive an assignment. The cost ($40.00) of the course is borne by the agency nurse or the employment service rather than by the hospital. On the same day that the course is taken, agency nurses also complete the National League for Nursing (NLN) medication administration test. If a passing score on the NLN test is not attained, the agency nurse follows the guidelines for independent remedial study and then

TABLE 6.9 • AGAPE INTERNATIONAL'S FIVE STAGES OF CULTURAL ADJUSTMENT*

Stage	Time Frame	Description
Honeymoon	1 to 3 months	Early encounter with new culture is associated with a sense of adventure; differences viewed as intriguing, exciting, and novel; individual may feel like a tourist
Culture shock	3 to 9 months	Excitement worn off; struggle with differences between the two cultures; social cues are hard to recognize and follow, making relationships difficult; feelings of isolation, alienation, and homesickness emerge and may be sufficient to precipitate return home if that option is available
Surface adjustment	After 1 year	Begins to recognize and employ some of the values, customs, and practices of the new culture; incipient relationships formed with local people; starts to feel more comfortable living and working there
Frustration	Variable	Fuller understanding of local culture leaves selected problems unresolved; frustration, boredom, isolation, and conflict may emerge
Genuine adjustment	Variable	Able to view new culture as an alternative; may not agree with or favor differences but understands them in context; forms deeper relationships with some local people

*From Williams J: *J Nurs Staff Development* 8(4):155, 1992.

must reschedule and retake the test at a later date. Although the consortium hospitals still must review any site-specific aspects of safety programs and medication administration procedures, this generic program design shifts much of the time and cost of agency nurse orientation to outside providers (the community college) and the individual agency nurse (or their agency).

Evaluating the Performance of Agency Nurses

In relation to agency nursing staff, JCAHO nursing care standards specify that "The performance of these nursing personnel [from outside sources] in the hospital is evaluated." In addition, hospital policy must define the responsibility for this evaluation. Thus, in order to fully comply with JCAHO requirements, hospitals that use independently contracted nurses must be able to document their competency on entry to the hospital, their completion of an orientation program, and the quality of the nursing care they actually provide in the work setting. The Joint Commission does not prescribe any specific method for this performance evaluation, so hospitals are free to design their own means for accomplishing this. Some type of clinical skills checklist is typically employed for this purpose.

International Nurses

Low salaries and limited employment and career opportunities for nurses in other parts of the world together with periodic shortages of nurses here at home have led to unprecedented immigration and recruitment of nurses from around the world into the United States. As a result, in many U.S. hospitals, the composition of hospital staff nurse orientees has been transformed from a relatively homogenous group of mostly white, middle-class persons of the same culture and educational system to an increasingly heterogeneous mixture of nurses from varying racial, ethnic, and socioeconomic subgroups, representing a wide array of cultures and educational systems.

Some 75% of foreign nurses come to the United States from only four countries: Great Britain, Ireland, Canada, and (the greatest number) the Philippines.[16] Others emigrate from various Asian countries or from one or more of the Spanish-speaking (Hispanic) areas of the world: Mexico, Cuba, Puerto Rico, and South or Central America. The settlement of these nurses in the United States creates the phenomenon of cultural diversity within the nursing profession. Madeline Leininger, a pioneer of transcultural nursing, defines *cultural diversity* as "the overt and covert differences among people of different population groups with respect to their values, beliefs, language, physical characteristics, and general patterns of behavior."[85] Welcoming, assisting, and educationally supporting these nurses has thus become a major consideration for many hospital staff development programs.

Webster defines the word *culture* as the "customary beliefs, social forms, and material traits of a racial, religious, or social group" and as an "integrated pattern of human behavior . . . (transmitted) to succeeding generations." Culture dictates the norms we live by, how we perceive and respond to life events, and affords our unwritten rules for living and behaving. Culture is an inclusive term that encompasses a myriad of elements, such as our beliefs, values, goals, priorities, behaviors, social mores and taboos, traditions, habits, rituals, family structures, communication patterns, etiquette, religious and dietary practices and preferences, educational and political systems, language, time and space orientations, and customs. The enveloping effects of culture have a pervasive influence on virtually every aspect of our lives, attitudes, and behavioral responses.[135]

When persons from different cultures are immersed in the same work setting, one of two scenarios may result. In

TABLE 6.10 • PILLETTE'S FOUR PHASES OF ADJUSTMENT FOR THE INTERNATIONAL NURSE*		
Phase	**Time Frame**	**Description**
Acquaintance	First 3 months (from overseas meeting to post-orientation)	First encounter with host hospital occurs overseas and includes interview and screening to match recruit's background and goals with needs of hospital. Realistic description of U.S. healthcare system and nursing practice needs to be shared.
		Second component begins with arrival in United States. Recruit's expectations of life and work may not be realistic, but energies focus on new activities, euphoria, and fascination with novel aspects of home and work life. Basic needs for housing, eating, and transportation often arranged and may be subsidized. Resource person designated and social support network established to minimize isolation and stressors. Orientation commences; orientee undergoes close scrutiny. If experienced, the foreign nurse may regress to learner role and resent close scrutiny of practice. Completion of orientation brings sense of achievement, regained independence, and often, significant financial gains.
Indignation	3 to 6 months	Contrasts between life and work at home and in United States become more striking, causing psychological, social, professional, and cultural dissonance. Discovery that one's accustomed ways of living and working are not necessarily the only or best ways lead to shock and disillusionment. As perceptions of life in the United States become more realistic, hopes and expectations may be dashed, leading to frustration and despair.
		Demands and pressures on nurses (legal concerns, accountability, documentation, sicker and older patients, demanding families, volume of skills and information to learn, etc.) may overwhelm and lead to anxiety and feelings of inadequacy. Prior beliefs and practices are called into question and may increase longing for home. Psychosomatic symptoms and behavioral effects may include fatigue or retreat to night shift. Psychological stress may lead to tension or guilt. Awaiting outcome of licensure examination creates uncertainty and stress. Emotions often intense but diffuse.
Conflict resolution	6 to 9 months	Emotions and decision making become focused. Outcome of RN licensure examination represents a benchmark. Those who fail it may feel suspended: going home represents failure while remaining adds additional uncertainty regarding the future. Those who pass experience relief, increased status to RN, and tendency to become more vocal regarding conflicts and contradictions they have noted. May change employer or even return home if conflicts cannot be resolved. Those who persist gradually become more fully absorbed into the local culture.
Integration	9 to 12 months	Personal tensions and conflicts diminish while enthusiasm and concern for peers increase. Nurses gradually feel that they are a part of the hospital, the unit, and its nursing staff.

*From Pilette PC: *J Cont Educ Nurs* 20(6):277, 1989.

the first scenario, the contrasting and divergent attitudes, values, beliefs, and behaviors lead to misunderstandings, misinterpretations, and conflict. In the second scenario, the cultural differences between the various groups are identified, compared, and acknowledged, leading to mutual understanding and clarification and more effective and harmonious working relationships.

In order to work effectively with a culturally diverse group of nurse orientees, hospitals need to acknowledge that cultural contrasts exist, understand and assist with the process, problems, and adjustments necessary when individuals enter a new culture, and make organizational and educational modifications that will facilitate accommodation of the needs of these nurses. When nurses whose homelands are outside of the United States enter this country, two parallel processes need to transpire: (1) our international colleagues need to become acquainted with the United States, its people and customs, and the U.S. health-

care industry, and (2) their U.S. counterparts need to become acquainted with the international nurses' respective countries, people, customs, and healthcare systems. For both groups of nurses, the initial step in the process of managing cultural diversity is to develop an awareness of cultural differences that may exist among and between persons of varying racial and ethnic heritages. As a result, the management of cultural diversity is a two-way street where each must try to walk in the other's footsteps for the common ground of understanding to be reached.

Development of Cultural Awareness

The development of cultural awareness is a sensitization process that includes both a full recognition of the attributes of one's own culture and a sensitization, appreciation, and respect for the attributes of cultures different from one's own. Individuals who are cognizant only of their

TABLE 6.11 • SUPPORTING THE INTERNATIONAL NURSE THROUGH CULTURAL ADJUSTMENT	
Adjustment Phase*	**Suggested Support**
Honeymoon/acquaintance	Hospitals that recruit international nurses should have a recruitment plan that specifies the number and types of nurses needed.
	Interviews need to be mutually informative; explanations of the U.S. healthcare system, nursing practice realities, opportunities, and potential obstacles need to be described to minimize illusions and unrealistic expectations. Trade-offs for high pay and working conditions need to be identified. Attempts should be made to estimate candidates' ability to adjust to work and cultural differences.
	Arrangements for provision of basic needs (housing, dietary, transportation, religious, etc.) need to be made.
	Social and professional support systems need to be integrated. If necessary, bilingual support staff may help with initial settlement.
	Learning how to greet and thank people in their native language can set a good precedent.
	Warm and cordial personal welcome and attention to jet lag and weather differences should precede the work of orientation.
	If possible, assign a mentor or preceptor to serve as the first-line contact and to initiate social and professional ties. Remember the primacy of establishing and nurturing relationships in other cultures.
	During orientation, reiterate the major differences international nurses are likely to experience and explain assistance to be provided for each. Explain our role as assisting them to be successful in their transition.
	Make every attempt to recognize and respect past nursing experience so that these nurses are not made to feel like novices or students. Portray differences in scope of nursing practice primarily *as* differences rather than implying that the U.S. system is better. Be matter-of-fact (this is how we do it here) rather than judgmental.
Culture shock/indignation	Anticipate the problems and conflicts that these nurses will experience. Provide ongoing support systems for identifying and resolving these issues insofar as possible. Remember that cultural dissonance is a natural and inevitable part of the adjustment process. The aim is not prevention but evaluation toward positive adjustment and adaptation.
	Schedule regular informal sessions for eliciting, discussing, and resolving problems as they become apparent.
	Provide as much information as needed to minimize problems and facilitate adaptation.
	Avoid becoming defensive; make every attempt to be open-minded regarding positive and negative aspects of nursing in the United States. Be curious about impressions and reactions to our healthcare system.
	Remember that frustration, withdrawal, and fatigue are commonly manifested during this stage.
	Proceed with orientation gradually; avoid overwhelming these nurses with large volumes of information to assimilate.
Surface adjustment; frustration/conflict resolution	Provide support of independent attempts to adapt to U.S. customs and practices. Maintain supportive ties without forcing relationships to develop.
	Maintain a healthy sense of perspective about local practices; see pluses and minuses.
	Encourage and support nurses before and after completion of the RN licensure examination.
	Recognize that the investment in these nurses is substantial for both the hospital and for the nurse.
	Understand that failure to pass the RN licensure examination may carry a devastating loss of face and dignity. Do everything possible to enhance performance on the test.
	Recognize that some of these nurses may not be able to make the adjustment necessary for long-term commitment to life in the United States.
	Lend support and encouragement without being intrusive on their decision to remain rather than return home.
	When possible, explain how frustration or disagreement over practices may be constructively resolved.
	Communicate in tones that are empathetic, respectful, and patient.

TABLE 6.11 • SUPPORTING THE INTERNATIONAL NURSE THROUGH CULTURAL ADJUSTMENT—cont'd	
Adjustment Phase*	**Suggested Support**
Genuine adjustment/ integration	Be realistic; don't expect others to discard their own culture and replace it with ours.
	Adaptation and adjustments are more likely to be selective and piecemeal.
	Continue support and nurturance in work and social structures.
	Enjoy the reduced tension, and stress interpersonal relationships. Build on foundations now established, and reawaken interests in opportunities available.
	Recognize that some nurses may remain in the United States despite their dissatisfactions. For some, acculturation may never be fully attained.
	Encourage their input and assistance in orienting other international nurses and, perhaps, in serving in an ongoing capacity with an intercultural awareness and assistance group.

*Phases reflect Agape International's five stages and Pilette's four phases of cultural adjustment.

own culture are vulnerable to the development of *ethnocentrism,* a tendency to believe and behave as though one's own values, beliefs, and customs are somehow superior to or better than those of others. Individuals who base their perceptions of others' cultures on oversimplified and often inaccurate generalizations are prone to stereotyping these individuals. A primary goal of cultural awareness is to avoid both ethnocentrism and stereotyping.[46,91] One way to accomplish these dual objectives is to identify culturally accurate information regarding both our own as well as others' cultures.

Table 6.8 lists a number of cultural attributes characteristic of the United States and contrasts each of these with differences that may exist for people from different countries. What this comparison illustrates is that striking contrasts may exist whenever individuals from different cultures interact with one another. As Copeland[34] points out, "Intercultural relationships are fragile. Countless hazards are created by communication problems, cultural differences in motivational and value systems, diverse codes of conduct, even differences in orientation to fundamentals such as perception of time and space." Differences in personal and social style that we take for granted as friendly or business discourse may, unintentionally, be considered rude or offensive and result in misinterpretation, embarrassment, or loss of face or dignity. American cultural preferences and practices, therefore, cannot be extended with impunity to persons from cultures different from our own but must be modified to accommodate the cultural preferences and practices of others.

As Table 6.8 indicates, elements of diversity for nurses from different cultures are not limited to broad areas of social influence but extend to their native healthcare systems, role of nursing, and nursing education systems as well. Given these contrasting sets of cultural attributes, the problems that foreign nurses encounter in the United States are both understandable and, to some extent, predictable. These problems may be somewhat less inclusive when the nurse comes from an English-speaking country such as Great Britain, but even British nurses must endure significant cultural adaptation because of differences in

word usage, idioms, and medical jargon that may stifle clear communication or because their experience in healthcare delivery is based on a socialized healthcare system. As a result, U.S. hospitals need to anticipate the cultural adaptations that nurses from other countries will have to make, recognize the problems and issues that are likely to arise, and use this information to modify staff development efforts accordingly.

Management of Culture Shock

In much the same way that newly graduated nurses experience reality shock when their school culture and values confront the hospital bureaucracy culture and values, nurses new to the United States experience *culture shock* when their accustomed ways of living, working, and relating to others confront American culture and values. In addition to their belongings, they carry their cultural baggage into the United States and experience identifiable phases or stages of adjustment while they learn and adapt to the new cultural rules of working, communicating, and living. Recognizing the phases of cultural adjustment and learning how we can support our colleagues at each phase is one way of assisting these nurses in this assimilation process.

PHASES OF CULTURAL ADJUSTMENT Williams and Rogers[143] incorporate the Agape International Training Program's five stages of cultural adjustment in preparing preceptors to work with nurses from other countries. A description of these stages is provided in Table 6.9.

Pilette[113] describes an alternative way of viewing this process that consists of four phases and includes events before the nurse's arrival in the United States. Her characterization of the adjustment process is summarized in Table 6.10.

Regardless of which of these descriptions one might prefer, their similarity and comparability to the phases of reality shock are readily apparent.

Supporting international nurses through the stages of cultural adjustment likewise has many corollaries with re-

Box 6.21

PROBLEMS EXPERIENCED WITH INTERNATIONAL NURSE ORIENTEES*

LANGUAGE

- English as a second language (ESL)
- Language difficulties may exist in the areas of speaking, listening, reading, and writing
- Language proficiency more difficult for adults
- American idioms, phraseology, dialects
- American medical terminology; nursing vocabulary, and jargon
- Standard and local medical abbreviations
- Lack of language facility limits ability to identify patient priorities, develop coherent care plans, and document patient care
- Fear of being misunderstood or misinterpreted may lead to avoidance in using telephone to call physician, reassure family, or give report
- Language difficulties may impair ability to read with speed and comprehension, to speak clearly, and to write concisely and coherently

INTERPERSONAL COMMUNICATION

- American expectations related to interpersonal behaviors may differ significantly from accustomed ways of relating
- Language and ESL problems tend to inhibit verbal exchanges and taking verbal orders from physicians
- Nurses may not admit they do not understand messages
- Nurses may not ask questions to avoid embarrassment of revealing lack of understanding
- Lack of assertiveness in communicating with peers, patients, physicians
- Lack of clear indication of understanding may leave others unsure regarding comprehension and learning
- Nurses may lack experience in working with LPNs and ancillary staff
- Nurses may be accustomed to more limited scope of responsibility for decision-making in patient care

CONTENT AREAS MISSING FROM BASIC NURSING EDUCATION

- Psychiatric–mental health nursing and therapeutic communication
- Brand names and side effects of drugs
- Phases of the nursing process and their application
- Physical assessment skills
- CPR and resuscitation team procedures
- Accountability for practice
- Time management: reporting to work on time, completing all tasks by end of shift
- Organizing and providing nursing care based on priorities
- Documentation: importance, detail required, organizing systems (nursing diagnosis, POMR, SOAP, etc.)

- Need for cost-effectiveness in delivery of nursing services
- Patient rights
- Patient/family education
- Nursing care delivery systems: primary nursing, case management
- Medications and IVs: unit-dose system, calculation of drip rates, titration, IV access devices
- Transcription of medical orders (manual, computer)
- Care of patients segregated in rooms vs. in open wards
- Ethical issues related to care of the dying and elderly
- Performance of technical procedures (done by physicians in their country)
- Legal aspects of nursing
- Risk management

STUDY SKILLS

- Reading and comprehension may be impaired by language difficulties
- Nurses may read more slowly and with less recall; reading assignments may be frustrating and time-consuming
- Note-taking skills may be limited, diminishing usefulness of lectures heavily laden with content
- Nurses may be unfamiliar with self-directed study; language difficulties may make self-directed study laborious and limited in value

TEST-TAKING SKILLS

- Lack of familiarity with multiple-choice test item format
- Lack of reading proficiency may cause misinterpretation of written problems, difficulty completing tests on time, neglect of nuances needed to locate correct answer

CLASSROOM LEARNING

- Nurses may be accustomed to highly structured learning environment
- Nurses may be used to receiving explicit details from teachers
- More time and effort may be required to assimilate all customary orientation content plus areas not covered in basic nursing program, especially if English is not the native language
- Ability to listen effectively and understand English may be limited and slow
- Self-consciousness about accent and accuracy of pronunciation
- Reluctance to participate in classroom setting for fear of being misunderstood, fear of loss of face if a mistake is made, desire not to be elevated above others in group, or out of respect for authority of teacher

*See references 45, 100, 112,. 132, 139, 140.

ality shock as well. Some of these forms of assistance and support that might be rendered are enumerated in Table 6.11.

In addition to recognizing and supporting international nurses through the phases of cultural adjustment, staff development departments can facilitate the assimilation of these nurses by becoming aware of problems frequently encountered when these nurses enter the U.S. healthcare system and by determining how the orientation process might be modified to accommodate the special needs of these nurses.

PROBLEMS EXPERIENCED BY INTERNATIONAL NURSE ORIENTEES   The difficulties faced by nurses who enter the United

States from foreign countries may be grouped into a number of different categories, including language problems, interpersonal communication problems, topics not included in nursing education programs, study skills, and test-taking skills. Box 6.21 enumerates a number of problems that often emerge in each of these categories.

MODIFYING ORIENTATION FOR INTERNATIONAL NURSES Cultural awareness and recognition of cultural contrasts and adjustment phases alone will not be sufficient for making a hospital responsive to the needs of international nurses unless other elements of our system also change in response to these realities. In addition to supporting these nurses through the cultural adjustment process and anticipating problems that are likely to arise, nursing staff development educators also need to consider ways in which each phase of the instructional process for the orientation program may need to be modified to make it more responsive to nurses from outside the United States. Some of the modifications are listed in Box 6.22.

Hospitals that have international nurses joining their staff will, of course, need to include these elements of cultural awareness, culture shock, and cultural adjustment into their preceptor training programs so that all those who relate to these nurses are familiar with these dynamics. Institution of a support group to assist international nurses may also be helpful in minimizing the anxiety, tension, frustrations, and problems that often accompany transition to

---

Box 6.22

TAILORING ORIENTATION PROGRAMS FOR INTERNATIONAL NURSES*

ASSESSMENT PHASE
- Explain how orientation expectations were derived
- Relate need to validate competency of all nurse orientees (not just international nurses)
- Describe how input and participation in the assessment of learning needs is necessary and valued
- Be explicit regarding the input you need related to assessment of learning needs for orientation
- Provide opportunities for orientees to describe and demonstrate how they are accustomed to doing things
- Include areas often neglected in basic nursing education programs in the assessment expectations

PLANNING PHASE
- Plan to begin with highly structured teaching sessions if these are most familiar to orientees
- Plan teaching methods to accommodate language barriers that exist: rather than using open discussions, question-and-answer sessions, or prolonged lectures, small groups, role modeling, and laboratory demonstration may be effective
- Design instruction that includes much hands-on clinical teaching
- Plan copious use of visual aids (charts, video, pictures, objects): secure audiovisual programs, design graphic handouts for class use and distribution
- Increase time allotments for instruction to allow for greater theory coverage of unfamiliar areas and to allow for longer time to process new information and customary orientation information in a second language
- Select preceptors who have been prepared to work with international nurse orientees
- Limit the information conveyed to essentials only; be selective
- If an orientee's native language is not English, plan learning experiences that minimize the need for extensive note taking and provide copies of visual aids as handouts; avoid reliance on heavy reading assignments
- Organize instruction to maximize understanding and provide easy transitions and applications; develop concrete examples to use in class
- Avoid the use of instructional strategies that focus attention on individual learners (making presentations, giving reports, leading discussions, etc.)
- Plan warm-ups and ice-breakers to increase social comfort for learners
- Consider the use of computer-assisted instruction as a nonthreatening means to provide teaching with visual reinforcement, immediate feedback, and no loss of face for mistakes or errors
- Mixed-culture study groups may be helpful for supporting language facility and study skills
- Kinesthetic and tactile learning experiences in laboratory and clinical areas may be particularly effective

Continued.

Box 6.22

TAILORING ORIENTATION PROGRAMS FOR INTERNATIONAL NURSES—cont'd*

IMPLEMENTATION PHASE

- Use structured learning experiences with explicit directions and steps in procedures
- Speak slowly and distinctly; avoid using unnecessary asides and parenthetical expressions
- Use nonverbal communication and speak in pleasant and nonthreatening tone
- Clarify and reiterate key words, terms, and phrases
- Summarize key points before changing topics
- Avoid slang, unfamiliar jargon, metaphors, anecdotes, and complex sentence structure
- Use concrete and specific examples to illustrate and emphasize
- Avoid putting any one orientee "in the spotlight" by calling on that individual
- Attempt to verify understanding by requesting orientee to paraphrase explanations or to demonstrate procedures
- Distribute copies of policies and procedures, employee benefits, and other relevant materials
- Be friendly, cordial, and respectful; avoid joking and teasing
- Allow orientees to tape class presentations for later review
- Be flexible and innovative; mix tours and social events with instruction
- In small group work, mix cultures to avoid segregation and expand social contacts
- Learn and use at least a few words or phrases in the native languages of the international nurses
- Include practice in areas likely to be unfamiliar or uncomfortable to orientees

EVALUATION PHASE

- Avoid use of (or develop nurses' skills in using) unfamiliar testing means such as the multiple-choice item
- Recognize that lack of familiarity with the item format and language difficulties may distort evaluation results
- Invite orientees to paraphrase theory or demonstrate procedures to evaluate their understanding
- Use self-evaluations and peer appraisals as much as possible
- Invite anonymous submission of written questions and suggestions for future programs
- Emphasize clinical performance evaluations
- Don't misinterpret verbatim reiterations or mirrored procedure performance as evidence of understanding; later repeat performance and application of theory in clinical area will be necessary
- When corrections are necessary, use plain, pleasant, and patient tone of voice
- Allot sufficient time for orientee to acquire and assimilate information before evaluation process commences
- Be sure that speed in performance is not a factor in evaluations
- Asking orientee to evaluate preceptor or other instructors may cause discomfort and be interpreted as rude and inappropriate; depersonalize program evaluations by evaluating attainment of objectives and program goals rather than instructors
- Be careful when interpreting results of program evaluations; orientees may not wish to offend hosts, teachers, or peers by criticizing any of them

*Modified from references 45, 100, 112, 132, 134, 139.

---

a new culture.[68] An international advisory panel composed of representatives from all cultural groups in the nursing department may also serve to keep diversity management and education initiatives on track.[113] Because international awareness develops in an evolutionary process, the BOMWGSAT (bunch of middle-class white guys/gals sitting around a table) method of cultural sensitivity is not likely to be very effective to that end.[39]

Historically, the United States has been viewed as a melting pot, a land where immigrants from diverse racial, ethnic, and cultural heritages are gradually assimilated into the American way of life.[58] Increasingly, however, the American melting pot image has been replaced by a mosaic, which not only recognizes and celebrates our common purpose and similarities to each other but also recognizes and celebrates the rich and distinct cultural heritages each group contributes to the whole. Hospital employers and nursing staff development departments must maintain responsiveness to this cultural mosaic.

PROGRAM EVALUATION

As mentioned in Chapter 5, evaluations are useful in staff development programs when they afford valid, reliable, and meaningful information that can be used to make necessary decisions about the program. The two major decisions that must be made in an orientation program relate to whether the orientation was *effective* and whether it was *efficient*. The first decision is reached by examining each of the three system components of the orientation program described earlier*:

- Input: Educational and administrative contexts in which orientation is provided
- Throughput: All facets of the program that relate to delivery of instruction to orientees
- Output: All results or outcomes attributable to the program.

Appraisals of program output, in turn, may be performed for any desired level of evaluation: satisfaction, learning, application, or impact.

The second decision is reached by examining the nature and amount of resources that were expended to provide the orientation program. In summary, then, the *effectiveness* of the orientation program is a function of whether the goals and outcomes established for the program were attained, and the *efficiency* of the orientation program is a function of what it cost the organization to provide the program.

An orientation program may be effective but not efficient, meaning that orientees attained the established outcomes but at a relatively or excessively high cost to the hospital. Orientation programs may also be efficient but not effective, implying that, although the costs were relatively low, the purposes and outcomes of the program were not attained. Of these two program evaluation factors, effectiveness takes priority over efficiency. Unless the outcomes of the orientation program are achieved, its relative cost is of secondary importance. Only after the program has been deemed effective should measures to improve its efficiency be considered.

EVALUATING THE EFFECTIVENESS OF AN ORIENTATION PROGRAM

Orientation programs for nursing staff nearly universally include evaluations at satisfaction, learning, and application levels. Ideally, but less often, such evaluations also en-

compass appraisal of their impact on the quality of patient care provided by nursing staff on the unit.

Satisfaction

Evaluations of orientation programs at the satisfaction level are typically secured from at least five different sources: (1) orientees, (2) preceptors, (3) other program faculty, (4) staff development educators, and (5) nurse managers.

Orientee

Evaluation of orientees' reaction or general satisfaction with various aspects of the orientation program may be obtained through informal or formal means and may be secured on an ongoing or summary basis. Informal determinations of orientees' reactions to the program may arise from serendipitous occasions when the preceptor, unit instructor, other nursing staff, educator, or nurse manager asks orientees about their impressions and experiences in the program. These queries often arise during the course of casual conversation on the unit or during breaks. Informal satisfaction appraisals may also be included at regularly scheduled meetings between the orientee and the preceptor, educator, and/or nurse manager as a means to keep communication channels open and to resolve any issues, problems, questions, or concerns that may arise. These ongoing informal evaluations might include inquiries such as the following:

- Did the self-learning package on patient admission procedures prepare you well for your first patient admission?
- Did the workshop on crisis intervention cover all of the questions you had?
- Are your patient assignments providing you with an adequate range of learning experiences?
- Are you progressing as quickly and smoothly as you had hoped?
- Do you need any additional instructional resources or practice sessions?

The orientee's responses to inquiries such as these can then be recorded on the learning contract or some other form used to document the orientation process.

Orientees are often asked to also provide more formal evaluations of the orientation program on an ongoing basis. These more formal appraisals may be related to specific learning experiences with classroom, laboratory, clinical, or self-directed instruction. The orientee's appraisal of individual learning activities in each of these settings provides immediate feedback for both the instructor and the program coordinator on how effective and useful the activity was from the orientee's perspective. An example of a sim-

---

*See initial discussion of these components in Chapter 5.

ple checklist that could be used for these evaluations is provided in Figure 6.5.

In addition to these ongoing appraisals of satisfaction, many hospitals also ask orientees to provide a summary evaluation of their reactions to the orientation program as a whole when they have completed all program requirements. Many of the same elements included in the ongoing evaluations are included here, but orientees are asked to generalize their appraisals to the overall program. Related features that may also be incorporated include the perceived degree of support they received from educators, other nursing staff on their unit, or nurse managers. An example of a checklist that might be used for this evaluation is provided in Figure 6.6. Some hospitals also provide follow-up evaluations of the orientation by requesting that orientees complete a similar appraisal at 6 to 12 months following completion of their orientation, when additional experience and perspective are available for reflection.

When a preceptorship format is employed for the orientation program, orientees are also asked to provide an evaluation of their experiences in the preceptorship and with their specific preceptor. An example of a form that could be used for the orientee's appraisal of the preceptorship process is provided in Figure 6.7.

Preceptor

Because of the pivotal role of preceptors in the orientation process, reactions and impressions regarding the program and the effectiveness of the preceptor-orientee relationship need to be determined. Figure 6.8 illustrates an evaluation form that could be used by preceptors for this purpose. Preceptor evaluations afford a wealth of information that can be used for planning future orientation programs as well as basic and advanced levels of the preceptor training program.

Other Program Faculty

Other program faculty who provide classroom or laboratory instruction may also be queried to determine their impressions regarding the orientation program. Faculty appraisals may include elements such as the adequacy of communication and support received before, during, and following their instruction period; their satisfaction with the learning experience provided; and identification of any problems or issues that arose from their presentation as well as any comments or suggestions they would like to offer for future programs. These evaluations are most easily obtained immediately after each learning activity they provide, when recollections are still full and readily identifiable.

Staff Development Educators

If staff development educators are division- or unit-based, they are likely to maintain close contact with both the or-

ientee and preceptor throughout the orientation program. Both ongoing and regularly scheduled meetings with these individuals provide the educator with input from each of these perspectives. In addition to monitoring and recording the effectiveness of the preceptor-orientee relationship and progress of the orientation, the educator may evaluate the need for staff development support of either or both members of this dyad. Documentation of the nature and extent of support requested or indicated can then be incorporated into future plans for the preceptor training program.

In the course of their ongoing monitoring of the preceptorship, educators may also be asked to look for indications that suggest needed changes in curriculum content coverage, sequencing, or time allotments; usefulness of audiovisual media and other instructional aids or reference materials; preparation or support of faculty; teaching methods employed; or evaluation tools or mechanisms. Thus, through their solicitation of the satisfaction of program providers and recipients as well as their monitoring of the orientation process as a whole, staff development educators can derive a considerable amount of useful information for program conduct and future curriculum planning.

Nurse Managers

Charge nurse, nurse manager, and division director input at the satisfaction level of evaluation affords a broad and necessary perspective regarding how well individual preceptor-orientee pairs are working as well as how the orientation affects the unit nursing staff and unit operations. Preceptorships often include regularly scheduled meetings of the unit nurse manager with the orientee and preceptor, alone and/or together to determine how each views the effectiveness and progress of this working group towards completion of the program's requirements. As a manager, the nurse manager is interested in determining the quality and effectiveness of this working relationship, eliciting any issues or problems that exist, and identifying ways in which support may be provided to either or both of these nurses. In addition, the manager will also determine whether the short- and long-term time frames established for completing the program are on schedule. Administrative assistance such as scheduling, patient assignments, unit rotations, and work load adjustments can also be identified and implemented at this time. The nurse manager's satisfaction with the effectiveness and efficiency of the orientation process can then be communicated to the educator so that any indicated educational support can be arranged.

Another important aspect for nurse manager evaluation is the determination of how the orientation program is affecting other nursing staff on the unit. Preceptors at times relate that they do not receive support from their peers when they function as preceptors. Some staff seem to resent preceptors not carrying their full patient work load when they precept, thereby leaving other nursing staff to assume

Topic: _____   Date: _____

Instructor: _____   Time: _____

Setting (check one):   ☐ classroom   ☐ laboratory   ☐ clinical   ☐ self-instruction

FEATURE	Excellent	Very Good	Good	Fair	Poor	Not Applicable
1. Content depth and scope						
2. Level of instruction						
3. Organization of instruction						
4. Clarity of instruction						
5. Teaching methods						
6. AV and instructional aids						
7. Usefulness of handouts, readings						
8. Personal objectives met						
9. Sufficient practice provided						
10. Sufficient time provided						

Comments or suggestions:

_____
Name (optional)

Figure 6.5 Evaluation of classroom learning experience.

a heavier patient assignment than usual to cover patient care needs. Disagreements over patient assignments or resentment that orientees leave the unit for classes or that preceptors leave the unit to teach classes may precipitate anything from subdued to angry reactions from the staff. Unless nurse managers take the initiative to plan staffing coverage that avoids or minimizes these situations, staff will continue to feel put upon. Keeping open lines of communication with staff, monitoring the effects of the orientation on smooth and safe work-flow patterns on the unit, and dealing proactively with fluctuations in staffing needs can keep these feelings of resentment and anger to a minimum. Expecting staff to accept burdensome or dangerously heavy workloads under the auspices of team spirit not only extinguishes *esprit de corps* but potentially jeopardizes quality patient care.

Orientee: _____   Date orientation started: _____

Unit: _____   Date orientation completed: _____

Instructions: Please rate each of the following features for your orientation experience.

FEATURE	Excellent	Very Good	Good	Fair	Poor	Comments
1. Quality of classroom instruction						
2. Quality of laboratory instruction						
3. Quality of clinical instruction						
4. Quality of self-instruction modules						
5. Depth and scope of instruction						
6. Level of instruction						
7. Clarity of instruction						
8. Teaching methods						
9. AV and instructional aids						
10. Usefulness of handouts, readings						
11. Personal objectives met						
12. Sufficient practice provided						
13. Sufficient time provided						
14. Support from educators						
15. Support from nursing staff						
16. Support from nurse managers						
17. Usefulness of written exercises						
18. Fairness of written tests						
19. Clarity of clinical skills list						
20. Helpfulness of meetings with preceptor(s)						
21. Helpfulness of meetings with nurse manager						
22. Helpfulness of meetings with educator(s)						

	NO	YES	If "yes," please explain below
23. Were any important areas/topics *missing* in your orientation?			
24. Did your orientation include any areas/topics that could be omitted?			

	YES	NO	If "no," please explain below
25. Did your orientation prepare you to function in a safe and effective manner as a staff nurse on your assigned unit?			

26. Please list those areas in which you need additional instruction or practice over the next 6 to 12 months:
    a. _____
    b. _____
    c. _____
    d. _____

27. If you have any other comments, critiques, or suggestions to offer in relation to your orientation program, please relate these here:

Figure 6.6 Orientee evaluation of orientation program.

Orientee: _____   Date orientation started: _____

Preceptor: _____   Date orientation completed: _____

Unit: _____

Instructions: Please rate each of the following features for the preceptorship and add any additional comments you wish to make.

FEATURE	Excellent	Very Good	Good	Fair	Poor	Comments
1. Preceptor as a role model: a. Demonstration of clinical procedures						
b. Demonstration of collaboration with other nursing staff						
c. Demonstration of collaboration with healthcare team						
d. Demonstration of collaboration with nurse managers						
e. Demonstration of professional role responsibilities (related to QA, standards, giving reports, etc.)						
2. Assistance with socialization a. Introduction to other staff						
b. Made to feel welcomed, accepted						
c. Helped to feel part of healthcare team						
3. Assistance with assessment of learning needs a. Recognized past experience, education						
b. Incorporated self-evaluations into assessments						
c. Validated learning needs						
4. Assistance with planning learning experiences a. Suitability of patient assignments to capability level						
b. Range of assignments offered						
c. Opportunities for increasingly more autonomous functioning commensurate with ability						
d. Assistance in drafting and updating learning contract terms						
e. Provision of shift rotations, as appropriate						

Continued.

Figure 6.7 Orientee evaluation of preceptorship.

FEATURE	Excellent	Very Good	Good	Fair	Poor	Comments
5. Assistance with implementing learning plan a. Quality (organization, clarity, sequence) of clinical instruction						
b. Effectiveness of clinical teaching methods						
c. Provision of sufficient clinical practice						
d. Explanations of physiology, pathophysiology, treatments, medications, etc.						
e. Accessibility and availability of preceptor when needed						
f. Support in attainment of program outcomes						
6. Assistance with evaluation of learning a. Helpfulness of daily reviews of performance						
b. Helpfulness of weekly progress meetings						
c. Clarity of feedback on performance						
d. Provision of both positive and negative feedback, as appropriate						
e. Provision of constructive feedback						
f. Provision of timely feedback						
g. Assistance in completing all entries in clinical skills checklist						
7. Overall quality of preceptorship						

Other comments or suggestions:

Figure 6.7—cont'd Orientee evaluation of preceptorship.

Learning

Orientation programs are evaluated at the learning level to determine whether the instruction provided resulted in the desired changes sought in the orientee's knowledge, attitudes, and/or skills. In a traditional approach to instruction, where the majority of behaviors contained in the instructional objectives are within the cognitive domain, a heavy reliance on written tests for evaluation of learning is typically employed. Affective behaviors are evaluated in written, simulated, or clinical settings, and psychomotor behaviors are usually appraised in either simulated or real clinical situations.

When a competency-based approach is used for the orientation program, a few adjustments in the types of evaluation employed are generally warranted. These changes include the following three modifications:

Preceptor: _____   Date orientation started: _____

Orientee: _____   Date orientation completed: _____

Unit: _____

Instructions: Please rate each of the following features for the preceptorship and add any additional comments you wish to make.

FEATURE	YES	NO	If "no," please explain below
1. In general, are you satisfied with the quality of this preceptorship?			
2. Did you have sufficient time with the orientee to complete all requirements of the orientation?			
3. During the preceptorship, were you sufficiently relieved from your normal workload to work with your orientee?			
4. Were you able to be immediately available when your orientee needed you?			
5. Did you understand the responsibilities of your role as a preceptor?			
6. Did the preceptor training program prepare you for your responsibilities as a preceptor?			
7. Did you receive adequate support from nursing staff development?			
8. Did you receive adequate support from other nursing staff on the unit?			
9. Did you receive adequate support from nurse managers?			
10. Did you receive adequate feedback on your performance as a preceptor?			
	YES	NO	If "yes," please explain below
11. Did you encounter any learning/teaching problems working with this orientee?			
12. Did you experience any interpersonal problems in working with this orientee?			
13. Did you experience any problems in using the clinical skills checklist?			
14. Did you encounter any problems with patient access for planning learning experiences?			
15. Did you experience any problems with use of learning contracts during this orientation?			

Other comments, critiques, or suggestions:

Figure 6.8 Preceptor evaluation of preceptorship.

- *Decreased reliance on written tests.* Because being knowledgeable in an area is not equivalent to being clinically competent in that area, CBO programs rely less on written tests since these evaluation tools only verify the cognitive component of clinical competence. Before nurses can function in a competent manner, they must first possess the knowledge base that underlies nursing practice. However, verification that this knowledge base exists affords no guarantee that the nurse can transfer and apply that knowledge to nursing practice in actual patient care situations. In CBO programs, therefore, appraisal of purely cognitive behaviors is usually reserved for a few areas. These might include the following:

> Areas that do not readily lend themselves to evaluation either in a clinical setting or in a simulated situation (e.g., evaluation of an orientee's knowledge of drug incompatibilities or side effects)

> Areas that have a limited direct clinical practice component (e.g., knowledge of the etiology or pathophysiology of various disease states or knowledge of the indications for hemodialysis or thoracentesis)

> Areas that relate to comprehending theories and principles that operate in patient care situations (e.g., principles of osmosis and diffusion operative in peritoneal dialysis, principles of cerebral autoregulation, or the principle of negative thoracic pressure in relation to chest tubes)

> Areas that are important for a nurse to know but that occur infrequently in the clinical setting (e.g., equipment malfunction)

For limited situations such as these, written tests remain an appropriate vehicle to validate the cognitive components of competency. These written tests are constructed and their test items are drafted using the same guidelines as described in Chapter 5. In addition, item analysis is performed in the same manner to verify the structural integrity of the evaluation tool. Assuming that the areas included as performance criteria were restricted to essential components of competency, the passing scores established for these written tests are usually set high (90% or higher). However, the passing score is not set at 100%, to allow for the possibility of measurement error and weaknesses either in the test blueprint or in test item construction. Since item analysis results rarely indicate ideal difficulty and discrimination indices for all test items, the educator needs to take these considerations into account in establishing the passing score.

- *Increased reliance on simulations for evaluation.* Evaluation of orientees in simulated situations affords a more valid and reliable measure of clinical competence than do written tests because simulated apprais-

als require orientees to actually perform as expected rather than merely to demonstrate that they are knowledgeable about a procedure. The artificiality of simulated situations, however, imposes a noteworthy admonition for the educator to bear in mind: although a simulated situation can be designed to resemble an actual clinical situation very closely, the two are not equivalent. Verifying that an orientee can perform correctly in a make-believe situation is, as with written tests, no absolute guarantee that they will do so in a real situation. But because of the closer parallels that exist between a simulated and a real situation, one can have commensurately greater confidence regarding clinical competency from the results of a simulation than one can have from a purely cognitive appraisal device. Rather than requiring only demonstration of knowledge, the simulation requires demonstration that orientees can apply their knowledge in practice.

The outcomes most suitably appraised in a simulated setting for a CBO program are determined by using the same general guidelines as previously described for simulations in Chapter 4. Thus simulated scenarios are appropriate for evaluation of an orientee's competency in situations that require control of environmental variables, in situations that involve a potential risk for patients or staff, or in specific emergency situations.

- *Maximal reliance on clinical evaluations.* The most valid means of evaluating orientees' clinical competence is achieved through appraisal of their performance in actual patient care situations on their assigned unit. Observation of a nurse's clinical practice in the normal work setting affords the most realistic circumstances for evaluation because all of the conditions and variables that normally exist for nursing practice on that unit are operative there. The contrived conditions characteristic of simulated situations (e.g., no patient or family interactions, no noise or other distractions or pressures) are now replaced by realistic conditions of everyday nursing practice. Rather than assuming that orientees will transfer and apply their knowledge, attitudes, and skills to real patient care situations, the preceptor or educator has a first-hand view of orientee performance under realistic circumstances. No assumptions regarding orientee abilities are necessary when reality is used to evaluate learning. For evaluations in both simulated and actual clinical settings, the evaluation tool employed is the performance checklist described earlier* and illustrated in Figure 6.2. As can be seen in this figure, the checklist includes all performance criteria as they were originally formulated during the assessment phase. Unlike traditional orientation programs, where instructional objectives need to be transformed and ex-

---

*See discussion of validation of orientee's educational needs in assessment section.

panded into a checklist such as this, in CBO this additional step is already accomplished at the time that the performance criteria are developed.

Application

Evaluation of orientation programs at the application level seeks to determine whether learning secured in the classroom, laboratory, or clinical setting is evidenced in the orientee's nursing practice. In contrast to verification of the orientee's performance on written tests or under simulated conditions, appraisals of learning at the application level verify that orientees are able to take what they have learned elsewhere and apply it to daily nursing care of real patients on their unit.

Application level evaluations may have either a short-term or long-term horizon. Short-term applications of learning are the type most often used in orientation programs. The time horizon is short-term because the time between the provision of instruction and conduct of the evaluation is brief—perhaps hours to days or a few weeks. All performance criteria and competency areas evaluated in the clinical setting can be categorized as short-term evaluations at the application level.

Hospitals that extend this evaluation to a long-term perspective accomplish this by conducting additional follow-up appraisals of orientee clinical performance at 6,[120] 12, and/or 18 months after completion of orientation. Appraisals of performance (either the full set or only selected competencies) using this longer time horizon verify whether learning and competence attained during the orientation have been maintained over time. Such appraisals answer the question of whether competency initially demonstrated has persisted over the time period selected.

Impact

Evaluation of an orientation program at the impact level seeks to determine whether the orientation process results in a measurable enhancement in the quality of nursing care delivered to patients. For reasons cited in Chapter 5 (cost, the large number of intervening variables, lack of resources to design and construct measurement tools, etc.), impact evaluations are rarely performed for orientation programs.

One way in which impact evaluation of orientation could be accomplished would be to join the outcomes of the CBO program with those used for the nursing department's total quality monitoring (TQM) and total quality improvement (TQI) program. The nursing department's TQI/TQM program could select performance criteria from the CBO program as quality indicators for nursing practice and establish threshold levels for each performance criterion statement. These indicators and thresholds could then be used to monitor the quality of patient care delivered by nurses who were at various lengths of service, following completion of their orientation program. A joint endeavor

such as this could simultaneously achieve three beneficial results:

- A reasonably easy mechanism would be established to provide impact evaluation of the orientation program for any desired time frame following completion of the orientation program.
- The effects of the orientation component of staff development would be linked directly with its ultimate purpose—that is, quality patient care.
- The endeavor would support compliance with JCAHO standards that require documentation that the effectiveness and appropriateness of orientation be evaluated through its quality assessment and improvement activities.

Rather than viewing evaluation of orientation programs as purely a staff development issue divorced from other hospital programs, a marriage of the orientation and TQM initiatives recognizes their inherent interrelatedness in contributing to optimal delivery of patient care services.

EVALUATING THE EFFICIENCY OF AN ORIENTATION PROGRAM

As mentioned earlier, the efficiency of an educational program relates to the amount of resources required to provide instruction. Every staff development program has certain fixed costs that are incurred regardless of the number of participants and other variable costs that change depending on the number of learners. Both fixed and variable expenses for an orientation program can be subdivided into a number of categories. A summary of these expenses is provided in Table 6.12.

Orientation programs can be made more efficient by reducing any of the costs associated with the program. One of the benefits of using a competency-based educational approach to orientation is the possibility of lowering a number of these costs. Because CBE allows for flexibility in the teaching strategies used for instruction, hospitals can reduce their instructional labor costs by instituting or expanding use of self-instructional materials such as self-learning packages, audiovisual programs, and computer-assisted instruction. Increased use of these self-teaching methods enables the institution to provide instruction with less labor-intensive means rather than paying salary and benefits for classroom teachers. Since orientees can take advantage of challenge mechanisms and use self-instruction only to the degree they require, the time necessary for completion of orientation can also be reduced. This will decrease the costs of labor not only for orientees' salaries but also for the salaries (and benefits) paid to their classroom and laboratory instructors as well as their clinical preceptors. Although the design and development of self-instructional materials increases program costs initially, the long-term benefits result in savings of subsequent instructional time for both orientees and faculty and are paid back as an

TABLE 6.12 • SUMMARY OF FIXED AND VARIABLE COSTS FOR ORIENTATION PROGRAMS

Category	Fixed Expenses	Variable Expenses
Labor	Salary and benefits: • Program development, planning, evaluation, and revision • In-house faculty (classroom, laboratory, clinical instructors) • Clerical staff support • Audiovisual staff support • Completing CEU (Continuing Education Unit) application forms (and application fee)	Salary and benefits: • Orientees: until orientation is completed • Preceptors: until orientee is able to function independently • Staffing coverage: until preceptors are able to resume normal workloads • Instructors: depends on amount of self-instruction used
Overhead	Use of facilities: rent, utilities, room setup, room cleaning Room rental: classroom or laboratory space	
Materials	Instructional materials: • Audiovisual hardware • Audiovisual software (slides, videotapes, audio tapes, etc.) • Teaching aids (charts, models, etc.) • Instructional supplies (overhead transparencies, easel paper, markers, chalk, etc)	Duplication of handouts, readings, and other instructional materials Folders, packets, or binders Name tags Printed CEU certificates, completion certificates
Time	Hospital orientation program (if fixed duration) Nursing department orientation (if fixed duration)	Depends on maximum length of time for completion of orientation Unit orientation depends on whether challenge mechanism, self-paced instruction are available
Food		Refreshments for breaks Meals provided

investment to the hospital in a relatively short period of time.

If self-directed instruction is used, costs associated with classroom rental or overhead expenses will decrease because orientees can use these materials wherever and whenever they find it convenient. Rather than incurring the expense of using large classrooms, individual study carrels in the hospital library or learning center can be employed. If large classes are not held, the costs for refreshments can also be avoided. Although use of a competency-based approach to orientation cannot guarantee greater program efficiency, the principal tenets of this approach open multiple windows of opportunity to achieve greater long-term program efficiency.

REFERENCES

1. Abbasi SM, Hollman KW: Managing cultural diversity: the challenge of the '90s, *Records Manage Quart* 10:24, 1991.
2. Aldrich S: A neuroscience internship and graduate nurse role conception, *J Neurosci Nurs* 20:377, 1988.
3. Alspach JG, ed.: *A competency-based orientation program for a medical/surgical intensive care unit,* Aliso Viejo, CA, 1990, American Association of Critical-Care Nurses.
4. Alspach JG: A critical care nursing internship program, *Superv Nurse* 9(9):31, 1978.
5. Alspach JG: Critical care orientation: a discussion of survey results, *Crit Care Nurse* 10(6):10, 1990.
6. Alspach JG: Critical care orientation programs: reader survey report, *Crit Care Nurse* 10(5):22, 1990.
7. Alspach JG: Designing a competency-based orientation for critical care nurses, *Heart Lung* 13(6):655, 1984.
8. Alspach JG: *How to develop a critical care internship program.* Paper presented at Chesapeake Bay Area Chapter and Greater Washington (DC) Area Chapter, American Association of Critical-Care Nurses, Critical Care Nursing Conference, Columbia, MD, February 28, 1992.
9. Alspach JG: Preceptor survey report: part I, *Crit Care Nurse* 9(5):2, 1989.
10. Alspach JG: Preceptor survey report: part II, *Crit Care Nurse* 9(6):2, 1989.
11. Alspach JG: *From staff nurse to preceptor: a preceptor training program—Instructor's manual* and *Preceptor handbook,* Aliso Viejo, CA, 1988, American Association of Critical-Care Nurses.
12. Alspach JG: The preceptor's bill of rights, *Crit Care Nurse* 7(1):1, 1987.
13. American Association of Critical-Care Nurses. *Integration of new graduates into critical care,* Newport Beach, CA, 1988, AACN.
14. American Nurses' Association: *Standards for nursing staff development,* Kansas City, Mo, 1990, ANA.
15. American Society for Healthcare Education and Training: *Compe-*

tency assessment: challenges and opportunities for health care educators, Chicago, 1992, American Hospital Association.

16. Arbeiter JS: The facts about foreign nurses, *RN* 51(9):56, 1988.

17. Archbold, CR: Our nurse-interns are a sound investment, *RN* 40(9):105, 1977.

18. Balacki MF: A competency-based tool for the clinical orientation and evaluation of psychiatric nurses, *N Y State Nurses Assoc Bull* 19(1):11, 1988.

19. Baylay EW, Ravreby AW: Development of competency-based orientation for burn nursing, *J Burn Care Rehab* 4(1):36, 1983.

20. Becker J, Ellson SK: How to develop a competency-based head nurse orientation program, *J Healthcare Educ Train* 4(3):32, 1990.

21. Benner P: *From novice to expert,* Menlo Park, CA, 1984, Addison-Wesley.

22. Bertucci RC: Orientation of temporary staff, *J Nurs Staff Develop* 4(1):34, 1988.

23. Bitgood, G: Critical care nurse-intern program, *Superv Nurse* 7(10):42, 1976.

24. Bliss JB, Alsdorf P: Generic orientation for agency nurses, *J Cont Educ Nurs* 23(2):60, 1992.

25. Borovies DL, Newman NA: Graduate nurse transition program, *Am J Nurs* 81(10):1832, 1981.

26. Brasler ME: Predictors of clinical performance of new graduate nurses participating in preceptor orientation programs, *J Cont Educ Nurs* 24(4):158, 1993.

27. Burrell B, Lally E, Wiklinski B: Internships for A.D. graduates, *Am J Nurs* 77(1):114, 1977.

28. Bushong N, Simms S: Externships: A way to bridge the gap, *Superv Nurse* 10(6):14, 1979.

29. Carroll P: Using personality styles to enhance preceptor programs, *Dimens Crit Care Nurs* 11(2):114, 1992.

30. Clark LE: A nurse educator's view of employing new graduates in critical care settings, *Focus Crit Care* 13(4):16, 1986.

31. Claytor KL: Working effectively with LPN-RN orientees, *J Cont Educ Nurs* 24(5):227, 1993.

32. Coco CD: A report on nurse internship programs, *Superv Nurse* 7(12):12, 1976.

33. Collins M, Moyer K. Integrating a critical care internship with a career ladder, *J Cont Educ Nurs* 18(2):51, 1987.

34. Copeland L: Cross-cultural training: the competitive edge, *Training* 22(7):49, 1985.

35. Cooney AT: An orientation program for new graduate nurses: the basis for staff development and retention, *J Cont Educ Nurs* 23(5):216, 1992.

36. Craver DM, Sullivan PP: Investigation of an internship program, *J Cont Educ Nurs* 16(4):114, 1985.

37. Dear ML, Celentano D, Weisman C et al: Evaluating a hospital nursing internship, *J Nurs Admin* 16(11):16, 1982.

38. deBlois CA: Adult preceptor education: a literature review, *J Nurs Staff Develop* 7(3):148, 1991.

39. Delatte AP, Baytos L: Guidelines for successful diversity training, *Training* 30(1):55, 1993.

40. del Bueno DJ, Quaife MC: Special orientation unit pays off, *Am J Nurs* 76:1629, 1976.

41. del Bueno DJ, Weeks L, Brown-Stewart P: Clinical assessment centers: a cost-effective alternative for competency development, *Nurs Econ* 5(1):21, 1987.

42. DiMauro K, Mack LB: A competency-based orientation program for the clinical nurse specialist, *J Cont Educ Nurs* 20(2):74, 1989.

43. Doherty MH: Preceptorship program for the small hospital, *Dimens Crit Care Nurs* 7:313, 1988.

44. Duffield C: Role competencies of first-line managers, *Nurs Manag* 23(6):49, 1992.

45. Eaton SM, Lowe T: Filipino GN to Filipino RN, *J Nurs Staff Develop* 7(5):225, 1991.

46. Eliason MJ, Macy NJ: A classroom activity to introduce cultural diversity, *Nurs Educator* 17(3):32, 1992.

47. Farmer ML: Competency-based orientation proved effective, *J Nurs Staff Develop* 2(3):126, 1986.

48. Faulhaber JA, Coleman JA, Cardwell RL: Orthopedic orientation: a guide for new nurses, *AORN J* 46(4):706, 1987.

49. Fenton MV: Identifying competencies of clinical nurse specialists, *J Nurs Admin* 15:31, 1985.

50. Ferraro AR: Developing a competency-based orientation program: the challenge of a multidisciplinary pediatric unit, *J Pediatr Nurs* 4(5):325, 1989.

51. Ferris L: Continuing education module for developing staff skills in precepting and staff development, *J Cont Educ Nurs* 19(1):28, 1988.

52. Fleming BW, Woodcock AG, Boyd BT: From student to staff nurse: a nurse internship program, *Am J Nurs* 75(4):595, 1975.

53. Frederiksen LW, Myers JB, Riley AW: A case for cross-training, *Training* 23(2):37, 1986.

54. Freeman A, McMaster D, Hamilton L: Staff development program for critical care nurses, *Crit Care Nurse* 3(2):86, 1983.

55. Fritsch-deBruyn RR: A process for determining content for a nurse internship program, *J Cont Educ Nurs* 21(3):118, 1990.

56. Gaffney TM, Anselmi-Majoros K, Vitello-Cicciu J: Competency-based education in thrombolytic therapy: a modular approach, *J Cardiovasc Nurs* 4(1):57, 1989.

57. Giles PF, Moran V: Preceptor program evaluation demonstrates improved orientation, *J Nurs Staff Develop* 5(1):17, 1989.

58. Glynn NJ, Bishop GR: Multiculturalism in nursing: implications for faculty development, *J Nurs Educ* 25(1):39, 1986.

59. Greipp ME: Nursing preceptors: looking back, looking ahead, *J Nurs Staff Develop* 5:183, 1989.

60. Hagerty BK: A competency-based orientation program for psychiatric nursing, *J Cont Educ Nurs* 16(5):157, 1986.

61. Haggard A: *Hospital orientation handbook,* Rockville, MD, 1984, Aspen Systems Corporation.

62. Hamilton EM, Murray MK, Lindholm LH et al: Effects of mentoring on job satisfaction, leadership behaviors, and job retention of new graduate nurses, *J Nurs Staff Develop* 5(4):159, 1989.

63. Hartshorn JC: Characteristics of critical care nursing internship programs, *J Nurs Staff Develop* 8(5):218, 1992.

64. Hast AS, Naser-Knapik M, Fasnacht-Allison CJ: Orienting occasional staff to critical care, *Crit Care Nurs* 9(5):86, 1989.

65. Hast AS, Serish A: Cross-training programs in critical care, *Crit Care Nurs* 6(6):74, 1986.

66. Hilliard M: *Orientation and evaluation of the professional nurse,* St Louis, 1974, Mosby.

67. Hitchings KS: Preceptors promote competence and retention: strategies to achieve success, *J Cont Educ Nurs* 20(6):255, 1989.

68. Holtz C, Wilson C: The culturally diverse student: a model for empowerment, *Nurs Educator* 17(6):28, 1992.

69. Houge MC, Deines ES: Verifying clinical competency in critical care, *Dimens Crit Care Nurs* 6:102, 1987.

70. Hudgins CL: Critical care competency-based orientation, *Crit Care Nurse* 11(8):78, 11(9):5870; 11(10):11, 1991.

71. Hughes L: Employment of new graduates: implications for critical care nursing practice, *Focus Crit Care* 14(4):9, 1987.

72. Inman L, Haugen C: Six criteria to evaluate skill competency documentation, *Dimens Crit Care Nurs* 10(4):238, 1991.

73. Jackson BS: Agency nursing: costs and quality, *J Nurs Admin* 19(6):5, 1989.

74. James LA: Orientation through self-study, *J Nurs Staff Develop* 9(5):85, 1993.

75. Joint Commission on Accreditation of Healthcare Organizations: *Accreditation manual for hospitals,* vol 1, Oakbrook Terrace, IL, 1994, JCAHO.

76. Kaeter M: Cross-training: the tactical view, *Training* 30(3):35, 1993.

77. Kasprisin C, Young W: Nurse internship program reduces turnover, raises commitment, *Nurs Health Care* 6:137, 1985.

78. Keller C, Bowen M: CBE for first-line managers, *Nurse Manage* 15(11):63, 1984.

79. Kopp MEA, Laskowski-Jones L, Morelli PK et al: Critical care nurse internship: in theory and practice, *Crit Care Nurse* 13(4): in press, 1993.

80. Kramer M: *Reality shock: why nurses leave nursing,* St Louis, 1974, Mosby.

81. Lachance-Everhart R: Transfer orientation: developing a retraining program, *J Nurs Staff Develop* 17(4):122, 1986.

82. Lawinger SJ: Competency-based orientation program for a surgical intensive therapy unit, *Crit Care Nurse* 11(4):36; 11(5):52; 11(6):20; 11(7):44, 1991.

83. Lee C: Cross-cultural training: don't leave home without it, *Training* 20(7):20, 1983.

84. Leidy K: Effective screening and orientation of independent contract nurses, *J Cont Educ Nurs* 23(2):64, 1992.

85. Leininger M: Cultural diversity in health and nursing care, *Nurs Clin N Am* 12(1):9, 1977.

86. Lewis KE: University-based preceptor programs: solving the problems, *J Nurs Staff Develop* 6(1):17, 1990.

87. Lewison D, Gibbons LK: Nursing internships: a comprehensive review of the literature, *J Cont Educ Nurs* 11(2):32, 1980.

88. Lohrman JM, Kinkade SL: *Competency-based orientation for critical care nursing,* St Louis, 1992, Mosby.

89. Martin B: Developing retention strategies within your internship program, *Dimens Crit Care Nurs* 8(1):50, 1989.

90. Maslow AH: *Toward a psychology of being,* Princeton, MA, 1968, VanNostrand.

91. Mattson S: The need for cultural concepts in nursing curricula, *J Nurs Educ* 26(5):206, 1987.

92. May L: Clinical preceptors for new nurses, *Am J Nurs* 80:1824, 1980.

93. McGrath BJ, Princeton JC: Evaluation of a clinical preceptor program for new graduates—eight years later, *J Cont Educ Nurs* 18(4):133, 1987.

94. McGregor RJ: A framework for developing staff competencies, *J Nurs Staff Develop* 6(2):79, 1990.

95. Metzger NJ: Revising the preceptor concept: cross training nursing staff, *J Nurs Staff Develop* 2(2):70, 1986.

96. Miller DM, Brosovich DL: Maintaining an effective preceptor program, *Focus Crit Care* 19(1):81, 1991.

97. Mims B. A critical care internship program, *Dimens Crit Care Nurs* 13(1):53, 1984.

98. Mirabile R, Caldwell D, O'Reilly C: Soft skills, hard numbers, *Training* 24(8):53, 1987.

99. Modic MB, Bowman C: Developing a preceptor program: what are the ingredients? *J Nurs Staff Develop* 5(2):78, 1989.

100. Morton HR, Himes JK, Stevens B: The foreign nurse program: an innovative NCLEX review, *J Nurs Staff Develop* 23(2):81, 1992.

101. Murphy ML, Hammerstad SM: Preparing a staff nurse for precepting, *Nurse Educator* 6(5):17, 1981.

102. Myrick F: Preceptorship: is it the answer to the problems in clinical teaching? *J Nurs Educ* 27:136, 1988.

103. Nederveld ME: Preceptorship: one step beyond, *J Nurs Staff Develop* 6(4):186, 1990.

104. Neumark AI, Flaherty MA, Girard FA: Individualized orientation in critical care, *Focus Crit Care* 14(5):35, 1987.

105. O'Connor CT: Competency-based orientation, *J Nurs Staff Develop* 5(6):286, 1989.

106. O'Friel JAB: The nurse internship experience, *J Nurs Staff Develop* 9(1):24, 1993.

107. O'Neal EA: An orientation designed for nurses in an ambulatory care setting, *J Cont Educ Nurs* 17(1):32, 1986.

108. Parker BK: The tie that binds: new employee orientation (module IV). In American Hospital Association: *American society for healthcare education and training resource manual,* Chicago, 1992, AHA.

109. Paterniti AP: Using Montessori's concepts on a transitional orientation nursing unit, *J Nurs Staff Develop* 3(2):71, 1987.

110. Payette E, Porter Y: Preceptor training: a practical approach, *J Cont Educ Nurs* 20:188, 1989.

111. Peterson KJ: Competency-based orientation program for a cardiovascular surgery unit, *Crit Care Nurse* 11(2):32; 11(3):17, 1991.

112. Phillips S, Hartley JT: Teaching students for whom English is a second language, *Nurse Educator* 15(5):29, 1990.

113. Pilette PC: Recruitment and retention of international nurses aided by recognition of phases of the adjustment process, *J Cont Educ Nurs* 20(6):277, 1989.

114. Plasse NJ, Lederer JR: Preceptors: a resource for new nurses, *Superv Nurse* 12(6):35, 1981.

115. Porter SF: Ensuring competency: toward a competency-based orientation format, *Crit Care Quar* 7:42, 1984.

116. Prociuk JL: Self-directed learning and nursing orientation programs: are they compatible? *J Cont Educ Nurs* 21(6):252, 1990.

117. Ressler KA, Kruger NR, Herb TA: Evaluating a critical care internship program, *Dimens Crit Care Nurs* 10(3):176, 1991.

118. Roberson JE: Providing support for preceptors in a community hospital, *J Nurs Staff Develop* 8(1):11, 1992.

119. Roell SM. Nurse-intern programs: how they're working, *J Nurs Admin* 11(10):33, 1981.

120. Rottet SM, Cervero RM: Clinical evaluation of a nursing orientation program, *J Nurs Staff Develop* 2(3):110, 1986.

121. Sams L, Baxter K, Palmer-Smith P: A competency-based model for nurse internships, *J Nurs Staff Develop* 6(2):93, 1990.

122. Schempp CM, Rompre RM: Transition programs for new graduates—how effective are they? *J Nurs Staff Develop* 2(4):150, 1986.

123. Schmaus D: Competency-based education—its implementation in the OR, *AORN J* 45(2):474, 1987.

124. Selfridge J: A competency-based orientation for the emergency department, *J Emer Nurs* 10(5): 246, 1984.

125. Shogan JO, Prior MM, Kolski BJ: A preceptor program: nurses helping nurses, *J Cont Educ Nurs* 16(4):139, 1985.

126. Smith MF, Altieri MJ: Competence based assessment of critical care nurses, *Focus Crit Care* 15(6):17, 1988.

127. Snyder-Halperin R, Buczkowski E: Performance-based staff development: a baseline for clinical competency, *J Nurs Staff Develop* 6(1):7, 1990.

128. Spicer JG: Pitfalls in developing nurse internship programs, *Nurs Admin Q* 3(3):69, 1979.

129. Stewart SL, Vitello-Cicciu JM: Designing a competency-based orientation program for the care of cardiac surgical patients, *J Cardiovasc Nurs* 3(3):34, 1989.

130. Stokes RA: Streamlining orientation for hemodialysis nursing: a competency-based approach, *ANNA J* 18(1) 33, 1991.

131. Strauser CJ: An internship with academic credit, *Am J Nurs* 79(6):1071, 1979.

132. Thiederman S: *Bridging cultural barriers for corporate success: how to manage the multicultural work force,* New York, 1991, Lexington Books.

133. Treloar DM: Strategies for bridging the knowledge/practice gap, *Focus AACN* 9(1):12, 1982.

134. Training foreign professionals: a case of mismatched agendas, *Training* 28(10):18, 1991.

135. Tuck I, Harris LH: Teaching students transcultural concepts, *Nurse Educator* 13(3):36, 1988.

136. Young S, Theriault J, Collins D: The nurse preceptor: preparation and needs, *J Nurs Staff Develop* 5(3):127, 1989.

137. Wallace PL, Mundie GE: Contract learning in orientation, *J Nurs Staff Develop* 3(4):143, 1987.

138. Weiss SJ, Ramsey E. An interagency internship: a key to transitional adaptation, *J Nurs Admin* 7(10):36, 1977.

139. Westra RJ, Graziano MJ: Preceptors: a comparison of their perceived needs before and after the preceptor experience, *J Cont Educ Nurs* 23(5):212, 1992.

140. Willey SP, Gillis DM: Orienting British Isle nurses to the American healthcare system, *J Cont Educ Nurs* 20(3):124, 1989.

141. Williams J: Orienting foreign nurse graduates through preceptors, *J Nurs Staff Develop* 8(4):155, 1992.

142. Williams J, Baker G, Clark B et al: Collaborative preceptor training: a creative approach in tough times, *J Cont Educ Nurs* 24(4):153, 1993.

143. Williams J, Rogers S: The multicultural workplace: preparing preceptors, *J Cont Educ Nurs* 24(3):101, 1993.

In-Service Education and Continuing Education

IN-SERVICE EDUCATION

DEFINITION

The American Nurses' Association (ANA) *Standards for Nursing Staff Development*[5] defines *in-service education* as "activities intended to assist the professional nurse in acquiring, maintaining, and/or increasing competence in fulfilling the assigned responsibilities specific to the expectations of the employer." The American Society for Healthcare Education and Training (ASHET)[6] defines it as "instruction relating to the education and training necessary to perform job-related duties." As mentioned in Chapter 1, the goal of in-service education is to ensure that all nursing personnel maintain competency in their respective positions following completion of their orientation and throughout their employment at that facility

CHARACTERISTICS

In contrast to orientation programs, in-service education programs typically have the following characteristics:

- Shorter duration (15 to 60 minutes per session)
- More informal structure and presentation styles
- Conducted in or immediately adjacent to the work site
- Shorter interval between instruction and evaluation of learning
- May involve faculty who are not hospital staff members
- Often involve only small groups of learners

DIMENSIONS

The ANA definition of in-service education can be used to distinguish the three important dimensions of this component of staff development:

- *Acquisition of competency.* Refers to acquiring competency in areas such as new policies, procedures, equipment, treatments, medications, products, monitoring systems, and the like that were introduced after the nurse's completion of orientation. This dimension may also include areas that are considered important to the nurse's assigned job responsibilities but not covered within the orientation program.
- *Maintenance of competency.* Refers to verification that competency has persisted in practice areas deemed important by the hospital or by various accrediting or regulating agencies. Examples would include all of the safety areas, such as fire safety, electrical safety, and universal precautions mandated by the Joint Commission on Accreditation of Healthcare Organizations (JCAHO) or by the Occupational Safety and Health Administration (OSHA).
- *Increase of competency.* Refers to the development of additional competency areas for nursing practice. These areas may include any local programs the hospital may use to certify or credential nurses to perform specific functions at the agency (such as defibrillation, endotracheal intubation, or arterial puncture) and that are added to the customary job responsibilities of someone occupying that role.

Acquisition of Competency
Acquisition of New Information

In-service education devoted to the acquisition of competency is an essential ingredient in professional competence because the knowledge base and rate of new developments in healthcare far outpace the ability of most healthcare professionals to "keep up." It is estimated that the volume of biomedical information made available to healthcare professionals doubles every 3 to 5 years.[100] A related estimate is that the half-life of knowledge for any given profession may be as brief as 2 to 3 years.[39] Because nursing is not immune to this information explosion in healthcare, it becomes imperative that nurses continue to acquire new areas of competency as contemporary understanding and revised or new health practices emerge.

Because the scientific and therapeutic bases of nursing practice are continually evolving, in-service offerings will always need to address these evolutionary changes so that nursing staff can keep apprised of developments that affect their practice and provide state-of-the-art levels of patient care. The range of possible inclusions for in-service offerings related to acquisition of competency consists of any of the following "new" elements:

- Hospital or nursing department policies
- Hospital or nursing department procedures
- Patient care protocols, routines, or standing orders
- Products
- Medications
- Therapies
- Technologies
- Equipment
- Patient care delivery systems
- Documentation formats or forms
- Monitoring systems
- Patient classification systems
- Disease entities
- Scientific findings or interpretations of findings
- Understandings related to the etiology, pathophysiology, diagnosis, or management of health problems

In-service offerings devoted to specific topics such as those listed enable nurses to keep up to date with new developments and continually refine their practice to meet current and future expectations of their employer.

Acquisition of "Good-to-Know" Areas

A second inclusion in this dimension of in-service offerings consists of additional areas considered relevant and important for nursing practice that are not covered in the orientation program. Because of the time and resource constraints that today's healthcare institutions may place on the provision of orientation programs, many content areas that were previously included in orientation have been de-

leted. When time and resources for orientation are particularly limited, the four factors used to establish educational priorities (fatal, fundamental, frequent, and fixed) must be assiduously applied. Dissecting out a short list of "essential-to-know" or "critical-to-know" content areas for coverage often results in leaving many "good-to-know," "useful-to-know," and "nice-to-know" areas on the cutting room floor. As mentioned in the last chapter, rather than deleting these practice areas entirely from the staff development program, pertinent areas can be carried over into program planning as offerings in the ongoing in-service program. Examples of these "useful-to-know" areas could include any of the following:

- How to perform comprehensive nutritional assessments (although it would probably not harm a patient [i.e., the *fatal* factor] if a nurse lacked this capability, nurses who can provide these assessments might be able to enhance their patients' recovery and healing to a greater extent than if only cursory nutritional assessments were performed)
- Understanding the genetic basis of health disorders (although this knowledge may not be essential to provide care to pediatric patients [i.e., the *fundamental* factor], familiarity with this content could facilitate the nurse's ability to allay parental fears and guilt regarding transmission of disorders to their child)
- Recognizing less common cardiac conduction disorders/providing care to surgical patients who are having less common surgical procedures performed/learning how to set up less commonly requested traction systems on an orthopedic unit (although none of these practice areas may be required to be performed on a daily basis [i.e., the *frequency* factor], the occasional need to provide these aspects of healthcare makes them worthwhile topics for instruction)
- Modifying customary procedures for application of dressings, for starting IVs, or for patient education (although there is no pressing need for nurses to know multiple ways to adapt procedures and treatments [i.e., the *fixed* factor], the potential patient benefits to be gained from a nurse's capability in these areas could be considerable)

Instruction in areas that do not qualify as absolutely essential or critical to everyday nursing practice can thereby be retained under the auspices of the in-service education program. These clinical practice areas are the ones that tend to distinguish experienced nurses from their inexperienced counterparts and represent development of the nurse along Benner's five stages in the novice-to-expert model.[13]

Two other inclusions related to the competency acquisition dimension of in-service education consist of informal but planned learning activities and incidental learning situations. The former includes in-service offerings such as patient care conferences, discharge planning conferences, nursing rounds, joint medical and nursing rounds, and other activities that can afford nursing staff numerous learning opportunities. Although the purpose of these activities may be primarily related to patient care, their concomitant educational benefits should not be overlooked. When professional nurses reflect on their clinical experiences, much learning can be deduced from these interactions with their peers, coworkers, patients, and families.

Incidental learning experiences occur serendipitously on every nursing unit. For example, a nurse may be familiar with the major actions of a particular medication but, through careful patient observation and assessment, that nurse now recognizes side or adverse effects that are rarely mentioned in the pharmacology literature. An emergency department nurse may have read about the signs and symptoms of combined alcohol and drug withdrawal, but individual patients may demonstrate highly unique patterns of clinical presentation that are instructive to the nurse and not found in any standard reference book. Incidental learning experiences such as these afford an enriched experience base for nursing practice that can enhance that nurse's clinical competency more than any classroom or laboratory activity can. As can be seen from the description of these four inclusions related to the dimension of in-service education, the acquisition of competency exists as an ongoing and pervasive process throughout one's professional career. Orientation programs initiate this process, but in-service education offerings must maintain the learning momentum.

Accommodation of Off-Shift Staff

A particularly challenging aspect of providing for competency acquisition is the need to accommodate off-shift nursing staff so that in-service offerings are as convenient and accessible to them as they are for day shift personnel. Morton[79] describes use of a monthly audio tape to keep evening and night staff informed about new medications and treatments, drug alerts, trends in nursing practice and management, journal articles, and research findings. Each topic was accompanied by learning objectives, pertinent handouts, summaries of important information, and an attendance sheet. Continuing education units (CEUs) were also awarded to participants.

Djupe[33] also found the use of self-directed learning methods helpful for meeting the in-service needs of off-shift nurses. In order to meet the night shift's preferences for independent study at times convenient to their schedule and staffing situations (2 AM to 4 AM was the best time), independent study packets (consisting of purpose, objectives, directions for use, journal articles, handouts or outlines, posttest and evaluation tools) and closed-circuit television programs were developed to accommodate

requested in-service topics, necessary updates, and mandatory coverage of areas such as fire safety, CPR, and disaster management.

Diaz's[29] work with evening and night shift staff suggested that relatively brief (30 to 45 minutes) programs on specific topics, held at certain shift-specific times (dinner time for brown bag in-services or 10 PM for evening shift staff and 2 to 4 AM for night shift staff) worked best, especially if conducted adjacent to the units. Self-learning packages and videotaped and closed-circuit television programs are other effective and efficient means to reach these staff. Vendor representatives may also be required to provide in-services to off-shift staff when new drugs, equipment, or supplies are introduced.

Maintenance of Competency

Certain aspects or functions of a nurse's role are sufficiently important in providing safe and effective patient care that healthcare agencies, or the organizations that accredit and regulate them, require that those areas of performance be evaluated on a regular basis to determine whether nursing staff have maintained competency. Thus the maintenance of competency typically includes coverage of areas required by the hospital, the state, or various accrediting or regulating organizations such as the JCAHO or OSHA. Many healthcare institutions label this set of expectations as "the mandatories" to distinguish them from in-service offerings on topics requested or otherwise locally necessitated. The "mandatory" label most often refers to requirements emanating from JCAHO or OSHA safety issues (CPR, fire safety, electrical safety, disaster management, infection control, universal precautions, and the like). Hospital standards may impose comparable or more stringent requirements on nursing staff compared to these external standards and regulations. For example, many hospitals require annual certification/recertification in basic cardiac life support (BCLS) by all nursing personnel, whereas the current JCAHO standards[58] require that this be completed no less often than every other year. In addition, some states such as Florida impose additional requirements on nursing staff that need to be incorporated into the maintenance of the competency segment of in-service.

A number of issues related to these competency maintenance areas deserve consideration. These include the following:

- *The number of maintenance areas is likely to continue to increase in the future.* Healthcare agencies and regulatory and accrediting bodies have heightened our awareness of accountability for providing safe and effective patient care. The high cost of healthcare has set the stage for the continued need to verify the accountability of healthcare professionals to the public in these areas.

- *The resources available for providing in-service education for maintenance areas are likely to continue to decrease in the future.* The number of staff development personnel, the size of staff development departments and budgets, and the time available for providing instruction have all decreased substantially over the past few years in many hospitals. Cost containment measures for the hospital industry can be expected to escalate with future healthcare reform measures. As a result, this form of in-service education must, of necessity, be made more efficient.
- *The need to document verification of competency maintenance is very likely to persist.* Hospital risk management programs, quality monitoring, and legal issues will provide continued impetus for documented competency verification mechanisms beyond that already afforded by JCAHO and OSHA requirements. Documentation of quality in these performance areas is a major component of accountability in the healthcare system.
- *Nursing personnel who are the participants in these competency maintenance activities will be increasingly less available during work hours for instruction in large groups.* Now that nursing staff scheduling patterns can range from 8- to 10- to 12-hour shifts, split shifts, weekend alternative schedules, shared positions, and self-scheduling, the predictable three-shift work pattern can no longer be used as a basis for scheduling in-service offerings. Attempts at scheduling specific lecture times for traditional in-service instruction, therefore, is often useless because it neglects whether staff will be available for instruction. At some hospitals, the nursing shortage of a few years ago has now been replaced by nursing layoffs. Pendular swings in staffing adequacy (either shortages or excesses) are not amenable to rigid scheduling of in-service classes—regardless of whether these classes are mandatory or voluntary.

As an outgrowth of issues such as these, current in-service programming aimed at the maintenance of competency has developed the following adaptive goals:

- Minimal learner time to complete instruction
- Minimal or no learner time away from patient care areas
- Available and accessible instruction when learner wishes and is able to use it
- Learner able to complete instruction at own pace
- Minimal instructor time required to provide instruction
- Standardization in instructional quality and content
- Maximal staff participation and compliance rates

- Provision of documentation of satisfactory performance
- Minimal or no boredom (for both learners and instructors) associated with repetition of the same material at ongoing intervals

In the face of increased demands for maintenance in-service offerings with no increase in resources or persisting demands with dwindling resources, staff development personnel have considered a wide variety of alternatives to the traditional lecture and lecture/demonstration methods of providing instruction for this purpose. Some of these instructional alternatives are described following.

All-Day Marathon In-Service

Some hospitals* favor the all-day (marathon, blitz, education day) approach to providing maintenance in-services. Many of these programs require nursing staff to come prepared by reviewing background information before the education day. The education day is then used to review highlights of this information, answer questions, and complete evaluations at various stops/stations throughout the day. Education days are usually conducted at various time intervals throughout the year or may be held annually. Both mandatory and other (optional) topics can be addressed during the course of the day. The cited advantages of this approach include increased attendance and compliance rates, enabling large numbers of staff to meet requirements in a brief time, the ability to use multiple teaching methods, use of a nonthreatening learning climate, no distractions by the unit, and lower costs per participant. Bethel[15] compared the direct, indirect, and overhead costs of providing in-service education for both unit-based and all-day methods over a 1-year period and concluded that the all-day method was more efficient both quantitatively and qualitatively.

Mobile In-Services

Rather than concentrating and centralizing the time and location when these in-services are offered, other hospitals have made these offerings movable and portable via so-called roving in-services[70] and mobile education carts.[127] This approach involves designing a cart with self-explanatory directions and instructional materials for a specific topic area, leaving the cart on the nursing unit for a defined period of time, and providing mechanisms for feedback and evaluation of learning as well as documentation of participation. The advantages of these mobile mechanisms are that staff do not need to leave their units at all, staff can complete the learning experience when this is convenient, no instructor is needed once the offering is developed and

*See references 10, 15, 21, 27, 28, 76, 88, 132.

refined, and all staff could use and complete the program in as brief or long a time as they required. Williams[127] described application of this approach to provide in-service and practice in use of the emergency crash cart for cardiopulmonary resuscitation.

Self-Directed Study

An increasing number of hospitals have initiated some form of self-directed study for some or all of their maintenance area in-service offerings. Goldrick[44] developed a programmed instruction module related to infection control and found that this teaching method resulted in statistically significant higher posttest scores compared to the lecture teaching method. Haggard[48] describes the employment of reusable self-study packets with instruction limited to the essentials necessary to meet JCAHO requirements and open-book tests consisting of objective test items related to the packet's objectives. Answer sheets can be scored quickly by clerical personnel, and records are computerized. The packets are designed so that all levels of employees who need to complete the same packet are able to read and understand the language and terms used. Problems with staff procrastination are minimized because all requirements in the program must be completed to secure a satisfactory performance evaluation. Information obtained from monitoring staff performance and from safety meetings, fire drills, and incident reports suggests that this approach is effective in maintaining and enhancing safety-related staff performance.

Educational Games

A number of hospitals have attempted to overcome the attendance, boredom, and repetition problems often associated with mandatory in-services by injecting some fun into learning. Instructional games patterned after television game shows such as *Jeopardy* and *Wheel of Fortune,*[53,97,101] board games such as *Life®*, and word games (puzzles, word scrambles, and word searches)[57] have all been employed as creative, enjoyable, and effective ways to enjoin staff to complete these maintenance in-service requirements.

One particularly creative innovation described by Proctor[97] was a "hazard hunt" consisting of 20 manufactured hazards in a simulated patient room that are designed as a "risk manager's nightmare." Nursing staff must list the 20 hazards within 15 minutes using a "what's wrong with this room?" approach. Moralejo and Gaese described a similar program using a mock isolation room to identify and review infection control infractions.[78]

Hudson[53] combined a multiple-game format together with the all-day approach in designing a "JCAHO Carnival" that lasted 3 days and enabled 867 of 1000 employees to complete all six mandatory safety areas.

One admonition in relation to the use of games for these requirements is that evidence of each staff member's attainment of all educational objectives needs to exist. This may be difficult when the game uses groups of participants as team members. A second caution in the use of games is that the fun element of the game cannot supersede the ability to verify the competency of each staff member. Games can be enjoyable, but they must also be effective in meeting the educational outcomes specified.

Combined Teaching Methods

Seigel[108] designed a comprehensive educational program for meeting regulatory and accrediting agency requirements that includes a diversity of teaching methods:

- *Self-learning packets* for requirements related to patient rights, incident reports, disaster policies, risk management, and confidentiality
- *In-service posters* for requirements related to organ procurement and use of restraints policy
- *Closed-circuit television* for requirements related to fire and electrical safety, infection control, and universal precautions
- *Marathon classes* for CPR certification and recertification
- *Hands-on experiences* for resuscitation procedures and use of emergency equipment and medications

Ford, Wickham, and Colver[38] described a skills fair workshop for verifying the competency of critical care nurses. The skills fair incorporated numerous decorated booths for selected skills and included the following teaching methods: brief presentation, videotapes, handouts, poster presentations, hands-on performance, demonstrations, and discussion groups.

CPR Recertification Programs

Of all the competency maintenance areas, the time- and labor-intensive requirements of CPR recertification seems to bring this area the greatest amount of attention in the literature. Patten[90] developed a "CPR Jeopardy" game so that staff from various healthcare fields could review background information related to resuscitation in an enjoyable and efficient manner. However, because this approach used teams rather than individual players as participants, it did not provide the ability to verify individual performance.

Moysenko[80] described a "CPR Marathon" for basic cardiac life support (BCLS) recertification that represented a modified version of the blitz technique described earlier. Four elements were incorporated into this 16-hour (7 AM to 11 PM) marathon:

- Reviewing a self-study booklet of background materials (risk factors, prudent heart living, etc.) *before* the marathon day

- Viewing a 40-minute videotape on all BCLS procedures (if the participant chooses to)
- Practicing CPR resuscitation procedures on infant, child, and adult mannequins with an instructor in attendance
- Completing the written and performance tests

Participants who came to the marathon well prepared were able to complete the recertification process in 2 to 2½ hours. Another attractive feature of the marathon was provision of free child care for all off-duty personnel.

A considerable amount of in-service program design in this area has examined the relative effectiveness of self-directed, self-paced teaching methods compared to the traditional lecture/demonstration method. Friesen and Stotts[41] reported that there were no significant differences between the lecture-demonstration/return demonstration and self-paced groups (using an American Heart Association slide-tape program, programmed instruction workbooks, and videocassette) of baccalaureate nursing students in either initial mastery or retention 8 weeks later for cognitive knowledge in BCLS (written test results) or psychomotor skill performance. While cognitive knowledge and skill performance were not significantly different between the two groups at either time interval and both groups maintained mastery of cognitive information at the 8-week time period, both groups fell below mastery in the skill performance. The cost for providing this instruction was calculated as $23.88 per participant for the lecture demonstration/return demonstration method and $38.48 per participant for the initial use of the self-paced method (included start-up and development expenses). Subsequent use of the self-paced method would be able to delete all costs related to initial design and purchase of the instructional materials. The average amount of time required to complete the learning activities was nearly 7 hours for the lecture-demonstration/return demonstration method and approximately 5 hours for the self-paced method.

Research findings from Coleman, Dracup, and Moser[22] and Nelson and Brown[84] supported those of Friesen and Stotts. The Coleman study reported little difference in CPR cognitive knowledge or skill performance between the traditional (lecture-practice) didactic method and a modular (self-paced, self-directed) teaching method immediately following or at 3 months following instruction. Retention of skill performance declined as it did in the Friesen study. Modular, self-paced instruction was again found to be an effective alternative to the conventional, time- and labor-consuming didactic method of CPR instruction and allowed savings of both instructor time and participant costs. These savings might enable the hospital to provide CPR skill practice and testing sessions more often to offset the erosion of competency that is revealed in these studies. O'Connor[86] also reported that a self-paced modular approach to CPR instruction provided comparable scores in both written and skill performance areas over 3- to 12-

month intervals. Plank[95] reported that the traditional (lecture-demonstration-practice) approach resulted in better CPR knowledge retention at 6 to 8 weeks after instruction than the self-paced approach (using videotape and independent practice without an instructor) but no difference in performance of psychomotor skills at the same retention period.

In contrast to studies that report a comparable amount of learning and retention in CPR knowledge and skills when either self-directed or traditional didactic instruction is used, Mueller and Glaser[81] found significantly higher cognitive and skill performances when the self-directed approach was used for CPR training compared to the traditional lecture-demonstration approach. The average cost per learner was also better with the self-directed approach: the average cost per learner was $13.63 in the self-directed methods compared to $33.10 in the lecture-demonstration group. DiPietro[32] also reported satisfaction with use of a self-directed learning module for CPR recertification, wherein the self-directed module required a maximum of 1 hour away from the unit to complete and cost $15.00 per learner while the traditional approach required 6 hours away from the job and cost an average of $67.35 per learner. The self-directed learning module was judged as effective as the traditional approach and considerably more efficient in terms of time and labor costs.

Although the effectiveness and efficiency of self-directed instructional approaches to CPR recertification are well supported in the literature, the findings in these studies concerning retention of these cognitive and psychomotor skills should not be ignored in the discussion on the relative efficacy of the teaching methods employed. The results of these studies suggest that retention of CPR knowledge and psychomotor skills is a major concern. While both cognitive and psychomotor skills erode steadily following instruction and fall to preinstructional (below mastery, unsatisfactory) levels within 1 year or less,[35] the deterioration in psychomotor skill performance is considerably faster and more precipitous than the loss of cognitive skills. Kaye et al.[61] found a notable loss of CPR skills within only 2 weeks following initial CPR training. Despite technological and educational innovations, such as the use of computer-assisted interactive videodisc CPR learning systems,[49,109,119] the erosion of competence in performance of CPR skills, particularly the psychomotor skills, persisted.[26,36,71] The clear implication of these findings for staff development is that competency in CPR/BCLS knowledge and skills erodes significantly within a few weeks to months, especially for the psychomotor skills. The maintenance of staff competency in CPR requires more frequent and vigilant attention than it has received to date. Even if the knowledge component of competence is retained better and longer, the loss of mastery in performance of resuscitation skills suggests that even shortly after being recertified in CPR, nursing staff may not be able to administer optimal resuscitation to patients who suffer a cardiopulmonary arrest. Standards that require verification of competency in CPR every 2 years are obviously inadequate to address the timing aspect of this skill erosion. Annual recertification may be adequate for the cognitive component of competence in CPR, but these studies suggest that a year is much too long for recertifying the psychomotor component of competency in this area. In-service support for the maintenance of competency in advanced cardiac life support (ACLS) knowledge and skills[91] is probably vulnerable to the same retention problems as have been identified for BCLS.

Since actual rehearsal and application of CPR/BCLS procedures can help to reinforce learning and thereby maintain skill performance levels, the use of "mock code" drills may represent an effective means of competency maintenance in this area.[43] Likewise, drill rehearsal can be an invaluable in-service device for retaining necessary skills in managing large-scale situations such as evacuation procedures for a fire or other emergency.[118]

Centralized vs. Decentralized Provision

Another consideration related to assessing maintenance of competency is the extent to which these competency validations and in-service offerings are provided in a centralized vs. decentralized manner. As described earlier in this chapter, clinical assessment centers can provide an effective and efficient centralized mechanism for larger healthcare institutions to provide instruction and verify competency in these maintenance areas.[111] An alternative means of centralized support for these programs is described by Dickerson.[30] This approach consists of the centralized provision of all audiovisual hardware and software, mannequins, and other instructional materials necessary for completing requirements in each area (fire safety, electrical safety, CPR, disaster management, and infection control) together with a decentralized implementation mechanism. A "mandatory" in-service manual developed by the nursing education department for use on each nursing unit enables nurse managers to access the centralized resources and then arrange for program provision on a decentralized basis. The in-service manual describes how to secure instructional materials and use audiovisual hardware, how to contact speakers for specific topics, and how to direct staff to complete documentation requirements.

The initial acquisition of nursing staff competency is a necessary prerequisite for effective nursing practice. Once past orientation, however, and for the vast majority of nursing staff, maintenance of their clinical competency becomes the paramount staff development concern.

Increase of Competency

In addition to the initial acquisition of competency associated with innovations and the maintenance of competency in areas related to accreditation and regulatory re-

quirements, in-service education should also address instruction for areas that represent extensions of a nurse's customary role. For example, certain nurses may complete a special training program that enables them to perform endotracheal intubation or defibrillation without a physician in attendance. Another group might receive special instruction that enables them to administer selected chemotherapeutic agents. Others may be prepared to provide hemodialysis or to manage patients on an intra-aortic balloon pump. Because these functions require special advanced knowledge and skills, hospitals typically restrict performance of these procedures to only those nurses who have received instruction in the area, who have successfully completed all program requirements, and who meet the explicit performance criteria established for competent performance in that area. Programs such as these that certify a nurse to provide selected functions are often referred to as *privileging* or *credentialing* programs.

Credentialing mechanisms generally have entry or eligibility requirements that may include a stated number of years of experience in nursing or in care of specific types of patients, a specific instructional program, an evaluation process that verifies knowledge and skills necessary for competent performance, and requirements for reappraisal of competency at specified time intervals.[2] For example, in order for certain nurses to be granted privileges to defibrillate patients without a physician in attendance, the nurse might have to meet the following requirements:

- *Entry/ eligibility:* Graduate of an NLN accredited school of nursing
  Current valid RN license
  Two years of staff nurse experience in CCU
  One year of code team experience
- *Education:* Successful completion of defibrillation
  In-service program based on current ACLS guidelines:
  Course attendance
  Skill practice sessions
  Completion of written test
  Completion of performance testing
- *Evaluation process:* Passing score (90% or higher) in defibrillation written test
  Attainment of all performance criteria in defibrillation procedure skills checklist
- *Reappraisal:* Annual recertification via written test and performance checklist required to retain privileges

Before the nurse would be authorized to provide defibrillation, then, each of these expectations would have to be met. The restricted nature of these clinical privileges reflects both the advanced knowledge and skills required of the nurse and the additional concern for patient safety involved in these functions. Many of the areas of nursing practice for which hospitals credential nurses are areas formerly provided by physicians and now delegated to select and specially trained cadres of nurses.

Educational Process

In-service education programs employ the four steps of the educational process in a manner quite comparable to that of other staff development endeavors. A few points specific to these steps for in-service offerings are summarized following.

Assessment

Assessment of learning needs for in-service education can be divided into programs related to acquisition of competency, maintenance of competency, and increase of competency.

Acquisition of Competency

Learning needs assessment for in-service education that focuses on competency acquisition is typically accomplished by three primary means: (1) recognition that a new policy, procedure, or product (or some other novel situation or event) exists and needs to be disseminated to nursing staff; (2) review of content and learning experiences provided during orientation to determine if other pertinent areas merit instruction; and (3) monitoring of current and anticipated future nursing practice to identify needs for ongoing in-service programming.

Other useful sources of information regarding the needs of nursing staff for in-service education are suggested in the JCAHO's *Standards for Orientation, Training, and Education of Staff*.[58] Standard SE 2 in this group relates that "The organization provides for education and training designed to maintain and improve the knowledge and skills of all personnel." The requirements of this standard stipulate that the needs identified for this training may be derived from one or more of the following sources:

- Needs of the patient population served (the type of nursing care required)
- Needs of individual staff members
- Results of quality assurance and quality improvement activities
- Needs generated by advances in medical and/or nursing sciences
- Results of staff performance appraisals
- Findings from peer review activities
- Findings from safety management programs
- Findings from infection control programs

One distinctive facet of needs assessment for this dimension of in-service education involves inclusion of product

representatives and vendors in the process. Many healthcare pharmaceutical, supply, and equipment companies have full-time staff who work with hospital nursing staff and staff development departments to determine and provide on-site offerings related to their company's products. A number of these vendors employ nurses as educators to assist hospital nursing staff in using these products.

As with any learning needs assessment, the larger the number of sources tapped for the assessment, the more comprehensive and thorough the appraisal and the greater the likelihood that the conclusions reached will represent worthy topic areas for instruction. This is particularly important for in-service education because it is the most open-ended in terms of the potential scope of content area that could be included.

Maintenance of Competency

Learning needs assessment for the in-service education that deals with maintenance of competency is considerably more limited than for competency acquisition. Because the JCAHO, OSHA, hospital, and nursing department requirements that need to be verified on an ongoing basis are already identified in hospital policies, the scope of this assessment is accordingly restricted to those areas. However, new or revised policies can be added, so nurse educators need to periodically review the list, content, and time frames required to ensure that updates or additions are made and communicated to all nursing staff.

Increase of Competency

The learning needs assessment related to hospital credentialing of nursing staff for particular functions is the most circumscribed of the three dimensions of in-service education. Small- and medium-size hospitals may have no credentialing of nurses at all, and even large healthcare institutions may offer only a limited number of these programs. As a result, monitoring and updating the learning needs of these staff members is typically not an onerous process.

As with needs assessment related to orientation, these assessments for the in-service program also need to have priorities established, competency statements formulated, and performance criteria developed. Often, a single competency statement (e.g., *Demonstrates the current procedure for instituting patient-controlled analgesia*) will suffice for the in-service educational component. The competency statement and performance criteria for that area of nursing practice can then be used as the basis for planning the offering.

Planning

Because in-service offerings, unlike orientation programs, are highly focused on a specific topic or competency area, the work involved in planning instruction is more restricted but consists of the same general elements. These planning elements include content selection, organization and sequencing of content, allotment of instructional time, selection of appropriate instructional media, and managing program faculty. All but the last element proceed as described in earlier sections.

Staff Nurse Faculty

In the past, staff nurses may have functioned as in-service instructors occasionally, if they enjoyed teaching their peers or new staff. When unit-based nurse educators and clinical nurse specialists were plentiful, the need or opportunity for staff nurses to serve in this capacity was greatly diminished. In today's healthcare facilities, however, two forces have combined to return more staff nurses to the role of in-service instructor: (1) the downsizing or elimination of many nurse educator and clinical nurse specialist positions and (2) the institution of clinical progression (clinical advancement or clinical ladder) systems and/or performance evaluation systems that require staff nurses to function as in-service instructors in order to advance or to receive a satisfactory performance appraisal. As a result, preparing and assisting staff nurses with their teaching skills may become an increasingly important staff development function.

Chapter 3 provides detailed descriptions of how staff nurses can be supported for this responsibility before, during, and following the instruction they provide. In addition, the principles of teaching and learning, principles of adult education, teaching and learning style preferences, and teaching methods for classroom, laboratory, and clinical settings in Chapter 4 can be incorporated as time permits. Provision of this support to staff nurses is important so that the experience is effective as an educational offering and, ideally, is also satisfying and edifying to the staff nurse who serves in this capacity. Inglis[55] suggests ten "common-sense teaching strategies" for effective in-service presentations by staff nurses. These are summarized in Box 7.1.

Product Representatives and Vendor Faculty

As mentioned earlier, many healthcare manufacturers and vendors employ their own staff to provide in-service training related to their products. Rather than being sales staff, an increasing number of these instructors are nurses who are specially prepared to provide this service to the company's customers.

Planning in-service offerings with these vendor representatives can be a smooth and satisfying experience. Many of the manufacturers provide an extensive array of high-quality instructional media (computer-assisted instruction, interactive videodiscs, videotapes, slide sets, etc.) in addition to printed monographs or other related literature, simulation exercises, and well-informed, experienced instructors. Although the hospital's nurse educator will need to coordinate scheduling, locations, and other logistical details with the product representative, the representatives will typically assume the major planning responsibility for the in-service program. Two planning areas that should not be overlooked are the need for documentation of the in-service provision and the need for any necessary follow-up or reinforcement. If the vendor representative will not be available for return visits, the nurse educator will need to be sufficiently proficient with the in-service session to provide ongoing staff support and follow-up. In some cases, vendor presentations can be unduly biased toward their own product. Educators would be well advised to audit at least the initial vendor program to monitor the information provided and ensure its accuracy and fairness.

Implementation

In general, implementation of in-service education programs employs the same guiding principles (teaching, learning, adult education, teaching and learning style preferences) and teaching method considerations as those described for orientation programs. In addition, since all in-service offerings are, by definition, directed at nurses who have already completed orientation, the special implications for working with experienced staff nurses that were

---

Box 7.1
TEACHING STRATEGIES FOR IN-SERVICE PRESENTATIONS BY STAFF NURSES

- Select a topic of interest to the staff nurse
- Establish goals for the session
- Set clear objectives [performance criteria in CBE]
- Organize the presentation
- Gear delivery to the intended audience
- Select an appropriate teaching strategy
- Use teaching aids as appropriate
- Provide a climate conducive to learning
- Convey enthusiasm
- Incorporate humor

From Inglis AD: *J Cont Educ Nurs* 23(6):263, 1992.

enumerated in Table 6.7 also apply for in-service programs. In relation to teaching methods, however, one noteworthy distinction needs to be emphasized: unlike the topics in orientation programs that emphasize the "essentials" of everyday nursing practice that should already be very familiar to experienced nurses, the topics covered in in-service programs may be totally familiar or totally unfamiliar to the nursing staff. As a result, the teaching methods selected for use with a particular in-service offering are not always those appropriate for experienced nurses at the competent, proficient, or expert levels of Benner's model. Rather, the teaching method employed needs to be tailored to the appropriate stage of clinical skill development. At times, the nature of the topic for a particular in-service offering may require that teaching methods suitable for the novice or advanced beginner be used for these experienced nurses.

A few examples might illustrate this point more fully:

- If the in-service education relates to competency maintenance areas such as CPR, fire safety, or infection control, teaching methods appropriate for nurses at the upper three levels of Benner's model can be used because experienced staff have high degrees of familiarity and expertise with these topics after many years of ongoing instruction and repeated verifications of their competency in those areas. Although a few subtle nuances may be added or refined each year, there is usually a limited amount of truly new information to learn and master.
- Teaching methods for the competent, proficient, and expert levels can also be used for most elements of competency acquisition. These might include updates or revisions to policies, procedures, or equipment operation; classes on the "good-to-know" areas not covered during orientation; and informal learning activities such as patient care conferences or nursing rounds. This type of in-service education represents a fine opportunity to apply the precepts of Benner's model to selection of teaching methods most suitable for highly experienced nurses who are approaching or at the uppermost levels of clinical skill development.
- An exception to this situation exists when competency acquisition is implemented for topics that staff have no background knowledge of or experience with. As mentioned in Chapter 6, when nurses are confronted with novel and/or unfamiliar clinical situations, they will tend to revert to novice and advanced beginner levels of skill development and need teaching strategies that are more analytical, rule-oriented, and principle-based. Examples of such learning situations occur whenever new health disorders are identified (such as when AIDS was first recognized as a clinical entity), when new classes of drugs are introduced (such as when monoclonal antibodies were first used), or when

new forms of technology are initiated (such as when pulse oximetry was introduced).

- After their initial credentialing process, experienced nurses whose knowledge and skills are being reappraised to verify their competence in special functions they provide may also need teaching methods for the three highest levels of Benner's model used for recredentialing sessions. Gradual progression in teaching methods (from the competent to the proficient to the expert level) can be used with each successive recredentialing session when review and instruction are needed.

Tailoring teaching methods to the appropriate level of instruction for those attending the in-service sessions can significantly influence the effectiveness of that instruction.[74] In addition to keeping this point in mind for the in-service education they provide, educators will also need to work with staff nurses and vendors who may serve as in-service instructors to ensure that this consideration is taken into account for other in-service providers as well.

Evaluation

Following the initial determination of a staff nurse's competency provided by the orientation program, the evaluation afforded by the in-service program verifies whether nursing staff have acquired, maintained, and increased their competency. In relation to the four levels of evaluation, in-service programs need to include evaluations of participant satisfaction, learning, and application to clinical practice. These appraisals are typically secured on completion of the in-service offering or very shortly thereafter. Evaluation at the impact level to determine outcomes in patient care can be performed in conjunction with either follow-up evaluation of a specific offering or as part of the quality monitoring and improvement program. The evaluations of competency included in an in-service program fall into one of two general categories: immediate and ongoing.

Immediate Competency Evaluations

Immediate evaluations of in-service education are performed coincident with the provision of instruction and typically are timed to immediately follow that instruction. Once the instructor has finished the teaching portion of the session, review, practice, and reinforcement are provided as warranted, and the evaluation segment commences. Depending on the nature and number of instructional outcomes established for the in-service, the evaluation tools may include only a performance checklist or both a performance checklist and a written test. Owing to the restricted scope of content usually covered in an in-service offering, both types of evaluation devices are usually brief and feedback on written and clinical performance is often provided immediately or shortly thereafter. The emphasis of this immediate feedback is on evaluation of learning.

When a competency-based approach is used for the provision of in-service programs, appraisals may be performed before instruction if the content of the program is already familiar to nursing staff. For nurses who do need instruction, evaluations can then be completed following the offering with the emphasis on verifying that all performance criteria established for the offering have been attained. Immediate evaluations are used for all components in the competency acquisition dimension of the in-service program. The design and construction of performance checklists and written tests and test items for this purpose are completed in the same manner as they would be for any other type of staff development program.

A second application of these evaluations occurs in the competency increase dimension of in-service education when staff nurses are initially credentialed to perform specialized functions. In much the same way that nurses who take BCLS and ACLS courses undergo evaluation of their knowledge and skills at the end of these programs, so nurses who seek to be credentialed in a particular area usually undergo appraisal of their capabilities at the termination of the instructional segment of these courses.

Ongoing Competency Evaluations

Although hospitals have been doing forms of ongoing competency appraisals via their in-service programs from nursing staff development and their performance evaluations from nursing management, the JCAHO brought this evaluation area to the forefront with its revised standards of nursing care and standards for orientation, training, and education of staff.[58] As Box 7.2 indicates, the Joint Commission requires that the competence of each member of the nursing staff be evaluated both initially to determine their current competence before they can be assigned patient care responsibilities and at "defined intervals throughout the individual's association with the hospital."

INITIAL COMPETENCY ASSESSMENT   The initial competency assessment program can be viewed in relation to two groups of nursing staff: new staff and existing staff.

New Nursing Staff   For new members of the nursing staff, the baseline or initial competency assessment is accomplished on entry as employees via the orientation program. In effect, then, the instructional outcomes (competency statements and performance criteria) used for the CBO can constitute the initial competency assessment mechanism as well. For most hospitals, the initial compe-

---

Box 7.2

JCAHO STANDARDS RELATED TO COMPETENCY ASSESSMENT

NURSING CARE STANDARDS

NC 2   All nursing staff members are competent to fulfill their assigned responsibilities.

NC 2.1 Each nursing staff member is assigned clinical and/or managerial responsibilities based on educational preparation, applicable licensing laws and regulations, and an assessment of current competence.

NC 2.1.1 An evaluation of each nursing staff member's competence is conducted at defined intervals* throughout the individual's association with the hospital.

NC 2.1.1.1 The evaluation includes an objective assessment of the individual's performance in delivering patient care services in accordance with patient needs.

NC 2.1.1.2 The process for evaluating competence is defined in policy and procedure.

ORIENTATION, TRAINING AND EDUCATION OF STAFF STANDARDS

SE 4 Each individual in the organization is competent, as appropriate to his/her responsibilities in the

SE 4.1 knowledge and skills required to perform his/her responsibilities;

SE 4.2 effective and safe use of all equipment used in his/her activities;

SE 4.3 prevention of contamination and transfer of infection; and

SE 4.4 cardiopulmonary resuscitation and other lifesaving interventions.

*The Joint Commission's publication titled *An Introduction to the Joint Commission Nursing Care Standards,* 1991, clarifies that "defined intervals" includes the following: "nursing staff members have their competence assessed as part of the initial employment and orientation process; the competence of nursing staff members is maintained through a combination of ongoing competence assessment and educational activities . . ." (p. 91).

From Joint Commission on Accreditation of Healthcare Organizations (JCAHO): *Accreditation Manual for Hospitals: Standards,* vol 1, Oakbrook Terrace, IL, 1994, JCAHO.

tency assessment of new nursing staff poses no significant problems, especially when a competency-based approach is already used for the nursing orientation program. Because the outcomes for the orientation program include all essential aspects of the nurse's job responsibilities on the assigned unit, these outcomes are functionally synonymous with competent performance in the assigned role. But what about existing staff who may have completed their orientation to the unit years or a decade earlier? How is their initial competency determined?

Existing Nursing Staff If the stated intent behind standard NC 2 is that "In order to provide quality patient care, those who deliver patient care services must be competent to do so," and if daily assignments must be based on "an assessment of current competency," then it would seem rather obvious that the competence of existing staff can neither be assumed nor automatically granted (grandfathered) on the basis of their years of nursing experience on the unit. Rather, the Joint Commission requires that clinical competence be demonstrated and documented for all nursing staff.

The mechanism for initial competency assessment of existing nursing staff can be described according to the what, why, how, who, when, and where aspects of concern:

What: The mechanism for initial competency assessment of existing staff can employ the same competency areas and performance criteria as those used for the orientation program.

Why: The rationale for this mechanism is that the essential or critical behaviors required of a nurse on a particular unit are the same for all nursing staff who occupy the same position on that unit. Holding existing staff to a different set of performance expectations would be inconsistent with the unit's definition of competency as embodied by its orientation program.

How: Because senior staff may feel uncomfortable and threatened when subjected to an appraisal, it should be accomplished as informally, discretely, and unobtrusively as possible. For example, the competency assessments might be performed when patient census is low, when the unit is quiet, possibly on off-shifts when fewer people are on the unit. It may also be useful to communicate the need to meet this JCAHO requirement in a matter-of-fact manner, as something that just needs to be done. It may also be helpful to characterize this effort as a competency *validation* program, rather than as a "test" of competency to minimize the negative connotations often associated with evaluations. If the hospital is in the process of developing or revising its CBO program, it may also be less threatening to staff if their com-

petency validation is performed as a pilot test of the CBO program. Any strategy that can accomplish the competency determination and diminish its stressful effects on senior staff is likely to be well received.

Who: Those who will perform staff appraisals should already have been deemed as "competent" themselves and have some experience using the evaluation tool designed for this purpose. Potential evaluators include the unit's nurse manager, clinical specialists, nurse educators, or other nursing staff. Senior nursing staff may be most comfortable having peers provide the validations. As long as the performance criteria are rigorously applied, the evaluator can be any nurse already designated as competent who knows how to do the evaluation.

When: As mentioned under the "how" aspect, the timing of these appraisals is probably best when the unit is relatively quiet and less densely populated with staff. In order for this process to be completed in a timely manner, it would be helpful if the nurse manager and educator could agree on a maximal time limit for completion of all baseline validations of staff competency. Staff can then be held accountable for completing their validations by that date. The time frame specified needs to be feasible so that unwarranted pressure to complete the appraisal is avoided and planning can proceed smoothly and comfortably for both members of the nursing staff and the evaluators.

Where: Just as with orientation, the baseline determination of staff competency is best determined on the clinical unit. Although some areas may be evaluated in a simulated situation or in a classroom setting, the majority of performance expectations should be demonstrated on the nursing unit.

Once the baseline evaluation of staff nurse competence has been accomplished, the hospital needs to determine what will be included in the ongoing competency assessment program and how often these evaluations will be done.

Ongoing Competency Assessment Once the initial competency validation process has been completed, the Joint Commission does not require staff nurses to be evaluated in relation to the full set of orientation competencies on an ongoing basis. Because the nurse manager has the opportunity to observe staff performance on virtually a daily basis and incorporates appraisals of specific areas of performance as part of the process of evaluation, there is no need for an ongoing competency assessment program to duplicate these evaluations.

Since the revised JCAHO standards neither prescribe the specific elements to be included in an ongoing competency assessment nor require that all inclusions be evaluated at the same "defined intervals," hospitals may exercise considerable discretion in determining what elements they wish to include in this mechanism and how often each element is evaluated. For example, the hospital, nursing department, or individual unit might reach consensus on which elements they would like to include for a 2-year period. These elements might be derived from quality assurance findings or recent in-service sessions on new products or procedures or from risk management findings. Some elements may be assessed hospital-wide, while others may only apply to certain nursing divisions, and still others may be unit-based. It might be decided that for the next 2 years, six different nursing practice elements will be examined on an ongoing basis. Of these six elements, two might be assessed after 18 months, two might be appraised annually, and two might be examined every 6 months during that 2-year period. What the Joint Commission does require in this regard is written policies and procedures that describe the competency assessment mechanism and documentation to verify that these assessments are completed.

There should be some rational basis for the decision regarding the frequency of ongoing competency assessments. In general, if staff compliance rates are high or nearly universally attained for a particular practice element, the hospital might consider extending the time interval for for the subsequent assessment. Conversely, the lower the attainment rate, the shorter the time interval for the next assessment could be. If the aim here is to ensure that all nursing staff are competent in certain areas of performance, then the results of these ongoing competency assessments can be used as the basis for determining the frequency intervals of subsequent assessments.

The mechanism used for ongoing competency assessments related to credentialing programs can operate in much the same manner as that for ongoing staff appraisals. One important difference, however, is that the scoring guidelines for orientation competency SE 4.1 stipulate that an individual's competence "to perform a particular procedure or task in a high-risk, problem-prone patient care process" must be verified and documented "at least every 2 years. . . ."[59] This 2-year maximum time interval also applies to the Joint Commission's requirements for competence in performing CPR and "other designated life safety interventions."

In nursing staff development, in-service education literally picks up where orientation ends and supports nursing staff in competent performance of their job responsibilities throughout their career. With orientation affording the foundation for competent nursing practice, in-service education builds on this foundation toward development of the nurse from the competent to the proficient, and, ideally, to the expert level of practice. Acquiring, maintaining, and increasing the competence of nursing staff are necessary ingredients to optimal staff development and to an optimal quality of patient care.

CONTINUING EDUCATION

DEFINITION

The American Nurses' Association[5] defines *continuing education (CE)* in nursing as "planned educational activities intended to build upon the educational and experiential bases of the professional nurse for the enhancement of practice, education, administration, research, or theory development to the end of improving the health of the public." The American Society for Healthcare Education and Training (ASHET)[6] defines it in a similar manner, as "education that is broad in scope and designed to build upon previously learned knowledge and skills."

CHARACTERISTICS

The attributes of continuing education include the content embraced by CE programs, program duration, formats, accreditation of offerings, providers, responsibilities for CE, and the relationship of CE to competency-based education.

Program Content

The ANA *Standards for Nursing Staff Development*[5] relate that the content of continuing education programs consists of concepts, principles, research findings, or theories related to nursing that build on the nurse's previously acquired knowledge, attitudes, and skills. In addition to content that ultimately improves patient care, the content of CE programs may also afford nurses the more general benefit of improved professional development as well as career advancement.

Tobin[117] relates that CE offerings generally can be classified as those that have a clinical emphasis or those that focus on one or more areas of leadership development. Clinical topics for CE are usually selected for their broad appeal across all clinical areas of nursing practice. Examples of these generic clinical topics might include areas such as working more effectively with families, creative approaches to discharge planning, modifying dressings for unique patient needs, working collaboratively with other hospital departments, simplified methods of dosage calculations, or reducing the potential for legal liabilities. Continuing education topics related to leadership development also need to be widely applicable. Leadership topics appropriate for CE might include problem-solving, decision-making, delegation, critical thinking, organizing work loads, or establishing priorities of nursing care.

Program Duration

In general, continuing education offerings are shorter in duration than orientation programs and longer than in-service offerings. The duration of a CE offering is usually related to the scope of content covered and the format used to present the learning experience.

Program Format

As mentioned in Chapter 6, the format of an education program refers to its general organizational structure. The encompassing nature of continuing education lends itself to a wide variety of formats that include brief sessions (lasting less than 1 hour) or more lengthy formats such as a workshop, seminar, conference, course, institute, symposium, or self-study.

A *workshop* is a brief (often only a single day) but in-depth educational program for a relatively small group of participants that emphasizes active learner participation. The focus of the workshop may be on detailed study of a particular topic, on development of a particular set of skills or abilities, or on solving a particular problem. Skill-based workshops often involve a considerable amount of hands-on learning experience using the equipment and supplies normally employed for that skill. Teaching strategies such as small group exercises, group discussion, case studies, role plays, and various forms of audiovisual media may also be used.

A *seminar* consists of a small group of learners who come to the learning experience prepared to exchange information about a specific topic. The subject for the seminar is determined in advance, and participants are expected to come prepared to discuss the topic following their own reading and study. A seminar leader manages and coordinates the group discussion and keeps it focused on addressing relevant issues and/or problems. The effectiveness and outcome of a seminar depend highly on the amount of preseminar preparation by participants and on the quality and effectiveness of the seminar leader.

A *conference* is another short-term group process format that involves participant discussion related to a single problem, situation, or issue. The purpose of a conference is to exchange points of view related to an area of common concern for participants. A conference leader or coordinator may facilitate exchanges among and between groups and subgroups in attendance. Conferences may last for several days if the issues to be discussed are complex or particularly problematic.

A *course* usually consists of an ordered series of classes or other learning experiences related to the same topic area. In contrast to academic courses that last for a number of months, short-term CE courses may last only a few days. During that time, however, intensive and comprehensive study of that topic area can be achieved.

An *institute* consists of an intensive program of instruction related to a particular field in which expert consultants present information to participants. Institutes are often multiday programs that involve limited learner participation and more formal learning experiences than with other CE program formats.

A *symposium* usually involves two or more experts presenting content related to an identified theme, followed by a summary of their comments by a symposium moderator, and then a question-and-answer period. A symposium can accommodate a fairly large audience but often aims for 10 to 20 audience members.

Self-study formats can include any of those described in Chapter 4. These formats may include programmed instruction, self-learning packages, reading books or journals, or using audiovisuals or computer-assisted instructional programs.

Accreditation

In contrast to orientation and in-service programs that typically do not seek accreditation, the continuing education component of staff development is frequently accredited by professional approval bodies (national, regional, state, or professional associations) so that continuing education units (CEUs) can be awarded for participation in the program. This feature is especially pertinent in states that require continuing education for nurse relicensure.

Providers

Except in rare instances, all nursing orientation and in-service programs are sponsored by a single provider, the employing healthcare facility. The major providers of continuing education, by contrast, comprise four broad categories and innumerable individual sponsors within each of those categories. The four major provider groups for continuing education are the following:

- Universities and professional schools at those institutions
- Professional associations
- Employers
- Independent providers[19]

In nursing, these CE provider groups encompass hundreds of schools and colleges of nursing and/or their continuing education divisions, hundreds of professional nursing organizations (such as national and state nursing organizations and national and local specialty nursing organizations), thousands of healthcare employers, and thousands of proprietary businesses and nonprofit organizations whose primary or major mission is provision of educational services to healthcare professionals.

Because the focus of this book is limited to continuing nursing education only within the context of nursing staff development (rather than to the entire field of continuing nursing education), the provider group considered here will be confined to healthcare employers. Readers interested in exploring the larger field of continuing professional education beyond that provided by healthcare facilities may wish to consult any of the numerous references that address that area.*

*See references 8, 17, 19, 34, 52, 98, 99, 128.

Responsibility for CE

The primary responsibility for continuing education rests with the professional nurse.[5] As a professional, the nurse has an implicit obligation to secure and participate in continuing education that enhances his/her professional practice.

Healthcare agencies that employ nurses often support this endeavor since it is consistent with their mission and philosophy of nursing staff development to do so. Support may be evidenced by the hospital's determination of CE learning needs as well as by planning, providing, and evaluating the effectiveness of these offerings. In states that require evidence of continuing education for relicensure of nurses, employer support for the CE needs of its nurses may be especially generous.

Educators in healthcare settings need to be mindful, however, that the primary mission of a healthcare facility is to provide patient care services. Staff education, particularly instruction that by definition is *not* directly linked to the nurse's present job responsibilities, represents a clearly secondary or even tertiary interest. In short, hospitals may support continuing education but have no implicit obligation to do so. This point has not been lost on many healthcare agencies which, in the face of declining revenues, downsizing, and other fiscal constraints, have discontinued or greatly diminished their financial largesse in this area.

CE and Competency-Based Education

For healthcare settings that use a competency-based approach to staff development, the continuing education component of staff development may be viewed as the enhancement of a nurse's competence in areas that lie outside or beyond present job requirements. In this context, then, nurses who develop additional or advanced competence in nursing practice, administration, education, or research that is not directly related to their current work responsibilities are participating in the CE component of nursing staff development. Although continuing education may well result in improved job performance, when the CE offering does not directly and immediately relate to that nurse's work, it may be classified as continuing education.

DIMENSIONS

The ANA's definition of continuing education in nursing[4] indicates that the dimensions that make up CE include any area(s) of nursing practice, education, administration, research or theory generation that may improve patient care. In general, specialty organizations (within and outside of nursing) devoted to the functional areas of education, administration, or research concentrate their programming resources in their respective areas of interest in CE. Hospitals that provide CE for nursing staff, by contrast, typically concentrate their support in the nursing practice dimension.

Three examples of continuing education topics that are frequently of interest within this area are enhancement of nurses' competency in problem-solving, decision making, and critical thinking. Some considerations and suggestions related to each of these CE topics follow.

Problem-Solving

Relevance to CE

The capacity to solve problems is one of the hallmarks of professional practice. As Houle[52] notes, "The nurse . . . (and every other professional) confronts one problem after another and is required, with the insight, skill, and knowledge available, to do the best he or she can do to deal with each confronted situation . . . The ultimate test of the success of a professional is the ability to solve problems. . . ."

Within the profession of nursing, the pivotal role of problem-solving in nursing practice is also acknowledged. Holbert and Abraham[50] and others[65,89] emphasize the analogous relationship between problem-solving and the nursing process: "The nursing process has been widely acclaimed as the prevailing model for nursing practice. This model, in essence, is a model for problem-solving." Berger,[14] concurs with this assertion regarding the relevance of problem-solving to nursing: "The ability to solve problems creatively is the hallmark of the modern nursing practitioner."

Description of the Process

The nature, definition, and components of what constitutes problem-solving are not universally agreed on. Different conceptions of the process and its components have been offered,[65] and some elements of general agreement exist among these. The basic steps involved in the problem-solving process as well as correlation to the steps of the nursing process are enumerated in Table 7.1.

Problem-solving involves a complex interplay of both content and process skills. The content skills reflect a combination of both the theoretical and specialized body of knowledge required for practice within one's particular profession together with the wisdom of practical knowledge derived from experience in practicing that profession. This blend of theoretical and practical knowledge must then be merged with the process skills involved with using the steps in the problem-solving procedure. Effective problem-solving results when theoretical and practical knowledge are then joined with a network of cognitive processes (reflection, integration of old and new learning with present experience, inductive and deductive reasoning, creative thinking, brainstorming), which enable the nurse to organize information meaningfully, consider alternatives, and arrive at plausible solutions to resolve a problem.

As Houle[52] points out, professionals at the start of their career tend to employ this process with a slow, rather tedious attention to each component part and serial execution of each required step. As experience is gained, the

TABLE 7.1 • STEPS IN THE PROBLEM-SOLVING PROCESS

Steps in the Problem-Solving Process	Steps in the Nursing Process
1. Define the nature of the problem	Assessment/Nursing Diagnosis
2. Distinguish possible causes of the problem	
3. Identify a number of possible solutions for each cause	Planning
4. Select the best solution among the possible solutions	
5. Determine the actions necessary to implement that solution	
6. Implement the proposed solution	Implementation
7. Evaluate the results and effects of that solution	Evaluation
8. Evaluate whether the solution needs modification	

steps are completed with greater speed and facility until, with the highly experienced practitioner, the component parts become virtually indistinguishable as the practitioner focuses on the patterns rather than the parts involved in the process. Houle's description of how facility in the problem-solving process becomes refined with professional experience is analogous to Benner's[13] description of how novice nurses progress from detail- and step-oriented followers of rules to proficient and then expert nurses who focus on holistic and intuitive patterns of clinical situations rather than solely on specific details of a situation to determine their practice.

Although this characterization of problem-solving is admittedly an oversimplification of a myriad of complex cognitive processes, there is emerging support for the view that the abilities involved in problem-solving can be taught. It should be noted here that the emphasis in instruction is aimed at the generic process of problem-solving rather than at teaching the "right answers" to problems that nurses will encounter in their practice.

Teaching Strategies

Holbert and Abraham[50] described a competency-based problem-solving seminar designed for graduate students majoring in nursing education. This seminar was based on Woditsch's[130] contention that generic skills such as problem-solving (Woditsch's "life-related competencies") can be used as the foundation on which role-related skills (such as those required of the nurse educator) can be constructed for professional practice rather than teaching a rigid set of

role behaviors. A second concept underlying the seminar was Bloom and Broder's[16] model for ideal problem-solving; the third component was Whimbey's[124] "cognitive therapy" approach to problem-solving, the components of which are:

Assessment:	Thinking aloud to develop awareness of your own and others' thought processes in problem-solving
Guided practice:	In using the problem-solving process
Evaluation:	By peers and experts/faculty

Students in the seminar completed the Whimbey Analytic Skills Inventory (WASI)[125] at the initial class meeting to provide objective pretest scores of problem-solving ability. During the eight 2-hour seminar sessions, students were given increasingly more complex problem-solving situations, practiced verbalization of their thinking with a peer, and received alternating peer and instructor-led group feedback on the effectiveness of their reasoning. At the end of the seminar, the WASI was again completed to provide posttest comparisons. Although no statistical data were offered in the report, the authors concluded that students in the seminar demonstrated substantial improvement in their problem-solving ability, greater flexibility in problem-solving approaches, and a greater number of approaches considered in problem-solving. This experience was also perceived as enhancing the nurses' awareness of their own habitual modes of thinking that, as Houle[52] relates, can have the "deadly effect" of leading to routinization of thought, automatic rather than contemplated solutions, and failure to recognize and appreciate the nuances of apparently routine problems or situations confronted in daily practice.

In addition to the seminar just described, other teaching strategies that can help to develop problem-solving include the following[68]:

- Written problem case studies for learners to analyze and solve in pairs or small groups
- Videotaped vignettes of both common and less frequently encountered clinical problem situations for small or large group resolution
- Computer simulations,[65] including situations correlated with Benner's levels of skill development[116]
- Soliciting actual problem situations from members of the audience for individual or small group analysis
- Multiple debate teams organized around controversial issues in nurse-physician relationships, patient vs. family wishes, ethical or legal issues, staff nurse and nurse manager relationships, or peer conflicts
- Written exercises for analysis and articulation of all sides of an issue
- Comparing the outcomes of practice exercises

wherein different groups of learners use habitual responses to common clinical problems vs. those who use an "ideal" model for problem-solving

Regardless of the teaching method(s) selected for use, it is evident that enhancing a nurse's problem-solving abilities can contribute substantially both to the quality of that nurse's practice and to the quality of patient care. Continuing education that enhances problem-solving abilities can ameliorate the mid-career nurse's vulnerability to automatic responses to everyday practice problems and keep those nurses progressing along the novice-to-expert continuum.

Decision-Making
Relevance to CE

The quality of nursing practice and, ultimately, patient care delivery is contingent on the nurse's ability to make sound clinical decisions. Effective clinical decision-making has been characterized as "a critical component of nursing practice,"[89] "the cornerstone of professional nursing practice," the "principal criterion by which expertise is judged," and "the skill that separates professional nursing personnel from technical or ancillary personnel."[54] Every step in the nursing process requires astute decision-making so that sound decisions can be reached regarding the relative importance and interpretation of various assessment data, the most appropriate nursing diagnoses, the optimal plan for nursing care, how implementation of the plan of care should proceed, and whether the outcomes of care were achieved. While the knowledge base underlying nursing practice grows and becomes rapidly obsolete in a few years, and the medications, treatments, and procedures needed for patient care undergo continued evolution, decision-making remains one of the few constants in nursing practice. Because of the centrality and importance of decision-making for nursing care at all levels of experience and in any clinical setting, enhancing a nurse's competency in this area represents a worthwhile topic area for continuing education.

Description of the Process

The general steps included in the decision-making process are listed in Table 7.2. As this table illustrates, the decision-making process, like the problem-solving process, has many parallels to the steps of the nursing process. A comparison of the decision-making process (Table 7.2) with the problem-solving process (see Table 7.1) reveals the similarity between these two phenomena as well.

Effective decision-making, like effective problem-solving, requires the union of both factual/theoretical knowledge (that is, "knowing *that*") and the practical knowledge ("knowing *how*") that experience provides. Knowing *that* a decision needs to be made is one thing; knowing *how* to proceed is something else again.

TABLE 7.2 • STEPS IN THE DECISION-MAKING PROCESS

Steps in the Decision-Making Process	Steps in the Nursing Process
1. Recognize the existence of a situation that requires a decision	Assessment
2. Gather information about possible causes of the situation	
3. Specify the precise nature of the necessary decision(s)	Nursing diagnosis
4. Identify the options available for decision-making	Planning
5. Weigh the potential outcomes (risks and benefits) of each decision option	
6. Select the best decision based on the available options	
7. Implement that decision	Implementation
8. Evaluate the outcomes of the decision taken	Evaluation

Benner's[13] description of how the decision-making ability of nurses develops with experience along the novice-to-expert continuum provides not only a means to understand the range of what the term *decision-making* includes but also affords a means to understand how staff development may assist nurses in learning and refining their capabilities in this area.

In Benner's model the **novice** nurse makes decisions by using a set of fixed rules. (*When a new patient is admitted to the unit, always follow this procedure: take vital signs and complete all sections on the nursing admission form.*) Novices will then tend to execute decisions in a more or less rote or automatic fashion that is often slow and labored, especially if their memory of the rules is faulty or incomplete. **Advanced beginners** cannot distinguish the most relevant aspects of clinical situations but make decisions on the basis of some general guidelines or principles they have derived from their experience. (*When a new patient is admitted to the unit, I know that I have to complete the nursing assessment form, but my experience says that sometimes I'll have to determine if the patient has any needs that require immediate attention and meet those needs first before I complete the admission assessment form.*) **Competent** nurses base their decisions on a more holistic view of the patient that enables them to focus on long-term as well as short-term interventions. (*When a new patient is admitted to the unit, it is often a good time to begin the early phase of patient and family education while I am obtaining the assessment data.*) **Proficient** nurses no longer need explicit rules or principles to guide their decisions but base their judgments on whether patients "fit" their anticipated pattern of how comparable patients should look and respond. Proficient nurses constantly compare a given patient to this composite to determine whether any data are present that should not be present or whether something that should be present is missing. Different types of patients are viewed in different ways, so a clinical context is always necessary for their judgments. *(When a new CHF patient is admitted to the unit, I always first assess whether he/she is dyspneic and whether the level of consciousness seems diminished. If these findings are present, I may defer completing some areas of the admission assessment form until the patient has stabilized and I have a clearer picture of his/her status.)* **Expert** nurses no longer base their clinical decisions on rules, principles, or even discrete patterns of clinical findings but operate by means of an intuitive grasp of the entirety of a clinical situation. Their perceptual acuity is also context-dependent and often difficult to articulate and explicate in any analytic way. *(When Mrs. Thompson was admitted to the unit with hypertension, her admission assessment data were within normal limits for her, but something wasn't quite right. Although her BP was high, it was beginning to respond to the medications; her pulse was regular but felt somewhat weak to me; her color was neither cyanotic nor pale, but I didn't like it; she was responsive and oriented but appeared lethargic at times. Her admission orders were for Q2 hour vital signs, but I'm going to check them every 30 minutes for awhile until my instincts tell me she is stabilized. I just don't have a good feeling about her. I'm concerned that she may have had or is having a CVA.)*

The succeeding stages of this practice model illustrate how the decision-making process is not only honed by a nurse's clinical experiences but is qualitatively transformed from a system based on rigid procedural steps and fixed rules to one rooted in professional instincts and intuition that do not even exist in the novice or advanced beginner's repertoire of capability. It should also be noted that as increased capability in this process proceeds, nurses are less likely to continue following the serial and simplistic route delineated by the nursing process. As Benner[13] points out, "In contrast to the situation-based, interpretive approach, the linear nursing process model can actually obscure the knowledge embedded in actual clinical practice because the model oversimplifies and necessarily leaves out the context and content of nursing transactions. . . . experts do not make decisions in this elemental, procedural way. . . . rather, they grasp the whole."

Although the discrete "steps" in the decision-making process enumerated in Table 7.2 are no longer used by nurses at the proficient or expert levels of practice, they represent the basic building blocks of "rules" that novices and advanced beginners need to master in the formative stages of developing competency in this skill. Only after these steps are successfully acquired and integrated will the nurse be ready for higher-order decision-making characteristic of proficient and expert practitioners. Failure to master any of these steps can lead to faulty or ineffective decision-making. As a result, the causes of ineffective decision-making can include any of the following:

- *Inability to recognize situations that require a decision.* The nurse may not be attentive for clues that a situation requiring a decision exists or may not know what to look for as cues that a decision is warranted, necessary, or useful.
- *Failure to solicit or inadequately soliciting information related to the situation.* The nurse may not gather enough information that bears on the situation or may gather irrelevant information.
- *Inability to clearly define the decisions necessary.* Because of insufficient or extraneous information or misinterpretation of that information, the nurse may formulate an inaccurate or premature conclusion regarding the decision that needs to be made. The inability to synthesize relevant information may lead to inaccurate determination of the nature of the decision that needs to be rendered.
- *Inability to consider the full range of alternative decisions that could be rendered.* Use of reflex responses to situations rather than contemplation of all possible options may limit the potential range of decisions. The nurse may neither be aware of nor solicit help from others regarding the potential decisions that could be employed or may be too disinterested to contemplate alternatives not immediately apparent.
- *Lack of weighing risks and benefits of each possible decision option.* The nurse may be unable or unwilling to take the time and effort to consider each possible option and weigh its pros and cons or likely outcomes. Failure to complete this step leaves all options equally plausible or risky.
- *Delayed or poor judgment in selection of optimal decisions.* Uncertainty or anxiety may cause the nurse to defer making any decisions and possibly allow the situation to become more pressing in the interim. If the relative benefits/risks of various options were not fully considered, whatever prompts the selection made may represent an invalid basis for the decision reached.
- *Faulty follow-through in implementing the decision.* Even if the optimal decision is selected, its execution may be of poor quality. Sound decisions can also be made but for the wrong reason (e.g., a nurse assesses the patient's neurologic status more often than ordered, when there really is no sound clinical basis to warrant this).
- *Faulty conclusions regarding outcomes of implemented decisions.* If the rationale for the decision was not sound, evaluation of the effectiveness of that decision will not be valid. The same results may be produced if any of the preceding stages were faulty, erroneous, or only partially completed.

The complexity of the decision-making process is one reason why it is difficult to teach and appraise in educational programs. Another source of difficulty related to providing instruction in this area is the duplicity of factors that may affect the quality, processes, or outcomes of decision-making. In addition to the influence of experience, some other influences on decision-making that have been identified include intelligence, knowledge, personal values and beliefs, tolerance for risk, situational stress, the urgency of the decision, its potential consequences, the complexity of the decision, and the environment within which decisions must be rendered.[54,89] Each of these factors has the potential of enhancing or diminishing a nurse's decision-making ability. For example, a healthcare facility where risk-taking is encouraged; where nurses' opinions and judgments are welcomed, respected, and supported by administration; where professionalism, autonomy, and accountability are promoted; and where communication channels among healthcare professionals are open is an environment in which professional discretion may thrive.[54,56] By contrast, the healthcare agency that is risk averse, that neither solicits, acknowledges, or respects nurses' opinions; where nurse dependency and subservience predominate; and where communication is stifled or unilateral tends to extinguish the potential benefits of nurses' decision-making.

It should also be noted that the association between clinical experience and decision-making is predicated on the assumption that "experience" denotes the "continued refinement of preconceived notions and theory through encounters with many actual practical situations that add nuances or shades of differences to theory." The term *experience* as Benner[13] uses it here "does not refer to the mere passage of time or longevity" in one's position. Unless professional experiences continually reshape and refine the nurse's understanding and practice, even decades of work may result only in development of reflex responses to clinical situations rather than to expert decision-making.

Teaching Strategies

In a competency-based approach to staff development, the primacy of teaching (and also evaluation) from real clinical situations remains the most effective instructional device. Therefore, whenever possible, clinical decision-making is best taught through the use of actual patient care situations that require nursing decisions. Once novice nurses and advanced beginners are familiar with the general procedural steps that make up the decision-making process, the educator needs to supplement this factual knowledge with the practical realities of actual patient situations. Asking these nurses to reflect on their patient assignments, to recount personal experiences, and to cite instances that need nursing decisions can be a fruitful starting point for determining how sound clinical decisions are reached.

Continued reflection and refinement of this process and its myriad of influences can then produce the "principles" that advanced beginners use to make clinical judgments. Small group work with nurses at comparable skill levels can then be employed for practice in distinguishing between salient and extraneous information and in identifying the essential aspects of the situation that demand decisions. Pairs of nurses can then appraise the relative pros and cons of alternative decisions to determine the optimal choice. Results from these deliberations can be compared to the actual decisions made in order to distinguish their similarities and differences and to reach conclusions regarding the effectiveness and wisdom of those decisions. Continued practice and sharing of experiences with more progressively complex decision-making and the broadening of insights to view patients more holistically rather than as the embodiment of innumerable masses of clinical data can assist the competent nurse toward proficient and expert levels of clinical discretion.

A second approach to instruction is through the use of simulations. As mentioned earlier, simulations—even ones that closely resemble reality—are not as effective as teaching strategies because of the element of artificiality they impose on learning nursing practice. Even the best simulations lack the urgency, potential risks, stress, and complexity of variables found in most real clinical events. Making sound decisions in a learning laboratory is no guarantee that the nurse will perform well under the fire of reality.

Despite these recognized limitations, simulations of various types (simulated patients, videotaped vignettes, teaching stations, role plays, games,[106] and the like) that require the nurse to demonstrate decision-making prowess at least afford an opportunity to observe that nurse's ability in a decision-making situation that uses circumstances comparable to those encountered in real life. Simulations also provide a safe haven to make mistakes while learning and afford both standardized types of situations that the nurse should be able to manage and control over the number and nature of variables operating in that situation. Scenarios can then be constructed for teaching and evaluating the nurse's ability to manage specific types of clinical or leadership decisions (e.g., making decisions in the following situations: acute shock syndrome, acute dyspneic episode, managing anaphylactic reactions, crisis intervention with a trauma patient's family, working with an irate coworker, delegation of nursing functions, and the like). Models could then be constructed to reflect how nurses at each of the five practice levels might approach, analyze, and arrive at decisions for these situations. An element of stress and urgency could be injected by using role plays to present cases and their evolution more realistically and by imposing a time limit on rendering the decision. Peer analysis and feedback could then be offered to broaden perspectives and practice consideration of a wider range of alternative courses of action.

The least effective but easiest teaching strategy is to merely describe cases and ask the nurse to verbally describe their process of decision-making. Although this approach removes all risks to the patient and can highly structure the types of decisions reviewed, it also erases professional experience and personal involvement with the decisions reached. In addition, this approach neglects all of the nuances of real situations as well as the multiple influences operative in most decision-making experiences. In relation to competency, this approach only addresses the cognitive element—that is, "knowing *that*"—and neglects the equally important "knowing *how*."

In addition to its importance for staff nurses, decision-making is also an appropriate CE topic for nurse managers,[37] clinical nurse specialists, preceptors, and unit educators.

Critical Thinking

Relevance to CE

Thinking may be conceptualized as the cognitive ability to organize new information and reorganize previously learned information into forms that can then be generalized and applied to new situations. Thinking, in turn, involves *reasoning*, the systematic and logical use of information to arrive at a conclusion or decision. According to Berger,[14] *critical thinking* is the product of reasoning and logic. Frederickson[40] defines critical thinking in a similar manner as the ability to analyze and solve problems logically. Other educators describe critical thinking as a skill that selects and guides the cognitive processes involved with defining and solving novel problems.[104]

From these definitions, the interrelationship among critical thinking, decision-making, and problem-solving seem readily apparent. Precisely how these concepts interrelate, however, is not universally agreed on. As Pardue[89] relates, some educators view critical thinking ability and decision-making skills as closely related cognitive processes, while others view critical thinking as one component of effective decision-making. Other authors appear to equate these cognitive processes or to combine thinking and problem-solving as the components of critical thinking.[65]

Regardless of the exact relationship these twin concepts have with one another, there does appear to be a high degree of agreement in two related areas: (1) that critical thinking is an essential ability for contemporary nursing practice and (2) that the majority of traditional college-age students (including student nurses) function at cognitive levels considerably below that required for critical thinking. White et al.[126] assert that "critical thinking is essential to nursing practice and should be represented as a basic theme throughout undergraduate curricula." Bauwens and Gerhard[12] relate that "the ability to think critically and analytically underlies much of competent nursing practice." Schank[104] conveys much the same sentiment: "The diversity and complexity of nursing practice make it necessary

to prepare nurses who can think critically. . . ." Professional recognition of the importance of critical thinking to nursing practice is also reflected in the accreditation requirements for baccalaureate programs in nursing where the National League for Nursing[83] accreditation criteria require schools of nursing to provide evidence that the curriculum content and teaching strategies emphasize critical thinking, decision-making, and independent judgment.

Critical thinking is also widely considered as an integral complement and/or as a parallel to use of the nursing process.[72] Pardue[89] describes this relationship very specifically: "In the nursing process . . . the nurse collects data utilizing both inductive and deductive reasoning, makes hypotheses . . . and plans, implements, and evaluates patient care. Many of the mental processes needed to successfully implement the nursing process are analogous to the mental processes defined as critical thinking ability." White et al.[126] relate that ". . . the nursing process may well represent the primary link between education and practice; it is the instrument that promotes and fine tunes critical thinking skills. . . ."

If critical thinking is, as has been described, so integral to nursing practice, is this skill well developed in new graduates by the time they enter the work site? The evidence in this area is admittedly incomplete, but some preliminary findings suggest that the answer to this question is "no." Malek[72] cites a number of public reports on education[85,114] that indicate the need for greater emphasis on critical thinking in schools at the high school level. The unsettling national report titled *A Nation At Risk* published by the National Commission on Excellence in Education[82] identified as one of the indications of risk that "many 17-year-olds do not possess the higher order intellectual skills we should expect of them. Nearly 40 percent cannot draw inferences from written material; only one fifth can write a persuasive essay; and only one third can solve a mathematics problem requiring several steps."

Confirmation of these findings among college students continues to support the commission's report. Klaasens[65] cites a number of sources[7,42,47,93,94] that indicated that significant numbers of college students function at cognitive developmental levels far below those necessary for effective critical thinking, problem-solving, and decision-making. Despite the fact that college courses may appear to require higher cognitive function levels, a majority of college students operate at concrete and elementary levels of cognitive development that preclude effective use of abstract and relativistic discrimination. If colleges and schools of nursing are inheriting high school students who are unable to think critically, how successful have these institutions of higher education been in initiating and developing critical thinking skills by the time these nursing students graduate?

Although many schools of nursing have been making great strides in attempting to fill in these gaps in cognitive development, the findings to date are unclear and equivocal at best. Both Berger[14] and Frederickson[40] found that critical thinking ability improved among baccalaureate nursing students over the course of their program, but Frederickson's pilot study's small sample limits the generalizability of its findings. Keeley, Browne, and Kreutzer[62] reported both good news and bad news: although senior nursing students scored higher in critical evaluation skills than freshmen, some 40% to 60% of these seniors could not detect illogical flow, ambiguity, or misuse of information contained in the written material they critiqued. In Sullivan's research,[112] registered nurses who were graduates of associate degree and diploma programs enrolled in a baccalaureate program were tested for critical thinking ability at the start and end of their program. The findings indicated that entry and exit critical thinking scores showed no significant differences—that is, critical thinking ability did not improve throughout their baccalaureate program. One significant correlation did emerge from Sullivan's study, however: the longer the time between nurses' graduation from the diploma or associate degree program and their entry into the baccalaureate program, the higher their critical thinking score. If neither high schools nor colleges are successful in developing critical thinking skills, and, if critical thinking is truly essential for effective nursing practice, then staff development educators will increasingly need to devote educational time and resources to this area if nurses are to eventually be able to demonstrate ability in this area. Sullivan's one significant finding, together with Benner's model, suggests, however, that critical thinking ability as well as higher-order decision-making may require some years of experience in nursing practice before these attributes are amenable to development.

Description of the Process

Classic cognitive theorists such as Piaget and Perry have devised detailed schemes of cognitive development. In Piaget's framework,[94] cognitive development begins at a primitive and reflex response level, progresses to an egocentric level where only one's own point of view influences thinking, develops to a concrete level of thinking where others' points of view can at least be acknowledged, and eventually matures to an abstract level where logical conceptual processes can resolve even seemingly contradictory and ambiguous issues.

In William Perry's framework,[93] cognitive development begins with a black-and-white (dualistic) view of issues where thinking tends to be very absolute and easily categorized as right or wrong, progresses to a gradually increasing openness to the relativity and multiplicity of issues and opinions, and matures to a level where the individual is willing to take actions or make commitments based on their own analysis of possible alternative responses. Effective critical thinking requires the individual to cognitively function at the highest levels in either of these two characterizations of cognitive development.

The specific components of critical thinking are described differently by various authors but, in general, are consistent with the definitions of critical thinking mentioned earlier. Bandman and Bandman's[9] conceptualization of critical thinking includes the ability to analyze and scrutinize issues and ideas; to distinguish among assumptions, inferences, and facts; to isolate issues, principles, beliefs, and values; to develop plausible arguments; and to reach logical conclusions and actions. Matthews and Gaul[73] identify the cognitive components of critical thinking as comprehension, analysis, synthesis, application, and evaluation.

The Watson-Glaser Critical Thinking Appraisal (CTA) instrument[123] is a widely used test for measuring critical thinking ability. This self-administered test consists of a series of 80 test items that require application of critical thinking abilities either to neutral content such as the weather or to controversial issues where emotions or prejudices may exist. The CTA measures five components of critical thinking that include the ability to recognize assumptions, make inferences, use deduction, make interpretations, and offer evaluations of various arguments. The set of abilities tested by this instrument is comparable to those used in problem-solving and decision-making and consists of the following:

- To recognize the existence of a problem
- To select relevant information for solution of the problem
- To recognize and distinguish between stated and unstated assumptions
- To formulate and select reasonable hypotheses
- To draw valid conclusions and judgments regarding the validity and generalizability of inferences made.

If the capability and abilities that make up critical thinking are developmental rather than innate (as Piaget and Perry's models contend), then understanding which abilities are important to foster and understanding how these attributes might be enhanced can afford the basis for devising instructional strategies for this purpose.

If readers recall the earlier discussion related to the difference between theoretical (knowing *that*) and practical (knowing *how*) knowledge, it is obvious that effective critical thinking—as with effective problem-solving or decision-making—requires a combination of both types of knowledge. Nurses must learn both the content relevant to problems and issues they confront in everyday nursing practice and the process of using the cognitive abilities that make up critical thinking.

Schank[104] suggests that the constituents of critical thinking must be practiced and acquired gradually and progressively in an integrated manner rather than as a single course or at a single time. Learning how to pay attention to relevant information, sift out extraneous information, follow the construction of an argument, detect illogical or false assertions, brainstorm possible solutions, and organize impressions into logical conclusions and decisions takes time and maturity. Maturity includes not only chronological age, but the maturity gained by actually practicing one's profession for a number of years.

If basic nursing education programs primarily focus on developing a nurse's theoretical knowledge base and have limited time or ability to develop a nurse's practical knowledge base, then the continuing education component of nursing staff development may rightfully need to assume a much greater responsibility in fostering and refining this capability. To the extent that nurses need experience in nursing practice to prepare them for this level of cognitive functioning, it may be unrealistic and inappropriate to expect that either nursing students or new graduates would be able to demonstrate effective critical thinking abilities. In this regard, the continuing education component of nursing staff development may be the more appropriate locus for development and refinement of this crucial skill.

Teaching Strategies

The teaching strategies for promoting critical thinking suggested in the literature range from general guidelines to highly specific suggestions. Some strategies are appropriate for classroom use, and others are intended for use in clinical instruction. All of these approaches to instruction in this area are predicated on progressive development of the cognitive skills that make up critical thinking ability. A sampling of these is described following.

Schank[104] suggests that nurse educators consider the use of Arons's[7] six processes that underlie analysis and inquiry in order to promote critical thinking. These six processes include the following:

- Raising questions when a body of information is studied or a problem is considered (to identify facts, how facts are derived, the source and reliability of data, and the relevance of information)
- Identifying gaps in needed information (rather than accepting information at face value)
- Probing for assumptions that underlie a line of reasoning
- Drawing inferences from data, observations, or other evidence when these can be derived
- Envisioning plausible outcomes that might result from various changes in a situation
- Distinguishing between inductive (from particular to general) and deductive (from general to particular) reasoning

Nurse educators can facilitate critical thinking by helping nurses to verify assumptions and speculations before using these as a basis for interventions, by encouraging the use of divergent thinking, by evaluation of their interventions, and by creating a work environment where questioning, curiosity, and open communication are fostered and supported.

White et al.[126] described the use of four teaching strategies to promote development of critical thinking skills in nursing students. These teaching methods include a nonclinical application of the nursing process, argument and debate, use of ethnographic techniques, and practice with ethical decision-making. The nonclinical application of the nursing process consists of a written description of a particular condition, its signs and symptoms, incidence, etiology, prognosis; comparison of the relative effectiveness of various treatments; and identification of a nursing diagnosis with several alternative nursing interventions. This assignment is given to students in their initial nursing theory course to assist them in using the nursing process and in organizing their thoughts in a nonthreatening environment. Practice in constructing and using argumentation and debate affords an opportunity to use reasoned judgment on one or a set of propositions, to distinguish relevant aspects of issues, including the social context, and to organize and present one's opinion and position relative to that issue in a coherent fashion. Ethnographic interviews teach students how to solicit, analyze, and evaluate information and perceptions from clients as a basis for identifying generalized problems and issues that exist in the healthcare delivery system as experienced by healthcare consumers. Practice in ethical decision-making offers students an opportunity to examine the complex interplay of ethical, moral, legal, and professional issues that are embedded in contemporary healthcare and to practice resolution of ethical dilemmas where there is no "right" answer and where decisions will not satisfy all concerned parties. Dealing with uncertainty, ambiguity, and conflicting value systems and beliefs makes this instruction especially meaningful to more experienced nurses as well.

Pond, Bradshaw, and Turner[96] advocate the use of case studies, computer-assisted instruction (especially interactive programs and simulations), guided design, and Barrow and Tamblyn's[11] "Portable Patient Problem Pack (P_4)." Guided design incorporates five steps in guiding the learner through the problem-resolution process. These steps include (1) identification of the problem, (2) elaboration of alternatives, (3) clarification through examples, (4) practice in testing selected decisions, and (5) weighing the outcomes of decisions made. The Portable Patient strategy employs a deck of color-coded and numbered cards that learners select from and order in terms of their importance for assessment, treatment, and evaluation of a particular patient problem. Each card contains written feedback for the learner and card numbers are tabulated to provide feedback regarding the appropriateness and priority of that information for the problem. The P4 technique was developed to help medical and nursing students develop inquiry skills and integrate facts in a problem-oriented, nonthreatening environment.

Both Pond et al.[96] as well as Lantz and Meyers[69] recommend the use of writing to foster critical thinking skills. Writing actively engages learners in understanding, processing, and transforming information in a logical and rational way and requires skills in generalization, elaboration, interpretation, and integration of information from diverse sources. One creative instructional technique based on writing that the authors described was personification: pharmacodynamics was taught by having each student assume the character of a particular drug, write a creative description of their "personal" attributes (actions, indications, dosing, side effects, and the like), and present this personal portrayal to their peers.

Malek[72] described a highly structured approach for fostering critical thinking based on Taba's[113,115] teaching model. This approach incorporates development of a written teacher's guide that lists sets of predetermined learning activities (progressive clinical experiences) as well as predetermined questions based on those learning situations to guide learners through the following four steps related to cognitive and affective skills in critical thinking: (1) concept formation, (2) data interpretation, (3) application of principles, and (4) interpretation of feelings, attitudes, and values. Two essential elements of Taba's approach are the twin principles of question sequencing and question pacing. The sequencing of questions posed by the instructor is intended to assist the nurse in eliciting relevant information and to foster inductive rather than deductive approaches to thinking and clinical problem-solving. Unlike deductive questions (such as "Is this a normal serum potassium level?") that tend to solicit "right answers" derived from textbook knowledge of facts, inductive questions (such as "What factors in this patient might contribute to an abnormal serum potassium level?") require learners to analyze and sift through a full range of clinical data, interpret the data, apply principles of physiology and pathophysiology to generalize their judgments in a coherent fashion. The pacing of questions reflects the need to challenge learners at a level of questioning appropriate for their cognitive development and to give learners sufficient time to assimilate, integrate, and synthesize data before offering their response. In contrast to purely classroom challenges that may require only reflex facts to be regurgitated, Malek[72] emphasizes that the development of critical thinking related to nursing practice requires learning experiences in the clinical setting, an approach consistent with competency-based precepts of instruction.

EDUCATIONAL PROCESS

As mentioned earlier in this chapter, the focus of this discussion is limited to continuing education provided by healthcare employers under the auspices of nursing staff development. In these days of hospital cost containment, the scope and volume of staff development that are devoted to continuing education may represent a dwindling resource as well. Increasingly, hospitals may be expected to allocate their CE resources to topics that can offer the prospect of enriching both individual nursing staff as well as patient care. For these selected CE offerings, the steps of the educational process are employed in much the same manner as they are for any staff development program. A few considerations that pertain to the CE component of staff development are discussed below. Because the staff development component of CE represents only a small fraction of what the larger field of continuing nursing education embraces, readers are again referred to the numerous sources already available in that field that describe each phase of the educational process in much greater detail than is appropriate here.*

Assessment

Sources

The sources consulted to determine the CE needs of nursing staff can be virtually the same as those used for other staff development offerings. However, because CE is not primarily directed towards a nurse's current job responsibilities, the needs assessment process may allocate less reliance on that nurse's job description and greater attention to the nurse's vision of his/her future professional and career plans. The nurse manager or educator may also be instrumental in the counseling and guidance of nursing staff toward potential areas of professional and career enhancement.

Methods

All of the methods previously described for determining the learning needs of nursing staff may be used for CE purposes as well. Because hospital-based CE is usually directed at areas of interest common to the majority of nursing staff, group methods of assessment (such as focus groups or questionnaires/surveys) may be employed more often than individual methods such as direct observation. If CE program offerings will be marketed to nurses who are not hospital employees, the learning needs appraisal may include assessment methods not used with either orientation or in-service programs. These methods could include direct mail surveys, telephone surveys, or computer-processed surveys.[110,129]

Validation

For both orientation and in-service programs, the focus of the learning needs assessment was placed squarely on dis-

*See references 8, 17, 19, 34, 52, 98, 99, 128.

tinguishing nurses' true educational needs in contrast to their felt or perceived need or their educational interests. For the CE component of staff development, however, the scope of the learning needs assessment can be extended to include nurses' educational interests related to their careers and to felt needs that can be confirmed as deficiencies, desires, or just areas they would like to explore.

Priorities

Because the potential number and scope of topics that might be included as learning needs for a CE program are relatively infinite and the resources available to meet those needs are finite, educators will find it necessary to work with nurse managers to establish priorities among the identified needs. Since the mere identification of a learning need does not constitute an obligation by the hospital to respond to that expressed need, educators and managers will have to collaborate to jointly determine the priority and relevance among the needs expressed so that direction can be set for the CE program endeavors. In making these value judgments related to the relative importance of an array of identified CE needs, educators and managers also need to guard against imposing their own value systems and opinions on the list of needs considered so that staff interests remain the focus of this process.[66] These priorities for CE can be established at the department, division, or unit level but most often are distinguished for department-wide interests. Division, unit, and individual desires for CE may be supported by educational leave and/or tuition reimbursement for academic or outside CE provider programs.

Guiding Selection of Relevant Programs

When identified CE needs are beyond those the hospital is able or willing to provide for, the educator's role may convert to guiding nursing staff in the selection of relevant and appropriate CE provided by one of the other three categories of providers. In this regard, the learning needs assessment process is directed externally to judging the quality of CE programs offered by colleges and universities, professional associations, and other nonprofit organizations as well as proprietary providers. Some areas that can be examined and questions that may be asked in reviewing brochures or catalogs for these offerings are summarized in Table 7.3. These considerations may be used by the educator to help nursing staff become informed and discriminating consumers of continuing education. Consumer consciousness is particularly necessary if individual nurses are increasingly paying more of the costs for CE rather than their employer. A few maxims in this regard may be useful to keep in mind:

- *In CE, as with most other purchases, you usually get what you pay for.* Top-quality CE programs provided by the best in their field and held at convenient and

comfortable locations cost money to plan and provide. With a little good fortune and intelligent planning, you will typically get your money's worth.
- *The most expensive CE programs are not necessarily the best.* Cost, unfortunately, is no guarantee of quality or satisfaction. The more you know about the sponsor, faculty, and facilities of programs you consider, the less likely you are to pay more than it is worth. Doing your homework is important.
- *The least expensive CE programs are not necessarily a bargain.* Compromising the quality of the program, speaker, or facility may result in enrollment at mediocre offerings that waste both time and money. Unless a program receives substantial financial underwriting from some grant, foundation, or other supporter, be very discriminating in program selection when the costs seem too good to be true.

Planning

Program planning for continuing education requires completion of all elements involved with planning any staff development program. These elements include decisions related to instructional content, organization of the curriculum, allotment of instructional time, selection of instructional media, determination of program format(s), management of program faculty, and preparation of an instructional schedule.

In addition to these general aspects of program planning, educators who work at healthcare institutions that provide CE would do well to review the accumulated research literature on factors that enhance or diminish nurses' participation in continuing education. Although most of these findings pertain to CE provided by sponsors other than hospital employers, much of this information has relevance to hospital-sponsored CE as well.

A number of authors have attempted to summarize and categorize the multiple reasons why professionals pursue continuing education. Cervero[19] reported that one extensive compilation using the Participation Reasons Scale (PRS) developed by Groeteleuschen, Harnish, and Kenny[46] shows that across professions, the most important reasons for pursuit of CE relates to the learner's desire for professional improvement and development. Other clusters of reasons for participation in CE, in order of their importance, relate to professional service, learning and interacting with colleagues, professional commitment, personal benefits, and job security. These findings are consistent with those of Houle[52] and others[24] as reasons for participation in continuing professional education both within and outside of the nursing profession. For nurses, participation in CE may be enhanced when the topic involves practical and hands-on aspects of patient care that improve clinical competence.[66] Other frequently cited reasons include personal enrichment, help getting a new job or to advance in one's present job, promotion, to meet other people, perceived quality and relevance of the program, the desire to reach a personal or professional goal, to become better informed, or for social interaction.

An equally informative group of studies have identified the barriers to participation in continuing education. The barriers identified include program cost, time constraints (insufficient time, amount of time to complete or attend program, geographical distance from program site, home and job responsibilities, lack of interest in topic, lack of sufficient information about program, lack of availability of desired programs, and a general apathy towards CE.*

Thus planning for CE needs to take into account the need for careful consideration of a number of factors that reflect the myriad of reasons why nurses may or may not participate in continuing education. Attention to features such as topic relevance, program location, day of week, total time involved, cost, sufficient time for networking and social interactions, and the like represent important features in program planning.[131] The goal of planning is to maximize elements that enhance participation and to minimize barriers to participation in continuing education. When the general elements of program planning are viewed in relation to these facilitators and barriers to participation in CE, further direction for the planning process can be discerned more readily.

Instructional Content

The instructional content for CE offerings needs to include topics of high interest for promoting competency in job performance beyond the fundamentals required to complete assignments. Nurses seek continuing education opportunities that will augment and extend their practice beyond the basics, promote career advancement, and/or prepare them for new positions. In order to accomplish these, CE programs need to be tailored specifically for certain roles: the staff nurse audience seeking clinical topics related to direct, practical, hands-on aspects of patient care, therapies, or medications, or the clinical nurse specialist audience seeking a clinical focus as well but with fuller attention to various aspects of their subroles as mentors, researchers, educators, patient advocates, or advanced level practitioners. Just as with the basic precepts of competency-based education, the content of CE offerings needs to be tailored to the anticipated positions and roles of the intended audience, their interests, experience, and career aspirations.

Curriculum Organization and Sequencing

When the CE program consists of multiple courses or offerings, these may be organized and sequenced by clinical area, functional area (practice, education, management, research), or broad areas of mutual interest (such as patient care, quality assurance, ethical issues, or patient education). Unless a series of interrelated topics is planned, however, separate offerings within the program can be sequenced as creatively and practically as desired. In this instance a wide range of sequencing flexibility is available to the educator.

Instructional Time Allotment

Allotments of instructional time are chiefly determined by two decisions: the total number of hours planned for instruction and whether concurrent (breakout) sessions will be used in addition to general sessions for the entire audience. Space availability (e.g., the number and seating capacity of breakout rooms at the facility, any constraints imposed by the facility on times for breaks and/or meals, traffic and transportation patterns, etc.) may also affect the time frames established for general and concurrent sessions. If a larger number of topics is desired, the time for individual sessions (both general and concurrent) will need to be reduced. Social gatherings and networking opportunities will also need to be included in the time allotment and sequencing decisions. Because most adult learners enjoy meeting new people and exchanging ideas with colleagues who work in similar areas, it is important to plan time for these activities.[110]

Media Selection

Although the general principles for media selection and use follow the guidelines described in Chapter 3, larger, multiday CE programs may entail a few additional considerations. If numerous sessions will be offered, the number and types of audiovisual equipment required may easily exceed the hospital's inventory. It may then be necessary to arrange procurement with an audiovisual service company or with the facility where the program is held. In addition, the cost of renting certain types of audiovisual equipment may be prohibitively high or some types of media may not be available for use. Clearly communicating these constraints to faculty so that they are aware of them before they prepare their presentations can help to avoid problems and misunderstandings later on.

Selection of Program Format

Any of the CE program formats described earlier may be used for single instructional offerings. When the program includes numerous sessions, a variety of formats is often advisable so that multiple learning style preferences as well as variation in teaching methods can be afforded to participants to enhance interest and active learner participation and to avoid boredom and monotony. The combination of

*See references 1, 19, 25, 52, 66, 105.

TABLE 7.3 • CONSIDERATIONS FOR SELECTING RELEVANT CONTINUING EDUCATION PROGRAMS: A CONSUMER'S GUIDE*

Program Feature	Considerations
Personal and/or professional learning needs or interests *(Is this program right for me?)*	• What am I interested in learning about: a clinical area (such as cardiovascular or pulmonary nursing), a functional area (such as management, education, or research), or an area of professional growth (such as collaborative practice)? • Do the purpose and objectives of the program match my needs and interests? • Does the content of the program coincide with the scope of my needs, or is it more or less than I want? • Is the content of the program consistent with the stated objectives? • Are the program objectives realistic and feasible for the time available?
Intended audience *(Am I right for this program?)*	• Who is the intended audience for this program? • Do I match the characteristics (experience, education level, etc.) of the intended audience? • If prerequisites are stated, do I have these capabilities or experiences? • Is the perspective of the program (e.g., care of renal patients for staff nurses vs. for nurse practitioners) appropriate for me? • Will the audience size be small enough so that some individual attention from the instructor would be possible? • If the program is advertised "for all healthcare workers," do the content and objectives seem more directed at professional groups *other than* nurses? Is a clear nursing perspective evident?
Learning activities	• What type(s) of teaching methods will be employed in the program? • Are the teaching methods compatible with my preferred ways of learning? • Will the size of the audience enhance or diminish my active participation? • Is there likely to be sufficient time to have my questions answered? • If the program relates to development of skills, do the learning activities include the opportunity to begin development and practice of these skills?
Time frames	• What day(s), date(s), and time(s) are planned for the program? • Are these days, dates, and times feasible for me to attend the program? • Would I be attending on work or personal time? • Would additional days for travel be necessary? • Are the time frames established for the program sufficient to achieve the program objectives as well as my personal objectives?
Faculty	• Who will be teaching the program? • Is this speaker knowledgeable and experienced in this topic area? • What are the speaker's credentials and qualifications for this topic? • Will the speaker be able to relate the content to my area of interest? • If the instructor is a recognized authority in this area, is his/her reputation equally good as a speaker? • If the instructor is a relative "unknown," does he/she have the potential to speak with authority on this topic? • Have any of my peers attended a program given by this speaker? If so, what are their opinions regarding the quality of this individual as a speaker?
Program sponsor	• Is the program sponsored by a reputable organization? • If colleagues have attended other programs provided by this sponsor, are their opinions of the sponsor favorable? • If the sponsor is not a nursing organization, is there evidence of nursing input into program planning? • Does this sponsor provide any means of guaranteeing my satisfaction with the program?
CEU approval	• Has the program already been approved for CEUs? If so, by which organizations? • How many and what category of CEUs will be awarded for attendance at this program? • If I work in a state where CEUs are required for relicensure, have the appropriate accrediting organizations approved the program?

Program Feature	Considerations
Location	• Where will the program be held? • Is this location convenient and accessible to me? • Are the meeting rooms at this facility comfortable and conducive to learning? • Does the facility offer services (free parking, meals, child care, lodging) that I need or want?
Cost	• What is the cost of tuition/registration for this program? • Are breaks and meals included in the cost of registration? • Would I incur associated travel costs (airfare, lodging, meals, ground transportation, etc.) to attend this program? If so, what would be the total cost? • How much work and personal time would my attendance at this program cost? • Is the total cost comparable for similar programs at similar facilities? • Are the anticipated benefits for attending this program worth the costs? • How much of the total cost would be borne by my employer? How much would be borne by me?
Social and professional interactions	• Will the program offer an opportunity to network with colleagues? To meet leaders in the field? To establish a professional support system? To advance my career? To secure a needed consultant?

TABLE 7.3 • CONSIDERATIONS FOR SELECTING RELEVANT CONTINUING EDUCATION PROGRAMS: A CONSUMER'S GUIDE*—cont'd

*Modified from American Nurses Association: *Continuing education in nursing—a consumer's guide,* Kansas City, MO, 1984, ANA, and Craft MJ, Heick M, Richards B et al: *J Cont Educ Nurs* 23(6):245, 1992.

creative and varied topics, creative and varied media, and creative and varied instructional formats enables the largest number of participants to find sessions and learning activities suitable for both their needs and preferences. Continuing education program planners need to be mindful that a balanced menu of active, passive, interactive, solitary, small and large group activities should be sought so that as many cognitive styles and learning styles as possible can be accommodated in the program.

Selection of Faculty

Faculty selection aims at designation of knowledgeable and experienced instructors who are effective educators in their areas of expertise. Local faculty who meet these criteria can be included in addition to those who have national reputations. Although "big names" may draw an audience to the program, planners should first verify that these individuals present well and have established track records of quality performance in providing CE programs before they are invited to serve in this capacity. Attending sessions that these individuals provide at other conferences is one good way to verify first hand whether your institution would like to invite them as a speaker. Another avenue is by soliciting the appraisals of associates, colleagues, and other organizations that have used these individuals as speakers. If neither of these methods is possible, a third approach would be to ask prospective speakers to provide a list of references so that these may be verified before the invitation is issued.

Instructional Schedules

The basic principles of preparing an instructional schedule for a CE program are the same as for any other component of staff development. These planning devices can be considerably more complex when numerous sessions are planned over multiple days, but the increased complexity of the procedure does not materially affect the process used. The schedules may be prepared either in the traditional vertical enumeration of sessions or as a grid that illustrates choices among concurrent sessions.

Faculty Support

Communicating with and supporting faculty before, during, and after their presentation follows a process comparable to that described in Chapter 3. The only notable exceptions to this process are that CE programs more often involve working with only experienced faculty who require less instructional support, working with some or many faculty who may be from out of town and unfamiliar with your facility, and the possibility of working with more faculty members simultaneously than for other staff development programs.

Experienced faculty will typically require only focused instructional support before, during, and after the program. Before the program, eliciting their needs and preferences for room size, room seating arrangements (Figure 7.1), number and types of audiovisual equipment and microphones, handout duplication, and travel arrangements is usually all that is necessary. During the presentation, staff need to be available for introducing the speaker; for audiovisual setup, use, and troubleshooting; for adjustments to room lighting and temperature; for resolving logistical issues (such as adding chairs or answering participant questions unrelated to the presentation or CEU procedures); and for collecting evaluation forms. Particularly when there are multiple concurrent sessions, speakers should not be left stranded if problems arise during their session. Staff support needs to be immediately available to keep things running smoothly. Some speakers may also need assistance in staying within their time limits by signs that indicate the amount of time remaining in the session.

Out-of-town faculty may need assistance before the program with making travel, lodging, and transportation arrangements.[60] Planning some time for these newcomers to meet local staff and key persons in the organization adds a nice social and professional dimension to their visit that enhances mutual networking.

Following the presentation, staff may assist speakers by making any necessary adjustments to room lighting, by retrieving the speaker's audiovisual media, and by offering directions to them for the location of their next session, the location of break or dining areas, or the speaker's lounge. Faculty are usually also asked to complete an evaluation of their experience at the program so that their impressions can be taken into account for future program planning.

Additional Aspects

Continuing education programs that will be marketed to nurses outside your facility pose some unique challenges to

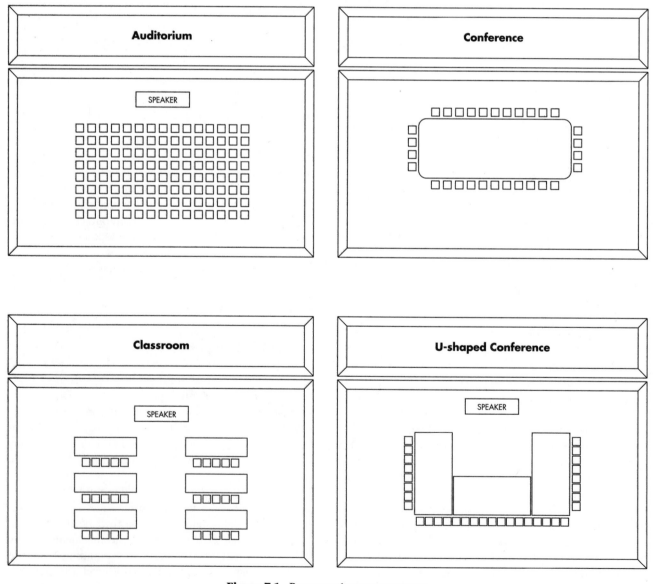

Figure 7.1 Room seating arrangements.

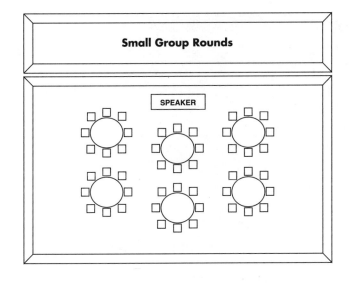

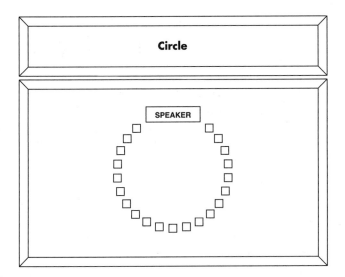

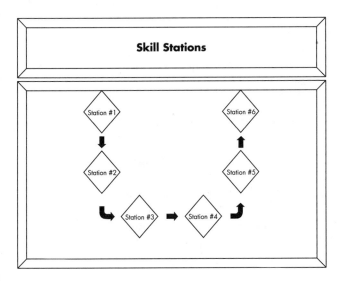

Figure 7.1—cont'd Room seating arrangements.

the educators who coordinate and plan these offerings. In addition to all of the customary planning that must be done for any CE offering, externally marketed programs often require a number of other planning features to be completed. A summary of these distinctive planning elements is enumerated below.

- More elaborate budget development*
- Promotion: design and duplication or printing of materials to advertise the program
- Marketing*: development of a marketing plan, creating or obtaining mailing lists, mailing brochures
- Reservation of facilities: classrooms (and lodging, if appropriate)
- Decisions related to exhibitors: whether to include, fees, exhibit space, registration
- Design, duplication, collation, and transport of program materials to facility
- Ordering food and refreshments for breaks, meals
- Reservation of audiovisual equipment and supplies
- Development of registration list
- Design and operation of registration process and procedures
- Design, construction, and placement of signs to designate registration and session locations
- Design and implementation of record-keeping system* related to attendance and CEUs awarded

Implementation

The implementation of continuing education programs includes two primary facets: provision of the individual instructional sessions and operational aspects of providing the program.

Instructional Aspects

The instructional aspects of program provision follow the same guiding principles (teaching, learning, adult education; cognitive, learning, and teaching style preferences) and teaching methodologies as for any other component of nursing staff development. Except for staff monitoring of the quality and conduct of each session during its presentation, there are no substantive differences for the CE component related to speakers' provision of instruction.

Operational Aspects

The operational aspects of program provision can be more complex with CE programs than with orientation and in-service programs. Some highlights of these distinctive and additional elements for continuing education are summarized in Box 7.3.

*These areas will be discussed more fully in Chapter 8.
*See references 23, 31, 63, 67, 75, 87, 92, 103, 120.

Box 7.3

OPERATIONAL ASPECTS OF PROGRAM IMPLEMENTATION IN CONTINUING EDUCATION

- Verifying room set up and seating capacity
- Verifying placement and operation of audiovisual equipment
- Setting up registration area for distribution of name tags, handouts/proceedings, and related materials
- Confirming catering needs and times
- Placement of signs for directions and room locations
- Greeting and assistance to speakers
- Opening general session:
  - Starting on time
  - Welcoming participants
  - Describing overview of program
  - Relating schedule and arrangements for breaks, meals
  - Mentioning location of telephones, restrooms, dining areas
  - Explaining use and submission of evaluation forms
  - Describing CEU information
  - Introducing the speaker
- Troubleshooting problems for participants, speakers

When multiple sessions and speakers are used, the educator (or designee) responsible for coordinating the CE program needs to remain available to both faculty and participants (and exhibitors) in case problems arise during the proceedings. Speakers may require assistance with adjusting the room lighting and turning the audiovisual equipment on/off at desired times, with seating late arrivals, placement of audience microphones, staying within the allotted time limits for their presentation, or locating other support staff. Potential problems that may arise and need attention can include audiovisual or microphone malfunctions or failures, extremes of room temperature, noise in adjacent rooms of the facility, or participant or speaker illness.

Following large CE programs, the educator will also have some additional responsibilities to complete. These may include any or all of the following:

- Thanking speakers and participants at the closing session
- Collecting and collating participant, speaker, and exhibitor evaluations
- Distributing attendance and/or CEU certificates
- Mailing thank-you letters and session evaluations to speakers
- Paying faculty, vendors, and the facility for services provided
- Finalizing record keeping related to the list of registrants
- Summarizing program costs and evaluations

Provision of a single CE offering of a few hours duration may entail no more effort than that required for implementation of an in-service offering. However, provision of large-scale CE programs that include many sessions over multiple days as well as large numbers of participants and faculty can represent a major educational undertaking that taxes the full complement of staff development resources. Although most of the instructional aspects of these larger endeavors are comparable to other components of staff development, the complexity and number of operational features can add considerably to the demands placed on the staff development department.

Evaluation

Evaluation of continuing education program effectiveness virtually always includes appraisal at the satisfaction level, often includes appraisal of learning, sometimes encompasses application to practice, but rarely includes impact evaluation. As mentioned in Chapter 5, this distribution in the frequency along the four levels of educational evaluation is typical of the entire fields of staff development and continuing professional education. Evaluation of the efficiency of continuing education programs, by contrast, is virtually always determined to a greater or less degree of detail.

Evaluation of Satisfaction

CE programs are concerned with determining the satisfaction of both participants and faculty.

PARTICIPANT SATISFACTION   Participants are most often surveyed regarding their satisfaction with general features of the program such as the following:

- Overall content
- Level of instruction
- Quality of faculty

- Teaching methods employed
- Program materials (proceedings, handouts, bibliographies)
- Usefulness of media
- Quality and comfort of the facility
- Accessibility of location
- Refreshments and meals

In addition, participants are usually asked to indicate both the degree to which the objectives of each session were met and the degree to which their personal objectives for attending the program were attained. Participants may also be asked to describe polar impressions such as which aspects of the program they liked most and which they liked least, their suggestions for program improvements, or their suggestions (topics, faculty) for future programs.

When the CE program includes numerous sessions and instructors, participants are typically asked to indicate their satisfaction with each session they attend. These appraisals are usually brief and directed at attainment of the objectives, the teaching strategies used, audiovisual quality, and faculty performance. An evaluation form such as that shown in Figure 6-5 could be used for this purpose.

FACULTY SATISFACTION   The faculty of CE programs need to be included in program evaluations in order to determine how satisfying the experience was from the provider perspective. The educator may divide the questionnaire for faculty into three phases: staff support and assistance prior to, during, and following the program. In addition to general ratings of the degree of their satisfaction, faculty may also be asked to identify any problems they encountered with either the instructional or operational aspects of the program. For out-of-town speakers, it may also be useful to determine their satisfaction with the travel, transportation, lodging, and dining arrangements they experienced.

Evaluation of Learning

Continuing education programs frequently include appraisals of learning for either one or both of two reasons: (1) the sponsor wishes to provide an opportunity to offer feedback related to learning to participants and (2) the sponsor needs to include an evaluation of learning in order to secure CEU approval for the program.

When CE programs include evaluation of learning, this is frequently achieved via learner-controlled, written self-assessment. A few open-ended questions may be posed or a few multiple-choice items may be given as well as an answer key for those items. Learners may then secure feedback on their learning if they desire to do so. The more rigorous learning appraisals characteristic of orientation and in-service education programs are usually not employed in continuing education. One reason for this may be because the knowledge, attitudes, and skills sought in

CE programs are not required for the nurse's present job, so less rigorous appraisal of this learning appears more appropriate. Adults' natural aversion to "testing" might also dissuade enrollment in CE courses if formal evaluations of learning were mandated. Of the three components of staff development, continuing education most approximates "learning for the sake of learning," so the need for exacting evaluation methods is open to question. The means of evaluation generally focus instead on whether nurses who participate in CE programs eventually apply this learning in their nursing practice or whether this learning results in a measurable impact on the quality of patient care. When a competency-based approach is used for CE programs, these applications and patient outcomes would be expressed as competency statements and performance criteria.

Evaluation of Application

The application of learning from a CE program to nursing practice may be viewed from either the learner's perspective or the provider's perspective and may be performed in any of three different time frames: immediate, short-term, or long-term.

FROM THE LEARNER'S PERSPECTIVE   Since learners enroll in CE to meet their own needs for learning, their impressions of the degree to which they are able to apply this learning can have significant personal and professional importance to the nurse. Some CE programs incorporate elements of immediate application in the evaluation form completed upon program completion. These forms may solicit participants' views and intentions regarding application of learning to their practice by posing the following types of questions:

- Please describe how the content of this program relates to your future practice of nursing
- Please name five specific ways in which you intend to apply what you learned in this program to your future practice in nursing
- Please estimate about how long you believe it would take for each of these applications to be incorporated in your practice

Short-term evaluations of learning application can be completed for learning applications anticipated to occur within a few weeks or months following the CE program.[63] These evaluations would involve identifying the intended applications that should have occurred within those time frames and determining the degree to which each was actually accomplished.

The long-term evaluation of learning application could encompass either of two elements: (1) initial appraisal of outcomes that were estimated to require many months (9 to 12 months) to complete, and/or (2) follow-up appraisal of the degree to which short-term applications have persisted following their earlier evaluation.

Evaluation of learning applications from the participant's perspective are generally based on self-reports rather than on more objective criteria such as direct observation of practice or audit findings. As a result, the validity and reliability of these subjective evaluations is open to question. A second issue related to this type of evaluation is the difficulty inherent in having the resources to follow up CE programs with the extended evaluation time frames necessary for appraising both short- and long-term applications to practice. Although the value of doing this type of evaluation may be recognized and affirmed, the resources for accomplishing this may be quite limited.

FROM THE PROVIDER'S PERSPECTIVE   When a CE program is planned, the provider may identify a number of desired instructional outcomes that reflect application of learning to nursing practice. Since these outcomes cannot be determined at the time of the program, they represent either short- or long-term appraisals of applications of learning to practice.

The CE program provider may use an evaluation procedure similar to that used to determine the participant's perspective. The only significant differences between these two approaches would be that the anticipated applications and time frames would be identified by the provider before the program rather than be identified by the learner at the time of program completion and that the evaluation procedure would employ an objective appraisal (e.g., via direct observation, checklist of performance behaviors, or audit process criteria) rather than a subjective survey.

Some additional areas that may be explored regarding evaluation of application to nursing practice relate to the extent to which the work environment supports and facilitates these applications. In addition to identifying the degree to which the participant was successful in applying learning to practice, information may be solicited regarding any of the following:

- The degree to which the participants' supervisors expected them to apply the learning acquired in the program
- The degree to which supervisors supported and facilitated applications of learning to practice
- The degree to which peers supported applications of learning to practice
- The participants' perception of work setting features that enabled them to apply learning to practice
- The participants' perception of work setting features that hindered or obstructed their application of learning to practice

This group of factors is often analyzed in relation to both the application and impact levels of evaluation. Because the influence of these variables represents the ultimate effect of CE on nursing practice and, in turn, quality patient care, they are considered under the discussion of educational evaluation at the impact level.

Evaluation of Impact

Although the assumed association between continuing professional education in nursing and quality patient care has persisted for decades, the empirical linkage of cause and effect or even association has been considerably more difficult to establish. Research and literature on the relationship among continuing education, nursing practice, and improved patient care accelerated when states began adopting requirements for mandatory CE for nurse relicensure. Since that time, research and experiential attempts to establish and support these relationships have proliferated. Of late, however, increased attention has been accorded to recognition that the quality of the CE program itself is only one ingredient, albeit an important ingredient, in the constellation of variables that may influence whether and to what extent learning acquired in a CE program finds its way into nursing practice and improved patient care. The difficulty, cost, and resources demanded by impact evaluation discussed in Chapter 5 notwithstanding, the section that follows provides an overview of current thinking in the area of application and impact evaluations of continuing nursing education.

A number of different models have been proposed for describing the effects of continuing education on nursing practice.[18,45,51,77,122] Of these, the inclusive and multidimensional nature of Cervero's model[18] currently seems to offer the greatest potential for recognizing the interrelated complexity of factors that may determine whether and to what degree CE affects the practice of nursing. Rather than isolating the CE program as the sole influence on changes in nursing practice, Cervero's model proposes that four different but interrelated categories of influence determine whether changes in practice result following a CE program. These four categories of potential influence include:

- Attributes or characteristics of the individual learner
- Attributes or characteristics of the CE offering
- The nature of the proposed behavioral change/improvement
- The environment or social system within which the learner works

With this model, changes in nursing practice and patient care could be explained on the basis of the relative degree to which each of these factors contributes to or hinders improvements in practice and patient care.

CHARACTERISTICS OF THE LEARNER   Many traits and attributes of the nurses who attend CE programs may conceivably affect whether these nurses take what they have learned in the program, apply their learning to changes in their practice, and thereby improve their quality of patient care. Nurses' motivation and initiative to participate in CE and their personal motivation and commitment to alter practice[20] may influence the degree to which practice changes are implemented. Nurses' attitudes toward potential practice changes (favorable vs. unfavorable, feasible or not feasible to achieve) and the perceived congruence between practice changes and their own beliefs and opinions[64] may affect the changes they initiate. The knowledge, attitude, and skill changes in nurses that result from a CE offering will affect their actual and perceived ability to implement the practice changes they envision. These capabilities, in turn, may be affected by the knowledge, attitudes, and skills that nurses bring to the CE offering, the amount of learning they actually gain there, as well as the degree to which they actively participate in learning activities.[19]

Factors in the learner that may potentially inhibit implementation of practice and patient care changes following a CE program represent the obverse of those mentioned previously. In spite of possessing the knowledge, attitudes, and skills related to the proposed change, nurses may lack facility with implementing the change process within an organizational setting. Waddell's[120] meta-analysis of the literature in this area revealed a few factors that do **not** appear to be associated with the effects of CE on nursing practice: whether the CE participants are all RNs or a multidisciplinary group, the nurse's age, or the number of years of nursing experience. Ruder[102] also found that nurses who attended CE programs voluntarily implemented changes in practice more frequently than those who attended on a mandatory basis.

CHARACTERISTICS OF THE CE OFFERING   Some of the influences on the effectiveness of a CE offering potentially include the content, design, and implementation of the educational program, the motivation and effectiveness of faculty, as well as the degree to which the instructional environment facilitates learning.[19] Although educators are accustomed to viewing program outcomes pretty much exclusively on the basis of the design of the instructional program itself, Waddell's[120] analysis revealed that changes in nursing practice following a CE program were *not* necessarily associated with the program content, the types or number of teaching/learning strategies used, program length, or the quality of the educational design (operationally defined as a rating based on the ANA's accreditation criteria for approval of a CE offering). The rating was completed using reported information submitted for CEU approval rather than on an appraisal of what was actually provided to participants. This latter finding regarding rating of a CE program is less surprising if educators recall that even well-planned educational offerings can go awry during implementation and result in a significant discrepancy between what was designed and what was actually delivered to participants.

NATURE OF PROPOSED CHANGE(S) IN PRACTICE   The desirability and complexity of proposed changes in practice may influence whether they are adopted. In general, highly desired changes that are relatively easy to implement,[121] that require minimal time and/or disruption of current procedures, and that involve little threat to those making the change are more likely to be effected than others.[18,92] Conversely, practice changes that staff find difficult to comprehend, that are inherently complex,[64] that affect more people, that are difficult to implement, or that are inconsistent or incompatible with staff beliefs and values may be considerably more difficult to bring about.

SOCIAL SYSTEM OF THE WORK ENVIRONMENT   The social system of the CE participant's work setting may exert a significant influence on whether that nurse is able to bring about improved practice and patient care following the educational activity. Systems theory suggests that some of the major components of a hospital social system incorporate both individuals and groups (patients, staff peers, supervisors, administrators), operational procedures and processes, communication patterns, and resources.

Potential influences on the impact of CE may include[19,64,92,120,121] the attitudes of peers, supervisors, and administrators regarding the institution of practice changes; the support or obstacles the system's players offer towards proposed changes; the character of the hospital in relation to openness to change and innovation, empowerment of staff, role of staff in decision-making, and whether maintenance of the status quo is valued over the instability of the change process. The degree of organizational support may also be associated with the degree to which the proposed change is viewed as consistent with the organization's mission and goals or the nurse's present work load. Apathy, resistance to change, and limited resources may all diminish the likelihood of changes in nursing practice.[64]

Waddell's[120] analysis of studies related to changes in nursing practice following CE found that, although practice changes were not associated with the type of healthcare facility (community vs. teaching hospital), or with the practice setting (home care vs. clinic), there was a significant relationship between the implementation of practice changes and the number of learners from the same healthcare institution: changes in practice were more likely to occur when the audience came from the same rather than from different facilities. This finding suggests that a captive audience of nurses from the same agency may be more successful in initiating improvements in nursing practice than if learners come from different work sites. Waddell suggested that educators who teach groups of nurses from different facilities include some basic tenets of change theory and suggestions for making changes happen in their presentations.

Readers will note that much of the previous discussion actually focuses on what has been described here as the "application" rather than the "impact" of continuing education. Although a number of the more than 250 research studies in this area generally support the contention that CE can and does result in improvements in nursing practice that persist over time,* systematic examination of the influence of continuing nursing education on patient outcomes is, as yet, more often assumed from changes observed in nursing practice than verified from actual patient data. The multiplicity of potential variables in this process that would need to be controlled in research, as only highlighted previously, contributes greatly to this information void. As a result, true impact evaluation of CE in nursing still awaits the development of research designs that can identify and control the effect of some of these variables so that the potential effects of a few can be examined with confidence. In that case all of the potential influences that might affect patient care and patient outcomes would need to be added to the confluence of influences already highlighted. Although impact evaluation is, as Cervero[19] calls it, "the Holy Grail of evaluation questions," it is presently at only the inceptual stage of conceptualization. Impact evaluation represents an ultimate aim for staff development, but our path to that target is not yet clearly in sight.

PROPOSED MODEL   In addition to the four categories of variables identified in Cervero's model, four additional categories might be added to more fully reflect the multivariate nature of factors that may influence whether a nurse's participation in CE offerings creates an impact on patient outcomes (Figure 7.2). These additional areas include the influence of the following:

- *Other healthcare workers.* The individual nurse is only one of many healthcare workers who interact with the patient. The actions and ministrations of other nursing staff, physicians, specialists (dietary, pharmacy, etc.), therapists (occupational, physical, respiratory, and the like), social workers, and many other professional and ancillary workers may positively or negatively affect patient outcomes.
- *The patient's health problem(s).* Although some aspects of the patient's health status are amenable to influence by the individual nurse, other aspects that reflect the nature, course, severity, and prognosis of these problems will vary in the degree of influence the nurse or any other healthcare worker can have. Some of these factors may persist regardless of the quality

*See references 23, 31, 63, 67, 75, 87, 92, 103, 120.

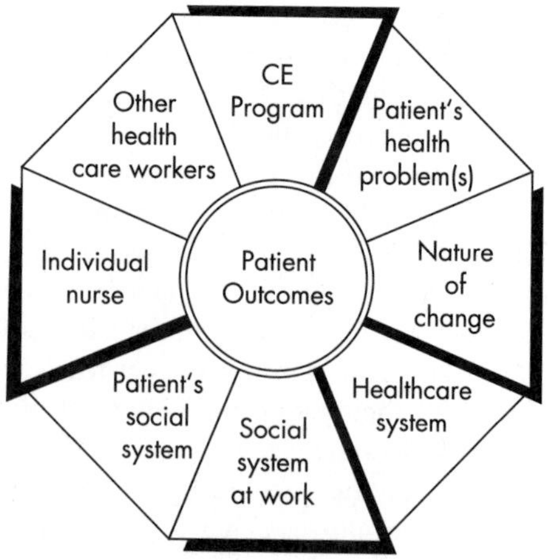

Figure 7.2 Factors affecting impact evaluation.
(Modified from Cervero RM: *J Cont Educ Nurs* 16(3):85, 1985.)

of nursing practice provided, and they may favorably or unfavorably affect patient outcome.

- *The patient's social system.* The patient's family and other social support as well as their cultural beliefs, attitudes, values, and health practices may enhance or retard positive patient outcomes in combination with or apart from the care provided by an individual nurse.
- *The healthcare system.* In addition to the social system of the work environment, other features of the healthcare system may impinge on patient outcomes. Some of these factors include the cost of healthcare services; the location, availability, and accessibility of healthcare services; pressures to reduce length of stay and healthcare costs; as well as whether the patient has adequate health insurance coverage. Each of these elements may facilitate or impede the realization of optimal patient outcomes independent of the quality of nursing care provided.

This somewhat enlarged perspective of impact on the patient suggests that isolation of the role of a continuing nursing education program in determining patient outcomes is not only a complex undertaking both conceptually and practically but may represent an overly simplistic view of the relationship between CE and patient outcomes. It also serves to remind educators that the competence of the nurse is only one of innumerable elements that may affect patient outcome, but it is an essential contributing element to which nursing staff development may contribute and sustain.

REFERENCES

1. Alspach JG: *The self-directed learning readiness of baccalaureate nursing students,* doctoral dissertation, College Park, MD, 1991, University of Maryland.
2. Ament LA: Competency assessment versus credentialing: promoting professional nursing practice, *J Nurs Staff Develop* 9(3):157, 1993.
3. American Nurses' Association (ANA): *Continuing education in nursing—a consumer's guide,* Kansas City, MO, 1984, ANA.
4. American Nurses' Association (ANA): *Standards for continuing education in nursing,* Kansas City, MO, 1984, ANA.
5. American Nurses' Association (ANA): *Standards for nursing staff development,* Kansas City, MO, 1990, ANA.

6. American Society for Healthcare Education and Training: *Standards for healthcare education and training,* Chicago, 1990, American Hospital Association.

7. Arons B: Critical thinking and the baccalaureate curriculum, *Liberal Educ* 71(2):141, 1985.

8. Austin EK: *Guidelines for the development of continuing education offerings for nurses,* New York, NY, 1981, Appleton-Century-Crofts.

9. Bandman EL, Bandman B: *Critical thinking in nursing,* East Norwalk, CT, 1988, Appleton & Lange.

10. Barako J, Reichert A, Nunez A: The N.Y.P.E.N. method: meeting learning needs and satisfying educational requirements, *J Nurs Staff Develop* 5(3):132, 1989.

11. Barrows HS, Tamblyn RM: *Problem-based learning: an approach to medical education,* New York, NY, 1980, Springer.

12. Bauwens EE, Gerhard GG: The use of the Watson-Glaser critical thinking appraisal to predict success in a baccalaureate nursing program, *J Nurs Educ* 26(7):278, 1987.

13. Benner P: *From novice to expert,* Menlo Park, CA, 1984, Addison-Wesley.

14. Berger MC: Clinical thinking ability and nursing students, *J Nurs Educ* 23(7):306, 1984.

15. Bethel PL: Inservice education: calculating the cost, *J Cont Educ Nurs* 21(3):105, 1990.

16. Bloom BS, Broder LJ: *Problem-solving processes of college students: an exploratory investigation,* Chicago, IL, 1950, University of Chicago.

17. Boissoneau R: *Continuing education in the health professions,* Rockville, Md, 1980, Aspen Systems.

18. Cervero RM: Continuing professional education and behavioral change: a model for research and evaluation, *J Cont Educ Nurs* 16(3):85, 1985.

19. Cervero RM: *Effective continuing education for professionals,* San Francisco, CA, 1988, Jossey-Bass.

20. Cervero RM, Rottett S, Dimmock KH: Analyzing the effectiveness of continuing education at the workplace, *Adult Educ Q* 36(2):78, 1986.

21. Cherry B, Howard J: CPR by blitz: an intense campaign for annual certification, *Focus Crit Care* 14(1):30, 1987.

22. Coleman S, Dracup K, Moser CK: Comparing methods of cardiopulmonary resuscitation instruction on learning and retention, *J Nurs Staff Develop* 7(2):82, 1991.

23. Connors HR: Impact evaluation of a statewide continuing education program, *J Cont Educ Nurs* 20(2):64, 1989.

24. Craft MJ, Heick M, Richards B et al: Program characteristics influencing nurse selection of CE offerings, *J Cont Educ Nurs* 23(6):245, 1992.

25. Cross KP: *Adults as learners,* San Francisco, CA, 1984, Jossey-Bass.

26. Curry L, Gass D: Effects of training in cardiopulmonary resuscitation on competence and outcome, *Can Med J* 137:491, 1987.

27. D'Aurizio P: Education day: concentration improves compliance, *Nursing Manage* 16(7):12, 1985.

28. D'Aurizio P, Bender J, Wormack S et al: Education days: mandatory reviews plus staff development, *J Nurs Staff Develop* 3(1):42, 1987.

29. Diaz DP: Promote recruitment and retention by meeting the unique learning needs of the off shifts, *J Cont Educ Nurs* 20(6):249, 1989.

30. Dickerson M: Mandatory educational programs: a decentralized approach, *J Nurs Staff Develop* 3(2):84, 1987.

31. Dickinson GR, Holzemer WL, Nichols E: Evaluation of an arthritis continuing education program, *J Cont Educ Nurs* 16(4):127, 1985.

32. DiPietro CM: A cost effective plan for CPR recertification, *J Nurs Staff Develop* 5(1):45, 1989.

33. Djupe AM: Night owl inservice: at your own pace, in your own place, *J Cont Educ Nurs* 18(5):154, 1987.

34. Dolphin P, Holtzclaw BJ: *Continuing education in nursing,* Reston, VA, 1983, Reston.

35. Dracup K, Breu C: Teaching and retention of cardiopulmonary resuscitation skills for families of high risk patients with cardiac disease, *Focus on Crit Care* 14(1):67, 1987.

36. Edwards MJ, Hannah KJ: An examination of the use of interactive videodisc cardiopulmonary resuscitation instruction for the lay community, *Computers Nurs* 3(6):250, 1985.

37. Flynn JP: Evaluation of two staff development programs for teaching decision techniques to first line nurse managers, *J Cont Educ Nurs* 20(5):237, 1989.

38. Ford LA, Wickham VA, Colver C: Developing a skills fair workshop: enhancing competency performance, *Dimens Crit Care Nurs* 11(6):340, 1992.

39. Frandson PE: Continuing education for the professions. In EJ Boone, RW Shearon, EE White, editors: *Serving personal and community needs through adult education,* San Francisco, 1980, Jossey-Bass, pp 61–82.

40. Frederickson K: Critical thinking ability and academic achievement, *J N Y Student Nurses Assoc* 10(1):40, 1979.

41. Friesen L, Stotts N: Retention of basic cardiac life support content: the effect of two teaching methods, *J Nurs Educ* 23(5):184, 1984.

42. Frisch N: Cognitive maturity of nursing students, *Image* 19(1):25, 1987.

43. Funkhouser MJ, Hayward MF: Multidisciplinary mock codes, *J Nurs Staff Develop* 5(5):231, 1989.

44. Goldrick BA: Programmed instruction revisited: a solution to infection control inservice education, *J Cont Educ Nurs* 20(5):222, 1989.

45. Gosnell D: Evaluating continuing nursing education, *J Cont Educ Nurs* 15(1):9, 1984.

46. Groteleuschen AD, Harnisch DL, Kenny WR: *An analysis of the Participation Reasons Scale administered to business professionals,* Occasional paper no 7, Urbana, IL, 1979, Office for the Study of Continuing Professional Education, University of Illinois at Urbana-Champaign.

47. Guardo C: Designing curricula for imaginary students, *Liberal Educ* 72(3):213, 1986.

48. Haggard A: Using self-studies to meet JCAHO requirements, *J Nurs Staff Develop* 8(4):170, 1992.

49. Hekelman FP, Phillips JA, Bierer LA: An interactive videodisk training program in basic cardiac life support: implications for staff development, *J Cont Educ Nurs* 21(6):245, 1990.

50. Holbert CM, Abraham C: Reflections on teaching generic thinking and problem-solving, *Nurse Educator* 13(2):23, 1988.

51. Holzemer WL: Evaluation methods in continuing education, *J Cont Educ Nurs* 23(4):174, 1992.

52. Houle CO: *Continuing learning in the professions,* San Francisco, CA, 1981, Jossey-Bass.

53. Hudson M: An innovative approach to mandatory inservice offerings, *J Cont Educ Nurs* 20(1):16, 1989.

54. Hughes KK, Young WB: Decision-making stability of clinical decisions, *Nurs Educator* 17(3):12, 1992.

55. Inglis AD: Ten common-sense teaching strategies for effective inservice presentation by staff nurses, *J Cont Educ Nurs* 23(6):263, 1992.

56. Jenkins HM: Improving clinical decision making in nursing, *J Nurs Educ* 24(6):242, 1985.

57. Johnson DM: A creative safety program, *J Nurs Staff Develop* 5(3):111, 1989.

58. Joint Commission on Accreditation of Healthcare Organizations (JCAHO): *Accreditation manual for hospitals: vol 1, Standards,* Oakbrook Terrace, IL, 1993, JCAHO.

59. Joint Commission on Accreditation of Healthcare Organizations (JCAHO): *Accreditation manual for hospitals: vol 2, Scoring guidelines,* Oakbrook Terrace, IL, 1993, JCAHO.

60. Kaeter M: The care and feeding of VIPs, *Training,* 30(suppl 7):13, 1993.

61. Kaye W, Mancini M, Rallis S et al.: Can better basic and advanced cardiac life support improve outcome from cardiac arrest? *Crit Care Med* 13:916, 1985.

62. Keeley SM, Browne MN, Kreutzer JS: A comparison of freshmen and seniors on general and specific essay tests on critical thinking, *Res Higher Educ* 17:139, 1982.

63. Kellmer-Langan DM, Hunter C, Nottingham JP: Knowledge retention and clinical application after continuing education, *J Nurs Staff Develop* 8(1):5, 1992.

64. Kiener ME, Hentschel D: What happens to learning when the workshop is over? *J Cont Educ Nurs* 23(4):169, 1992.

65. Klaasens E: Strategies to enhance problem solving, *Nurs Educator* 17(3):28, 1992.

66. Kristjanson LJ, Scanlan JM: Assessment of continuing nursing education needs: a literature review, *J Cont Educ Nurs* 23(4):156, 1992.

67. Kuramoto AM: Research on continuing education in nursing, *Ann Rev Nurs Res* 3:149, 1985.

68. Kurfiss J: The reasoning-centered classroom: approaches that work, *Amer Assoc High Educ Bull* 39:12, 1987.

69. Lantz JM, Meyers GD: Critical thinking through writing: using personification to teach pharmacodynamics, *J Nurs Educ* 25(2):64, 1986.

70. Lesher DC, Bomberger AS: The roving inservice—an innovative approach to learning, *J Cont Educ Nurs* 14(3):19, 1983.

71. Lewis FH, Kee CC, Minick MP: Revisiting CPR knowledge and skills among registered nurses, *J Cont Educ Nurs* 24(4):174, 1993.

72. Malek CJ: A model for teaching critical thinking, *Nurse Educator* 11(6):20, 1986.

73. Matthews CA, Gaul AL: Nursing diagnosis from the perspective of concept attainment and critical thinking, *Advan Nurs Sci* 2(11):17, 1979.

74. McGregor RJ: Advancing staff nurse competencies, *J Nurs Staff Develop* 6(6):287, 1990.

75. Meservy D, Manson MA: Impact of continuing education on nursing practice and quality of patient care, *J Cont Educ Nurs* 18(6):214, 1987.

76. Miley H, Foley MA: Critical care blitz weekend: fun for all, *J Nurs Staff Develop* 8(2):85, 1992.

77. Mitsunaga B, Shores L: Evaluation in continuing education: is it practical? *J Cont Educ Nurs* 8(6):7, 1977.

78. Moralejo D, Gaese C: The mock isolation room: a fun way to review infection control, *J Cont Educ Nurs* 24(4):185, 1993.

79. Morton PG: Providing CE to evening and night staff, *J Cont Educ Nurs* 21(5):230, 1990.

80. Moysenko PT: A practice approach to CPR recertification, *J Cont Educ Nurs* 23(5):238, 1992.

81. Mueller SJ, Glaser D: Cost-effective methods of implementing CPR training, *J Cont Educ Nurs* 21(4):186, 1990.

82. National Commission on Excellence in Education: *A nation at risk,* Washington, DC, 1983, U.S. Government Printing Office.

83. National League for Nursing: *Criteria for evaluation of baccalaureate and higher degree programs in nursing,* New York, NY, 1983, National League for Nursing.

84. Nelson M, Brown C: CPR instruction: modular versus lecture course, *Ann Emerg Med* 13(2):72, 1984.

85. Norris S: Synthesis of research on critical thinking, *Educ Leader* 5:40, 1985.

86. O'Connor CT: Brief: evaluation of a modular method of cardiopulmonary resuscitation instruction, *J Cont Educ Nurs* 21(6):271, 1990.

87. Oliver SK: The effects of continuing education on the clinical behavior of nurses, *J Cont Educ Nurs* 15(4):130, 1984.

88. Pack JT, Chamberlain JA, Johantgen MA et al: Education day: the evolution of a learning experience, *J Nurs Staff Develop* 8(3):119, 1992.

89. Pardue SF: Decision-making skills and critical thinking ability among associate degree, diploma, baccalaureate, and master's-prepared nurses, *J Nurs Educ* 26(9):354, 1987.

90. Patten BC: Brief: when to place your staff in "Jeopardy"—a CPR teaching strategy, *J Cont Educ Nurs* 20(3):136, 1989.

91. Patterson NG: Preparation techniques for ACLS exam, *Dimens Crit Care Nurs* 8(4):244, 1989.

92. Peden AR, Rose H, Smith M: Transfer of continuing education to practice: testing an evaluation model, *J Cont Educ Nurs* 23(4):152, 1992.

93. Perry W: *Forms of intellectual and ethical development in the college years,* New York, NY, 1970, Rinehart & Winston.

94. Piaget I: *The theory and stages in cognitive development,* New York, 1986, McGraw-Hill.

95. Plank CH: Effect of two teaching methods on CPR retention, *J Nurs Staff Develop* 5(3):145, 1989.

96. Pond EF, Bradshaw MJ, Turner SL: Teaching strategies for critical thinking, *Nurs Educator* 16(6):18, 1991.

97. Proctor ME: Creative methods of meeting JCAHO inservice requirements for hospital staff, *J Nurs Staff Develop* 5(6):285, 1989.

98. Puetz BE: *Continuing education in nursing,* Rockville, MD, 1987, Aspen.

99. Puetz BE, Peters FL: *Continuing education for nurses,* Rockville, MD, 1981, Aspen.

100. Riegelman RK, Povar GJ, Ott JE et al: A strategy for the education of 21st century physicians, *Med Teach* 7(3):279, 1985.

101. Roberts C, Rondestvedt J: Don't go 'way, it's time to play . . . the safety game! *J Cont Educ Nurs* 24(4):189, 1993.

102. Ruder SK: The comparison of mandatory and voluntary participation in continuing education on nursing performance. Doctoral dissertation, Northern Illinois University, 1987, *Dissertation Abstracts International* 49, 187A.

103. Sakalys J, Carter M: Outcome evaluation: continuing education in rheumatology for nurses, *J Cont Educ Nurs* 16(5):170, 1986.

104. Schank MJ: Wanted: nurses with critical thinking skills, *J Cont Educ Nurs* 21(2):86, 1990.

105. Schlosser SP, Jones JT, Whatley JH: Continuing education needs of hospital-based nurses in Alabama, *J Cont Educ Nurs* 24(3):135, 1993.

106. Schmitz BD, MacLean SL, Shidler HM: An emergency Pursuit game: a method for teaching emergency decision-making skills, *J Cont Educ Nurs* 22(4):152, 1991.

107. Schoessler M, Yount S, Marshall D et al: Safety First©—a board game for safety education, *J Cont Educ Nurs* 22(6):263, 1991.

108. Seigel H: Innovative approaches to inservice education, *J Cont Educ Nurs* 22(4):147, 1991.

109. Shehee A: Computer-certified CPR, *Am J Nurs* 89(4):548, 1989.

110. Simerly RG: *Planning and marketing conferences and workshops,* San Francisco, CA, 1990, Jossey-Bass.

111. Snyder-Halpern R, Buczkowski E: Performance-based staff development, *J Nurs Staff Develop* 6(1):7, 1990.

112. Sullivan EJ: Critical thinking, creativity, clinical performance, and achievement in RN students, *Nurse Educator* 12(2):12, 1987.

113. Taba H: *Teaching strategies and cognitive functioning in elementary school children* (cooperative research project 2404), Palo Alto, CA, 1966, San Francisco State College.

114. Taba H: The problem in developing critical thinking, *Progress Educ* 28:45, 1950.

115. Taba H, Durkin M, Fraenkel J et al: *A teacher's handbook to elementary social studies: an inductive approach,* Reading, MA, 1971, Addison-Wesley.

116. Thiele J: Identifying decision-making levels of simulations, *Nurs Educators Microworld* 5(4):30, 1991.

117. Tobin HM, Yoder Wise PS, Hull PK: *The process of staff development,* ed 2, St Louis, 1979, CV Mosby.

118. Turner SJ: Preparation for a fire disaster in a long-term care facility, *J Nurs Staff Develop* 7(3):134, 1991.

119. Umlauf MG: How to provide around-the-clock CPR certification without losing any sleep, *J Cont Educ Nurs* 21(6):248, 1990.

120. Waddell DL: The effects of continuing education on nursing practice: a meta-analysis, *J Cont Educ Nurs* 23(4):164, 1992.

121. Wake M: Effective instruction in continuing nursing education, *J Cont Educ Nurs* 18(0):188, 1987.

122. Warmuth JF: In search of the impact of continuing education, *J Cont Educ Nurs* 18(1):4, 1987.

123. Watson G, Glaser EM: *Critical thinking appraisal manual,* Dallas, TX, 1980, The Psychological Corporation.

124. Whimbey A: *Intelligence can be taught,* New York, 1975, EP Dutton.

125. Whimbey A, Lochhead J: *Problem solving and comprehension,* ed 3, Hillsdale, NJ, 1982, Lawrence Erlbaum.

126. White NE, Beardslee NQ, Peters D et al: Promoting critical thinking skills, *Nurs Educator* 15(5):16, 1990.

127. Williams J: The mobile educational crash cart: self-directed learning supplement that meets staff needs, *J Cont Educ Nurs* 17(2):59, 1986.

128. Willis SL, Dubin SS: *Maintaining professional competence,* San Francisco, CA, 1990, Jossey-Bass.

129. Wilson SG: Market research techniques—a synopsis for CE providers, *J Cont Educ Nurs* 23(4):182, 1992.

130. Woditsch G: Specifying and achieving competencies. In Milton O, editor:, *On college teaching,* San Francisco, CA, 1975, Jossey-Bass.

131. Wyatt G, Dimmer SA: A planning model for continuing education presenters, *J Cont Educ Nurs* 23(4):161, 1992.

132. Zellinger MJ: An alternative method for annual skills certification in the critical care unit, *Focus Crit Care* 18(5):422, 1991.

UNIT 4

Managing Nursing Staff Development Programs

CHAPTER 8

Managing Selected Staff Development Functions

In addition to coordinating all phases of the educational process, educators in nursing staff development are also responsible for managing a number of organizational and operational functions related to orientation, in-service, and continuing education programs. These managerial functions include the monitoring and improvement of organizational performance in nursing staff development, the development of policies and procedures related to nursing staff development, the maintenance of educational records, the preparation of budgets, and the marketing of staff development offerings.

MONITORING AND IMPROVING ORGANIZATIONAL PERFORMANCE

The management area formerly designated as *quality assurance (QA)*, *quality improvement (QI)*, *continuous quality improvement (CQI)*, or *total quality management (TQM)* continues to undergo evolutionary changes not only in nomenclature but also in understanding and approach. The current JCAHO standards[37] characterize this area as the improvement of organizational performance. Within this context, a healthcare organization's **performance** includes both what and how well it provides patient care services. The degree to which an organization does the right things and does them well, moreover, is "influenced strongly by the way it designs and carries out a number of important functions. . . ."[37] The Joint Commission considers **important functions** as those that most directly and significantly influence the quality of patient care. Some important functions, such as patient and family education, are highly visible and directly experienced by patients, whereas others are less visible but necessary to support the provision of patient care. The latter category includes all of the organizational support functions related to nursing staff development as well as its counterpart from the field of training called *human resource development*.

The ultimate goal of all segments of the department of nursing is delivery of high-quality patient care. The Joint Commission on Accreditation of Healthcare Organizations (JCAHO)[37] defines *quality of care* as "the degree to which health services for individuals and populations increase the likelihood of desired health outcomes and are consistent with current professional knowledge." Nursing practice, nursing administration, nursing staff development, and nursing research each contribute toward this ultimate goal in its own unique yet interrelated way. The management of organizational performance in the department of nursing encompasses the combined effects of all four of these department segments on the quality of nursing care delivered to patients.

Although the JCAHO accreditation requirements do not mandate that each separate hospital department have its own plan for monitoring and improving organizational performance, the standards do require evidence that all departments, services, and disciplines collaborate in this plan. In addition, standard SE 3 requires that the effectiveness and appropriateness of orientation, training, and other education provided by the hospital be evaluated *through its quality assessment and improvement activities.* If this rationale is extended to the nursing staff development segment of the nursing department, it follows that a written description of the staff development plan for improving organizational performance could be useful for documenting how staff development contributes to this collaborative process. Such a plan would then link nursing staff development activities to both the nursing department and the hospital performance improvement process.

STAFF DEVELOPMENT'S CONTRIBUTION TO IMPROVING ORGANIZATIONAL PERFORMANCE

As discussed in Chapter 1, nursing staff development contributes to quality patient care primarily by ensuring that all nursing staff are competent to fulfill their assigned responsibilities. This contribution is achieved through staff development's provision of orientation, in-service, and continuing education offerings that are designed to assist nursing staff in acquiring, validating, maintaining, and developing their competency on a current and ongoing basis. Rather than providing direct patient care services as nursing practice does, providing and managing patient care resources as nursing administration does, or generating and performing investigations related to patient care as nursing research does, nursing staff development makes its contribution via instructional programs on the knowledge, attitudes, and skills that underlie nursing practice and quality patient care.

COMPONENTS OF PERFORMANCE IMPROVEMENT IN STAFF DEVELOPMENT

The improvement of organizational performance in nursing staff development includes three basic components: (1) the identification of standards that define "quality in nursing staff development," (2) the monitoring of compliance with those standards, and (3) the institution of improvements in performance where these are indicated. Each of these components is more fully described below.

Definition of Quality in Nursing Staff Development

How a healthcare institution defines quality in nursing staff development depends on how it operationally defines what a "standard" is and what it adopts or creates as its own performance standards for staff development.

Standards

A *standard* is variously defined as a statement of quality, a statement of expectation . . . that must be in place in an organization to enhance . . . the quality of care[37]; an agreed-upon level of excellence[3]; an authoritative statement . . . by

which the quality of practice, service, or education can be judged[4]; or an explicit statement about the quality or quantity of an element.[6]

Standards related to nursing staff development may be established locally and/or may be adopted from nationally promulgated sets of standards. In either case, these statements reflect the organization's definition of what constitutes "quality" in nursing staff development.

In order for standards to be amenable to monitoring, they must be written in observable, measurable terms. These terms may describe certain physical or organizational elements (the hospital's mission, goals, and philosophy; human, financial, material, and human resources) that must be in place (structure standards); certain activities, protocols, or procedures that must occur (process standards); or certain results or effects that must be produced (outcome standards). Because standards are stated in broad, encompassing terms, they are often accompanied by a set of criteria that define expectations more explicitly and facilitate determination of compliance with the standard.*

Relevant Sets of Standards Related to Nursing Staff Development

Until rather recently, hospital-based nurse educators had no recourse but to develop their own standards for nursing staff development because nationally recognized statements of quality in this area did not exist. Over the past few years, however, a number of sets of standard statements pertinent to nursing staff development have been developed. These include the newly released American Nurses' Association (ANA) *Standards for Nursing Professional Development: Continuing Education and Staff Development*[4] (Box 8.1), which combines the ANA *Standards for Continuing Education in Nursing*[3] with the ANA *Standards for Nursing Staff Development*[5] (Box 8.2); the JCAHO *Standards for Orientation, Training, and Education of Staff*[37] (Box 8.3) and its successor, the newly drafted *Management of Human Resources Standards*[49] (Box 8.4); and the American Society for Healthcare Education and Training (ASHET) *Standards for Health-Care Education and Training*[6] (Box 8.5), as well as standards emanating from specialty nursing organizations such as the American Association of Critical-Care Nurses' *Education Standards for Critical Care Nursing*.[1]

A review of these standards (Boxes 8.1 to 8.5) reveals two pertinent findings. First, in terms of applicability, the ANA *Standards of Nursing Staff Development* are specific to the nursing staff development department whereas the JCAHO and ASHET standards could also apply to hospitalwide education or human resource development departments. Second, considerable overlap exists among the areas addressed by each set of standards. Hospitals that

---

*Readers will note that the relationship between standards and criteria is comparable to the relationship between competency statements and performance criteria in a CBE program.

Box 8.1

**ANA STANDARDS FOR NURSING PROFESSIONAL DEVELOPMENT:
CONTINUING EDUCATION AND STAFF DEVELOPMENT***

Standard 1. Administration

Administration of the provider unit is consistent with the organization's mission, philosophy, purpose, and goals. The organizational structure facilitates the provision of learning activities for nurses.

Standard 2. Human Resources

Qualified administrative, educational, and support personnel are responsible for achieving the goals of the provider unit.

Standard 3. Material Resources and Facilities

Material resources and facilities are adequate to achieve the goals and implement the functions of the provider unit.

Standard 4. Educational Design

Principles of education and adult learning are used to design educational activities.

Standard 5. Records and Reports

The provider unit establishes and maintains a record keeping and report system.

Standard 6. Professional Practice

The professional development educator role is practiced in a manner that enhances learners' competence to provide quality health care and enhance their contributions to the profession.

*Criteria for each standard can be found in the original reference document. From American Nurses' Association (ANA): *Standards for nursing professional development: continuing education and staff development,* Washington, DC, 1994, ANA.

---

wish to adopt more than one set of standards for their institution, therefore, might merge these sets of standards into a single set that reflects this consolidation and minimizes repetition in coverage. In addition, healthcare agencies may reword, add, or delete criteria or standard statements to tailor these to local needs, preferences, and circumstances.

Monitoring Organizational Performance

The Joint Commission's standards related to improving organizational performance (its PI standards) address hospital activities designed to appraise and improve the quality of patient care. In this group of standards, standard PI 1 requires that hospitals use a "planned, systematic, organizationwide approach to design, measure, assess, and improve performance." The current JCAHO accreditation manual[38] defines the term *systematic* as "pursuing a defined objective(s) in a planned, step-by-step manner." The 10-step quality monitoring and evaluation process for healthcare agencies designed by JCAHO[39] is presented in Box 8.6 and is described in greater detail later with applications to nursing staff development. Although the Joint Commission does **not** require hospitals to use this specific 10-step approach, adaptation of this model for nursing staff devel-

opment can afford a systematic approach for monitoring and improving performance.

Step 1: Assign Responsibility

This step requires a decision regarding the individual who will be vested with overall authority, responsibility, and accountability for monitoring and improving organizational performance in nursing staff development at the facility. The specific assignment of this responsibility is influenced by how the organizational and administrative structure of the hospital hierarchy is divided and the degree to which service line functions are centralized or decentralized. Hospitals that have large staff development departments may assign this responsibility to the director of nursing staff development, the director of nursing education, the director of human resources, or to some other administrative position. It is also possible that the department head might delegate this responsibility to an individual within the staff development or human resource department. If the facility has no nursing staff development unit, the nurse responsible for coordinating staff development may be given this assignment or the responsibility may be shared among a number of nurses in various positions (educator, nurse manager, and clinical nurse spe-

Box 8.2

ANA STANDARDS FOR NURSING STAFF DEVELOPMENT*

Standard I. Organization and Administration
The nursing service department and the nursing staff development unit philosophy, purpose, and goals address the staff development needs of nursing personnel. The organizational structure facilitates the provision of learning experiences for nursing service personnel.

Standard II. Human Resources
Qualified administrative, educational, and support personnel are provided to meet the learning and developmental needs of nursing service personnel.

Standard III. Learner
Nursing staff development educators assist nursing personnel in identifying their learning needs and planning learning activities to meet those needs.

Standard IV. Program Planning
The provider unit systematically plans and evaluates the overall nursing staff development program in response to health care needs, health care trends, nursing personnel's learning needs, and organizational needs and goals.

Standard V. Educational Design
Educational offerings and learning experiences are designed through the use of educational processes and incorporate adult education and learning principles.

Standard VI. Material Resources and Facilities
Material resources and facilities are adequate to achieve the goals and implement the functions of the overall nursing staff development unit.

Standard VII. Records and Reports
The nursing staff development unit establishes and maintains a record keeping and report system.

Standard VIII. Evaluation
Evaluation is an integral, ongoing, and systematic process which includes measuring its impact on the learner, patient, and organization.

Standard IX. Consultation
Nursing staff development educators use the consultation process to facilitate and enhance achievement of individual, departmental, and organizational goals.

Standard X. Climate
Nursing staff development educators foster a climate which promotes open communication, learning, and professional growth.

Standard XI. Systematic Inquiry
Nursing staff development educators encourage systematic inquiry and application of the results into nursing practice.

*Criteria for each standard can be found in the original reference document. From American Nurses' Association (ANA): *Standards for nursing staff development*, Kansas City, MO, 1990, ANA.

cialist). Some staff development units may have a single individual within the unit who provides this function and serves as the unit's representative to a centralized quality assurance department or council.

If the individual responsible for overall quality management for nursing staff development delegates one or more of the remaining steps of the monitoring and improvement process to other individuals or groups, those responsible for each step of the process should be identified. For example, the director of nursing staff development may be responsible for designing the committee structure for the performance improvement plan, coordinating its development and analysis, and communicating its findings to the nursing department. Nurse educators may work with clinical nurse specialists to determine relevant aspects of service to be monitored, to identify pertinent indicators for

---

Box 8.3

JCAHO Standards for Orientation, Training, and Education of Staff*

SE 1 The organization provides an individual who is new to the organization or to a department/service with an orientation of sufficient scope and duration to inform the individual about his/her responsibilities and how to fulfill them within the organization or department/service.

    SE 1.1 An individual's orientation includes, at least, information about

        SE 1.1.1 organizational mission, governance, policies, and procedures;

        SE 1.1.2 department/service policies and procedures;

        SE 1.1.3 the individual's job description;

        SE 1.1.4 performance expectations;

        SE 1.1.5 the organization's plant, technology, and safety management programs and the individual's safety responsibilities;

        SE 1.1.6 the organization's infection control program and the individual's role in the prevention of infection; and

        SE 1.1.7 the organization's quality assessment and improvement activities and the individual's role in these activities.

SE 2 The organization provides for education and training designed to maintain and improve the knowledge and skills of all personnel.

    SE 2.1 The needs identified for training and education are based on, as appropriate,

        SE 2.1.1 the patient population served and type and nature of care provided by the hospital and the department/service;

        SE 2.1.2 individual staff member needs;

        SE 2.1.3 information from quality assessment and improvement activities;

        SE 2.1.4 needs generated by advances made in health care management, and health care science and technology;

        SE 2.1.5 findings from department/service performance appraisals of individuals;

        SE 2.1.6 findings from review activities by peers, if appropriate;

        SE 2.1.7 findings from the organization's plant, technology, and safety management programs; and

        SE 2.1.8 findings from infection control activities.

    SE 2.2 Learning objectives are based on performance expectations and address the knowledge, skills, and behaviors appropriate to the individual's job responsibilities and needed to maintain and improve his/her job performance.

    SE 2.3 The design of the education and training provided is based on effective instructional strategies to accomplish the specified learning objectives.

SE 3 The effectiveness and appropriateness of orientation, training, and education provided for by the organization are evaluated through its quality assessment and improvement activities.

SE 4 Each individual in the organization is competent, as appropriate to his/her responsibilities in the

    SE 4.1 knowledge and skills required to perform his/her responsibilities;

    SE 4.2 effective and safe use of all equipment used in his/her activities;

    SE 4.3 prevention of contamination and transfer of infection; and

    SE 4.4 cardiopulmonary resuscitation and other lifesaving interventions.

*See also JCAHO standards related to competency (Box 7-2) and Special Care Unit Standards. From Joint Commission on Accreditation of Healthcare Organization (JCAHO): *Accreditation Manual for hospitals*, vol 1, Oakbrook Terrace, IL, 1994, JCAHO.

---

those services, and to establish thresholds of evaluation. Data collection and evaluation may be delegated to a smaller task force within the department, and improvements may be implemented by specially designated individuals. Whatever division of responsibilities is decided on, these should be summarized in writing so that all individuals who participate in this process understand their respective roles and obligations.

Step 2: Delineate the Scope of Service

The scope of service statement for a nursing staff development unit encompasses description of the general services provided, the clients served, the programs offered, providers, times, locations, and access to services. A list of the potential inclusions for the scope of service statement is enumerated in Box 8.7.

Box 8.4

JCAHO STANDARDS FOR MANAGEMENT OF HUMAN RESOURCES*

HR 1 **The organization's leaders define for their respective areas the qualifications, competencies, and numbers of staff needed to fulfill the organization's mission.**

HR 2 **The organization provides staff whose qualifications are commensurate with anticipated job responsibilities and applicable licensure, law and regulation, and/or certification.**

HR 3 **Processes are designed to assure that the competence of all staff members is assessed, maintained, demonstrated, and improved on a continuing basis.**

   HR 3.1 An orientation process includes initial training and information and includes an initial competence asessment.

   HR 3.2 Ongoing inservice and/or other education and training maintains and improves staff competence.

   HR 3.3 The organization collects aggregate data on a continuing basis regarding staff competence patterns and trends to identify and act on staff learning needs.

HR 4 **The organization assesses an individual's ability to achieve job expectations as stated in his/her job description.**

*Because the Human Resources standards were still in draft form and undergoing final development when this book went to press, the final wording of these standards may differ somewhat from what appears here. From Patterson CH: New Joint Commission draft standards for management of the human resources function, *Healthcare Education Dateline,* Summer-Fall, 4, 1993.

Step 3: Identify Important Aspects of Service

In order to afford greater focus for performance improvement, it is necessary to distinguish which areas included in the scope of service are the most important. The relative importance of certain aspects of service should be determined because it establishes the relative priority of these aspects within the staff development unit. Since resources do not allow for the entire scope of service to be monitored, only the areas of highest priority merit this appraisal.

One potential problem in reaching a consensus regarding the most important aspects of staff development services is the inherent subjectivity of the decision. Some of this subjectivity can be reduced by employing the Joint Commission's descriptions of what constitutes an "important aspect" of care or service. If JCAHO standards PI 3.4.1.1 through PI 3.4.1.3 are reworded for nursing staff development, they specify that an important aspect is one that affects a large percentage of staff;* that places patients or staff at risk of serious consequences if it is not provided correctly, not provided when indicated, or provided when it is not indicated; or one that has or is likely to produce problems for patients or staff.[37] Thus "important aspects" include those that are high-frequency (high-volume), high-risk, or problem-prone areas of service.

Some examples of high-frequency aspects of staff development include programs such as the so-called

"JCAHO mandatories" that are provided frequently for orientation and competency assessment programs that affect large numbers of nursing staff.

Examples of high-risk aspects of staff development may be viewed in relation to patients, staff, or the hospital. High-risk areas related to patients would include the correct, timely, and appropriate execution of basic or advanced cardiac life support (BCLS or ACLS). High-risk areas related to staff would include programs on electrical safety and universal precautions. High-risk areas related to the hospital organization might include programs on risk management of legal liabilities, on legal aspects of documentation, or on the management of large-scale continuing education programs, which incur substantial financial risks to the hospital if minimum enrollment requirements are not reached.

Problem-prone aspects of staff development can be identified from a review of incident reports or from the findings of prior quality appraisal or risk management activities. The problem-prone areas revealed might include deficiencies in documentation, execution of procedures, adherence to policies, problem-solving, or other areas of staff performance or educational operations.

An initial determination of these important aspects of nursing staff development might generate a large number of areas that could be monitored. In order to keep the

---

*To apply the JCAHO standards to staff development, references to patients as the recipients of services have been reworded to recognize nursing staff as the major recipients of staff development services.

Box 8.5

ASHET STANDARDS FOR HEALTH-CARE EDUCATION AND TRAINING*

PHILOSOPHY AND MISSION

Standard: There is a concise statement of the philosophy and mission of the education services department that reflects the department's values and purpose.

ORGANIZATION AND STRUCTURE

Standard I: There is an identifiable education and training function positioned within the structure of the healthcare organization.

Standard II: There is a written description of the structural and collaborative relationships between the education services department, the healthcare organization, and the corporate system.

Standard III: The education services department is staffed with sufficient, competent individuals who are able to implement an organized schedule of educational programs, services, and activities.

Standard IV: The education services department manager and staff are empowered and accountable to administer an organized schedule of educational programs and activities.

Standard V: The education services department has a 3- to-5-year plan that defines the business of the department (e.g., internal markets, customers, mission) and the organization of the department (e.g., structures, communications, etc.).

FUNCTIONS

Standard I: Education services department staff function as adult educators in a variety of settings and with a variety of audiences.

Standard II: Education staff function in the area of human resource development.

Standard III: Education staff function as internal consultants and change agents in organizational activities.

FACILITIES AND EQUIPMENT

Standard: Educational facilities, equipment, and resources are provided to achieve the education mission and to enhance the individual's learning experience.

FINANCIAL MANAGEMENT

Standard I: A budget is developed by the manager of education services department that supports the department's mission.

Standard II: Approved funds are monitored and managed in a fiscally responsible, professional manner.

Standard III: Promotion and advertising provide full and accurate information regarding the program's fees.

POLICY AND PROCEDURE

Standard: The provision for education and training services is guided by written policies and procedures.

PRODUCTIVITY MEASUREMENT

Standard: The education services department has a productivity measuring system.

CLINICAL AFFILIATIONS/CONTRACTS

Standard: A current contract/letter of agreement exists for affiliations with organizations that define the responsibilities for student experiences.

---

quality monitoring process realistic for the time and resources available, it may be necessary to scrutinize this initial list of aspects and devise a second list of top priorities selected for monitoring for a given period of time. This second list of priorities can be very selective and change over time as the needs and resources of the nursing staff development unit, the nursing department, and the hospital change.

Step 4: Identify Indicators Related to the Important Aspects of Service

Indicators are "data-driven monitoring tools"[39] used to measure the quality of the aspects of service considered

most important. As with any other measurement tool, indicators need to possess the three benchmarks of measurement: validity, reliability, and usefulness. In order for an indicator to be valid, it must reflect current knowledge and state-of-the-art practice in the field. In order for an indicator to be reliable, it must provide consistent measurement results. In order for an indicator to be useful, it must be objective, measurable, and easy to interpret.

The JCAHO states that indicators are "measurable variables related to a structure, process, or outcome" of care or service.[39] Indicators are tools the healthcare organization uses to measure processes, outcomes, and the performance of functions over time.[37] *Structure indicators*, such as resources, equipment, instructional aids, or the number and

---

Box 8.5

ASHET STANDARDS FOR HEALTHCARE EDUCATION AND TRAINING*—cont'd

---

RECORD KEEPING
Standard: Educational records are maintained for each program sponsored by the organization, and participation is documented.

PROFESSIONAL DEVELOPMENT
Standard: Professional and technical education staff conducting education and training activities shall possess appropriate competencies and credentials by virtue of academic background, occupational experience, and continuing education.

RESEARCH
Standard: The education services department regularly reads and/or conducts research and uses the results of research activities to improve the current level of practice.

QUALITY IMPROVEMENT
Standard I: A process to ensure continuous quality of services has been implemented for education services.
Standard II: A quality assurance (QA) program has been formulated for the education services department.

EDUCATIONAL PROCESS
Assessment
Standard: The education services department utilizes a variety of methods to define and identify issue(s) or problem(s) of individuals and/or the organization for the purpose of assessing learning needs.

Design
Standard I: There are clear, concise written statements of intended learning outcomes. The learning activity is designed to utilize the principles of adult education and current research on educational methodology.
Standard II: Educational facilities, equipment, and resources are provided to achieve the education mission and to enhance the individual's learning experience.

Delivery
Standard I: The educational activity is designed and delivered to facilitate learning. Instructional methods and materials are based on the learning objectives.
Standard II: Instructional staff are qualified by education and/or experience to provide instruction in the relevant content area.

Evaluation
Standard: Evaluation is an integral, ongoing, and systematic process of the education services department.

*Criteria for each standard can be found in the original reference document. From American Society for Healthcare Education and Training: *Standards for healthcare education and training*, Chicago, 1990, American Hospital Association.

Box 8.6

JCAHO TEN-STEP QUALITY MONITORING AND EVALUATION PROCESS

---

1. Assign responsibility
2. Delineate scope of service*
3. Identify important aspects of service*
4. Identify indicators related to the important aspects of service*
5. Establish thresholds for evaluation
6. Collect and organize data
7. Evaluate service* when indicated by the threshold
8. Take action when opportunities for improvement or problems are identified
9. Assess the effectiveness of actions
10. Communicate relevant information to the organization-wide program for continuous improvement in performance

*In order to tailor this process for nursing staff development, JCAHO references to patient "care" have been reworded to reflect the "service" provided by staff development. From Joint Commission on Accreditation of Healthcare Organizations: *An Introduction to Joint Commission nursing care standards*, Oakbrook Terrace, IL, 1991, JCAHO.

Box 8.7

SCOPE OF SERVICE FOR NURSING STAFF DEVELOPMENT

GENERAL SERVICES:

- Primary service provided: Staff education
- Education services include: Learning needs assessments
      Program planning and design
      Program implementation
      Program evaluation
- Other services may include: Patient/family education
      Community education
      Career guidance and development
      Internal and external consulting
      Program collaboration and coordination
      Credentialing of selected nursing staff
      Regional educational program planning
      Staff educational record keeping and tracking
      Coordination of student affiliations

CLIENTS SERVED:

- Types of staff: Only nurses
      Nurses and ancillary nursing staff
      Nonstaff (e.g., student nurses)
- Levels of staff: Professional, technical
      Ancillary, volunteer
- Number of staff: Estimated number of each type of staff served
      Total number of staff served annually

PROGRAMS:

- General programs: Hospital orientation   Competency assessment
      Nursing orientation   Leadership development
      Unit orientation   Basic cardiac life support
      In-service education   Advanced cardiac life support
      Continuing education   New graduate program
- Specialized programs: Nurse internship program
      Preceptor training program
      International nurse program
      Specialty clinical areas: OB, pediatrics, critical care,
        maternal-child, OR, trauma
      Credentialing programs: intubation, defibrillation,
        hemodialysis

---

qualifications of educational staff, facilitate the provision of services. *Process indicators*, such as activities related to any phase of the educational process, represent how staff development services are to be provided. *Outcome indicators*, such as applications of staff development to nursing practice changes or to patient care improvements, reflect the results of services provided. As this description suggests, the standards and criteria adopted or developed for staff development can be employed as indicators for the quality monitoring and improvement process. The National Nursing Staff Development Organization's (NNSDO) recent publication entitled *Quality Indicators for Nursing Staff Development*[34] affords a comprehensive array of quality indicators based on the ANA *Standards for Nursing Staff Development*. The indicators offered are referenced to the specific ANA standards and criteria to

which they correspond. Educators can then add, delete, or modify the indicators suggested to suit their own institution's needs and situation.

Indicators are the means employed to collect information about the quality of staff development services and to direct attention toward areas of these services that warrant improvement. Consensus regarding the indicators for staff development is important because indicators represent the salient and measurable attributes of staff development services that become the focus for the performance improvement process.

Step 5: Establish Thresholds for Evaluation

A *threshold for evaluation* is a level or point at which further investigation of performance in relation to that indi-

---

Box 8.7

SCOPE OF SERVICE FOR NURSING STAFF DEVELOPMENT—cont'd

SERVICE PROVIDERS:

- Number and types of education staff: Unit instructors
  Division instructors
  Central education instructors
  Clinical nurse specialists
  Nurse therapists (IV, nutrition support,
  enterostomal therapy)
- Roles and responsibilities of staff: Distinguished for each type of staff

SERVICE TIMES:

- Office hours for department management and staff
- Additional shifts, days, and times of availability for program and service provision

LOCATION OF SERVICES:

- Classroom
- Temporary or permanent learning laboratories
- (Audiovisual) learning centers
- Clinical assessment center
- Clinical units
- Offsite: meeting facilities (conference center, hotels, healthcare agencies)

ACCESSING SERVICES:

- Mechanism(s) for requesting educational services
- Mechanism for processing requests for educational services
- Standards used in provision of services

---

cator is indicated. Once the threshold is reached or crossed, the investigation may involve a fuller evaluation, more detailed auditing, or peer review to determine why the threshold was reached. Each indicator used in the performance improvement process needs to have a threshold established so that opportunities to improve performance relative to that indicator can be readily identified. Threshold levels may be expressed as a ratio but are most often expressed as a percentage ranging from 0% to 100%. Thresholds for some indictors may be set at 0% so that every occurrence of an "important indicator" is investigated. For example, if a threshold of 0% were established for an indicator related to "medication errors that result in harm to the patient," then every instance of such a situation would trigger a further examination as to why this situation occurred. Other indicators may have thresholds of 100% so that every instance of *non*compliance with the indicator is investigated further. An example of the latter would be using a threshold of 100% for an indicator related to "the percentage of staff RNs who are currently certified in CPR." The level at which a threshold is established is most often based on factors such as potential risk or consequences to the patient, staff, or the hospital; national norms of acceptable incidence (e.g., the national incidence of nosocomial infections); or locally established performance levels (e.g., "coronary care unit nurses who have

completed the basic ECG course will recognize potentially lethal cardiac dysrhythmias and conduction defects in 97% of cases").

The basic consideration in setting the threshold is: at what point is a potential problem or a need for improvement warranted? Although thresholds need to be stringent in establishing quality levels of service or performance, they also need to be realistic and feasible to attain. If the quality monitoring and evaluation process is to be perceived as constructive and helpful in making improvements rather than being viewed as chastising staff by holding them to unrealistic levels of performance, reasonable levels of performance must be used in defining thresholds.

Step 6: Collect and Organize Data

The data collection and compilation step involves a number of decisions related to the indicators and thresholds already established. These decisions include what data will be collected, which data sources will be used, which tool(s) and methods will be used for data collection, how much data will be collected, and how often data will be collected and compiled.

The *nature of the data* to be obtained relates directly to the indicator and its threshold level. For example, if the nursing staff development unit were monitoring the number of instances in which a nurse's medication error caused a patient harm, that data would consist of any "incident" of this situation over a specified period of time. If it were monitoring completion of all competency assessments of RNs, the data would consist of the entry in individual RN staff education records that pertained to assessment of current competency.

The *data sources* depend on the specific type of data to be monitored. In many instances, data related to staff development activities already exist and can be retrieved from educational records, program evaluations, test score results, competency assessment checklists, the policy and procedure manual, and other sources. In other instances, the data must be generated from surveys of staff, chart audits, or peer reviews. An example of the latter would be if CCU nurses who had completed a basic ECG course were monitored for their ability to identify lethal cardiac dysrhythmias and conduction defects 6 weeks following course completion. A chart audit of posted hourly and prn ECG rhythm strips (or review of computerized monitoring tapes) and the nurse's interpretation of each rhythm in the nursing notes could be used to determine the number of instances when nurses who had completed the course correctly recognized these disorders. Sources of data for staff development indicators include various forms of documentation and records, the policy and procedure manual, direct observation, incident reports, nursing notes, medication and flow sheets, staff or patient surveys, and written or clinical performance evaluations.

The *data collection tool(s)* or instrument(s) is usually designed with clarity and simplicity in mind. Simple checklists or grids can be constructed to allow for easy recording of findings and straightforward tabulation of whether or not the threshold level is attained for each indicator. In order to keep the monitoring process constructive rather than punitive, data are obtained in an anonymous fashion so that individuals are not identifiable. The tool should enable each entry to be designed in a categorical way regarding whether it reaches the established threshold level or it does not. A simple *yes/no* or *met/not met* column heading can be used so that check marks under the appropriate category can be readily counted to calculate the compliance percentage for that indicator.

The *data collection method(s)* varies with the type and sources of data to be obtained. Data may be collected either retrospectively or concurrently, or some combination of the two methods may be employed. For example, orientees' performance on a written test related to patient education could be tabulated retrospectively together with a concurrent chart audit of their documentation in that area.

The decision related to *how much data needs to be collected* relates to how large the sampling of data must be to sufficiently reflect a valid and representative appraisal. That is, how many orientees should be examined to judge the quality of the orientation program? How many charts need to be audited to determine the outcomes of an in-service on documentation? Do all instances (the entire population)

have to be considered, or can a smaller representative group (a sample) be surveyed to determine quality? The Joint Commission recommends that the hospital's computer information management system be consulted to assist in determining appropriate sampling methods and size where high-volume aspects of service are being monitored.[39] Where information management support services are not available, some preestablished sampling percentage (such as 5%, 10%, or 20%) could be selected and adjusted as circumstances and results warrant. As a guideline, enough instances need to be examined so that a reasonably valid and reliable appraisal is produced but not so many that the sampling exceeds the time and resources available for data collection procedures. If virtually the same results can be obtained after auditing 25 charts as for 50 charts, the smaller number would suffice for data collection purposes.

Data collection frequency refers to how often data will be secured. Although some indicators (e.g., whether all staff have completed JCAHO safety requirements within the past year) may require only a single episode of data collection, other indicators may be more appropriately monitored on an ongoing weekly, monthly, quarterly, or semiannual basis for a certain period of time. For example, an in-service program on a recently revised procedure might be monitored every week for a 6-week period by direct observation of staff or by asking staff to complete self-assessments of their own performance of the procedure to determine if the revisions are being implemented correctly and consistently. Ongoing quality monitoring intervals are also less likely to be viewed as "one-time shots" and are more consistent with the philosophy of continuous improvement in organizational performance.

In addition to the frequency of obtaining data, the *frequency of data tabulation* must also be considered. How often the accumulated data are compiled and summarized will depend on a number of factors. In general, the higher the elements of risk, volume, and potential problems related to that indicator, the more frequently data need to be aggregated and summarized. Collection, organization, and summarization of the data set the stage for its analysis in step 7. The NNSDO publication[34] mentioned earlier offers a useful example of a grid for organizing, collecting, and summarizing quality monitoring data for a nursing staff development department.

Step 7: Evaluate Service When Indicated by the Threshold

Once the data collection procedure and frequency are determined, periodic appraisal and analysis of the data may be completed to decide whether performance monitoring findings indicate that staff development services are satisfactory or need improvement. When data indicate deviation from established or desired thresholds (i.e., when the percentages tabulated exceed or fall below the threshold levels for a given indicator), the reasons or causes need to be investigated and possible remedies to improve performance in those areas need to be identified.

The process used for analysis and evaluation of performance data needs to be a balanced one: areas where compliance is attained need to be recognized and praised, just as areas where compliance was not achieved need to be recognized and improved on. If the monitoring process ignores successes and focuses solely on noting and "punishing" failures, the nursing staff's commitment to the performance improvement program can be extinguished.

The search for possible causes of noted deficiencies in performance needs to consider a wide array of potential categories of causes. The discussion and model (Chapter 7, Figure 7-2) of factors that affect the results of impact evaluation can serve to remind educators that appraisal of the effectiveness of staff development activities can be influenced by many factors other than the attributes and quality of a selected educational program. Although some performance deficiencies may occur as a result of problems in the design or execution of staff development offerings, others may be the result of problems on the clinical unit, problems related to unit operations, problems with some element in the hospital social system, problems with administrative support or staffing levels, or even problems with an individual nurse. Unless all possible causes of the deficiency are considered, the actions selected to remedy the deficiency are not likely to be on target. The full range of possible causes is more likely to be elicited when all relevant nursing and educational staff participate in the evaluation process.

Step 8: Take Action When Opportunities for Improvement or Problems Are Identified

When the evaluation indicates the existence of one or more opportunities for improving the quality of staff development services, the next step is to determine which corrective action(s) to take, who needs to initiate the action(s), when and how these corrective actions need to be taken, and when the improvement should be evidenced. When the cause of the noted deficiency is attributable to a need for instruction, an educational offering can be designed and implemented to address this performance area. When the cause of a deficiency is a hospital system problem, possible courses of action include the initiation or modification of a policy or procedure, the establishment or reopening of communication channels, increasing resource allocations, adjusting staffing coverage, or enhancing a documentation system. When the deficiency is attributable to some attribute of an individual nurse other than a need for instruction or educational support, possible courses of action include counseling or a change in assignment. If the hospital's threshold for compliance with the JCAHO or OSHA safety areas specifies that "95% of all nursing staff have completed these requirements within the last year" and evaluation reveals that only 87% of staff are compliant in this area, any number of possible courses of action could

be taken, but the only action that will improve the compliance rate would be the one directed at the true cause of the situation. Compliance might be deficient because no written policy exists in this area or because the policy that does exist is vague or ambiguous regarding how often these requirements need to be met (system problem). Compliance may be deficient because the program designed by staff development uses ineffective or inefficient teaching methods or poorly prepared instructors (instructional problem). Compliance may be deficient because staff coverage is never sufficient to enable nurses to attend the instructional programs (system problem) or because nursing staff view the requirements as a waste of their time (individual behavior problem). Unless the root cause is accurately isolated, the actions taken are not likely to succeed in improving performance in that area.

Step 9: Assess the Effectiveness of Actions

After a remedial action is taken to improve an area of performance, that area needs to be monitored again to determine whether the action taken was successful in improving performance relative to the established threshold level. The evaluation procedure used in this step is the same as that employed for step 7 and is repeated as often as warranted to achieve improvements.

If performance in the area has not improved within the expected time frame, a number of explanations should be explored to determine the reason. Sufficient time may not have been allowed for improvement to be evidenced. The action(s) selected may not have been effective. The cause of the deficiency may not have been correctly identified, or the threshold may not have been set at a realistic level of expectation. This follow-up procedure may then prompt different responses, depending on the results of this analysis. If this process is viewed as an ongoing means of enhancing the quality of staff development services, then these temporary deficiencies can be perceived as stepping stones to achieving improved performance rather than as setbacks or failures.

Step 10: Communicate Relevant Information to the Organizationwide Program for Continuous Improvement in Performance

The performance monitoring and evaluation program of the staff development department is only one component of this endeavor within the nursing department. The nursing department's performance improvement program, in turn, is only one component of the hospital's program in this area. In order for organizational performance improvement to be an integrated and coordinated process at the institution, relevant results of the efforts of all participating groups within the hospital community need to be communicated to other segments of the hospital system.

A detailed report of the mechanisms, conclusions, follow-up and outcomes of performance improvement in nursing staff development should be circulated among all members of that unit. A summary of the indicators, findings, and changes implemented should be forwarded to the director of nursing. The nursing director's office may then prepare a synopsis of that report for submission along with the nursing department's documentation of performance improvement activities in its communication to the hospitalwide program. Regardless of the form in which these reports are prepared (minutes of meetings, narrative descriptions, summary data tables, and the like), they need to communicate conclusions reached, recommendations made, actions taken, and the follow-up results.

Improving Organizational Performance

The systematic approach to monitoring and evaluating performance described previously is the primary means by which a healthcare institution's definition of quality patient care is translated and operationalized by staff into a mechanism that enables performance to be improved on an ongoing basis. In that 10-step process, the first five steps establish the mechanism to be used for monitoring and evaluation, the sixth and seventh steps encompass collection and evaluation of relevant data, and the last three steps reflect attempts to improve the provision of services rendered.

The Joint Commission defines *performance improvement* as "the continuous study and adaptation of functions and processes of a healthcare organization to increase the probability of achieving desired outcomes and to better meet the needs of patients and other users of services."[37] When this definition is applied to nursing staff development, it implies that performance improvement will be an ongoing study and enhancement of the processes of providing staff development services to nursing staff, patients, and others.

The notion of continuous performance improvement represents the desired product of the total quality management process. Recognizing the importance of defining, monitoring, and evaluating performance in staff development services is an important support element in this process. Managing performance is a means; continually improving performance in staff development services is its end. High-quality staff development is not a static destination to be reached, but a dynamic entity toward which we continually strive.

DEVELOPING POLICIES AND PROCEDURES

DEFINITIONS
Policy

A *policy* establishes an organization's position relative to a particular issue or situation. Policies serve as guideposts for the agency's employees to understand how the organization views that issue and what parameters it has estab-

lished for that situation. Policy statements are used as the basis for decision-making and actions. A well-developed hospital policy includes general descriptions of the hospital's position, identifies accountability for policy implementation, and distinguishes any pertinent limits the institution wishes to impose in relation to a specific issue. For example, a hospital policy related to tuition assistance might include the following elements:

- *Position:* A statement expressing the hospital's opinion regarding the value of providing employees with a tuition assistance program
- *Accountability:* Identification of who is responsible for administering and managing the tuition assistance program
- *Parameters:*
    Which employees are eligible for tuition assistance
    Types of tuition assistance available (academic, and nonacademic offerings)
    Limits of assistance: annual and aggregate amounts
    Form of payments: employee reimbursement vs. direct payment to sponsor

The purpose of an organizational policy is to establish broad guidelines that will influence the performance and actions of employees for a given situation.

Procedure

A *procedure* is an established way of doing something. Organizational procedures describe the "how-tos" for implementation and operationalization of a policy at that agency. For example, a procedure for the tuition assistance policy defined earlier could include the following elements of how that policy is to be implemented:

- How to apply for tuition assistance
- How requests for tuition assistance are to be processed
- How tuition assistance applicants will be notified regarding disposition of their requests
- How payments for tuition assistance are to be made

Policies define the organization's stance in a specific area, and procedures describe how employees are to proceed with implementation of that policy.

BENEFITS OF POLICIES AND PROCEDURES

The major benefits of written policy statements are to identify areas where the organization has an expressed opinion or stance on an issue and to clarify the nature of that opinion. The primary benefits of written procedures are to establish guidelines for practice that afford consistency in how certain situations are managed at that agency. Taken together, policies and procedures offer the following benefits[63]:

Box 8.8

PROCESS FOR DEVELOPING STAFF DEVELOPMENT POLICIES AND PROCEDURES

- Identify a situation or practice that needs to be standardized so that it is handled in a consistent manner.
- Communicate the need for policy development to the appropriate nurse managers and administrators for their concurrence.
- Convene a task force for policy-making that includes representatives of nursing administration as well as all groups who would be affected by the new policy and procedure
- Draft the policy and procedure so that it is consistent in content and format with other nursing department policies and procedures.
- Distribute copies of the draft policy and procedure to all relevant groups for their comments, corrections, and suggestions.
- Submit the finalized version of the policy and procedure to all appropriate individuals and groups for their approval and written endorsement.
- Disseminate the policy and procedure through customary communication channels to all applicable staff.

Box 8.9

STAFF DEVELOPMENT POLICIES AND PROCEDURES

- Administrative support for attendance at staff development programs
- Application for continuing education unit (CEU) approval
- Awarding of continuing education units (CEUs)
- Budget development and management
- Co-providership of programs
- Co-sponsorship of programs
- Competency assessments (initial and ongoing) for new, current, float, and agency nursing staff
- Continuing education program
- Contracts for student affiliations
- Contracts with external organizations and vendors
- Credentialing of nursing staff
- CPR certification and recertification
- Educational leave
- Educational records: department, individual
- Ethical practice: confidentiality, copyright, revenue sources, fees, truth in advertising
- Exhibitors at programs
- General vs. specialty area programming
- Honoraria for outside faculty
- Hospital orientation program
- In-service education program
- Mandatory vs. voluntary program attendance
- Marketing programs
- Nursing department orientation program
- On-duty vs. off-duty participation
- Participant registration
- Patient and community education
- Planning conferences marketed to nurses in the community
- Program advertising
- Program cancellation
- Program development process
- Program evaluation process
- Program fees for employees and nonemployees
- Quality monitoring and improvement
- Selection and use of outside faculty
- Student affiliations
- Tuition assistance
- Unit orientation

- Afford a quick and valid reference for communicating and meeting expectations of the employer
- Afford a means to meet expectations and requirements of various accrediting and regulatory agencies
- Afford consistency and continuity in how certain routine situations are implemented at that institution
- Facilitate smooth and predictable management of certain situations and activities
- Minimize the need for repeated decision-making on routine matters

DEVELOPING AND REVIEWING POLICIES AND PROCEDURES

Policies and procedures may be written at various levels of applicability; some will apply hospitalwide, others will apply throughout the nursing service, and others may apply only within the staff development department. Because the nursing staff development unit operates under the auspices of the nursing department, staff development policies and procedures must be developed in a collaborative, cooperative, and consistent manner with those of the nursing department. The policy-making process generally consists of the steps enumerated in Box 8.8.

Existing policies and procedures need to be reviewed on a periodic basis to determine their continued accuracy, relevancy, and applicability. The director of nursing staff development may perform this review alone or enlist the participation of educators and other nursing staff to make any necessary updates, additions, deletions, or other changes to keep the set of staff development policies and procedures current and complete.

The policy and procedure review process can be more readily accomplished when all policies and procedures pertaining to staff development are compiled into a single manual.[48] Because policies and procedures are influenced by and need to be consistent with many other existing staff development statements and documents, the contents of the nursing staff development manual often include the following items:

- Mission, philosophy, and goals of nursing staff development
- Nursing department and staff development organizational charts
- Scope of services statement (for inclusions, see Box 8.7)
- Staff development position descriptions
- Standards of nursing staff development
- Staff development quality monitoring and improvement program
- Staff development policies and procedures
- Staff development documentation and processing forms
- Educational record and reporting system

STAFF DEVELOPMENT POLICIES AND PROCEDURES

The number and nature of policies and procedures related to nursing staff development depend on the requirements of external accrediting and regulatory agencies as well as internal needs and preferences. For example, the JCAHO standards require that all healthcare institutions have written policies and procedures related to the competency assessment process. Individual hospitals may determine whether these policies and procedures related to competency assessment are summarized in a single document or whether they are divided into separate policies and procedures for new nursing staff, existing nursing staff, float nurses, and agency nurses. A list of some of the policies and procedures that may be developed for nursing staff development is provided in Box 8.9.

RECORDKEEPING AND REPORTS

USES

The documentation of staff development activities is a necessary function for both professional and practical reasons. Professional reasons include the need to monitor instructional programs for their effectiveness, relevance, and efficiency as well as the need to comply with established educational standards, accreditation standards, and state laws and licensing regulations. Practical reasons for this documentation include the need to communicate information related to staff development in a clear, concise, and timely manner to relevant groups within the hospital who use this information for planning, managing, and decision-making purposes.

A well-designed recordkeeping system enables the staff development department to provide the types of information required or requested by various users and present this information with that audience in mind. The section that follows addresses the variety of audiences that exist for staff development records/reports and the types of information each audience may seek. Additional considerations include the use of computerized recordkeeping management systems as well as the length of time that records are maintained.

AUDIENCES

Staff development records/reports are prepared according to the information needs of specific individuals or groups external or internal to the healthcare agency. A good starting point for designing the recordkeeping system, then, is to determine who the relevant audiences are for these records/reports and what types of information these audiences require or are likely to request. The audiences for information related to staff development activities may be categorized into external and internal groups. External audiences may include national accrediting and regulatory organizations such as JCAHO or OSHA as well as state regulators such as the state board of nursing. Internal audiences may range from the hospital administrator, director of nursing services, various levels of nurse managers, and the staff development division itself to individual members of the nursing (and, with a human resource development structure, nonnursing) staff.

Federal and State Agencies and Regulators

Compliance with federal requirements and guidelines emanating from the Occupational Safety and Health Administration (OSHA) as well as the Centers for Disease Control (CDC) may need to be documented for verification. State nurse practice acts and boards of nursing may also influence the need for certain types of records and reports.

Statistical reports regarding verification of current nurse licensure and, in states where continuing education is required for nurse relicensure, documentation of continuing education unit earnings reports for individual nurses may be needed. Records pertaining to state statutes for nurse practitioners or nurse anesthetists may also need to be compiled. States such as Florida that impose additional requirements for specific instructional programs may also warrant summary reports of compliance with those mandates.

JCAHO Accreditation Surveyors

The Joint Commission standards for accreditation of healthcare organizations mandate documentation of a number of areas related to staff development. When the JCAHO surveyors arrive for the accreditation site visit, the reports and forms of documentation indicated in Box 8.10 need to be readily available for their inspection.

While some of these reports may summarize compliance rates and other information for the entire nursing department (professional and nonprofessional staff alike), others may be summarized by category of nursing staff (RN, LPN, nursing technicians, aides, unit clerks, etc.), by organizational division (medical-surgical units, critical care units, ambulatory care units, etc.), by individual nursing unit, or by individual staff member. In order to substantiate compliance with JCAHO standards, healthcare institutions should be prepared to provide various types of written evidence in any form that surveyors are likely to request. Review of the scoring guidelines for the JCAHO standards[38] can be helpful in suggesting the forms of report presentation that would most likely be solicited by the accreditation team.

Hospital and Nursing Administrators and Managers

Any requests for information related to nursing staff development that originate from the hospital administrator are likely to be channeled through the director of nursing. Reports at the hospital CEO level would most probably consist of an annual report of staff development activities. The *annual report* may request either a synopsis or a more detailed enumeration of all educational programs provided throughout the year (calendar or fiscal) sorted by staff development component (orientation, in-service education, continuing education), the number of nursing staff who participated in these programs (perhaps sorted by category of staff), the number of CEU/contact hours awarded for the programs, and a financial summary of budgetary expenditures. If staff development provides programming for and charges fees to participants who are not hospital employees, a summary of the revenues, expenses, and net profits realized for each applicable program may also be requested.

In addition to an annual report, the director of nursing may request *periodic reports*, consisting of a quarterly or monthly report of staff development activities. These ongoing reports might consist of information similar to that provided in the annual report, but be sorted by nursing division, nursing unit, or category of nursing staff and indicate year-to-date (YTD) figures in addition to the current reporting period (monthly, quarterly). The nurse executive may also be interested in knowing the compliance rates for federal, state, and JCAHO requirements; budget data for separate nursing divisions and units; and progress reports on current long-term projects. The degree of detail provided in these reports will be influenced by the size, complexity, and organizational structure of the nursing department.

The nurse executive may also request submission of an annual *strategic plan* for nursing staff development. In contrast to the retrospective view of most reports, a strategic plan considers the future trends, goals, and initiatives projected for nursing staff development over the next year, next 2 years, or next 5 years. Strategic plans consider current and projected trends and needs with an expressed vision of where staff development should be headed for the future. An important ingredient in this document is identification of current and foreseeable problems and obstacles that would impede progress toward realization of future goals, with recommendations regarding how those obstacles might be overcome.

Nurse managers at the division and unit levels may also request periodic monthly or quarterly reports of staff development activities specific to their areas of responsibility and sorted by category of nursing staff. Information regarding staff compliance rates for initial and ongoing competency assessments, for attendance at mandatory in-services, and for in-services on new or revised procedures or equipment use, as well as credentialing requirements, may be viewed as important elements in their reports. Other helpful forms of information would consist of the due dates for various staff certifications, recertifications, and valida-

---

Box 8.10

JCAHO DOCUMENTATION REQUIREMENTS RELATED TO STAFF DEVELOPMENT

STANDARD	REQUIRED DOCUMENTATION

Nursing Care Standards

NC 2.1   Completion of initial and ongoing competency assessments for all nursing staff: new, current, float, outside agency.

NC 5.4   Evidence that programs are developed, implemented, and evaluated to promote the recruitment, retention, development, and continuing education of nursing staff.

NC 5.6   Evidence that nursing leaders collaborate with educators from affiliating schools of nursing to influence curricula, including clinical and managerial learning experiences.

Orientation, Training, and Education Standards

SE 1.1   Evidence that staff orientation includes information related to the organization's mission, governance, policies and procedures; departmental/service policies and procedures; employee's job description; performance expectations; safety and infection control program responsibilities; and quality assessment and improvement responsibilities.

SE 2   Evidence that the hospital provides and tracks participation for instruction to maintain and improve the knowledge and skills of staff (in-service and continuing education).

SE 2.1   Evidence that the instruction provided is based on the patient populations served and the care they require; the needs of individual staff; the findings of quality assessment and improvement activities; advances in healthcare management, science, and technology; individual performance appraisals; peer review activities; safety management and infection control programs.

SE 2.2   Documentation of those for whom instruction was provided and specification of learning outcomes that relate directly to performance expectations of learners.

SE 2.3   Evidence that effective and appropriate teaching strategies are used to accomplish the specified learning outcomes.

SE 3   Evidence that the effectiveness and appropriateness of orientation, training, and education are evaluated through the organization's quality assessment and improvement activities.

SE 4.1   Evidence that the knowledge, skills, and instruction required for each position have been defined and demonstrated; that applicable licenses, registrations, and certifications have been verified at least every two years; that the competency assessment mechanism is described and that each staff member's competence has been verified.

SE 4.2   Evidence that staff competence to operate equipment in a safe and effective manner has been demonstrated.

SE 4.4   Evidence that staff who are designated to perform CPR and other lifesaving interventions have demonstrated competency to do so at least every 2 years

---

tion programs as well as highlighting of any staff members who are overdue on these requirements. Other possible areas of interest to the first- and second-line nurse manager are staff participation in continuing education programs sponsored within or outside the agency, staff participation in committee, task force, or volunteer work, awards or degrees received, and any other aspects of professional or career development. Provision of this type of information can assist the nurse manager in completion of performance appraisals, in deciding career ladder advancements or promotion decisions, or in the awarding of bonuses or other forms of staff recognition for continued professional growth.

Staff Development Unit

Within the staff development unit itself, certain types of records and reports will facilitate the smooth management and operation of daily endeavors. Some primary record-keeping areas include need assessment compilations, program files, faculty files, program evaluation compilations, status reports for ongoing projects, and a schedule or calendar of events.

Needs Assessment Compilations

In order for staff development to maintain a balanced and contemplative approach to program development and to

	Box 8.10

JCAHO DOCUMENTATION REQUIREMENTS RELATED TO STAFF DEVELOPMENT—
cont'd

STANDARD	**REQUIRED DOCUMENTATION**

Management of Human Resources Standards*

HR 1   Evidence that all staff positions have defined qualifications and job expectations, a job performance evaluation system related to those expectations, and a staffing plan to provide the required level of care.

HR 2   Documentation that verifies that each worker (employee or contracted) meets the educational requirements stipulated in applicable laws, regulations, or hospital policies and possesses appropriate licensure, certification, registration as well as the knowledge and experience needed for his or her assigned responsibilities.

HR 3.1   Evidence that prior to working in unsupervised situations, each staff member has completed an orientation that promotes safe and effective performance of their duties and completes an initial assessment of his or her competence to perform their job.

HR 3.2   Evidence that each staff member participates in inservice and other educational activities appropriate to his or her job responsibilities and patient population(s).

HR 3.3   Documentation of patterns and trends in ongoing appraisals of staff competence with evidence of inservice and other education that addresses identified areas of learning needs.

HR 4   Evidence that competence assessment mechanisms exist and that each staff member's competence to achieve the expectations stated in his or her job description has been demonstrated and documented.

*Because the Management of Human Resources standards were still in draft form and undergoing final development when this book went to press, these requirements may differ somewhat from the draft version presented here.

avoid reflex responses to requests for new or modified programs, the needs assessment process should be ongoing, thorough, well-documented, and cumulative. A deliberative and ongoing needs assessment affords more time to gather relevant information, verify and validate true educational needs, note recurring trends in needs, and establish clearer priorities among needs that compete for available resources. As the JCAHO orientation standard SE 2.1 specifies, educational needs are identified from numerous sources, including advances in care, patient populations, staff members' individual needs, and the findings of quality monitoring, performance appraisal, peer review, safety, and infection control activities. When these sources are coupled with those described in Chapters 2 (for any staff development program), 6 (for orientation), and 7 (for inservice and continuing education), the staff development unit can be easily overwhelmed by the sheer number and volume of input sources that need to be included in a comprehensive needs assessment. A reporting form that could be used to record and manage this information is illustrated in Table 8.1. Rather than attempting to consider and respond to each of these diverse input sources as they are individually generated throughout the year, it might be better to compile these separate sets of findings and recommendations into a single document that analyzes this in-

formation and identifies the trends and patterns of needs indicated.

Program Files

Recordkeeping related to staff development services may be rendered more useful by envisioning two levels of educational events: major programs and the individual offerings included within each program. The major programs in nursing staff development would include the three components of orientation, in-service education, and continuing education together with competency assessment, credentialing, patient/family education, and student education as appropriate.

The separate instructional events provided within each of these categories would constitute an individual educational offering. For example, during the course of a year, staff nurse orientation may be offered six times, nurse manager orientation may be provided twice, and nursing assistant orientation might be given twelve times. Each of these separate orientations would represent an orientation offering and the total of all orientation offerings over the course of a year would represent the orientation program.

Box 8.11 lists the various attributes of program offerings that may be documented for recordkeeping and storage/

TABLE 8.1 • NURSING STAFF DEVELOPMENT: NEEDS ASSESSMENT COMPILATION FOR 19___					
Date	Source(s)	Related Program*	Findings	Recommendations	Disposition

*Orientation, competency assessment, in-service: mandatory, in-service: voluntary, continuing education, credentialing, patient/family education, student education, consultation, other (specify).

filing purposes. The separate documentation of each offering within a program can then be summarized to produce a composite record of all offerings in that program. Merging of program records then affords a complete report of all instructional services provided by the staff development unit. The value of recordkeeping that allows for the distinction of separate offerings lies in the ability to scrutinize not only average trends from the aggregated data but also the specific qualities of each educational event that may be similar to or very different from the averaged statistics.

Two entries in the offering attributes may be coded to supply more definitive data for accreditation purposes. The program code number could consist of a six-digit code that distinguished the year of the data, the program the offering belongs to, and the number of the offering in that program series. Box 8.12 illustrates how a coding system could be developed for this purpose.

Box 8.13 shows how a second coded entry might be used to distinguish the basis for providing the instruction.

Identification of the reason and/or source for origination of the instruction affords a rationale for why it was provided and assists in documenting compliance with JCAHO standard SE 2.1. Coding systems such as these would be particularly useful for making statistical comparisons and analyses of staff development services and/or for computerizing the recordkeeping system.

Faculty Files

In addition to securing a copy of each faculty member's curriculum vita, some demographic and descriptive data related to each instructor may be useful to maintain. This data might include the faculty member's full name, credentials (degrees, licenses, certifications), and current position and area(s) of expertise as well as a summary of participant evaluations of that instructor. For faculty who are not employees, additional data would include their current employer, work and mailing addresses, telephone and fax

---

Box 8.11

DOCUMENTATION OF INDIVIDUAL PROGRAM OFFERINGS

Audiovisual equipment used
Audiovisual software/media used
Basis/source of program
Brochure
Budget
CEU approval application
Content outline
Coordinator
Correspondence
Date(s) provided
Description
Evaluation tools
Evaluation findings
Faculty
Fee(s) charged
Handouts
Honoraria paid
Instructional outcomes
Net income
Number of CEUs/contact hours awarded
Participant roster
Place provided
Problems encountered
Program code number
Program designers
Staff support needed
Supplies used
Teaching methods
Time provided
Title
Total number of participants (employee, nonemployee)

Box 8.12

CODING SYSTEM FOR PROGRAM CODE

PROGRAM CODE NUMBER	PROGRAMS
1st two digits = year	01 = Orientation
2nd two digits = program	02 = Competency assessment
3rd two digits = offering	03 = In-service education
	04 = Continuing education
	05 = Credentialing
	06 = Patient/family education
	07 = Student education
	08 = Consultation
	09 = Other

---

numbers, social security number (for tax purposes), and honorarium requirements.

Internally, faculty files may be used to review the effectiveness, performance quality, and productivity of each staff member and to analyze staff work loads. Review of data related to outside or guest faculty can assist in decisions regarding future use of that individual as an instructor.

Program Evaluation Compilations

In much the same way that aggregated needs assessments can afford improved management of the program assessment, planning, and implementation phases of the educational process, compilations of evaluation data can afford a fuller and more integrated approach to appraisals of staff development activities. Rather than viewing and reacting to evaluations of each separate offering as it is provided,

---

Box 8.13

CODING SYSTEM FOR BASIS/SOURCE FOR PROVISION OF OFFERING

PROGRAM BASIS/
SOURCE CODE NUMBER
01 = New development
02 = Patient population/needs for care
03 = Individual staff member's need
04 = Performance appraisal
05 = Findings from quality monitoring
06 = Findings from peer review
07 = Findings from safety program
08 = Findings from infection control program
09 = Findings from risk management
10 = Followup to incident report
11 = Mandatory offering
12 = Other

---

cumulative and summary evaluative data can be analyzed for emerging trends and patterns that these data reveal. With this more deliberative approach, major modifications of programs (additions, deletions, or other substantive alteration of the curriculum or faculty) would be based on recurring rather than isolated instances of a situation that suggests the need for improvement. Table 8.2 shows a form that could be used to record and summarize evaluative data.

Ongoing Projects

Each offering provided by staff development requires the tracking and coordination of numerous instructional and operational aspects that need to be managed individually and collectively. The number of features that require management will vary with the size and complexity of the offering but typically involves aspects such as processing course registrations; scheduling rooms, audiovisual equipment, and catering services; corresponding with participants, faculty, and exhibitors or hotels; monitoring and tabulating expenses and revenues; photocopying course materials and handouts; applying for continuing education units (CEUs); preparing rosters and name tags; preparing attendance or CEU certificates for distribution; and a myriad of other details. Manual tracking of the ongoing status of each of these separate activities can be a burdensome, time-consuming, and tedious task. Automating these tasks (and many other related ones) is one of the major benefits obtained by using a computerized educational management system.

Schedule or Calendar of Events

Larger staff development units often find it both useful and necessary to keep track of all educational activities by summarizing these in either a printed schedule or calendar of events. A schedule of events simply lists all of the instructional activities for a specified time period. The schedule might include the following information in separate columns: date, time(s), title of offering, location, instructor(s), and appropriate audience(s). A calendar format presents much the same information but, because of space restrictions, may truncate or abbreviate session titles and use a coding system to designate audiences or instructors. The schedule or calendar could be used internally as a reference for staff development educators and could be distributed to all nursing units as an announcement of offerings to all prospective participants. If offerings are available to healthcare workers who are not hospital employees, the schedule or calendar could also be used for marketing these programs to the local area.

Individual Nursing Staff

A record of the staff development activities of each member of the nursing staff is useful for a number of purposes. If the healthcare agency is located in a state where a specified number of units or contact hours of continuing education are required for relicensure of nurses, these individual staff development records can be used to provide a transcript to the state board of nursing for substantiation purposes. License renewals and state-mandated certifications can be documented in a similar manner.

Nurses who attain voluntary certifications through the American Nurses' Association Credentialing Center or through various other specialty nursing organizations (including designations such as C, CCRN, CDE, CEN, CNOR, CPAN, OCN, and the like), may also request transcripts of this educational record to document their compliance with recertification requirements. In addition to documenting past accomplishments, educational records may also include notation of due dates for renewal of licenses, certifications, and credentialing privileges.

			Written Tests		Performance Checklists		Recommen-dations	Disposition
Date	Program Code #	Program Title	Passing Score	% Attained	% Required	% Attained		

TABLE 8.2 • NURSING STAFF DEVELOPMENT: EVALUATION DATA COMPILATION FOR 19_____

Individual staff members may review their educational record to monitor continuing professional development, and nurse managers may use these records to assist in performance evaluations and promotion decisions. A sample form of an educational record is provided in Figure 8.1.

COMPUTERIZED RECORDS AND REPORTS

The escalating complexity and volume of requirements for timely recordkeeping, reporting, and documentation of staff development activities together with the need to manage educational programs more efficiently have caused healthcare institutions to reexamine the inefficiencies of their manual systems for these functions. As a result, staff development departments are increasingly converting their time-consuming, labor-intensive, and duplicative manual recordkeeping tasks to computerized data management systems. Once the decision for computerizing this function has been reached, hospitals need to decide whether to design a system tailor-made for recordkeeping needs of their staff development unit or to purchase a commercially designed software system for this purpose.

Designing a Tailor-Made System

Hospitals that decide to design their own computerized educational recordkeeping systems are confronted by two possible alternatives: either linking with the hospital's existing mainframe computer or using a personal computer (PC) system. When staff development recordkeeping is integrated with the mainframe computer, software programming expertise can usually be secured from the hospital or

Nursing staff development educational record

Name: _____ Date of hire: _____

Employee ID #: _____ Position: _____
Unit: _____

Type of License	License #	**Expiration Date**	Comments

Employer-Sponsored

PROGRAM	OFFERING	CONTACT HRS	COMPLETED	RENEW DATE
Orientation:	Mission, governance, policies, procedures	NA		
	Unit policies, procedures	NA		
	Job description	NA		
	Performance expectations	NA		
	Quality monitoring	NA		
In-service:		NA		
Safety programs:	Fire safety			
	Electrical safety	NA		
	Hazardous wastes	NA		
	Infection control	NA		
	CPR	NA		
	ACLS	NA		
Competency:	Initial	NA		
	Ongoing	NA		
Other in-services:				
Credentialing:	Code team	NA		
	Defibrillation	NA		
	Intubation	NA		
Continuing ed:				

Figure 8.1   Nursing staff development educational record.

Outside-Sponsor

PROGRAM	TOPIC	CONTACT HOURS	COMPLETED	EMPLOYER SUPPORT GIVEN

Academic Courses

INSTITUTION	COURSE TITLE	CREDIT HOURS	COMPLETED	EMPLOYER SUPPORT GIVEN

Certifications

Organization	Credential	Effective Date(s)	Recertification Date

Figure 8.1—cont'd Nursing staff development educational record.

management information services (HIS/MIS) division of the hospital who will work collaboratively with the nurse educators to determine the necessary features, database elements, tracking records, and reports desired and the formats most suitable for each. Screen design, layouts, ease of entry, and system flexibility are refined over time to make the system as user friendly as possible. Explicit and detailed reports can be generated to meet the varying needs of both internal and external audiences.[9,32,52] Integration of nursing staff development recordkeeping with the hospital mainframe computer offers the additional feature of linking these records and database with the hospital's personnel or human resource databases. When staff change positions or work areas, their educational records automatically follow them.

Some hospitals that wish to design their own educational recordkeeping software experience dissatisfaction with one or more aspects of the existing hospital mainframe system and opt to use a decentralized personal computer system instead. Custom design of software for the personal computer will require either hiring of outside consultants to develop the necessary programs[13] or having one or more of the educator staff write the programs. The former option may be costly and leave persisting problems of support for revisions, refinements, and additions as concerns. The latter option requires that at least one educator be very knowledgeable and adept at computer programming and be able to be released for the time it takes to develop the software. Although this can be accomplished,[46] it may not be a feasible alternative for many healthcare agencies.

Purchasing a Commercially Produced System

Over the past few years, a number of commercial software products for educational recordkeeping have been developed. Many of the currently available systems are designed for use in any training, human resource development, or continuing education setting.* A smaller number of products have been developed for hospital-based settings.† Some of the features and capabilities available with these products are enumerated in Box 8.14.

A few caveats should be kept in mind before purchasing any of these commercial systems:

- *Identify the features, capabilities, and requirements necessary to meet your current and anticipated needs before examining any product.* Be as explicit and detailed as possible in enumerating your needs. Your list of

"must-haves" and "must-be-able-to-do's" can assist in focusing your search among the products available and leave you less vulnerable to distraction by flashy features that are creative but not useful. A good starting place is to examine the reports you currently produce to see if these can be readily duplicated or improved upon by the commercial system.[30] Then add your wish list of capabilities (things you have always wanted) and those you will need to show to accrediting and regulatory agencies.

- *Try out any software you are considering for purchase before investing in it.* Secure a working preview copy of the program (usually available for a nominal fee) so that you can experience using the software and documentation. Demonstration disks that only present some of the screens in the software will be of little value here because they do not enable the customer to actually try out the software. Use the working copy to evaluate screen and menu layouts for clarity of meaning and visibility. Have the persons who will do data entry practice using those screens to check ease of entry and the ability to correct or delete entered records. Practice processing and printing reports that match those you expect to use. Check the system for versatility, flexibility, user friendliness, and ease of use.

- *Carefully review the hardware, memory, disk storage, and printer requirements of the product.* See if you would need to purchase new computers, modems, disks with greater storage capacity, or printers in order to use the product. Determine if the new system would be compatible with existing hardware and software already in place. Calculate the cost that any new hardware would impose.

- If your staff development department is large, *check whether multi-user and local area network (LAN) capabilities are available for the product.* If these features cost extra, find out what the additional cost would be.

- *Determine the security features available in the system.* Check whether user access and/or data access can be limited so that confidentiality of records is maintained.

- *Check the customizing capability of the product.* No software system is likely to possess every capability you might need. Inevitably, some area of need is overlooked, not anticipated, or arises long after the product is purchased. Be sure the product allows you to create and customize reports to meet your needs.

- *Just because a product is "created by hospital educators for use in hospitals" does not necessarily mean it is bet-*

---

*ED-U-KEEP II© from The Edukeep Co, Bedford, IN; EDU-RECORDS and TR (Training Records) PLUS from HRD Software, Amherst, MA; INGENIUM™ for Windows™ from Meliora Systems, Rochester, NY; Registrar,® Scheduler,™ ANALYZER,™ HISTORIAN,™ and TUITION REIMBURSEMENT ADMINISTRATOR™ from Silton-Bookman Systems, Cupertino, CA; TRAINING ADMINISTRATOR™ from Gyrus Systems, Midlothian, VA.

†EDUCATION TRACKER from Business Management Solutions, Acampo, CA; CE-TRAK© from Marker Systems, Severna Park, MD; STAFF DEVELOPMENT MANAGER from Vision Medical Systems, Amherst, NY.

Box 8.14

**CAPABILITIES OF COMMERCIAL SOFTWARE PACKAGES NEEDED FOR
EDUCATIONAL RECORDKEEPING**

Software packages are able to:

- Analyze expenditures and revenues per offering or program
- Automatically enroll previously wait-listed registrants
- Automatically generate billing invoices
- Automatically generate correspondence to participants, faculty, and others
- Automatically generate reminders to enroll in mandatory classes before lapse of certification
- Automatically generate to-do lists
- Automatically schedule for required recertifications
- Calculate and sort compliance rates for mandatory instruction
- Compute and summarize employee course and skill completion rates
- Create calendar of instructional events
- Customize input screens, databases, and reports using simple, menu-driven instructions
- Download data to spreadsheets or word-processors
- Enroll groups of staff into a course by batch (vs. individual) entry
- Generate telephone numbers or letters for all registrants for notification of course cancellation
- Identify staff who did not complete required training/recertification programs
- Import data or files from other sources
- Keep track of faculty schedules
- List all staff with licenses due to expire for any given target date
- Maintain individual employee education records
- Provide ongoing software maintenance and support services
- Check for prerequisites and conflicts in scheduling
- Print attendance/CEU certificates

- Print class registrant rosters
- Print course catalogs
- Print mailing lists, mailing labels, and name tags
- Print training reports by job category, EEO classification, department, or any variable of interest
- Purge files of outdated information
- Register participants for courses
- Relate classes and skills required to a specific job
- Schedule classes
- Schedule rooms, faculty, supplies, and audiovisual resources for specific classes
- Search on any variable in database files
- Select from over 100 standard reports
- Show offerings open for enrollment
- Sort staff development activities by department, category of staff, class, or any variable of interest
- Store and retrieve evaluation data on programs and instructors
- Summarize data on monthly, quarterly, or annual basis
- Track actual vs. budgeted expenses for offering or program budgets
- Track demographic profiles of participants for marketing or evaluation purposes
- Track instructor work loads and evaluations
- Track ongoing training needs analysis
- Track room and resource utilization rates
- Track test scores and skill completion rates by learner, department, or job category
- Wait-list participants automatically for offerings
- Perform Windows™ interface with extensive use of icons for rapid inputs and reports

---

ter, more suitable, or more cost-effective than the more generic training/HRD software. Because most of the generic programs can be easily tailored to distinguish records for competency assessments, CPR and safety mandatory requirements of JCAHO, and the like, be sure that a full and balanced critique is given for all products considered. The versatility, visual layouts, ease of use, and relational database features of some of the newer products on the market (e.g., those that use the Windows environment and icon-based com-

mands) make them more than even competitors with many of the products designed for hospitals.

- *Determine the amount of training and user support that will be available after purchase and its cost.* Look for detailed and clear documentation (user manual) with troubleshooting explanations. Find out if in-service training of all end-users will be provided. See whether the system offers on-line help or tutorials. Check if an 800 telephone number is provided for extended support services. When updates and new versions of the software are developed, these should be available to previous purchasers at a reduced cost.

- *Be wary of first releases (version 1.0) of software.* Initial releases of software may have numerous programming faults and other "bugs" that should be corrected in subsequent releases of the program. Ask for references of other hospitals that have used the program for at least 1 year to determine their satisfaction with the product and any problems they might have experienced.

In the past, recordkeeping in nursing staff development entailed maintaining a few files of attendance rosters and CPR certification records. Today's extensive requirements for documentation of so many aspects of educational activities demands a sophisticated, versatile, and flexible system of data and record management and retrieval. Whether your institution decides to design its own system or purchase a commercial product, recordkeeping in nursing staff development will remain an essential managerial function.

LENGTH OF TIME TO RETAIN RECORDS

There is some variation regarding the length of time that various authors advocate for retaining educational records. Austin[8] suggests that records be kept for staff throughout their employment plus 3 years. Bell, Bowen, and Dilling[9] relate that this information should be retained for at least 5 years. The ANA *Standards for Nursing Staff Development* do not specify any time frame for record retention, but the ASHET *Standards for Health Care Education and Training* require that:

- Program records be retained for at least 5 years, or as required by regulatory agencies
- Active employee records be retained for the length of employment

- Records of terminated employees be merged with personnel files and retained for the duration of that file

Although the JCAHO standards do not specify a particular time period for retention or archiving of educational records, their requirements for historical data related to staff orientation, initial competency assessment, and the like, as well as their 2-year time frame for verification of CPR and other lifesaving interventions (standard SE 4.4), suggest that relevant historical data and documentation need to be available to surveyors regardless of when those activities were actually completed.

BUDGETING

DEFINITION

A *budget* is a financial management tool used to plan, monitor, evaluate, and control the allocation of fiscal resources within an organization. Just as the program goals, curriculum, and instructional outcomes represent an education plan for instructional activities, the budget reflects the fiscal plan for these activities. Budgets represent a financial expression of how the goals and objectives of the staff development unit will be attained over a specified period of time.

USES

A budget can be used in a number of ways for management of nursing staff development activities. Some of the uses for a budget are listed in Box 8.15.

RELEVANCE

The fiscal environment of today's nursing staff development unit makes effective budgeting of educational activ-

---

Box 8.15

USES FOR A BUDGET

- To document fiscal accountability of the staff development unit
- To identify the financial support required for meeting agency needs related to staff development
- To promote and improve operational efficiency in the use of resources
- To control fiscal outlays
- To assist in decision-making regarding the feasibility and efficiency of instructional activities
- To assist in determination of priorities for allocating limited financial resources
- To project costs for new programs and initiatives
- To assess the costs of current programs and activities
- To provide services within the constraints of current financial allocations
- To identify and monitor trends in resource utilization
- To evaluate offerings, programs, and departmental functions from a financial perspective

ities a managerial imperative. The reasons for this situation are numerous and interrelated but can be roughly divided into three categories: a decreased supply of resources for nursing staff development, an increased demand for staff development services and programs, and the costs of hospital education.

Decreased Supply of Staff Development Resources

The replacement of a retrospective reimbursement system with a prospective payment system for healthcare services more than a decade ago has perpetrated an inalterable series of changes in the structure, operation, and management of healthcare services. Government, insurance industry, employer, and public pressures to control the escalating costs of health care have led to an evolving system of healthcare reforms aimed at curbing and reducing costs. The financial impact of these changes to hospitals has included decreased reimbursements for patient care services, fewer patient admissions, decreased lengths of stay, decreased occupancy rates, and heightened competition for patients among healthcare providers.

The loss of substantial hospital revenues, in turn, has led to organizational restructuring, downsizing of departments and staff, regrouping of functions under flattened organizational hierarchies, greater competition among all hospital departments for fewer budget dollars, and heightened pressure on all segments of the hospital to do more with less. The direct trickle-down effect of these events on departments of nursing and nursing staff development are all too familiar now and include the following[11,16,17,24,33]:

- Fewer staff development instructors
- Reduced staff development budget allotments
- Layoff of support staff
- Reduced funding for outside educational programs
- Loss of entire staff development departments or units

Some indirect effects of dwindling resources for staff development are also apparent. These indirect effects include the following[16,17]:

- Inability to purchase instructional materials or media to update or augment existing programs
- Less time available to educators to update courses or develop new offerings or programs
- Decreased availability of nursing staff to attend educational programs due to greater use of part-time nurses, sicker patients, higher nurse:patient ratios, reduced numbers of nursing staff from layoffs, and lack of overtime pay
- Less vendor and pharmaceutical company support for educational activities owing to reduced revenues

These effects are only compounded by a national economy strapped with a long-standing recession, high levels of un-employment, lack of job security, and reduced salary and benefits for many workers. Nurses themselves, their spouses, and their children are all affected by these economic realities.

In a supply-demand equation, this diminished supply of resources available for nursing staff development is only half the problem. If the demand for staff development were proportionately reduced to a level commensurate with the reduced supply, the equation could remain balanced. Unfortunately, this is not the case.

Increased Demand for Staff Development Services

The continual introduction of changes in healthcare technologies, treatments, delivery systems, pharmaceuticals, and therapies has increased demands for staff development services. A larger proportion of more acutely ill patients who require high-tech equipment and more intensive care on units previously unaccustomed to these patients has added to the instructional burden for nursing staff. Even the purchase of systems aimed at improving staff productivity, such as patient acuity/classification systems, computerized monitoring and documentation systems, and the like, increase the need for staff development programming.

In addition to demands that emanate from patients and the care they require, compliance with accreditation and regulatory requirements mandate that specific types of offerings be made available. Hospital, nursing department, or staff development policies and/or standards may also require certain types of instructional programs and activities.

Because nurses often view staff development as an important employment benefit,[54] increased availability of educational programming may be necessary as a recruitment and retention vehicle in areas where competition for nursing staff is high. Union contracts may also specify that certain numbers and types of learning opportunities be provided to nursing staff. Contracts with area schools of nursing may dictate certain educational support as necessary for student affiliation at that facility. If the hospital is located in a state where continuing education is required for relicensure of nurses, the hospital may be committed or obliged to offer an augmented program of educational offerings to retain nurses.

The restructuring process at some healthcare facilities has resulted in the regrouping of functions that may add new areas of responsibility to the staff development unit. Functions such as quality assurance, community education, special projects, and the training of nonnursing personnel may be assigned to nursing staff development. In hospitals where patient education is also a staff development responsibility, the abbreviated lengths of stay of sicker patients create a situation where patient and family needs for instruction are greatly increased while the time available to complete patient education may be severely limited for both inpatient and outpatient populations. The cumulative effects of decreased resources in the face of increased demands for nursing staff development are untenable to manage without a budget to guide resolution of these competing forces.

Cost of Hospital Education

The 1993 annual survey of the training industry[20] found that among U.S. organizations with 100 or more employees, the total budget for formal training was $48 billion, an increase of 7% over the prior (1992) year. Health services organizations represented 8% in this sample of 2496 organizations surveyed. This figure represents only budgeted training expenditures and does not include either costs of any informal, on-the-job instruction or the costs of hidden expenses such as learners' salaries during periods of instruction. The average amounts budgeted by health service agencies for specific categories of expenses are summarized in Table 8.3.

In contrast with both the nursing staff development literature and anecdotal reports that indicate reduced budgets for hospital staff development units, this national survey found that in the health services sector of the training industry, 56% of survey participants reported having the same budget amount as they had received the year prior; 30% received a larger budget than the year before; and only 14% reported a smaller budget. The reasons for this discrepancy are not clear, but it may be that the "health services" category included many agencies that were not hospitals or that its sampling of 208 healthcare agencies represented a group of organizations somehow dissimilar to the "average hospital." In any event, it is apparent that education and training in the healthcare industry represents a major financial investment.[25]

Little information is available regarding the average size of nursing staff development budgets. A 1987 study[17] of eight medical centers found that a conservative estimate is that hospitals spend between 2% and 6% of their total annual operating expense on education and training, with an average of slightly more than 4%. In 1987 dollars, this reflects spending levels from $1.8 million to more than $3.9 million and includes both staff training and patient education, with staff education representing 44% to 73% of the total cost of education. When the "hidden costs" of education such as learner salaries during instruction and course preparation time were added in, the total education costs were found to be five to six times greater than the known, budgeted costs.

A more recent study of continuing education budgets[54] that included 661 hospitals and 685 nursing homes in the Midwest found that the average amounts that hospitals budgeted for outside continuing education ranged from $3037 for hospitals with fewer than 100 beds to $15,736 for hospitals with 100 to 500 beds and $13,271 for hospitals with more than 500 beds. In addition, it was found that educational support for staff nurses included payment of wages in 52% of cases and registration fees in 49% of cases, but lesser amounts of support for materials such as books (only 29% of cases), transportation expenses (25% of cases), meals (17% of cases), or lodging (12% of cases).

For hospitals, the price tag for nursing staff development and continuing education is substantial, especially when this funding must compete with reimbursable expenses related to the central mission of direct patient care services. For individual nurses, the residual expenses that they may be asked to bear can also be significant in an environment of economic recession, job insecurity (their own and their spouses, as well as those of family members), and unemployment.

TERMS USED IN BUDGETING

The budgetary process employs a number of terms that may not be familiar to nurse educators. A brief glossary of some of these terms is provided in Box 8.16.

TYPES OF BUDGETS

There are two basic types of budgets that are commonly used in healthcare settings: operational and capital. Each type of budget is described following.

Operational Budget

The *operational budget* (or general operating budget) for a nursing staff development unit consists of a financial plan of the expenses and revenues that will enable provision of staff development services on a daily basis over a particular period of time. The time period is typically a fiscal year rather than a calendar year (January-December). The time frame of the fiscal year may be any designated consecutive 12-month period: for example, July 1 of the current year

TABLE 8.3 • AVERAGE ANNUAL BUDGETS FOR HEALTH SERVICES ORGANIZATIONS WITH OVER 100 EMPLOYEES

Expense Category	Amount Budgeted ($)	Proportion of Budget (%)
Trainer salaries	206,050	75.3
Seminars/conferences	20,863	7.6
Hardware	11,127	4.1
Off-the-shelf materials	10,624	3.9
Facilities/overhead	9,129	3.3
Outside services	9,061	3.3
Custom materials	6,812	2.5
TOTALS:	273,666	100.0

From Filipczak B: *Training* 30 (10):37, 1993.

Box 8.16

TERMS USED IN BUDGETING

Accounting:	The collection, processing, and reporting of financial information.[22]
Capital budget:	The financial plan of major expenditures that supplement the organization's operational budget over a specified period of time. Expenses are usually projected over a multi-year (rather than single-year) time span.
Cost:	The outlay or expenditure made to achieve something; expense.[67] The amount paid or charged for a product or service.[22]
Direct costs:	Expenses that are directly attributable to a particular program or activity.
Encumbered costs:	Monies committed for expenditure but not yet spent
Fixed costs:	Costs that do not vary with the level of output (e.g., with the number of participants or programs)[22]
Indirect costs:	Costs (such as overhead) that are secondarily associated with a particular program or activity.
Operational budget:	The financial plan of projected expenditures and revenues for conducting day-to-day activities over a specified period of time (usually 1 fiscal year). Inclusions vary with how expense categories are designated at that institution.
Opportunity costs:	Reflect the profit contribution of the employee's lost time; the cost of opportunities that might have been realized if allocated resources had been directed toward other organizational needs (e.g., staff attending an in-service program might have been more productive if they had remained on their unit).[22]
Overhead costs:	Expenses or costs (such as rent, insurance, or heating) that are not chargeable to a particular part of the work or product of a business.[67] A percentage determined for each work area based on an analysis of indirect costs related to total direct costs.[62]
Revenue:	Income.
Sunk costs:	Fixed costs (such as advertising) that are nonrecoverable even though a program is canceled.[62]
Total cost:	Sum of all costs.
Variable costs:	Costs that vary with the level of output[22]; costs that vary with the level of participation.[62]

---

through June 30 of the following year, or October 1 through September 30.

Preparation

The hospital's finance department is likely to have standard forms for preparation of operational budgets that specify how anticipated expenses and revenues are to be defined and organized on the budget document. These forms are forwarded to the manager responsible for staff development some months before the budget draft is due. Although the manager is ultimately responsible for budget preparation, solicitation of the input of all educators is a valuable means for creating a more complete, accurate, and well-conceived planning tool that more fully coincides with departmental and organizational goals and objectives. Staff participation in the budget development process also enables educators to make a contribution that reflects their personal commitment to the plan.

If the staff development unit has prepared operating budgets previously, the prior fiscal year's budget serves as a good starting point for planning purposes because it contains an enumeration of the categories and amounts designated for particular expenses (and, in some cases, revenues) to be included. When the staff development unit's budget is new, however, these initial projections may need to be identified from past experience, discussion, and reflection.

Different institutions will require different degrees of detail and notation in recording of the operating budget. Some may request only an indication of total amounts for each major category of expense and income, while others may request much fuller detailing of the subtotals represented by those totals so that the cost or revenue basis for the figure is apparent. When formulas are used to establish a category total, the finance department may ask that the formulas used be specified as footnotes to the figure given. For example, if the costs for orientation were computed on the basis of having 100 orientees per fiscal year at a cost of $500 per orientee, the following formula could be added as a footnote notation:

$$\begin{array}{ccc} \text{Number of orientees} & \times \ \text{Cost per} & = \ \text{Anticipated cost} \\ \text{per year} & \text{orientee} & \text{of orientation} \\ (100) & \times \ (\$500) & = \ (\$50,000) \end{array}$$

Once the initial estimates of expenses and revenues are recorded, the draft budget document should be reviewed to ensure that it is succinct, clear, arithmetically accurate, fully substantiated, and consistent with the mission, goals, and objectives of the staff development unit, the parent department (nursing department or human resource development [HRD] department), and the healthcare facility. The proposed operational budget will then be forwarded to the staff development manager's administrator, who will review it, provide feedback, and indicate any necessary changes. After preliminary approval of the budget, it will be included within the parent department's budget and then forwarded to the hospital administrator for final approval.

Inclusions

The elements contained in the operating budget include the two general areas of expenses and revenues. If no revenues are anticipated, only expenses are detailed. Expenses are typically divided among a number of different categories. The finance department will usually define each category of expense; these definitions need to be followed closely in preparing the budget so that figures are allocated to the correct category.

The expense categories generally include salary and benefits, supplies, services, and travel, and, at some institutions, overhead. Salary figures may be designated as a total or be subdivided among different positions. If salary increments (merit, promotional, or tenure) are anticipated, these increases need to be included. New positions will also need to be added if hiring is planned during the next fiscal year. When a new position is proposed, a description of the position and its justification should be appended to the budget. If the agency anticipates the need to pay honoraria to outside faculty or consultants, the expected costs of these honoraria should be included as well. Because employee benefits are usually calculated as a percentage of the employee's base salary, benefit estimates can most readily be determined after all salary figures (including salary increases) have been projected.

The category of supplies refers to consumable items such as office supplies; instructional materials such as overhead transparency film, paper, and markers; reference materials such as books; small, disposable medical supplies; and postage. This category is sometimes designated as supplies and materials to reflect its inclusive nature.

The category of services may include the costs of photocopying, offset printing, telephone and facsimile charges, catering, and equipment repair and maintenance, as well as program advertising and promotion (if applicable). If the staff development unit is charged for overhead expenses, this figure can be obtained from the finance department and covers the unit's apportioned charges for facility space rental, utilities, building maintenance, and depreciation.

The travel section of the budget includes the costs incurred for staff travel to provide offerings at off-site locations as well as staff attendance at continuing education meetings. Travel items should be documented as explicitly as possible and include the date, location, and title of the conference and anticipated charges for registration fees, meals, transportation (air and ground), and related expenses, as well as the number of staff attending. Figure 8.2 illustrates an example of how an operational budget may be prepared.

Capital Budget

A *capital budget* for nursing staff development reflects the unit's needs for major expenditures that exceed some established cost level. Organizations set the threshold for capital expenses at varying amounts. Smaller institutions may use $250; medium-size agencies may use $500, and larger organizations might use $3000. Any anticipated expense that exceeds the preset level would need to be included on the capital (rather than on the operational) budget request.

Preparation

Because the costs for capital expenses are high and the funds available for them are limited, careful and thorough preparation of this budget is necessary. The process begins with a thoughtful review of the hospital's current goals and objectives, the nursing department's goals and objectives, and the staff development unit's goals and objectives for the next few years. If available, the hospital's strategic plan for the next 2 to 5 years would be good to review as well. With this context in mind, staff development's role in supporting and facilitating not only its own but its parent department's and hospital's objectives needs to be distinguished. Using this long view of the facility, educators can then begin to identify the capital items that staff development should procure to best contribute to attaining these sequential goals and objectives.

The capital budget form will be forwarded by the hospital's finance department to the manager of nursing staff development. The information requested on this form may include areas such as the following in relation to requested items or services:

- Description of the item or service
- Justification for expense
- Funding priority

- Cost estimate
- Approximate useful life span (in years)

Figure 8.3 provides an example of a capital budget request form.

As with operating budgets, the capital budget will be forwarded up to successively higher administrative levels for review, possible revision, resubmission, and eventual disposition. When healthcare agency balance sheets are already operating "in the red," capital expenditures may be severely limited, delayed for funding, or even curtailed completely until funds are available. Current cost constraints within the healthcare industry make it imperative that all requests for capital expenses reflect essential needs that make a clear contribution to the facility, its mission, and its goals.

Inclusions

Capital budgets for nursing staff development usually include requests for major purchases of office or instructional equipment such as computers, printers, video cameras, projectors, CPR mannequins, furniture (tables, desks, and chairs), or expensive software or audiovisual programs. Services that may be included in a capital budget consist of facility expansions or renovations of teaching, office, or storage spaces.

BUDGET FUNDING SOURCES

Historically, staff development has been viewed as a support service for nursing practice and nursing management. The costs associated with the provision of staff development have been borne by the nursing or HRD department with no expectation that revenue be generated to offset those costs. Over the past few years, however, an increasing number of healthcare facilities have not only reduced their budgetary allotments to staff development but suggested or expected that staff development be responsible for covering at least some of its costs to the institution. As a support service, staff development is not typically expected to serve as a revenue center, but the realities of the current hospital reimbursement system tend to make areas not involved with direct patient care vulnerable to pressures of this nature. To the extent that nursing staff development can improve its efficiency without compromising its central mission, it is worthwhile to consider various potential sources of revenue that staff development may be able to secure in order to make it more self-supporting. These potential funding sources fall into three categories: internal, participant, and external.

Internal Funding

Internal funding is the traditional source of revenue for nursing staff development. Operational and capital budgets are submitted and approved as previously described, and the parent organization or one of its subdivisions provides the approved funds. Depending on the facility's organizational structure, nursing staff development may be a distinct cost center that receives direct funding by the hospital via the finance department. More often, nursing staff development receives its budgetary allocation as one segment of the nursing or HRD department. In highly decentralized structures, funding may partially or wholly originate within the budget of a nursing division or even within an individual nursing unit. Internal funding may provide for coverage of all staff development expenses, or it may be supplemented by funding from participant or external sources.

Participant Funding

When certain types of offerings or an entire program (e.g., the continuing education program) must be able to cover its expenses, a commonly tapped avenue for revenue is the institution of fees charged to participants. Although hospital employees are not generally expected to pay for any mandatory staff development offerings, they may be asked to pay a small charge to cover the costs of CEU application fees, refreshments, and materials provided to them at the offering.

A more commonly employed means of participant funding involves the marketing of hospital offerings to outside participants. Outside participants may be drawn from the local community, the region, or even nationally. Registration fees for workshops and conferences may partially or completely cover costs for the offering and may also generate net profits that can be used to offset expenses of other offerings.

External Funding

External funding for staff development activities may be available from a number of sources: exhibitor fees, contributions, gifts, grants, and contracts for instruction or consultation services, as well as published works. When offerings are marketed to outside participants, enrollments are often sufficient to justify the inclusion of exhibitors at the meeting. When exhibitor space is planned, fees can then be assessed from exhibitors, based on the size of the exhibit area they wish to use.

Contributions may be derived from hospital auxiliaries, community organizations, civic and social service agencies, and foundations. Gifts received from patients, families, or the medical staff can be used to underwrite programs. Outright grants may be secured from healthcare product vendors, pharmaceutical companies, book publishers, private foundations, or even federal or state government agencies.

Larger staff development units often have a number of staff with considerable expertise to share. These individuals may be able to contract with other healthcare facilities

Operational Budget Form

Department/Unit Name: _____   **Fiscal Year** _____

Directions: Please attach copy of goals and objectives for your department for fiscal year _____ to this budget. Provide description and justification for all entries marked with an asterisk.*

Expenses

Salary & Benefits

Position	# Staff	Base Salary	Salary Increases* Merit	Tenure	Base Benefits	Benefit Increases*	Subtotal
Director of SD:							
Educators:							
Unit instructors:							
Part-time staff:*							
Secretary:							
Consultants:*							
Outside faculty:*							

Supplies (list specific inclusions)

Instruct materials:	
Medical items:	
Office supplies:	
Postage:	
Subscriptions:	
Other:	

Services (describe basis/formula for each estimate)

Catering:	
Maintenance:	
Photocopying:	
Printing:	
Promotion:	
Rental fees:	
Repairs:	
Telephone/fax:	
Other:	

Figure 8.2 Operational budget form.

Department/Unit Name: _____   **Fiscal Year** _____

Travel

Meeting	# Staff	Registration Fees	Meals	Airfares	Ground Transport	Other expenses	Subtotal
Hospital:							
Other sponsor:*							

Overhead

Dept/unit
charge: _____

Revenues

Sources

Source	Description	Amount

Total revenues = $ _____

Total expenses = $ _____

Net: $ _____

Figure 8.2—cont'd   Operational budget form.

Capital Budget Form

Department/Unit Name: _____   **Fiscal Year** _____

Directions: Please provide the information requested below for all expenses that exceed $_____.

Priority Ranking		Description of Item or Service	Estimated Life span	Cost/Unit	# Units	Justification
Dept	Unit					
Hosp						

Figure 8.3 Capital budget form.

to provide a range of educational consultation services.[70] The fees charged for these instructional or consulting services would reimburse the hospital for the educator's wages, benefits, and expenses, as well as allow a net profit.

A number of healthcare institutions have recognized the potential value and usefulness to other educators and organizations of materials they have developed. As a result, programs and materials such as policy and procedure manuals, self-instruction packets, curricula, CBO programs, and various types of media that were initially designed for internal use are made available for external purchase. Some facilities do their own design, production, marketing, and advertising, whereas others submit their material to established healthcare publishers for production and marketing. The former requires an internal system to provide support for design, printing, binding, packaging, advertising, order processing and fulfillment, shipping, and storage, and the latter approach leaves all of these concerns to the publisher. In relation to revenues, the internal approach will yield net revenues (gross receipts minus all associated direct and indirect costs), while the publisher approach centers on either a single lump payment for the project or a royalty percentage of net receipts.

Three caveats should be noted with regard to profit-generation and external funding. The first concern is an admonition regarding the various issues that need to be considered before in-house programs and materials are marketed externally. Although the decisions and process may appear to be straightforward, they require a considerable amount of deliberation, planning, and resources.[19,29] A second concern relates to the need to keep service as the central and predominant focus of the nursing staff development unit. Staff development exists to provide educational support for nursing practice and patient care. Its primary mission does not include generating profits for the facility. The third concern relates to the need to be vigilant regarding the tax treatment of so-called unrelated business income in nonprofit organizations.[24] Aggressive entrepreneurial activities in nonprofit corporations need to be carefully monitored so that tax regulations related to not-for-profit institutions are closely adhered to.

LEVELS OF BUDGETING

Budgets can be prepared at any of three different levels: individual offering, program, or unit. Each affords a means for fiscal management at that level so that an orderly monitoring and control of expenses and income (if any) can be guaranteed.

Single-Offering Budget

The lowest level of budgeting occurs with the financial planning for a single educational offering. Before the days of prospective reimbursement and drastically reduced hospital revenues, the costs of staff development offerings were sometimes not computed at all or only took into account the cost of instructor salaries during the period of instruction. Today's fiscal environment demands a much more thorough and detailed tracking of costs that accounts for the full financial impact of each offering and allows for an analysis of where expenses are incurred.

Figure 8.4 illustrates a form for summarizing the budget of a single staff development offering. Rather than merely tallying the cost of instructor time to provide the offering, it also includes entries for indicating the additional costs of program design and development (inclusive of all related learning needs assessments and program planning), a more comprehensive accounting of direct and indirect program delivery costs, and expenses related to evaluation.

One noteworthy element in the program delivery section of this budget is the cost of staff time away from their work area. These lost work hours, including the costs to replace attendees on their units, represent *opportunity costs* of having staff attend the offering rather than perform their customary duties. The true labor costs associated with staff development activities are a combination of instructor time and clerical and other staff time as well as employee learner time. Budgets that only recognize instructor time in teaching the offering neglect major expenses incurred in these activities. Except in instances where program design and development costs are high (as in design of a new, comprehensive offering), the largest single expense for any staff development offering is usually these lost work hours. Not only are wages and benefits paid to attendees, but their replacements on the unit are also paid, effectively doubling the costs involved. Two intriguing features of opportunity costs are that many hospitals neglect to include them in calculating offering costs[16] and that nurse attendees often do not perceive time lost from work as a cost.[64]

Program Budget

Program budgets reflect the combined accounting for all offerings included in that program. For example, the orientation program budget includes all offerings of the RN staff nurse orientation, the LPN and nursing assistant orientations, new graduate orientation, nurse manager orientation, and any other orientation offering provided during the fiscal year. The in-service program budget would include all in-service offerings for that fiscal year: each offering of the mandatory safety classes, CPR and ACLS certification and recertification courses, initial and ongoing competency assessment sessions, and any other planned in-services. The continuing education program would consist of all offerings within this category scheduled throughout the year. An example of a form for budgeting a staff development orientation program is provided in Figure 8.5. Rather than repeating all of the detailed analysis found in the single-offering budget, the program budget merely captures subtotals of the major subcategories of actual expenses and transfers these to the program budget. In ad-

Single staff development offering budget

Title: _____   Program category: ☐ orientation
Date: _____   (check one)   ☐ in-service education
Contact hrs: _____   ☐ continuing education
                                      ☐ other: _____

Expenses	Estimated	Actual	Total
*Development**			
Salary and benefits			
▪ SD director			
▪ Educators			
▪ Unit instructors			
▪ Secretary			
▪ Other:			
Materials & supplies			
Telephone, fax			
Promotion			
▪ Photocopying announcements			
▪ Printing brochures			
▪ Postage			
▪ Mailing list			
▪ Advertising			
CEU application fee			
Other:			
Delivery			
Salary and benefits			
▪ SD director			
▪ Educators			
▪ Unit instructors			
▪ Secretary			
▪ Staff time away from work**			
Outside faculty honoraria & expenses***			

* Includes all costs related to needs assessment and program planning
** Equals number of staff participants times their hourly wages and benefit costs
*** Costs of travel, lodging, air and ground transportation, meals

Figure 8.4   Budget for single staff development offering.

Materials & supplies			
• Handout photocopying			
• Folders, name tags, CEU certificates			
• Instructional materials			
• Misc.:			
Facility rental fees			
AV services and support			
Catering: breaks, meals			

Evaluation

Salary and benefits			
• SD director			
• Educators			
• Unit instructors			
• Secretary			
• Other:			
Materials & supplies			

Overhead

Revenues	Estimated	Actual	Total
Participant fees			
• Staff registrants			
• Outside registrants			
External funds			
• Exhibitor fees			
• Contributions, gifts			
• Grants			
• Consulting fees			
• Publications			

Summary

Net profit <loss>

Cost per participant

Cost per contact hour awarded

Figure 8.4—cont'd   Budget for single staff development offering.

dition, the program budget enables the manager to monitor the use of resources among all offerings within a given program.

Unit Budget

The highest level of budgeting provides a summary of financial information for all programs and related activities for which the staff development unit is responsible. In addition to the three customary program components of orientation, in-service, and continuing education, some staff development units are also responsible for areas such as quality improvement, internal consultation to staff, research,[2] patient and community education, as well as committee and task force collaboration, and student affiliations. If staff development's involvement with these activities requires a significant expenditure of resources, these activities need to be included in the unit budget. Figure 8.6 illustrates a unit budget for nursing staff development.

BUDGET ANALYSIS

Budget information can be analyzed in a number of different ways. These include ongoing monitoring as well as a series of more formal procedures that include break-even analysis, cost-benefit analysis, cost-effectiveness analysis, and productivity analysis.

Ongoing Monitoring

The manager of nursing staff development is responsible for reviewing budgetary data related to offerings, programs, and the unit as a whole on an ongoing basis to ensure that financial resources are being used effectively, efficiently, and appropriately. A systematic monthly review of offering budgets and interim program budgets as well as a quarterly review of the unit budget should enable the manager to make these determinations. These ongoing reviews can be used to identify the judicious use of funds, the sufficiency of funding, whether adjustments are necessary in how funds are distributed, and any significant discrepancies that may appear between expected and actual expenditures.

On a semiannual basis, the manager may also enlist the input of all staff development unit members to search for ways in which the outcomes of educational activities could be enhanced, the resources expended be reduced, or the quality of programs and services be improved. Major sources of expense (such as opportunity costs or the duration of instructional events) as well as potential but as yet untapped revenue sources need to be carefully scrutinized to see where enhancements could be instituted.

Because the volume of information (both financial and statistical) necessary and required for budget and record-keeping management can be extensive, managers will find a computerized recordkeeping system helpful in providing timely and targeted reports of required data. Automated systems can be useful not only for large staff development units but also for smaller units that have only one or two persons. Because these individuals usually spend the majority of their time providing educational offerings, little time is available to them to manually monitor data and prepare interim budget reports. Having software that tracks this information and generates these reports quickly and accurately can be an immense time-saving feature that enhances effective budget management.

Some of the more sophisticated and detailed methods of budget analysis are also most readily performed via computerized methods. Although some are amenable to manual calculation, the tedious and time-consuming nature of this activity is difficult to justify when computer programming can reduce the entry and processing times involved to a fraction of their manual requirements. Because most of these analyses represent rather complex endeavors that are just beginning to be used in nursing, they will only be highlighted here.

Break-Even Analysis

A *break-even analysis* refers to a calculation of the point at which an offering's revenues are equal to its expenses. It is a simple calculation that is useful in determining the number of registrants an offering needs to cover its expenses.

Educational offerings incur different types of costs: *fixed costs*, which remain the same regardless of the number of participants (e.g., printing and mailing brochures); *variable costs*, which change with the number of participants (e.g., meals or photocopies of handouts); *direct costs*, which are attributable to a specific offering (e.g., the CEU application fee); and *indirect costs*, which are not directly attributable to a particular offering (e.g., overhead).

Various forms of break-even analysis take different numbers and types of costs into account in determining the number of participants needed to cover those costs. The basic formula for calculating the break-even point (BEP) is as follows[61]:

$$BEP = \text{Expenses} \div ([\text{Registrant fee}] - [\text{Variable costs/registrant}])$$

An example of how to calculate the break-even point for covering all direct and fixed costs of an offering follows.

If the total of direct and fixed expenses for the offering was $3000, the registration fee was $100, and the variable costs were $40 per participant, the formula would be applied as follows:

BEP = Expenses ÷ ([Registrant fee] − [Variable costs per registrant])

BEP = $3000 ÷ ([$100] − [$40])

BEP = $3000 ÷ ($60)

BEP = 50 registrants

Staff Development Unit Budget

Fiscal Year: _____

Expenses	Orientation Program	In-service Program	Continuing Education Program	Other program: ___	Other program: ___	TOTALS
Development						
Salary and benefits						
Materials & supplies						
Telephone, fax						
Promotion						
CEU application fee						
Other:						
Delivery						
Salary and benefits						
Outside faculty honoraria & expenses						
Materials & supplies						
Facility rental fees						
AV services and support						
Catering: breaks, meals						
Evaluation						
Salary and benefits						
Materials & supplies						
Overhead						
TOTAL EXPENSES						

Revenues		
Participant fees		
External funds		
TOTAL REVENUES		
Net Revenue <expense>		

Figure 8.6 Staff development unit budget.

Staff Development Program Budget: ORIENTATION PROGRAM

Fiscal Year: _____

Expenses	Staff Nurse						Head Nurse		CNS		LPN				Nursing Assistant			GN		Totals
	Jan	Mar	May	July	Sept	Nov	Feb	Aug	Feb	Aug	Jan	Apr	July	Oct	Apr	Aug	Dec	Jan	July	
Development																				
Salary and benefits																				
Materials & supplies																				
Telephone, fax																				
Promotion																				
CEU application fee																				
Other:																				
Delivery																				
Salary and benefits																				
Outside faculty honoraria & expenses																				
Materials & supplies																				
Facility rental fees																				
AV services and support																				
Catering: breaks, meals																				
Evaluation																				
Salary and benefits																				
Materials & supplies																				
Overhead																				

Revenues			Totals
Participant fees			
External funds			

Figure 8.5 Staff development program budget: orientation program.

			TABLE 8.4 • EXPENSES					
Number of Participants	×	**Variable Cost/ Participant**	=	**Variable Costs**	+	**Fixed Costs**	=	**Expenses**
10	×	40	=	$ 400	+	$3000	=	$3400
20	×	40	=	$ 800	+	$3000	=	$3800
30	×	40	=	$1200	+	$3000	=	$4200
40	×	40	=	$1600	+	$3000	=	$4600
50	×	40	=	$2000	+	$3000	=	$5000
60	×	40	=	$2400	+	$3000	=	$5400
70	×	40	=	$2800	+	$3000	=	$5800
80	×	40	=	$3200	+	$3000	=	$6200
90	×	40	=	$3600	+	$3000	=	$6600
100	×	40	=	$4000	+	$3000	=	$7000

In order to break even with the direct and fixed expenses, 50 participants would need to register for the offering.

If one were interested in determining the BEP to cover *both* direct and indirect fixed costs, the figure used for "expenses" would be modified accordingly and the break-even point would indicate the greater amount of expenses necessary to cover both indirect and direct expenses.

If the total of direct and indirect fixed expenses for the offering was $4200, the registration fee $100, and the variable costs $40 per participant, the formula would be applied as follows:

BEP = Expenses ÷ ([Registrant fee] − [Variable costs per registrant])

BEP = $4200 ÷ ([$100] − [$40])

BEP = $4200 ÷ ($60)

BEP = 70 registrants

In order to cover both direct and indirect costs, then, a total of 70 registrants would be needed. The need for 10 additional registrants reflects the added burden of covering indirect as well as direct expenses.

Two additional sets of calculations can be made by developing a spreadsheet from this same basic formula. These calculations include the effect of different registration fees (higher or lower) on the break-even point and the effect of different levels of enrollment on the amount of profits or losses experienced. In the first case, the registration fee per participant will be inversely related to the break-even point, that is, a higher registration fee will reduce the number of registrants needed to break even and a lower registration fee will increase the number of registrants needed to break even.

The second calculation was nicely illustrated by Sheridan,[56] who showed how both the break-even point for fixed costs and the variable effects of different enrollment levels can be determined. Using increments of enrollment from 10 to 60 participants, the combined effects of variable costs and variable revenues can be observed. The expense elements were calculated as follows:

		TABLE 8.5 • REVENUES		
Number of Participants	×	**Registration Fee**	=	**Revenues**
10	×	100	=	$1000
20	×	100	=	$2000
30	×	100	=	$3000
40	×	100	=	$4000
50	×	100	=	$5000
60	×	100	=	$6000
70	×	100	=	$7000
80	×	100	=	$8000
90	×	100	=	$9000
100	×	100	=	$10,000

$$\text{Number of participants} \times \frac{\text{Variable cost/}}{\text{participant}} = \frac{\text{Variable}}{\text{costs}}$$

and

$$\text{Variable costs} + \text{Fixed costs} = \text{Expenses}$$

The revenue element was calculated as follows:

$$\text{Revenue} = \text{Number of participants} \times \frac{\text{Registration fee/}}{\text{participant}}$$

Substituting changes in the number of participants will influence both variable costs and revenues. Plotting these variables on a graph visually illustrates the relationships between expenses and revenues. Using the example given earlier, the spreadsheet data would appear as shown in Tables 8.4 and 8.5 when the variable cost per participant is $40, the fixed costs equal $3000, and the registration fee per participant is $100.

As Figure 8.7 illustrates, the break-even point of this sample budget would be 50 participants. If fewer than 50 participants enroll, the offering cannot cover its fixed expenses and a loss would be incurred. If more than 50 participants enroll, revenues will exceed fixed expenses and a profit would be realized for the offering. The value of making these calculations with spreadsheet software (such as Microsoft EXCEL or Lotus 1-2-3) is that the ripple effect of changes in any one variable in the formula can be immediately seen and graphically illustrated to answer all of the "what if . . . " areas of concern in managing the budget for that offering. The remaining types of budget analysis are considerably more complex than break-even analysis.

Cost-Benefit Analysis

Rossi and Freeman[54] define *cost-benefit analysis* as "the economic efficiency of a program expressed as the relationship between costs and outcomes, usually measured in monetary terms." This type of analysis requires estimation of the benefits of a program (both tangible and intangible) as well as the costs of the program (both direct and indirect). Once these elements have been identified, both the costs and benefits must be translated into a common measurement, which is usually monetary in nature. Costs are then compared with benefits to ascertain either the net benefits or, more commonly, the ratio of benefits to costs.[54]

Although the itemization of staff development program costs is, as previously described, quite feasible to accomplish, the itemization of program benefits in monetary terms poses conceptual and practical problems inasmuch as the outcomes of staff development programs are not typically viewed or expressed in monetary valuations. The need to "reduce" the benefits of staff development activities to a monetary common denominator limits the usefulness of this type of analysis.

Certain types of benefits that may be amenable to cost-benefit analysis include the comparison of staff development costs to each of the following:

- The costs of initiating a nurse internship program vs. the costs of recruitment and turnover of new graduates
- the costs of converting from a traditional to a competency-based orientation program vs. the savings realized from reducing the time required for experienced nurses to complete orientation
- The costs of increasing the volume and quality of continuing education offerings vs. the costs of turnover among experienced staff nurses
- The costs of developing and providing an inservice offering on organizing work loads vs. the cost of overtime attributable to poor organizational skills

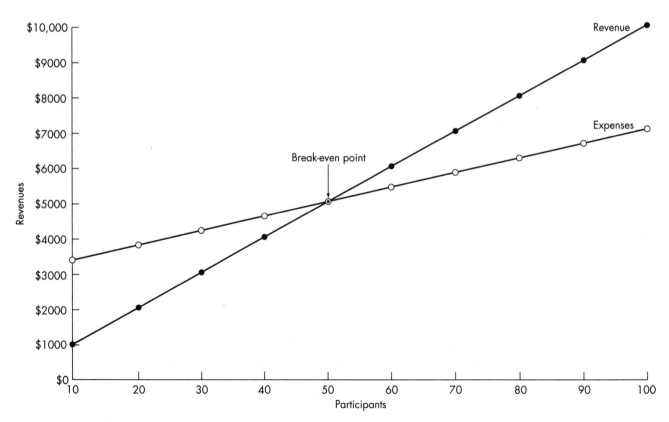

Figure 8.7 Break-even analysis.

As can be seen from these examples, some benefits of nursing staff development can indeed be translated into monetary terms. But many educational outcomes at the learning, application, and impact levels cannot readily be converted into dollar denominations. Readers interested in learning the specifics of performing a valid and meaningful cost-benefit analysis are referred to the work of Rossi and Freeman[54] and other sources,[22,27,57,61] which explain many of the details and alternatives involved.

Cost-Effectiveness Analysis

Cost-effectiveness analysis is defined as the efficacy of a program in achieving given outcomes in relation to program costs.[54] In contrast to cost-benefit analysis, which compares costs to monetary outcomes, cost-effectiveness analysis compares program costs to the attainment of specified program outcomes. With cost-effectiveness analysis, the costs of educational offerings with the same instructional outcomes can be compared to determine which achieves these outcomes at a lower (more efficient) cost. Comparing different methods for teaching CPR recertification courses or forming a consortium to regionalize and economize on staff development programs usually utilizes cost-effectiveness analysis. Cost-effectiveness is enhanced when the same outcomes can be attained at a lower program cost.

Rossi and Freeman[54] characterize cost-effectiveness analysis (as an extension of cost-benefit analysis) as more appropriate than cost-benefit analysis for health services. Both types of analysis are based on the same principles and assumptions, calculation methods, and procedures, but cost-effectiveness considers outcomes that go beyond merely monetary terms.[54,57] The three elements involved with computing cost-effectiveness include: (1) the identification of program objectives, (2) calculation of program costs, and (3) specification of instructional outcomes in observable and measurable terms.

The criteria used as a basis for judging cost-effectiveness may include comparisons between the attainment of program objectives and the costs per participant, the opportunity costs of lost work hours, the costs of program development and delivery, improved test scores, or audited clinical performance criteria. In contrast to cost-benefit analysis, which requires comparison of monetary units, cost-effectiveness analysis can embrace comparisons that examine observable behaviors and standard educational evaluation models such as written tests and completion of clinical skills checklists.[23] Although outcomes must still be quantifiable, they need not be monetary in nature. The dollar figures associated with cost benefits may be easier for hospital administrators to relate to, but cost-effectiveness computations may often be more meaningful in relation to the overall purpose, goals, and mission of the nursing staff development unit. Readers interested in performing the specific procedures required for analysis of cost-effectiveness may refer to a number of useful references.[14,35,54]

Productivity Analysis

Productivity is defined as a ratio of work input to work output that results from a given process over a specific period of time. In a hospital setting, work input includes the labor, materials, time, and financial resources used to provide patient care; the time frame is the patient's length of stay; and the work output or product is the health status of the patient at discharge.[10]

In nursing staff development, work input can be quantified with any of a number of resource categories used to provide educational services: labor (salary and benefits), materials and supplies, time, or budget allotments. The most commonly employed input measure is the time that staff spend on various educational activities. The time frame for evaluating productivity could be based on any preestablished period: a week, a month, a quarter, or a year. The work output or product could be measured via a number of possible output units: the attainment of predetermined goals and objectives, the number of offerings provided to staff, the number of continuing education units awarded in a year, and the like.[65]

Productivity analysis typically focuses on the relationship between work input and output. Analyses may be done to monitor and improve this relationship in a number of possible ways:

- Use *less* input to achieve *greater* output (do more with less)
- Use *less* input to achieve the *same* output (do the same with less)
- Use the *same* input to achieve *greater* output (do more with no more)

Productivity is enhanced whenever decreased input can achieve the same desired output, when the same input results in greater output, or when less input can achieve greater output. In a hospital setting, productivity relates to the contribution that each department makes toward achieving organizational goals and objectives. Productivity measurements attempt to quantify and substantiate that contribution.

As mentioned earlier, the productivity of a nursing staff development unit may be measured in a variety of ways but is most often measured in relation to how educators spend their work time.[15,33,40,65] *Time-based* approaches to productivity analysis involve the basic ingredients involved in so-called "time-and-motion" studies: how much time staff spend engaged in different work activities. Design of a time-based productivity analysis involves identification of the work activities to be measured; development of a system to tabulate input work units (e.g., converting 3 hours and 45 minutes of instructional time into 3.75 work units) and work output product units (e.g., attainment of organizational goals such as 100% compliance of all nursing staff in completing JCAHO safety requirements); determining the time period, frequency, and methods of data tabulation;

and determining the ratio of input (e.g., the time spent in providing instruction) to output (100% staff compliance with JCAHO safety requirements). Output measurements can be simple (100% compliance) or more complex (e.g., converting 100% compliance to an output unit of 3, greater than 75% compliance to an output unit of 2, 50% to 74% compliance to an output unit of 1, and less than 50% compliance to an output unit of 0).

Time-based approaches to productivity analysis provide useful information for making personnel and management decisions related to how efficiently educators use their time, how work loads are distributed among the educators and within the staff development unit, how to determine the average amount of time spent in various activities, how to plan realistic work loads, and how to determine where or whether increased work loads can be accommodated.[33,35] Thus the staff development manager is able to derive information for appraising both individual educator performance and performance of the entire staff development unit.

Two limitations of the time-based approach to productivity analysis are that (1) no standards exist to identify what constitutes an "acceptable level of productivity" for nursing staff development activities (for either work inputs or outputs) and that (2) time-based approaches neglect consideration of the relative importance or priority of that activity to the organization.

Kelly[40] addressed the lack of an organizationally defined acceptable level of productivity for judging the output of nursing staff development activities by devising a productivity measure of the "expected level of service." The expected level of service was operationally defined as the number of nursing staff who were expected to accrue contact hours *multiplied by* the required number of instructional hours per year. This expected level of staff development service was then adjusted for attendance and compared to the "actual level of service" (number of instructional hours in required areas actually provided over 1 year) to determine the ratio between expected and actual service levels.

Waterstradt and Phillips[66] addressed the issue of the relative importance of various educational activities by devising a value-based approach to productivity analysis. As these authors describe it, a *value-based approach* to productivity considers the value of educational activities to the organization where productivity units are calculated based on the contribution that activity makes toward meeting organizational goals. Development of a value-based system for staff development involves identifying educational activities that contribute to organizational goals, grouping activities into various importance or priority levels based on their contribution to attainment of those goals, and designing an objective method of calculating value-based units of productivity.

In their productivity system, Waterstradt and Phillips[66] gave high-priority activities a value of 3 to 4 units per hour (depending on the number of participants) and included all JCAHO and other regulatory agency requirements as well as instruction related to new information necessary for staff to perform competently. Medium-priority ratings were awarded a value of 2 to 3 units per hour (again, depending on the number of participants) and encompassed nonrequired offerings such as updates, skill and practice laboratory sessions that clarified procedures or explained pathophysiology, and preparing for or following through on committee assignments. Low-priority activities were assigned a value of 1 unit per hour and included educator rounds, selected projects, and attendance at committee meetings.

A value-based approach to productivity provides information on the extent to which educators are spending their time on high- vs. low-priority endeavors and encourages both staff and management to focus on maximizing their work in areas of greatest importance to institutional goals. As with time-based systems, value-based approaches also need consensus on what constitutes an acceptable productivity level for staff development and consensus on how input and output units will be defined, measured, and tabulated.

Although productivity analysis is yet in its formative stages for nursing staff development, its continued development paves the way not only for dealing with the cost-consciousness and cost-efficiency mandates of the current healthcare industry but also for identifying ways to substantiate and enhance the productivity of staff development efforts.

MARKETING

DEFINITIONS
Market

A *market* refers to a meeting of people for the purpose of trading valued goods or services. It is defined as "a course of commercial activity by which the exchange of commodities is effected"[67] or as "a distinct group of people or organizations that have resources which they want to exchange . . . for distinct benefits."[43] Just as a hospital markets healthcare services to prospective clients in the community it serves, nursing staff development departments market educational services to their prospective clients. Heightened competition for healthcare services, cost constraints on staff education departments, and an environment of educational consumerism combine to mandate that nursing staff development units develop a marketing mindset toward the educational services they provide for prospective learners.[47]

Marketing

Marketing is defined as "the analysis, planning, implementation, and control of programs designed to create, build, and maintain beneficial exchanges . . . with target markets for the purpose of achieving organizational objectives."[43]

In education, marketing is an ongoing process that uses consumer needs, interests, and motivations to help staff create programs and services that benefit the learner and enable the staff development unit to meet organizational goals and objectives. In nursing staff development, the "commodity" exchanged with target markets is educational services. The challenge for the staff development unit is to design its programs in such a way that prospective learners (that is, the target market) will avail themselves of those services.

Internal marketing (Box 8.17) refers to marketing directed to prospective learners within one's own institution, whereas *external marketing* refers to marketing of programs and services to prospective learners outside one's own institution. External marketing may be directed to the local geographic area or to a larger geographic region, nationally, or even internationally.

BENEFITS

The potential benefits of marketing for nursing staff development include the following:

- Simultaneously meets the needs of prospective learners while meeting organizational goals and objectives
- Links program providers and recipients as partners in program planning
- Keeps educational services focused on and responsive

to prospective learners' needs, interests, and motivations for learning
- Promotes the desirable educational attributes of competition and accountability[68]
- Enables allocation of resources based on market supply and demand principles[68]

THE MARKETING PROCESS

Based on the definition of marketing given previously, the marketing process can be viewed as including the following interrelated components: completion of a market analysis, development of a marketing plan, implementation of the marketing plan, and management of the overall marketing process.

Market Analysis

Market analysis (market audit or market research) consists of an investigation and scrutiny of both the internal and external environments of the staff development unit.[43] The internal environment includes attributes and conditions within the employing organization such as its mission, philosophy, priorities, and goals; its resources and constraints; its expectations of the staff development unit; and the number, types, and needs of its staff. The external environment includes salient attributes and conditions that exist outside

---

Box 8.17

ANALYSIS OF THE INTERNAL ENVIRONMENT

- Whether the hospital's mission, goals, strategic plans, and current objectives support both the internal and external marketing of staff development programs and services
- Whether nursing staff development services are perceived as a purely internal support activity or as both an internal and external service to the community
- Whether the nursing staff development scope of service statement supports the marketing of educational services both internally and externally
- The extent of resources (financial, facility, material, personnel, time, etc.) that currently exist to support internal marketing efforts and the extent to which additional resources would be available to support external marketing efforts
- Whether increased efforts directed toward marketing educational services externally would adversely impact other programs and services
- Whether the hospital presently has a marketing department
- The hospital's expectations related to the marketing of staff development services: if these services were to be provided, would they operate at a financial loss, at a break-even level, or as a revenue-generating activity? Would those expectations differ among different programs (e.g., orientation and in-service programs operating at a loss, but the continuing education program expected to break even or operate at a profit)?
- Who the intended consumers of nursing staff development services are and whether these consumers are limited to current nursing staff or include prospective nursing staff, nursing students, nurses in the surrounding community, state, region, or larger geographic area.
- The range and priority of needs for educational programs and services among hospital employees
- The characteristics and educational needs of prospective learners within that agency

the healthcare agency that may affect the marketing of staff development services.

Analysis of the Internal Environment

Analysis of the internal environment requires that educators make a careful and candid appraisal of the hospital's current and potential marketing position. Some of the issues that need to be addressed in such an analysis are listed in Box 8.17.

Before a healthcare institution ventures into external marketing, it needs to carefully consider some of the potentially adverse effects that could significantly affect its internal environment. These potential pitfalls of outside marketing include declining enrollments during the recession, handling large volumes of requests for training, competition between internal and external audiences for corporate resources, hidden costs, and limited experience in marketing procedures.[29] Before proceeding with substantial commitments to externally marketing educational services, the institution needs to ensure that its internal environment is truly able and willing to make that commitment without compromising its primary mission.

Information related to the educational needs of existing staff can be derived from any of the educational needs assessment sources and techniques described previously in this text. Answers to the remaining questions will require a close examination and communication with hospital and nursing department administrators to ensure that any proposed marketing plans are consistent with and cognizant of the hospital's goals and expectations for the staff development unit. The purpose of this internal analysis is to determine the hospital's goals and objectives related to educational services, to clarify the organization's strengths and weaknesses in relation to resource availability for educational services, and to identify its capabilities as well as its limitations in this area.

Analysis of the External Environment

If the hospital decides to market educational programs and services, to clients beyond its own employees, a number of additional factors need to be included in the market analysis. These factors include trends that may influence the marketing of educational services to healthcare workers, the boundaries targeted for marketing, and existing competitors.

TRENDS   Trend analysis is important for keeping educational efforts oriented toward both current and future needs. Thus an encompassing examination of developments related to trends in healthcare delivery systems; healthcare reform proposals; changes in nursing practice; technologic advances; fiscal, legislative, regulatory, and accrediting environments of the healthcare industry; and social and demographic issues are relevant areas of consideration. Nursing staff development marketing efforts are more likely to be successful if program planning aims at coverage of salient aspects of current and future trends affecting the healthcare industry and nursing practice.

BOUNDARIES   Deciding on the geographic or territorial boundaries of the market area focuses the marketing process as narrowly or broadly as desired and appropriate. At times, a scarcity of marketing resources may limit the provision of services to the immediate geographic area. In other instances, the hospital may be willing and able to extend services to a wider area ranging from the state to adjacent states, a designated region, or even the nation. Determination of the size of the marketing area is an important feature of market analysis because it influences the scope and outcomes of educational needs assessments and has a major influence on the cost and extent of resources required for marketing efforts and program planning.

COMPETITION   When staff development programs and services are marketed externally, it is essential that the staff development unit include an appraisal of current competition in its marketing analysis. Since the initiation of mandatory continuing education for nurse relicensure, numerous public and private, profit and nonprofit providers of continuing professional education have emerged both locally and nationally. This multiplicity of providers creates a marketing challenge because providers are all potentially competing for the same learners and educational dollars, thereby diminishing the marketing potential of any one provider. Surviving in the educational services marketplace requires a careful scrutiny of the competition so that one or more aspects of the hospital's programs or services distinguish it in some meaningful way(s) from its competitors.

Some of the means available for analysis of the competition include those suggested by Kuramoto[44]:

- *Get on their mailing lists.* Either directly or through a friend who will forward mailings to you
- *Call to request more information about a particular offering.* To determine how effectively the request is handled and how helpful staff are
- *Register for one or more offerings.* To identify how smoothly and effectively the registration process is managed by telephone, mail, or facsimile; to determine how easily various forms of payment such as credit cards may be used; and to experience the level and quality of customer service from initial contact through confirmation letter and receipt of program materials
- *Attend one or more of the competitor's offerings.* To experience and observe how effectively and efficiently the program is managed from the consumer's point of view and to judge the advertised vs. actual offering in relation to its overall quality, content, faculty, exhibitors, and operational aspects

Analysis of one's competitors will be more effective if this is performed in a fairly structured manner. Identifying who and how many competitors exist, how their current system operates, who they target as learners, and their practices and policies can assist the hospital staff development unit in determining each competitor's strengths and weaknesses and help in deciding a marketing approach that is both realistic and feasible in terms of attracting an audience. Figure 8.8 illustrates a grid that could be used for documenting this analysis of competition.

A thoughtful and comprehensive scrutiny of the competition enables the staff development unit to distinguish itself among its competitors. Analysis of its internal environment identifies the employer's expectations and needs for the staff development unit as well as its own resource strengths and limitations. This allows the staff development unit to position itself within the target market. Analysis of its external environment identifies prevalent trends within the healthcare industry and the geographic boundaries for the marketing effort. When the information derived from these two sources is then compared to the strengths and weaknesses of existing providers and to judgments regarding how and how well competitors are meeting educational needs, decisions can then be reached regarding which groups of learners and topics are already being accommodated well, which are underserved or neglected by competitors, and which of those remaining service areas would be desirable and feasible for the staff development unit to serve. Finding an appropriate niche within the existing marketplace allows the staff development unit to avoid planning offerings that are already well provided by competitors; to avoid planning programs that competitors could provide equally well, better, or at lower costs to participants; and to focus on audiences, content areas, formats, or other features that will make the offering unique, attractive, and desired by prospective learners. For example, a hospital staff development unit could market offerings that reflect unique services, procedures, or patient populations served at that facility. It might distinguish its niche by offering programs for less commonly served groups such as clinical specialists, nurse educators, case managers, or directors of nursing. It might aim only at nurses who are highly experienced and advanced in their practice or use creative formats that involve actual patients or families. Whatever market niche is selected, it needs to recognize as well as capitalize on competitors' strengths and weaknesses.

In contrast to a head-on approach to marketing against stiff competition, the hospital may also elect to cosponsor rather than compete with other providers. Joint efforts are especially useful when both agencies have only moderate or limited resources available but their combined resources could successfully complement each other.

A third possibility is that no direct competitors exist in the area and yet neighboring healthcare facilities (smaller hospitals, clinics, nursing homes, etc.) have few educational resources to provide for the educational needs of their staff. In this situation, one hospital's staff development unit may market its educational programs to neighboring facilities[70] and/or share revenues with those institutions.[21]

Market analysis is often compared to the needs assessment phase of the educational process[12,69] because its purpose is to determine which goods and services are needed by a particular group of people and to determine the ability and suitability of the provider to meet those needs. Wilson[69] describes a number of qualitative (personal interviews, focus groups, and nominal group process) and quantitative (direct mail or telephone surveys, computer questionnaires, and document and literature review) techniques that can be employed for market analysis. Market analysis sets the stage for more definitive market planning.

Market Planning

The second phase of the marketing process is development of a marketing plan. Market planning is typically described in relation to a *market mix*, that is, a set of elements or variables necessary for development of an effective market plan. The number of elements included in the mix varies somewhat among different authors but virtually always includes the four classical Ps of marketing: product, place, price, and promotion, and often includes a fifth P related to participants.* The aim of market planning is to design the right *promotion* to deliver the right *product* to the right *participant* at the right *price* and *place*.

Participants

The participants or prospective audience for educational programs and services represent a pivotal feature in market planning. Before a staff development unit can be successful in its marketing efforts, it must first know the participants it intends to reach and their needs. For both internal and external marketing, identification of the intended audience or target market and its characteristics represents an essential aspect of preliminary program planning.

TARGET MARKET CHARACTERISTICS

Once the general attributes of the target market have been determined (internal vs. both internal and external audiences, the geographic territory of the market), the staff development unit can examine more closely the salient personal and professional attributes of the participant group(s) it intends to reach in its marketing efforts.

Some personal or demographic traits that should be considered include the age range, gender, marital status, family status, and financial resources of prospective participants and their preferences for sites, formats, and local vs.

*See references 36, 42, 45, 51, 53, 60.

Feature	Hospital	Competitor #1	Competitor #2	Competitor #3
1. Name and address of competitor				
2. Audiences sought				
3. Advertising methods and frequency				
4. Registration process:				
a. overall effectiveness and efficiency				
b. methods offered: mail, telephone, fax				
c. payment options available				
d. confirmation procedure				
e. quality of customer service				
5. Costs charged to participants:				
a. one-day fee (average)				
b. multiple day/conference fee (average)				
c. reduced/discount fees available				
d. cancellation fee				
e. availability of refunds				
6. Program reputation:				
a. overall quality				
b. timeliness of content				
c. instructional level				
d. quality of faculty				
e. quality and convenience of location				
f. quality of AV services				
g. instructional methods used				
h. creative/innovative aspects				
i. credits awarded (CEUs, academic)				
7. Greatest strengths				
8. Greatest weaknesses				

Figure 8.8   Assessment grid for analysis of competition.

national faculty. The current economic recession, variable levels of employment for nurses in different parts of the country, and changing family patterns (such as more single-parent families) may translate into not only limited financial resources but limited time available for program attendance and absence from work or child care.

Some relevant professional characteristics of participants include the following:

- Category of nursing staff (RN, LPN, unlicensed staff)
- Position (staff nurse, nurse manager, clinical specialist, case manager, educator, etc.)
- Employment status (full-time, part-time, per diem, unemployed)
- Educational level
- Experience level (beginning, intermediate, advanced)
- Clinical area
- Perceived instructional priorities, needs, and interests
- Motivations to participate
- Barriers to participation (cost, release time, child care)
- Current vs. future educational needs
- Type and degree of employer support for attendance
- Where and how they usually learn about available educational offerings
- Degree of satisfaction with other education providers

In addition to identifying features that would enhance a participant's desire or ability to attend educational offerings, it is also useful to identify perceived or actual barriers to attendance so that marketing endeavors can reduce or eliminate as many of these as possible.[18] Fees might be lowered or discounted for hospitals that send more than one participant if financial resources are a deterrent; on-site child care might be provided if large numbers of participants need this support; or travel costs could be minimized by targeting only nurses in the local area.

DATABASE MARKETING

Some institutions have taken advantage of their computerized recordkeeping systems for registration of participants and have used this information to compile various profiles of their registrants. Because individuals who have attended programs in the past are likely candidates to attend future programs in their areas of interest, a database of information related to registrants can be used to target marketing efforts for particular programs.

Database marketing involves using an up-to-date and comprehensive system of data relevant to prospective clients for the purpose of generating repeat registrations and sending the right promotional materials to the right groups of people at the right time.[28] The categories of data that Havlicek[28] suggests retaining on adult learner registrants are as follows (in rank order of importance):

- Type of course(s) in which previously enrolled
- Occupation

- Income level
- Educational level
- Employer
- Age
- Gender
- Life cycle (starting career, mid-career, etc.)
- Avocational interests
- Marital status

Other data that may be relevant include registrants' preferences for time of year, month, day(s) of the week, course length, facility location, teaching method(s), inclusion of meals, and the like. Although Havlicek's data categories need to be modified somewhat to reflect personal and professional characteristics pertinent to nurses, they represent the type of database developed for this purpose.

Distinguishing various attributes of the potential participants allows for development of a profile of prospective participants and enables the educator to examine relevant subgroups or subdivisions within the target market. For example, the database might reveal that OB/GYN nurse managers prefer group teaching methods, 1-day courses at a nearby hospital, and Thursday course days, whereas critical care staff nurses prefer a mixture of lecture and interactive teaching methods, 2-day courses at a local hotel, and Monday and Tuesday course days.

MARKET SEGMENTATION

Market segmentation involves the identification of salient features or attributes that serve to distinguish various subgroups (segments) of the target market. For example, the target market of "nursing staff" could be segmented by the feature of "category of staff" into RNs, LPNs, nursing assistants, nurses' aides, and ward clerks. The target market of "RNs" could be further segmented by the attribute of "position" into staff nurse, nurse manager, clinical nurse specialist, nurse educator, case manager, supervisor, researcher, and assistant director of nursing. The RN market could also be segmented by clinical practice area into medical, surgical, pediatric, neonatal, OB/GYN, critical care, emergency, ambulatory surgery, operating room, geriatrics, and the like. Other variables that could be used for market segmentation include the nurse's employment setting, educational level, or any other relevant attribute.[60] The purpose of identifying market segments is to specify the target market(s) as clearly and precisely as possible so that their characteristics, needs, and interests can be known and used as a basis for marketing and program planning.[12]

Successful marketing efforts often involve the identification of multiple rather than single attributes of a target market. For example, program planning and marketing for "RNs who work as staff nurses in cardiac surgical units" would be very different from a target market of "RNs who work as staff nurses in pediatric critical care units." Because the patient populations and health problems of these two clinical areas differ from each other, the prospective audiences would also differ in a number of important ways.

Many staff development offerings have more than one potential audience. For example, an offering on physical assessment of the pulmonary system could draw participants from many different clinical areas and nursing positions. In these instances, it is often useful to distinguish between the primary and secondary market segments that marketing intends to reach. The *primary market segment* is the subgroup that marketing is most directed toward. The *secondary market segment* refers to other subgroups within the target market who may also find the program helpful or informative for their practice. For example, the primary market segment for the pulmonary physical assessment offering might be nurses with less than 1 year of clinical experience who work in critical care areas. If this were the primary market sought, the program would be designed to provide the fundamentals of pulmonary physical assessment that relatively inexperienced nurses need to learn to care for patients who are critically ill. Secondary markets might include nurses with less than 1 year of experience who work in emergency departments, step-down units, telemetry units, or postanesthesia units. Although the patient populations in the secondary market areas differ to varying degrees from those in the primary market area, many of the techniques and principles of pulmonary assessment would nonetheless apply for nurses in those areas as well. Secondary market areas are usually distinguished by the need for participants to transfer and adapt what they learn to the unique characteristics of their own work setting. Participants in the primary market segment, by contrast, should find the program content, examples, frame of reference, and emphasis directly and immediately applicable to their clinical setting.

Regardless of whether marketing is directed at the hospital's own staff or learners from outside the sponsor's institution, successful marketing requires that the target market and any relevant segment(s) of that market be identified so that their needs can be known and addressed in the program. The better one knows those markets, the more likely that marketing efforts will be successful in meeting their educational needs.

Product

A *marketing product* refers to the services or items that can be made available to the market. In nursing staff development, the marketing product most often consists of one or more educational offerings but may also include educational services such as consultation or counseling or even published works such as self-learning packages, modules, workbooks, games, videotapes, or videodiscs. The former group may be marketed either internally or externally, while the latter is primarily marketed externally. The focus of this discussion relates to the marketing of educational offerings.

In contrast to the internal marketing of obligatory programs, such as orientation and mandatory in-services, the marketing of other types of internal offerings and all external marketing require some special attention to the relationship between the educational product and its prospective audience. Some aspects that warrant this special attention include topic selection, product title, content, and instructors.

TOPIC SELECTION

The topic area(s) selected for the marketed product needs to be derived from the results of prior market analysis. This type of market-driven product will be useful in two important ways: (1) it will ensure that the target market's needs, desires, preferences, and constraints are used as the basis for program planning, and (2) it will ensure that marketing efforts and resources are not wasted on designing offerings that have little or no market potential—that is, offerings that will not be successful in inducing the target market to attend. Market analysis generates the information necessary to determine the needs and preferences of the prospective audience, and topic selection should follow these specifications as closely as possible.

Product topics must be timely and relevant to prospective learners. Every educational topic has a natural life span. Some topics (such as physical assessment, ethical issues, ECG monitoring, documentation, and medications) endure through generations of nurses, others (such as burnout and management by objectives) are now well past their prime, and some (such as case management) have more recently arrived on the healthcare scene. The planner's challenge is to select topics of immediate relevance, usefulness, and priority to the targeted market, preferably those that represent high-risk, high-frequency, and problem-prone areas of practice.

TITLE WORDING

How the product and topic area(s) are characterized in communicating these to the prospective audience can be a very important element in marketing success. In order for learners to be drawn to an educational offering, the title selected for the offering needs to be clear, informative, appealing, and provocative to the intended audience. For example, if the topic area for an offering was "abdominal surgery patients" and the proposed title for this offering was *Nursing Care of Abdominal Surgery Patients*, it might not be clear to readers whether this program was intended for OR nurses, PAR nurses, critical care nurses, or nurses who work on medical-surgical wards. The title is minimally informative because the emphasis of the offering is vague. Titles such as these are not particularly appealing because the "what's-in-it-for-me?" element is not readily evident for the learner's consideration. Given these points, the title is unlikely to provoke or motivate one to attend. A simple rewording of the title with addition of a subtitle, such as *Postoperative Care of Abdominal Surgery Patients: Compli-*

cations the *Unit Staff Nurse Can Prevent,* clarifies the focus and audience for the program and motivates that particular group to register for the program because it is designed with their special needs and interests in mind.

CONTENT

Once the general topc area and title of the product are determined, content for the offering can be developed. As the instructional outcomes and content outline are designed, it is important to pay particular attention to the nursing market targeted for the offering: their educational and experience levels, their particular areas of interest, and their position. An offering designed for beginning level nurses will not be satisfying or informative to experienced nurses; offerings that emphasize summaries of research methodology and statistical analysis may be wonderful learning experiences for nurse researchers with masters and doctoral degrees but will not be helpful to staff nurses without advanced degrees who are unfamiliar with research terminology. Offerings that emphasize acute, inpatient hospital care will be of very limited value to nurses who work exclusively in community settings. Product content needs to be tailored to the unique needs and desires of the primary target market.

INSTRUCTORS

The guidelines related to selection of instructors for marketed educational offerings are the same as those discussed for using local and outside speakers in continuing education offerings. Many faculty with established national reputations and demonstrated expertise in a particular area can indeed draw large audiences and offer state-of-the-art perspectives that reflect their acquaintance with issues at a national level. Because these individuals usually also command a premium honorarium, however, prudent market planning would need to first verify that they demonstrate excellent platform skills, good audience interactions, practical know-how, and solid content. A "big name" may be entertaining or impressive, but he/she should also be an informative and expert instructor before planners make an investment in that person. A mixture of local and national expertise represents a useful approach for faculty selection.

By following the customary process of educational program development and giving special attention to the areas mentioned here, the instructional product to be marketed begins to take definitive shape. Locating this product at the "right place" for the audience is the next step in the market planning process.

Place

Although the location of educational offerings marketed only to the hospital's employees may be dictated solely by the nature of the instructional outcomes and the facilities available at that agency, basic marketing (and adult education) precepts suggest that attention to features such as comfort, adequate seating, good lighting and ventilation, visibility of audiovisuals, and acoustic quality are also important in motivating staff to attend. Just because the audience consists of employees is no excuse for forgetting that they are also consumers of educational services.

When offerings are also marketed to external and often much larger audiences, many sponsors find it necessary to secure larger facilities for this purpose. Some healthcare agencies are fortunate to have cutting-edge conference facilities on site, but most need to locate these offerings to an off-site facility at an area hotel or convention center. In this case, the following features should be sought during the site selection process:

- *Accessibility*: Proximity and ease of arrival and departure for participants are important, especially for those who will be driving or using public transportation. Although location is usually considered less important than content and speakers, many programs are canceled as a result of their inconvenient location.[44]
- *Professional setting*: The professional image of the sponsoring organization should be enhanced by the selected location. Poorly maintained hotels with mildew odors, stained carpets, and marginal service will leave lasting impressions on participants that reflect poorly on the program and its sponsor.
- *Cost*: Insofar as possible, the costs of driving, parking, meals, and lodging need to be recognized and kept within reasonable limits for the targeted audience, especially when participants may be bearing more of the financial burden themselves. Cost considerations, however, also need to be balanced against quality issues: the cheapest is often not the best way to offer quality programs and surroundings. Just as a "big name" may double or triple the number of registrants, a serene and comfortable setting can provide the backdrop for an enjoyable and satisfying learning experience.
- *Security*: Unfortunately, safety issues are a growing concern among program sponsors, particularly in large urban areas that may be unfamiliar to out-of-town participants. In some cities, nurses may be hesitant to drive or use public transportation to reach a program site or may fear leaving the site if programs end in the evening hours.
- *Adjacent facilities*: Especially with multiple-day conferences, participants will often enjoy leaving the meeting site for some respite. Nearby recreational, dining, shopping, or tourist attractions can enhance interest in attendance at the meeting.

Although some program sponsors may avoid using resort locations so that their offerings are not misperceived as "vacations," many of today's busy professionals enjoy the opportunity to combine attendance at a professional meeting with some leisure time away from home. A recent study reported by Harrison[26] found that for continuing medical education programs in cardiology offered at resort locations, location of the meeting was second only to subject matter in participants' decisions to register for the program. In a consumer-oriented society, attention to program location is both a fact of life and a potentially potent marketing tool.

Price

Establishing the "right price" for an educational offering depends on a number of different factors. The primary goal is to establish a price that is satisfactory to the program sponsor as well as to the participant. What is "satisfactory" to the sponsor depends on the employer's pricing expectation: that is, whether the employer expects the program to operate at a loss, to break even with some or all direct and indirect expenses, or to generate a profit. Once the projected costs have been determined and the break-even point has been identified, sponsors can calculate the fee levels necessary for meeting the employer's pricing expectation. What is "satisfactory" to the target market depends on the agency's degree of financial support, their personal or family's financial resources, and local economic conditions and norms.

Factors to consider in setting the price include the probable salary level of the target market, the degree of employer support for program costs at hospitals in the area, the fees charged by competitors for comparable programs, the number of anticipated registrants, past experience related to enrollments at various pricing levels, an estimate of "what the market will bear," and estimated totals for direct and indirect costs.

Another consideration to bear in mind is that the perceived value of a particular program may be as or more important than its price. If participants perceive that they receive good value for their money, even a fairly steep price may still be acceptable to them. As mentioned earlier in this chapter, quality costs money. Even in recessionary times, nurses are educated consumers who seek value for their monetary investments. Successful marketing recognizes this point and seeks to offer true value at a reasonable price.

Promotion

DEFINITIONS AND PURPOSES

Promotion, the final element in development of a marketing plan, involves the communication of essential information about the product to the target audience at the appropriate time in such a way that the message motivates the audience to obtain that product. The aims or purposes of promotion are to inform, to generate interest, and to create desire for the product among members of the target market. In order to achieve these goals, promotion efforts attempt to provide the greatest degree of product exposure to the target market at the lowest possible cost.

INFLUENCES

The nature and extent of promotional efforts are influenced by two major categories of variables: the resources available and the scope or size of the target market. When the monetary, material, and manpower resources available for marketing are limited, marketing efforts and options must be scaled down accordingly. Although the customer-oriented drives at many healthcare institutions have hastened the rise of their marketing efforts, this market-driven approach to healthcare delivery does not always trickle down to the nursing staff development unit. Restricted marketing resources translate into restricted marketing options: although marketing efforts will proceed, the costlier methods will not be feasible and alternative means will need to be used.

The second category of influences on promotion relates to the scope and size of the target audience. When marketing is targeted only for the hospital's own nursing staff, the nature and extent of promotional activities are fairly circumscribed. When external marketing is added to internal marketing, however, both the nature and extent of promotion can be increased significantly. These increases tend to be proportionate to the size of the external market: local area promotion is the least expensive, state or regional promotion is more costly, and national promotions are the most expensive. The amount of logistical planning (for site selection, lodging, parking, meals, etc.) also tends to increase with a larger size and scope of the targeted market.

METHODS OF INTERNAL PROMOTION

Since the primary customer base of a nursing staff development unit is its own hospital's nursing staff, promotion of staff development offerings and services to staff represents an ongoing marketing priority. Even when a healthcare institution is interested in having outsiders attend its offerings, the primacy of the hospital's own staff, including their needs as well as their constraints, should never be lost in the promotion process.

Some of the more commonly employed methods for promoting staff attendance at educational offerings include the design of eye-catching flyers; the display of colorful and creative banner announcements; distribution of notices with paychecks; placement of tent cards on cafeteria, lounge, and meeting room tables; posting a monthly or quarterly calendar of events; drawing appealing posters; handing out door prizes; using unit attendance contests, public address announcements, hospital newsletter notices, games and friendly competition among participants; and the creative use of bulletin boards dedicated only to staff development promotions. Although these techniques are often effective, especially when variety is used, the single best promotional magnet is provision of a truly relevant offering tailored to staff needs and organizational goals and provided at a time and place convenient to staff.

METHODS OF EXTERNAL PROMOTION

When educational offerings and services are to be promoted to external as well as internal markets, internal promotional activities may proceed as described previously and external promotional efforts will represent supplements to those internal activities. The methods available for external promotion may be categorized into interpersonal means, broadcast media, and print media.

Interpersonal Means

Word-of-mouth promotion is the single best means of advertising an educational program. A satisfied customer is capable of communicating about the quality and usefulness of an educational program more effectively and with greater credibility than any paid form of promotion. Because satisfied consumers are likely to tell not just one but many of their colleagues about their experience with the program, this interpersonal form of promotion can easily have a multiplicative effect. In addition, communicating their satisfaction to their supervisor who approved the participation lays the groundwork for other colleagues' requests for attendance at that or related programs to be approved with confidence. Program sponsors also need to be mindful that the converse of this situation occurs just as readily: that is, dissatisfied consumers can adversely affect all subsequent promotional efforts.

Broadcast Media

Radio and television advertisements are rarely used for promotion of staff development offerings because of the prohibitively high costs of even limited air time. Unless a local station is willing to provide some public service time to nonprofit institutions for this purpose, the cost of paid broadcast advertising typically precludes its use in educational promotion efforts.

Print Media

Printed materials represent the most commonly employed medium for promotion of staff development offerings and services. Printed matter can be further subdivided into free print advertising, paid print advertising, and direct mail advertising. Before describing each of these different forms of print promotions, some general guidelines for any form of print advertising should first be considered.

General Guidelines

Hon and Caravatt[31] offer some suggestions for items that must be communicated to the target audience in any form of advertising. These four items include the following:

- What the product is
- What its value is
- How the value applies to the audience
- How to obtain or secure the product

Printed materials can be effective promotional vehicles if they communicate these message components in an eye-catching, informative, easy-to-read, and convincing manner to prospective participants.

Free Print Advertising

Free print advertising may be available in local, state, regional, or national newsletters published by various nursing or educational organizations. Local newspapers may also provide space for announcements or news releases as a public service to nonprofit organizations. Some hospitals join in cooperative efforts to publish bulletins of upcoming offerings in their regions, and state nurses association newspapers often include a column for these listings. National nursing journals owned by a professional nursing association or affiliated with a nursing organization may also be willing to provide space for this purpose if the offering is targeted to their membership.

Paid Print Advertising

Paid advertising of educational offerings and services is available through many nursing journals and magazines at fairly nominal rates and may also be available at less costly rates in association newsletters. Some nursing and educational organizations (e.g., the American Hospital Association's American Society of Healthcare Education and Training) also publish resource directories for their members that include listings paid for by various instructors, consultants, and vendors who provide services related to staff development.

Direct Mail Advertising

Much of the promotion of staff development to external markets is achieved through direct mail advertising. Direct mail items may include calendars, catalogs, or brochures that describe the educational products offered.

Calendars and Catalogs Calendars or catalogs of educational offerings may require considerable long-range planning on a quarterly, semiannual, or annual basis. Because of this long-range focus, these vehicles may be comprehensive but less detailed regarding the specific features of any one offering. Educational calendars and catalogs can be useful for alerting prospective participants to future offerings so that they may make arrangements to attend those of interest when the individual brochures for those offerings arrive. Calendars and catalogs may include only general information related to each offering such as its title, dates, and a brief description. When calendars or catalogs are sent many months in advance of programs, they often need to be followed by individual-offering brochures to rekindle interest and provide the detailed

information participants need to follow through with registration.

Offering Brochures   One of the most commonly employed methods of promotion is the direct mailing of individual-offering brochures to the target audience. This endeavor involves three major elements: (1) securing or developing a mailing list, (2) developing copy for the brochure contents, and (3) mailing the brochures to the target market.

Mailing Lists

The mailing list for promotion refers to the names and addresses of individuals and/or institutions who represent the target market for a particular offering. In order for a mailing list to be effective, it must be up to date, accurate, and complete. The options available to secure a mailing list are to develop and maintain one's own list, to rent or purchase one or more lists, or to use some combination of these approaches.

Developing One's Own Mailing List   In the past, development and maintenance of a mailing list could be a very laborious, time-consuming, and therefore costly endeavor. When these procedures had to be performed manually, the clerical time alone for typing, updating, filing, and printing labels could make it prohibitive for all but the very largest staff development departments. Today's computerized recordkeeping systems have greatly simplified this procedure and made hospital management of its own mailing lists both possible and cost-effective.

Development of the database for the mailing list is typically an integral component in the computerized recordkeeping systems and consists of converting class lists of previous attendees into mailing lists. The rationale here is that past participants are very likely to be future participants. Relevant data related to market segmentation variables (such as category of nurse, clinical area, position, mailing address, previous programs attended, etc.) allow for sorting and coding of both past participants and new registrants so that individuals are contacted only for programs of potential interest to them. In addition to individuals, hospitals that have sent their nurses to past programs can also be coded so that they are included (as appropriate). The software will often be able to check for duplicate entries so that these can be corrected and eliminated before mailing, thereby saving postage and handling costs. When the educational product is cosponsored with another institution, that organization will usually be willing to provide its own mailing list for promotional use. If lists are to be merged, duplicate entries should be deleted before the labels are printed.

Renting or Purchasing Mailing Lists   Mailing lists which are directed to the target market are available for rental or purchase from numerous sources. List rental is more common than purchase. List rental typically involves the one-time use of a list for a specific mailing. Rented lists cannot be copied because they remain the property of the organization that makes them available. Ordering a mailing list from a professional association or nursing organization usually involves rental rather than purchase of the list. List purchasing generally implies that the purchaser is able to copy and reuse the list at will.[58]

Lists may be secured from state boards of nursing, general or specialty area professional nursing associations and organizations, or educational organizations on a local, state, regional, or national level. In addition, many nursing journals and related healthcare periodicals make their readership lists available for educational uses.

The requirements, sorting capabilities, and costs for these mailing lists vary with different organizations. Some organizations require prior approval of the brochure, local chapter sponsorship, or CEU approval of the offering before the mailing list can be rented. Some associations will send the labels directly to the renter, while others require the use (and additional cost) of a mailing house to affix labels and mail the brochures.

Most professional associations can sort addresses by state, zip code, and chapter membership. Others can also sort addresses by specialty area, position, and functional area (manager, educator, researcher, and practitioner). The costs of mailing labels are usually calculated per orders of 1000 labels. Adhesive labels are somewhat more expensive than nonadhesive labels and peel-off labels are more costly than computer-affixed versions. Prices vary widely among different organizations but are usually less than $100 per 1000 labels, with larger volumes sold at a discounted rate. Some agencies also have minimum charges regardless of the volume requested.

Combined Approaches   Hospitals that do a moderate or extensive amount of external marketing for staff development offerings often find it useful to maintain their own mailing lists and to complement this with selective purchase of other lists as target audiences and program content dictate. The hospital's list may be used to reach local or regional nurses who have previously attended programs at that facility, while the purchased list(s) is used to reach a wider geographic area or to penetrate new market segments. This combined approach to mailing lists also affords flexibility as budgetary and other operational constraints and resources vary over time.

Brochure Copy

Developing an effective promotional brochure for a staff development offering involves attention to three major areas: (1) the general features of good brochure design, (2) the specific attributes of brochure sections, and (3) proofreading of copy before it goes to the printer or duplication service.

General Features of Good Brochure Design

Simerly[58] offers a number of useful suggestions related to important features of effective brochures. Some of these tips include the following:

- Employ a professional graphic designer
- Minimize the use of different typefaces
- Be sure the selected typefaces (fonts) are easy to read
- Select paper stock that complements the image and quality of the program
- White or buff-colored paper provides the best background for reading copy
- Dark ink colors are easier to read than pastels or metallic inks
- Use multiple ink colors judiciously and sparingly
- Never produce a direct-mail brochure that is smaller than $8\frac{1}{2} \times 11''$
- Always use graphic designs appropriate for the target audience
- Use blank (white space) areas to enhance readability and visual appeal

If the objectives of a promotional brochure are kept in mind (to capture the recipients' attention, stimulate and maintain their interest in the offering, motivate their desire to attend, and facilitate their registration), the guidelines for designing effective brochures are much easier to understand and follow.

Specific Attributes of Brochure Sections

In general, the brochure cover is responsible for capturing the reader's initial attention, the brochure interior must hold and build interest and desire to attend, and the registration process and form must make enrollment as easy as possible.

The *cover* of a brochure must be eye-catching and professional. Typeface, ink color, layout, and graphics need to announce the offering in clear and effective ways so that the reader can immediately see the most important preliminary elements of information. These include the title of the program, its date(s), location, and sponsoring organization(s). Some organizations require that their logo be incorporated on the cover of any promotional material. Unless the cover is successful in its mission, readers probably will not bother to examine the brochure any further.

Brochure cover artwork may be subdued or prominent, depending on the image to be conveyed, but needs to be professionally prepared. Harrison's[26] study on the effect of cover content on enrollment of physicians in cardiology courses found that when the conference was held at a resort location, brochures which provided a photograph of the resort on the cover resulted in twice as many registrations as those which used a stylized logo on the cover.

The *interior* pages of a brochure vary somewhat with the number of pages used and the length of the offering (single-day vs. multiple-day) but generally contain a common core of essential information designed to hold and enhance participant interest in the program. The elements typically included in the interior of a brochure are enumerated in Box 8.18.

The *description* and *purpose* of the offering need to be written in a clear, crisp writing style. Verbosity, ambiguity, and vague characterizations should be avoided so that readers can readily determine what the "product" is.

The *benefit profile* represents one of the most important inclusions in the brochure. For many educational programs, benefits are stated in terms of instructional objectives. Although these may well reflect the instructional intent of the program, they may at times convey a rather dry and "educationese" tone that addresses only what will be learned rather than what participants will be able to do with that learning. As Puetz and Peters[50] suggest, benefits to the participant are better stated so that they answer the "so whats?" that prospective participants or their supervisors may ponder. So what if staff nurses learn the basic principles of patient education? So what if nurse managers learn the differences between primary nursing and case management? So what if nurse educators learn the precepts of competency-based education? As Table 8.6 shows, instructional outcomes and the benefits of instruction are not synonymous. Benefits need to reflect how participants will be able to use what they have learned to better solve problems or manage situations encountered in their work setting.

Table 8-6 illustrates two other important aspects related

Box 8.18

INTERIOR BROCHURE ELEMENTS

- Description and purpose of offering
- Benefit profile
- Intended audience
- Schedule of topics (with dates and times)
- Speaker biographies
- Exhibit information
- Special features (creative teaching methods, tours, etc.)
- CEU accreditation information
- Fees
- Hotel and travel information
- Description of registration procedure
- Registration form
- Telephone number for questions or information

TABLE 8.6 • BROCHURE BENEFIT STATEMENTS

Sample Instructional Outcome	Benefit to Participant	Benefit to Organization
Participants will be able to describe the ten basic principles of patients education.	• You will develop your knowledge and skills in patient education. • You will have the opportunity to practice patient education skills.	• You will be able to improve your hospital's compliance in provision of patient education. • You will be able to better prepare patients for early discharge.
Participants will be able to distinguish between primary nursing and case management.	• You will enhance your understanding of the nurse's role in case management. • You will be better prepared to make the transition from primary nursing to case management.	• You will be able to assist in your hospital's conversion to nursing case management.
Participants will be able to identify the hallmark attributes of competency-based education.	• You will be prepared to convert your traditional orientation program to a competency-based orientation program. • You will develop the knowledge and skills necessary for designing a competency assesssment program.	• You will be able to improve the effectiveness and efficiency of your hospital's orientation program. • You will be able to meet the JCAHO's requirements related to competency assessment of new and existing nursing staff.

to the benefit profile. The enumerated benefits are best written in the second person and should include outcomes that the registrant's employer can anticipate. *You* statements communicate potential benefits in a more personalized manner so that the reader can relate to them more directly. Since interested nurses are likely to apply for educational leave and registration fee payment from their employer, the nurse's supervisor who will be reviewing and approving that request will also have "so whats" to ask and needs to be able to see how the program will not only benefit the employee, but the hospital as well.[59]

The *fee structure* established for the offering may be simple or complex. Some programs have a single fee. Some sponsors have different fees for members vs. nonmembers of particular organizations or for daily vs. full conference attendance. Some offer discounts for early registration (effectively imposing a penalty for later registration and, at times, an even greater penalty for on-site registration), and others offer discounts for groups from the same institution. Some also impose cancellation penalties (processing fees, administrative fees, or handling fees) after specified dates.

Despite the economic and operational incentives to institute discounts for early registration, Simerly[59] advises against using these because, he contends, early registration discounts meet the needs of the sponsor rather than the consumer and penalize the potential registrants for situations often beyond their control (e.g., a slow administrative approval process, late posting of the brochure, or vacations or reassignments causing delays in reading the brochure). Simerly also suggests abolishing all cancellation penalties for much the same reason: they penalize early registrants

who later find out that they are unable to attend. He suggests that consumer-oriented services need to be responsive to the realities that adult clients face and establish procedures and (mailing brochures earlier, second mailing of brochures, and providing a list of future programs when refunding fees) that benefit the prospective client rather than the sponsor.

The *registration process* and *form* need to be as easy and convenient to use as possible. The registration form should only request information that is absolutely necessary for processing the registration.[50] This information typically includes the following:

• Name
• Home address
• Employer
• Employer's address
• Home and work telephone numbers
• Social security number

Ideally, participants should be able to register by whatever method is most convenient for them, including by mail, telephone, or facsimile. Sponsors can track the number of registrants who use each method to determine which is the most preferred by their target audience. Telephone registrations can be entered directly into a computer to secure the same information as obtained with mailed registration forms. Telephone and fax registrations can be facilitated by enabling registrants to use credit cards for payment of fees. Rather than requiring the time-consuming process of organizational invoices and purchase orders to generate checks, using credit cards can greatly speed and simplify this process and afford good documentation for reimbursement of expenses.

To make the process maximally convenient for the prospective registrant, multiple payment options may be offered, including a hospital's corporate check, a personal check, money order, or credit card information. Once all of the payment and registration options and other content of the cover and interior for the brochure have been developed and formatted, the entire draft of the brochure needs to be proofread before it is submitted for photocopying or printing.

Proofreading Brochure Copy

Proofreading is an essential aspect of developing an effective promotional brochure and consists of carefully reading over a document in order to detect and correct errors, omissions, misstatements, or faulty design and layout. Proofreading may reveal errors in spelling, grammar, word usage, or formatting that need to be corrected. Essential information such as dates and times, telephone numbers, fees, deadlines, mailing addresses, and the like need to be double checked for inclusion and accuracy. General spell-checking software can help detect misspellings of commonly used words but will be less helpful for medical terms and not helpful to verify spelling of speakers' names and credentials.

Although proofreading can be a somewhat laborious task, its importance to the success of the offering cannot be overestimated. Missing or erroneous information can mandate expensive reprinting and/or remailing of brochures or error notices. Preventing mistakes is the key, and careful proofreading is the only way to accomplish this.

Because those who helped design the brochure are often too close to and familiar with it to easily detect needed corrections and omissions, it is always wise to have someone from the customer role perform the proofreading. He/she is much less likely to read in material that is not provided, to reinterpret vaguely worded sections, or to be biased by a favorite layout or typeface. Asking a few members of the program's target audience to read the brochure copy and offer their critique can be truly enlightening and invaluable for quality control.

Several individuals should be asked to proofread the brochure rather than just one.[7] Some individuals may be more sensitive to wording, others to the artwork and layout, and some to technical aspects such as spelling and clarity. A sufficient number of proof copies of the brochure need to be made so that each reader can make corrections and comments directly on the copy, using a bright ink or highlighter. If the brochure will be printed rather than photocopied, proofreading may be necessary at a number of stages in the production process to ensure that the brochure to be mailed is as flawless as possible in both form and substance.

Mailing Brochures

Although the mailing of program brochures only sounds as if it requires a simple trip to the post office or hospital mail room, it represents another crucial aspect of the promotion process. Some considerations that need to be taken into account in relation to brochure mailing are postal regulations, different mailing classes, and the timing of the mailing.

Postal Regulations The postal service has very specific requirements related to the minimum and maximum sizes and weights of mail items. Additional regulations govern the use of business mail permits and how these are to be indicated on each brochure. Unless all pieces of mail meet specifications, the postal service will not deliver the brochures.

Classes of Mail* First-class mail is the most expensive mail class but should provide delivery in 2 to 3 days within the continental United States. One advantage of using first-class mail is that mail will be forwarded if the addressee has moved (and provided a forwarding address) within the past year. If the forwarding notice period has expired, mail will be returned to the sender with the forwarding address attached (if one was provided) so that remailing can be done. The latter is useful in keeping mailing lists up to date. First-class mail can be used for individual items weighing 11 ounces or less.

Third class is a less expensive alternative for mailing. It is available either at regular rates or at special bulk rates to authorized users. Items weighing less than 16 ounces can be sent by third-class mail. Other means to reduce mailing costs include use of nine-digit zip codes, sorting and bundling mail by zip codes, and having a mailing house affix bar coding to addresses.

The obvious advantage to using bulk mail is the substantial savings it offers on postage, especially for nonprofit organizations. Two disadvantages of bulk mail also need to be kept in mind: (1) bulk mail delivery times are considerably slower than those for first-class mail and (2) bulk mail has the lowest priority for delivery at each post office through which it passes.[58] Rather than being delivered in 2 or 3 days, bulk mail can require 1 week for even local delivery, 1 to 2 weeks within the state, 2 weeks within adjoining states, and 3 to 4 weeks to reach across the continental United States.[58]

Some sponsors have experienced situations when their brochures have literally sat on a mailroom or postal service floor for weeks before being delivered or were delivered

---

*Because postal service regulations change over time, these guidelines need to be verified on a regular basis.

after the discount date or deadline for registration. Although such horror stories are relatively uncommon, they remind sponsors of the need to carefully manage the mailing process and to track all mailings to determine actual delivery times. Only by knowing the average times required for recipients to receive the brochures can planners determine how much time is required to initiate the mailing process. These concerns are less problematic for offerings marketed only to the local area but are major concerns for sponsors who market to wider regions, nationally, or internationally.

Mail Timing   The timing of brochure mailing represents another salient feature in the promotion process. Some times of the year such as holiday periods in November and December are so busy that brochures are not likely be read until long after the scheduled event. Other times to avoid mailings include the summer vacation months when many recipients will be away from home and work.

Certain months such as February and September seem to bring tidal waves of brochures at the same time that other bulk mailers are sending out catalogs and other materials. The easiest guidelines to follow here are to avoid mailing when the intended recipients are not likely to be available, when all of your competitors are mailing their brochures, or when unrelated mailings (such as holiday catalogs) are inundating the postal system. All of these situations reduce the chance that your intended audience will see your brochure in time to register. This rule also applies to day-of-the-week timing. Since the busiest days at post offices are usually Mondays and Fridays, mailings might be better delivered to the postal service on a slower day such as Tuesday.

Mailing needs to allow sufficient time for the target market to receive the brochure, make a decision regarding participation, secure approval and financial support for attendance, and arrange staffing and scheduling changes to obtain the time off and for sponsors to fully process registrations. A number of authors[41,50,59] recommend a minimum time frame of 8 weeks prior to the event as lead time for mailing program brochures. Mailing brochures after this time frame tends to reduce enrollments. Considering all of the effort that goes into planning the offering and its promotion, compromising its success with a late mailing would be a real tragedy.

Implementation and Management of the Marketing Process

Once the marketing plan has been completed, its implementation can proceed in an orderly and straightforward process. Implementation consists of converting each of the marketing mix elements into its full expression and operation. In marketing terms, promotion efforts result in joining participants and product together at the right place and price to exchange mutual benefits. In educational terms, learners participate in the planned learning experiences so that both the sponsor(s) and participants find the exchange satisfying and beneficial. Implementation involves all of the intermediary steps required between planning the educational event and completing its provision. This phase comprises everything from developing detailed content outlines and quality audiovisuals to making sure that room temperatures are comfortable for all of the break-out sessions. On-site management and evaluation of the offering are essentially the same as previously described for the implementation and evaluation phases of continuing education in Chapter 7.

One element of evaluation that does differ for externally marketed programs is appraisal of the relative success of various marketing strategies. Tracking of registrations, mailing lists, different classes of mail, or timing of mailings can provide a wealth of useful information related to maximizing enrollments and making the best use of marketing resources. Analysis of participant and faculty evaluations provides the information needed to ensure continued provision of quality educational offerings that reflect well on the staff development manager as well as the employer.

• • •

Effective management of the nursing staff development unit involves attention to a diverse yet interrelated array of issues. Quality improvement, policies and procedures, recordkeeping, budgeting, and marketing represent only a few of the more salient aspects involved with the organizational and operational facets of the unit's function. As the healthcare system evolves, nursing staff development must likewise adapt and mature so that it fulfills its support role to nursing practice and quality patient care.

REFERENCES

1. Alspach JG, Bell J, Canobbio MM et al, editors: *AACN education standards for critical care nursing*, St Louis, 1986, Mosby.
2. American Nurses' Association (ANA): *Roles and responsibilities for nursing professional development: continuing education and staff development across all settings*, Washington, DC, 1992, ANA.
3. American Nurses' Association (ANA): *Standards for continuing education in nursing*, Kansas City, MO, 1984, ANA.
4. American Nurses' Association (ANA): *Standards for nursing professional development: continuing education and staff development*, Washington, DC, 1994, ANA.
5. American Nurses' Association (ANA): *Standards for nursing staff development*, Kansas City, MO, 1990, ANA.
6. American Society for Healthcare Education and Training: *Standards for health care education and training*, Chicago, 1990, American Hospital Association.

7. Arlington BC: Designing quality brochures, *J Nurs Staff Develop* 8(1): 35, 1992.

8. Austin EK: *Guidelines for the development of continuing education offerings for nurses*, New York, NY, 1981, Appleton-Century-Crofts.

9. Bell D, Bowen T, Dilling D: Computerizing records for continuing education, *J Nurs Staff Develop* 7(1):36, 1991.

10. Bertz EJ: Hospital productivity plays key role under prospective pricing, *Hosp Manag* 13(6):7, 1983.

11. Bethel PL: Inservice education: calculating the cost, *J Cont Educ Nurs* 21(3):105, 1990.

12. Clark G: Healthcare educators as marketers, *J Healthcare Educ Train* 3(1):24, 1988.

13. Crucius L: An educational documentation system for a hospital nursing education department, *J Nurs Staff Develop* 7(2):71, 1991.

14. del Bueno DJ, Kelly KJ: How cost-effective is your staff development program? *J Nurs Admin* 10(4):31, 1980.

15. Dombro M: Using a computer data management system to measure hospital staff development productivity, *J Nurs Staff Develop* 1(2):52, 1985.

16. Farmer AP: Costs and benefits of hospital education programs. Part 1, *J Healthcare Educ Train* 2(1):32, 1987.

17. Farmer AP: Costs and benefits of hospital education programs. Part 2, *J Healthcare Educ Train* 3(1):17, 1988.

18. Faulkenberry J: Marketing strategies to increase participation in continuing education, *J Nurs Staff Develop* 2(3):98, 1986.

19. Feuer D: Taking your in-house training to market, *Training 22(1):41, 1985.*

20. Filipczak B: Training budgets boom, *Training* 30(10):37, 1993.

21. Fisher ML, Crawford MA: Marketing nursing programs, *J Nurs Staff Develop* 3(1):15, 1987.

22. Fogel DS: The role of the healthcare educator: relating success in business terms, *J Healthcare Educ Train* 1(1):6, 1986.

23. Godkewitsch M: The dollars and sense of corporate training, *Training* 24(5):79, 1987.

24. Grubb AW: Future hot spots for health care educators, *J Healthcare Educ Train* 2(2):1, 1987.

25. Haislip OL: How to treat training as an investment, *Training* 24(2): 63, 1987.

26. Harrison RV: The influence of brochure covers on CME enrollments, *J Cont Educ Health Prof* 11(3):265, 1991.

27. Hassett J: Simplifying ROI, *Training* 29(9):53, 1992.

28. Havlicek C: Demystifying database marketing, *Adult Learn* 2(1):13, 1990.

29. Hequet M: Selling in-house training outside, *Training* 28(9):51, 1991.

30. Holmes SA: Data management . . . recordkeeping, *J Nurs Staff Develop* 9(1):44, 1993.

31. Hon D, Caravatt P: Five surprisingly useful things trainers can learn from advertisers, *Training* 16(5):21, 1979.

32. Hoover JJ, Gillmore C: Using computers in administering a continuing education program, *J Cont Educ Nurs* 18(4):141, 1987.

33. Jazwiec RM: Economics, productivity and effectiveness, *J Cont Educ Nurs* 18(1):8, 1987.

34. Jeska SB, Fischer KJ, McClellan MG: *Quality indicators for nursing staff development*, Pensacola, FL, 1992, National Nursing Staff Development Organization.

35. Johnson JA: Cost, value and productivity: the bottom line in education, *J Nurs Staff Develop* 2(1):28, 1986.

36. Johnson SH: A model for marketing continuing education in a recession, *J Cont Educ Nurs* 16(1):19, 1985.

37. Joint Commission on Accreditation of Healthcare Organizations (JCAHO): *Accreditation manual for hospitals, vol 1, Standards*, Oakbrook Terrace, IL, 1994, JCAHO.

38. Joint Commission on Accreditation of Healthcare Organizations (JCAHO): *Accreditation manual for hospitals, vol 2, Scoring guidelines*, Oakbrook Terrace, IL, 1994, JCAHO.

39. Joint Commission on Accreditation of Healthcare Organizations: An introduction to Joint Commission nursing care standards, Oakbrook Terrace, IL, 1991, JCAHO.

40. Kelly KJ: A productivity measure for nursing staff development, *J Nurs Staff Develop* 6(2):65, 1990.

41. Kelly KJ: *Nursing staff development*, Philadelphia, 1992, JB Lippincott.

42. Kotecki CN: Marketing critical care education programs, *Dimens Crit Care Nurs* 10(2):108, 1991.

43. Kotler P: *Marketing management: analysis, planning and control*, ed 5, Englewood Cliffs, NJ, 1984, Prentice-Hall.

44. Kuramoto AM: Marketing university-based continuing education programs, *J Cont Educ Nurs* 24(2):61, 1993.

45. Lauffer A: *The practice of continuing education in the human services*, New York, 1977, McGraw-Hill.

46. McMurray AR: Educational administration enhanced by data-base management: programmable software for healthcare education records, *J Healthcare Educ Train* 3(1):1, 1988.

47. McVeety KM: Education and marketing: a new link to productivity, *J Healthcare Educ Train* 7(3):5, 1993.

48. Morton PG: A hospital nursing education manual, *J Nurs Staff Develop* 1(1):61, 1985.

49. Patterson CH: New Joint Commission draft standards for management of the human resources function, *Healthcare Education Dateline* Summer-Fall, 4, 1993.

50. Puetz BE, Peters FL: *Continuing education for nurses*, Rockville, MD, 1981, Aspen.

51. Renner JF: Healthcare marketing of community education programs, *J Healthcare Educ Train* 4(3)146, 1990.

52. Robinette JE, Weitzel PS: Design and development of a computerized education records system, *J Cont Educ Nurs* 20(4):174, 1989.

53. Rodriguez L: In-house marketing of staff development programs. In Abruzzese RS: *Nursing staff development: strategies for success*, St Louis, 1992, Mosby.

54. Rossi PH, Freeman HE: *Evaluation: a systematic approach*, ed 2, Beverly Hills, CA, 1982, Sage.

55. Schoenbeck SL, deSantis AT, Gessner BA: Continuing education policy and budgets, *J Nurs Staff Develop* 9(2):88, 1993.

56. Sheridan DR: Break-even analysis: an essential tool for financial success, *Nurs Staff Develop Insider* 1(6):5, 1992.

57. Shipp T: Cost-benefit/effectiveness analysis for continuing education, *J Cont Educ Nurs* 12(4):6, 1981.

58. Simerly RG: *Planning and marketing conferences and workshops*, San Francisco, 1990, Jossey-Bass.

59. Simerly RG: The top ten marketing mistakes and how to avoid them, *Adult Learn* 1(5):22, 1990.

60. Southern Regional Education Board: *Continuing education in nursing: a sampler of marketing and evaluation strategies*, Washington, DC, 1983, Division of Nursing, US Department of Health and Human Services.

61. Spencer LM: How to calculate the costs and benefits of an HRD program, *Training* 21(7):40, 1984.

62. Talbot GJ: Keys for successful program budgeting, *J Cont Educ Nurs* 14(3):8, 1983.

63. Tobin HM, Yoder Wise PS, Hull PK: *The process of staff development*, ed 2, St Louis, MO, 1979, CV Mosby.

64. Turner P: Benefits and costs of continuing nursing education: an analytical survey, *J Cont Educ Nurs* 22(3):104, 1991.

65. Ulschak F: *Creating the future of healthcare education*, Chicago, 1988, American Hospital Association.

66. Waterstradt CR, Phillips TL: A productivity system for a hospital education department, *J Nurs Staff Develop* 6(3):139, 1990.

67. *Webster's new collegiate dictionary*, Springfield, MA, 1993, G & C Merriam.

68. Welnitz K: Marketing a continuing education course for healthcare managers, *J Cont Educ Nurs* 21(2):62, 1990.

69. Wilson SG: Market research techniques—a synopsis for continuing education providers, *J Cont Educ Nurs* 23(4):182, 1992.

70. Wolgin FS, Cunningham M: Contracting, *J Nurs Staff Develop* 3(2): 54, 1987.

Index

A

Adult education
  cognitive style of adults, 64-66
  implications for educators, 62-64
  learning environment, 63, 64
  principles of, 61-64, 197
Affective domain, evaluation of learning
    in, 147-149
Agency nurses, 213-215, 217-218
  cost factors, 214-215, 217-218
American Nurses' Association (ANA), 8
  continuing education, definition of, 8,
    249, 251
  Credentialing Center, 296
  in-service education, definition of, 8,
    237
  nursing, definition of, 2
  nursing staff development, definition
    of, 8
  orientation, definition of, 8, 162
  *Standards for Nursing: Continuing
    Education and Staff
    Development,* 277
  *Standards for Nursing Staff
    Development,* 8, 237, 277, 284
  standards of practice, 166
American Society for Healthcare
    Education and Training (ASHET),
    8, 237, 249
  *Standards for Health-Care Education
    and Training,* 277, 302
Audiovisual media, 35, 45-47, 50, 73-74

B

Benefit profile, 331-332
Budget, defined, 302
Budgeting, 302-320
  break-even analysis, 314, 317-318
  budget analysis, 314, 317-318
  capital budget, 306-307
  cost-benefit analysis, 318-319
  cost-effectiveness analysis, 319

Budgeting—cont'd
  cost of hospital education, 304
  funding sources, 307, 311, 314
  glossary of budgeting terms, 304
  operational budget, 304-306
  opportunity costs, 311
  productivity analysis, 319-320
  program budget, 311, 314
  single-offering budget, 311
  staff development resources and
    services, 303-304
  unit budget, 314

C

Centers for Disease Control (CDC), 291
Class schedule, 52-54
Classroom learning, 61, 72
Clinical assessment center, 166-167, 243
Clinical expertise, 92-95
  scheduling activities, 94-95
  see also Clinical teaching methods
Clinical setting, 90-91
Clinical teaching methods, 90-99
  bedside nursing rounds, 96-97
  criterion-referenced performance
    checklists, 97-99
  developing clinical expertise, 92-95
  instructional outcomes, 91
  role model, 95-96
  see also Role playing; Simulations
Cognitive development, 257
Cognitive domain
  evaluation of learning in, 124-147
  written tests, 230
Cognitive style, 64-66
Competency areas of nursing, 8
Competency-based education (CBE),
    114-115, 162, 172
Competency-based orientation (CBO)
    programs, 164
  cognitive behaviors and, 172-173

Competency-based orientation (CBO)—
    cont'd
  collaboration with nursing
    management, 174, 177
  critical behavior checklist, 172
  emphasis of, 166, 168, 172
  learner-controlled, 179
  nurse manager's role, 168-169, 177
  performance criteria, 168-169; writing
    of, 171-173
  published programs, 173
  teaching methods, 201-202
  written tests for evaluation, 232
Competency statements, 168-169, 181
  writing of, 169-171
Competent nurse, defined, 208, 209
Computer-assisted instruction (CAI), 45-
    46, 47
  costs, 46
  self-paced learning, 71
Computerized market analysis, 325
Continuing education (CE)
  accreditation, 250
  application to nursing practice, 267-
    269
  assessment of needs, 259-260
  and competency-based education,
    251
  defined, 249
  dimensions of, 251-259
    critical thinking, 256-259
    decision making, 253-256
    problem-solving, 251-253
  evaluation, 266-270
  implementation, 265-266
  influence of work environment, 269
  planning, 260-261, 263-265
  program content and duration, 249
  program formats, 250
  providers of, 250
  responsibility for, 251
Core curriculum texts, 15

Correlation coefficient, 120-121
   reliability coefficient, 122
Critical thinking
   relevance to CE, 256-259
   test for measuring, 257
Cross-trained nurses, 211-213
Cultural diversity, defined, 218
Culture, defined, 218
Culture shock, defined, 221
   management of, 221-225
Curriculum development, 33-54
   allotting instructional time, 34-35
   definition of, 33
   developing faculty, 47-52
   organizing curriculum, 33-34
   preparing schedules, 52-54
   selection of content, 33
   selection of instructional media, 35-
      47; *see also* Instructional media,
      criteria for evaluating, 36;
      guidelines for use, 36, 38-39

D

Data collection and evaluation, 280,
   285-286
Data analysis, 286-287
Data sources, 286
Decision making
   ineffective, 254
   influences on, 255
   relevance to CE, 253-256
   teaching strategies, 255-256
Distractor, 132, 143
Distractor analysis, 147

E

Educational games, 241
Educational need, defined, 12
Educational needs
   categories of, 12, 13
   educational vs. "felt" needs, 19
   identifying needs, 13-16
      advisory committee functions, 15-
         16
      setting priorities, 19-20
      sources of information, 13-16
      validation of, 20, 22
   see also Needs assessment
Educational process, 244-249
   assessment, 244, 247-249
   evaluation, 246-249
   implementation, 245-246
   planning, 244-245
   see also In-service education
Ethnocentrism, defined, 221
Evaluation, defined, 112
   see also Program evaluation
Evaluation of learning
   analysis of group performance, 136-
      143
   criterion-referenced, 135-136

Evaluation of learning—cont'd
   measures of central tendency, 138-
      139
   measuring effectiveness, 117-124
      appraisal, 118
      benchmarks, 118-119, 124
      comparison, 117-118
      content validity, 119-122
      decision, 118
      face validity, 119-120
      measurement, 117
   norm-referenced, 135, 136
   reliability, 122-124
   test construction, 124-128
   written test items, 128, 130-135
   see also Learning; Learning style
Evaluations in simulated and clinical
   settings, 173, 232

F

Faculty
   acquiring and developing, 47-52
   feedback to, 52
   knowledge of subject matter, 49
   presentations, 49-52, 59, 60, 74
   responsibility of, 57
   role of, 107
   as role models, 50
   supporting faculty, 51-52, 263-264
   traits, 47
   see also Teaching-learning process
Faculty confirmation form, 52
Field-dependent (FD) learners, 65-67,
   197
Field-independent learners (FI), 65-67,
   197
   case method and, 77-78
Four *f*s, in in-service education, 20, 167-
   168, 238

G

Grading systems, 142-143

H

Health care costs, 239-240
Human resource development
   departments, 9

I

Indicators, defined, 282, 284
In-service education, 237-249
   characteristics of, 237
   competency and, 237-249
   cost factors, 242
   definition of, 237
   instructional alternatives, 240-243
      all-day marathon, 240
      combined teaching methods, 241
      CPR recertification programs, 241-
         243
      credentialing programs, 243
      educational games, 241

In-service education—cont'd
   self-directed learning and, 239, 241,
      242
Instruction, 48-54
   applying theory and principles to
      practice, 51
   appropriate level, 49
   instructional schedules, 52-54
   planning relevant activities, 48-50
   program syllabus, 53
   time and pacing of, 50
   see also Faculty; Learners; Other-
      directed teaching methods
Instructional media
   audio tapes, 49
   audiovisual media, 35, 47, 50, 73-74
   chalkboard, 39-40
   computer-assisted, 45-46
   films, 36, 43
   flip charts, 40
   marketboard, 40
   models, 42-43
   overhead transparencies, 41
   posters, 40-41
   print media, 41-42
   slides, 42
   sources of instructional media, 46-47
   television, 43-45
   uses, 35
   see also Curriculum development
Instructional objectives, 23-33
   components of, 27-29, 31
   definition of, 23, 26-27
   examples of, 31-32
   performance, 27-29, 31
   purposes of, 27
   uses of, 32-33
Instructional outcome statement, 124-
   125
   see also Instructional objectives
Interactive videodisc (IVD), 45-46
International nurses, 218-225
   cultural awareness and, 218, 219, 221
   problems of, 222-225
Internship, 185-188

J

Joint Commission on Accreditation of
   Healthcare Organization
   (JCAHO)
   accreditation manual, 278
   accreditation standard, 163
   accreditation surveyors, 291
   competency evaluations, 247-249
   cross-training programs, 212
   indicators, definition of, 282
   Management of Human Resources:
      Standards, 277
   "mandatories," 281
   performance improvement, definition
      of, 288

Joint Commission on Accreditation of Healthcare Organization (JCAHO)—cont'd
  quality of care, definition of, 276
  retention of records and, 302
  ruling on agency nurses, 214-215, 217-218
  safety areas, 237
  standard SE 2.1, 293, 294
  standard SE 3, 276
  standards, 22, 212, 239, 244, 276, 278; revised, 247-249
  standards of competency assessment, 281, 290
  Standards for Orientation, Training, and Education of Staff, 277
  ten-step monitoring and evaluation process, 278-288
  verification of clinical competency, 209

K

Kolb's Learning Style Inventory, 66 (Table 4.3)

L

Laboratory and clinical settings, 61, 72
Laboratory setting, 80-81, 95
Learner-directed teaching methods
  laboratory teaching methods, 80-90
  learning laboratory, 83-85
  seminar, 79-80
  see also Adult education
Learners
  evaluation of, 50, 51
  learning environment and, 51, 66
  see also Adult education; Teaching-learning process
Learning
  definition of, 26
  experience of success, 58, 60
  process, 60-61
  see also Teaching-learning process
Learning-style preferences, 66-68

M

Management of staff development, 276-288
  developing policies and procedures, 288-290
  high-risk aspects, 281
  monitoring and improving performance, 278-288
  model standards, 277-278
  reporting improved performance, 287-288
  scope of service statement, 280
  taking remedial action, 287
  ten-step process for, 278-288
  recordkeeping and reports, 290-302
  annual and periodic reports, 291-292

Management of staff development—cont'd
  audiences for 290-292
  calendar of events, 296
  computerizing the system, 294, 297, 300-302; *see also* Data collection and evaluation
  faculty personnel files, 294-295
  needs assessment compilations, 292-293
  nursing staff files, 296-297
  ongoing projects, 297
  program evaluation compilations, 295-296
  program files, 293-294
  retention of records, 302
  see also Budgeting; Marketing
Market, defined, 320
Market analysis, defined, 321-322
Marketing
  competition, 322-323
  defined, 320-321
  external environment, 321-323
  internal environment, 321-322
  marketing area, 322
  trends, 322
Marketing plan, 323, 325-326
  site selection, 327-328
Marketing educational product, 326-334
  determining price, 328, 332
  external promotion methods
    broadcast media, 329
    brochures, 330-334
    calendars and catalogs, 329-330
    direct mail, 329-330
    mailing lists, 330
    print media, 329
    word-of-mouth, 329
    writing brochure copy, 331-333
  internal promotion methods, 328-329
  target market characteristics, 323, 325, 328
Maxims, 209
Measurement method, 118
Measuring instrument (test), defined, 118
Mission statement, 3, 4-6, 23

N

National Audiovisual Center, 46
National League for Nursing, 47
  medication administration test, 217-218
National Library of Medicine's AVLINE (audiovisuals on-line), 46
  MEDLINE, 46, 49
National Nursing Staff Development Organization (NNSDO)'s *Quality Indicators for Nursing Staff Development*, 284, 286

Needs assessment, 12-22, 23
  categories of need, 12-13
  methods for assessing, 16-18
  process of, 23
  sources of information, 13-16
  see also Educational needs
Negative lessons, 76
Nurse
  advanced beginner, 253, 254
  competent, 208, 209, 253
  expert, 209, 254
  novice, 253, 254
  proficient, 209, 253-254
Nurse managers, 14, 163, 291-292
Nursing associations' standards, 166, 277
  core curriculum texts, 166
  records, 297
Nursing education priorities, four *f*s, 20, 167-168, 238
Nursing practice, educational foundation of, 2
Nursing staff
  causes of performance problems, 19
  self-assessment, 14
  standards of health care, 13, 14
Nursing staff development
  components of, 23, 26
  educators' evaluations, 226
  groups involved, 5
  monitoring activities, 2
  philosophical foundation, 2-6, 8
    mission, 3-4, 6, 23
    philosophy, defined, 4
  structural foundation, 8-9
  theoretical foundation, 2
Nursing staff development manual, 290
Nursing staff scheduling, 240

O

Occupational Safety and Healthcare Administration (OSHA), 163, 237, 239, 291
Orientation, defined, 162
Orientation programs
  goals of, 162
  implementation, 196-213
    cognitive styles, 197
    guiding principles, 197-201
    learning style preferences, 197-200
    teaching methods, 201-202
    teaching style preferences, 200-201
  needs assessment, 162-177
    methods for assessing, 166-167
    performance checklist, 173, 232
    role model method, 95
    setting priorities, 167-168
    sources for determining needs, 163-164, 166
    validation of needs, 173
    verification of needs, 173-174

Orientation programs—cont'd
  planning, 177-196, 202, 205-209, 211-215, 217-218
    assessing learner's capabilities, 177
    curriculum development 178-180
      selecting content, 178
      selecting media, 180
    preparing instructional schedules, 195-196
    selection of program format, 182-189
    sources of evaluation, 225-227, 230, 232-234
Other-directed teaching methods, 72-79
  brainstorming, 79
  case method, 77-78
  case study, 76, 95, 252
  group discussion, 74-75
  incident process, 78-79, 95
  lecture, 72-74
  nursing care conference, 75-76, 95

P

Performance domains, 28, 29, 69, 81, 82
Performance improvement
  components of, 277
  defined, 288
Pharmaceutical companies, 47
Policy, defined, 288
  statements and procedures, 288, 290
Preceptor, 95
  in orientation program, 163-164, 202, 207-208
  preceptorship, 184-185, 202
  supporting international nurses, 221-225
Preceptor training program (PTP), 191-192
  competency-based approach, 192
  learner evaluation, 192
  role of preceptor, 191-192
  support for, 193-195 202
Problem-solving skills, 74, 76, 77
  relevance to CE, 251-253
Procedure, defined, 288
Professional literature, 15, 329
Program evaluation
  components of, 113
  cost and difficulty of, 114, 117
  effectiveness and efficiency, 117
  evaluation, defined, 112-113
  functions of, 112
  levels of, 113-119
    application, 114
    impact, 114
    learning, 113-114
    satisfaction, 113
  model of program evaluation, 114-115
  participants in, 115
  time frames for, 114

Program evaluation—cont'd
  timing of, 116-117
  see also Evaluation of learning
Program implementation, 56-109, 196-213;
  cognitive styles, 197
  guiding principles, 56-61, 197-201
  learning style preferences, 197-200
  securing and managing faculty, 47-52, 190-195
  teaching methods, 201-202
  teaching style preferences, 200-201
  see also Instructional media
Program planning, 23-54
  components of, 27-29, 31
  preparing schedules, 52-54
  securing and supporting faculty, 47-52
  see also Instructional media, Instructional objectives
Program syllabus, 53
Psychomotor domain
  clinical or simulated situations, 230
  evaluation of learning in, 149-159
    construction of tools: anecdotal records, 158-159
      checklist, 155, 157-158
      rating scales, 153-155
      self-evaluation devices, 159
    evaluation instruments, 151-153
    setting, 152-153
Psychomotor skills, 82

R

Role playing, 89-90

S

Self-directed learning (SLD), 99-109
  learning contracts, 106-109
  management responsibilities, 106
  programmed instruction, 101-102
  self-learning packages (SLPs), 102-106
  suggestions for design, 104-106
Self-instructional materials, 233-234
Simulation games, 87-89
Simulations, 85-89, 252, 255
  advantages, 85-86
  used for evaluation, 232
Staff nurse position, 162-163
Standard, defined, 277-278
Standards for Healthcare Education and Training (ASHET), 8
Statistics
  descriptive, 136
  frequency distribution, 136-137
  inferential, 136
  measures of central tendency, 138-139
    mean, 138
    median, 139
    mode, 139

Statistics—cont'd
  measures of variability, 140-142
    interquartile range, 141
    range, 140-141
    standard deviation, 141-142
  types of distributions, 139-140

T

Taxonomics of performance, 28-29
Teacher-directed teaching methods, *see* Other-directed teaching methods
Teaching-learning process, 56-61
  feedback, 60
  guiding principles, 56-61
Teaching methods, 68-90
  defined, 68
  demonstration, 81-83
  laboratory teaching methods, 80-90
  selecting a teaching method, 68-90
    content to be covered, 69
    educators' expertise, 71-72
    resources available, 71
    teaching methods, 72-79
    techniques of creative teaching, 70-71
Television, 43-45
  cable network, 44, 45
  closed circuit, 43-45
  costs, 45
  limitations, 44-45
Test items, 118
  see also Written test items
Tests
  item analysis of test performance, 143-147
  performance tests, 118
  simulation device, 118
  written, 118
Theoretical expertise, 92
Theoretical (or declarative) knowledge, 92
Threshold for evaluation, defined, 284-285
Total quality improvement (TQI) program, 233
Total quality monitoring (TQM), 233

V

Validity (in educational measurement), 119-122
  construct validity, 121-122
  criterion-referenced, 120-121
  face validity, 119-120
  predictive, 120
Video teleconferencing, 43-45

W

Written test items, 128, 130-135
  analysis of performance, 143-147
  essays, 128, 130
  matching items, 132